Medico-legal Aspects of Dermatology and Plastic Surgery

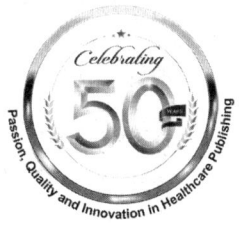

Disclaimer

This book is intended purely to create awareness of legal aspects as it applies to doctors particularly dermatologists and plastic surgeons. This book does not serve as a substitute to legal advice which must be taken in specific cases from your legal advisor. Laws are amended from time to time. The judgments of the courts may be reversed or modified by the higher courts in appeal or revision. Therefore, a referral to the latest laws and judgments is necessary. The book contains in many places individual opinions of authors, in given certain circumstances. They should not be construed as absolute OR infallible recommendations to be followed; rather the fast changing scenario of Medicolegal Guidelines makes it imperative for any reader to take professional opinion before proceeding on any specific matter. The authors and editors will not be liable in any way, for any legal claim arising out of applying the information in this book for any real life situations.

Medico-legal Aspects of Dermatology and Plastic Surgery

Chief Editors

Venkataram Mysore
MD DNB DipRCPath(Lond) FRCP (Glasgow) FISHRS
President, Dermatologists and Aesthetic Surgeons League (DASIL)
President, Indian Association of Dermatologists, Venereologists and Leprologists, 2015
President, Association of Hair Restoration Surgeons, India, 2013
President, Association of Cutaneous Surgeons of India, 2010–2013
Editor-in-Chief, Journal of Cutaneous and Aesthetic Surgery, 2007-2010
Consultant, Dermatologist, Dermatopathologist and Hair Transplant Surgeon
Director, Venkat Charmalaya, Centre for Advanced Dermatology and Postgraduate Teaching Centre
Bengaluru, Karnataka, India

Satish Bhat
MS DNB(Surg) MCh DNB(Plastic Surg) MRCS(Edin, UK)
Consultant Plastic and Cosmetic Surgeon
Linea Cosmetic Clinic
Mangalore, Karnataka, India

Subodh Permanand Sirur
MBBS DVD DNB LLM
Consulting Dermatologist
(Wockhardt Hospitals Mumbai Central)
Medical Law Consultant
Mumbai, Maharashtra, India

Associate Editors

Madhulika Mhatre
MD FRGUHS
Senior Consultant, Dermatologist
Wockhardt Hospitals, Mulekar Vitiligo Clinic
Mumbai, Maharashtra, India

Vivekanshu Verma
MBBS DFM
Associate Consultant and Fellow
Department of Emergency and Trauma Care
Medanta—The Medicity
Gurugram, Haryana, India

Aniketh Venkataram
MBBS MS MCH FDAFPRAS FASAPS
Plastic and Cosmetic Surgeon
Venkat Charmalaya Center
Bengaluru, Karnataka, India

Foreword
N Santosh Hegde

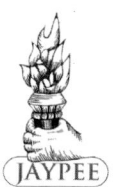

JAYPEE BROTHERS MEDICAL PUBLISHERS
The Health Sciences Publisher
New Delhi | London | Panama

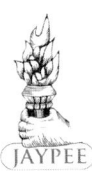 **Jaypee Brothers Medical Publishers (P) Ltd**

Headquarters
Jaypee Brothers Medical Publishers (P) Ltd
4838/24, Ansari Road, Daryaganj
New Delhi 110 002, India
Phone: +91-11-43574357
Fax: +91-11-43574314
E-mail: jaypee@jaypeebrothers.com

Overseas Offices

JP Medical Ltd
83 Victoria Street, London
SW1H 0HW (UK)
Phone: +44 20 3170 8910
Fax: +44 (0)20 3008 6180
E-mail: info@jpmedpub.com

Jaypee-Highlights Medical Publishers Inc
City of Knowledge, Bld. 235, 2nd Floor
Clayton, Panama City, Panama
Phone: +1 507-301-0496
Fax: +1 507-301-0499
E-mail: cservice@jphmedical.com

Jaypee Brothers Medical Publishers (P) Ltd
Bhotahity, Kathmandu, Nepal
Phone: +977-9741283608
E-mail: kathmandu@jaypeebrothers.com

Website: www.jaypeebrothers.com
Website: www.jaypeedigital.com

© 2019, Jaypee Brothers Medical Publishers

The views and opinions expressed in this book are solely those of the original contributor(s)/author(s) and do not necessarily represent those of editor(s) of the book.

All rights reserved. No part of this publication may be reproduced, stored or transmitted in any form or by any means, electronic, mechanical, photocopying, recording or otherwise, without the prior permission in writing of the publishers.

All brand names and product names used in this book are trade names, service marks, trademarks or registered trademarks of their respective owners. The publisher is not associated with any product or vendor mentioned in this book.

Medical knowledge and practice change constantly. This book is designed to provide accurate, authoritative information about the subject matter in question. However, readers are advised to check the most current information available on procedures included and check information from the manufacturer of each product to be administered, to verify the recommended dose, formula, method and duration of administration, adverse effects and contraindications. It is the responsibility of the practitioner to take all appropriate safety precautions. Neither the publisher nor the author(s)/editor(s) assume any liability for any injury and/or damage to persons or property arising from or related to use of material in this book.

This book is sold on the understanding that the publisher is not engaged in providing professional medical services. If such advice or services are required, the services of a competent medical professional should be sought.

Every effort has been made where necessary to contact holders of copyright to obtain permission to reproduce copyright material. If any have been inadvertently overlooked, the publisher will be pleased to make the necessary arrangements at the first opportunity. The **CD/DVD-ROM** (if any) provided in the sealed envelope with this book is complimentary and free of cost. **Not meant for sale.**

Inquiries for bulk sales may be solicited at: jaypee@jaypeebrothers.com

Medico-legal Aspects of Dermatology and Plastic Surgery

First Edition: **2019**

ISBN 978-93-5270-897-0

Printed at Sanat Printers

Contributors

Amarnath Munoli MBBS MS (General Surgery) MCh DNB (Plastic Surgery)
Associate Professor
Lokmanya Tilak Municipal General Hospital
Mumbai, Maharashtra, India

Ameesha Mahajan MD (Dermatology)
Consultant Dermatologist
RM Aesthetics
Amritsar, Punjab, India

Anant Patil MBBS MD (Pharmacology)
Assistant Professor
Dr DY Patil Medical College
Navi Mumbai, Maharashtra, India

Aseem Sharma MD DNB MNAMS MBA
Assistant Professor
Department of Dermatology
Lokmanya Tilak Municipal Medical College and General Hospital
Mumbai, Maharashtra, India

Atul Shah LLM (Gold Medal) MCh (Plastic and Reconstructive Surgery) MPhil (Cosmetology) MPhil (Health and Hospital Systems Management) PG Diploma in Medical Law and Ethics
Consultant
Cosmetic, Plastic, Reconstructive and Burns Surgery
Vadodara, Gujarat, India

Bhanu Prakash MBBS MD PGDHHM PGDMLE
Professor
Department of Dermatology
Vydehi Institute of Medical Sciences and Research Centre
Bengaluru, Karnataka, India

Chandrashekhar Sohoni MBBS DNB (Radiology)
Consultant Radiologist
Department of Radiology
NM Medical
Pune, Maharashtra, India

Charan JC MCh (Plastic Surgery)
Consultant Plastic Surgeon

DA Satish MBBS MD (AIIMS) FRCP (Glasg)
Senior Consultant Dermatologist
Sagar Hospitals and Skin
Cosmetic and ENT Care Center
Jayanagar, Bengaluru, India

Devendra Richhariya
MBBS MD (Internal Medicine) FICM IDCM
Associate Director
Emergency and Trauma Care
Medanta—The Medicity
Gurugram, Haryana, India

Dharmendra Arora MBA PGDBM (Masscom)
Professor of Media
(Masscom, Event Management and Advertising)
Secretariat, DERMASOURCEINDIA
Gurugram, Haryana, India

Dinesh Kumar Devaraj
MBBS MD MRCPS (Glasgow)
Consultant Dermatologist
Dr Dinesh's Skin and Hair Clinic
Chennai, Tamil Nadu, India

Feroze Kaliyadan MBBS MD DNB (European Board of Dermatology) SCE-RCP
Consultant Dermatologist
College of Medicine
King Faisal University
Al-Ahsa, Saudi Arabia

Govind S Mittal
MBBS MD DVL FRGUHS (Dermatosurgery)
Consultant Dermatologist
Therapeia Skin Hair and ENT Centre
Bengaluru, Karnataka, India

Kajal Mehta MBBS DVD
Senior Resident
Department of Skin and Venereal Diseases
Baroda Medical College
Vadodara, Gujarat, India

Karalikkattil T Ashique
MBBS DDVL PG Dip (Med Cosmetology)
Medical Director and Senior Consultant Dermatologist
Nahas Skin Clinic (Amanza Health Care)
Perinthalmanna, Kerala, India

Kiran Godse MD PhD FRCP(Glasg.)
Professor
Department of Dermatology
DY Patil University-School of Medicine
Navi Mumbai, Maharashtra, India

K Ramachandran MS MCh MNAMS
Senior Consultant and Cosmetic Surgeon
Apollo Spectra Hospitals
Chennai, Tamil Nadu, India

Lakshyajit D Dhami MS MCh (Plastic Surgery)
Consultant Cosmetic, Laser and Plastic Surgeon
Vasudhan Cosmetic
Laser and Plastic Surgery Centre
Mumbai, Maharashtra, India

Lalit Kapoor
Senior General and Gastrointestinal Surgeon
Medical Director
Shakuntala Memorial Hospital
Andheri, Mumbai
Senior Surgeon
Suchak Hospital and Research Centre
Malad East, Mumbai, Maharashtra, India

Lalit Kumar Gupta MD (Dermatology)
Senior Professor
Department of Dermatology
RNT Medical College
Udaipur, Rajasthan, India

Madhulika Mhatre
MD FRGUHS (Aesthetic Dermatology)
Consultant Dermatologist
Wockhardt Hospitals
Mulekar Vitiligo Clinic
Mumbai, Maharashtra, India

(Col) Manas Chatterjee
MD DNB (Dermatology and Venereology)
Professor and Head
Department of Dermatology
Institute of Naval Medicine
INHS Asvini
Mumbai, Maharashtra, India

Manish Khandare MBBS MD (Surg It Cdr)
Assistant Professor
Department of Dermatology
INHS Sanjivani, Naval Base
Kochi, Kerala, India

Manjot Marwah MBBS MD
Consultant Dermatologist and
Hair Transplant Surgeon
Dr Manjots Clinic
Jalandhar, Punjab, India

Manjunath R MD (Skin and VD) PGDMLE (NLSIU)
Consultant Dermatologist
Spoorthi Skin and Hair Care Clinic
Kollegal, Karnataka, India

Contributors

Maya Vedamurthy MD DD MAMS FRCP (Glas)
Consultant Apollo Hospitals, Chennai
Medical Director and Consultant Dermatologist
RSV Skin and Laser Center
Chennai, Tamil Nadu, India

Medha A Bhave (Khair)
MS DNB (General Surgery) MCh DNB (Plastic Surgery)
Plastic Surgeon
Lasercosmesis
Thane West, Maharashtra, India

Milan Doshi MCh (Plastic Surgery)
Cosmetic Plastic Surgeon and Director
Allure MedSpa
Mumbai, Maharashtra, India

Milind S Wagh
MS (General Surgery) MCh (Plastic Surgery)
Consultant Plastic Surgeon
Make-A-Change: A Centre for Cosmetic Surgery
Mumbai, Maharashtra, India

Mukund Jagannathan MB MS MCh (Plastic Surgery)
Professor
Department of Plastic Surgery
Lokmanya Tilak Municipal General Hospital
Mumbai, Maharashtra, India

Namitha Chathra MBBS MD FRGUHS
Consultant Dermatologist
Department of Dermatology
St John's Medical College
Bengaluru, Karnataka, India

Nanda B Kishore MD
Professor
Department of Dermatology, Venereology and Leprosy
Father Muller Medical College
Mangaluru, Karnataka, India

Narasimha Rao Kankanala
MBBS MS (Orth) PGDMLE
Consultant
Sai Care Hospital
Trichy, Tamil Nadu, India

Nayeem Sadath Haneef MBBS MD
Professor and Head
Department of Dermatology, Venereology and Leprology
Deccan College of Medical Sciences
Hyderabad, Telangana, India

Neeraj Nagpal MBBS MD (Medicine) FIMSA
Director
Hope Gastrointestinal Diagnostic Clinic
Convenor, Medicos Legal Action Group (MLAG)
Chandigarh, India

Priyadarshini P Gaddagimath
MBBS DDVL FRGUHS
Consultant and Pediatric Dermatologist
The Venkat Center for Skin and Plastic Surgery
Bengaluru, Karnataka, India

Putta Srinivas MD
Director
Government Medical College
Mahabubnagar, Telangana, India

Rajesh M Buddhadev MD (Dermatology)
Chief Dermatologist
NU SKIN WORLD©
Consultant Dermatologist
Mahavir Hospital
BAPS Hospital
Surat Mahanagar Seva Sadan
Surat, Gujarat, India

Rajesh Verma MD (Forensic Medicine)
Jaipur, Rajasthan, India

Rakesh Bharti MD
Consultant Dermatologist
Bharti Derma Care and Research Centre
Amritsar, Punjab, India

Rakesh Kalra
MBBS MS (General Surgery) MCh (Plastic Surgery)
Consultant Plastic Surgeon
Ashirwad Hospital
Dehradun, Uttarakhand, India

Rakesh Kumar Khazanchi
MS MCh PG Diploma (Medical Law)
Chairman
Department of Plastic, Aesthetic and Reconstructive Surgery
Medanta—The Medicity
Gurugram, Haryana, India

Rani Umul Khair Mulla MCh (Plastic Surgery)
Visiting Fellow in Cosmetic Surgery
Allure MedSpa
Mumbai, Maharashtra, India

Rasya Dixit
MBBS MD (Dermatology, Venereology and Leprosy)
Consultant Dermatologist
Dr Dixit Cosmetic Dermatology
Bengaluru, Karnataka, India

Reema Baxi MBBS
Postgraduate Student
Department of Skin and Venereal Diseases
Baroda Medical College
Vadodara, Gujarat, India

Sanjay Parashar
DNB (Plast) MCH (Plast) FICS (Plast) Fellowship Plastic and Craniofacial Surgery Australia)
CEO and Director
Consultant Plastic Surgeon and Laser Specialist
Cocoona Centre of Aesthetic Transformation
New Delhi, India

Sanjeev J Aurangabadkar MD
Consultant Dermatologist
Skin and Laser Clinic
Hyderabad, Telangana, India

Santosh Kumar Verma BSc LLB
Advocate
Rajasthan High Court
Superintendent, Central Excise (Retd)
Jaipur, Rajasthan, India

Satish Bhat MS DNB (Surgery) MCh DNB (Plastic Surgery) MRCS (Edin, UK)
Consultant (Plastic and Cosmetic Surgeon)
Linea Cosmetic Clinic
Mangaluru, Karnataka, India

Satyanarayana Rao KH
MD PGDMLE PGDHHM Dip STD/AIDS (Bangkok)
Principal Consultant (Dermatology)
Central Health Service
Bengaluru, Karnataka, India

Savitha AS MD DNB FRGUHS
Associate Professor
Department of Dermatology
Sapthagiri Institute of Medical Sciences
Bengaluru, Karnataka, India

Shilpa K MBBS MD FRGUHS (Dermatosurgery)
Associate Professor
Bangalore Medical College
Bengaluru, Karnataka, India

Shrirang Pandit
MS (General Surgery) MCh (Plastic Surgery)
Project Director and Lead Surgeon
Smile Train Project at Poona Hospital and Research Center, Pune
Head (Plastic Surgery)
Pandit Clinic
Professor of Plastic Surgery
Bharati Vidyapeeth
Pune, Maharashtra, India

Sidharth Sonthalia MD DNB MNAMS FISD
Medical Director and Senior Consultant Dermatologist
Skinnocence: The Skin Clinic and Research Center
Gurugram, Haryana, India

Sneha Gandhi MBBS MD
Senior Resident
Gulbarga Institute of Medical Sciences
Kalaburagi, Karnataka, India

Contributors

Subodh Premanand Sirur MBBS DVD DNB LLM
Consulting Dermatologist and Medical Law Consultant
(Wockhardt Hospitals Mumbai Central)
Mumbai, Maharashtra, India

Sunil Keswani MS (Surg) MCh (Plastic Surgery)
Consultant Plastic and Cosmetic Surgeon
National Burns Centre
Navi Mumbai, Maharashtra, India

Vaishali Masatkar MBBS MD (DVL)
Assistant Professor
Ananta Institute of Medical Sciences and Research Centre
Rajsamand, Rajasthan, India

Venkataram Mysore MD DNB DipRCPath (Lond) FRCP (Glasgow) FISHRS
Director
Consultant Dermatologist
Hair Transplant Surgeon
Dermatopathologist
The Venkat Center for Skin, Plastic Surgery and Postgraduate Training (RGUHS)
Bengaluru, Karnataka, India

Vipan Bhasin
Senior Advocate
Amritsar, Punjab, India

Virender Pal Singh MD (Forensic Medicine), LLB
Dayanand Medical College
Ludhiana, Punjab, India

Vivekanshu Verma MBBS DFM
Associate Consultant and Fellow
Department of Emergency and Trauma Care
Medanta—The Medicity
Gurugram, Haryana, India

Yogesh S Marfatia MBBS MD (Skin-VD)
Professor and Head
Department of Skin Venereal Diseases
Baroda Medical College
Vadodara, Gujarat, India

Foreword

Doctor is a Healer and has been held in high esteem for centuries. This high esteem for doctors has also meant a high standard of conduct and ethical behavior. However, in recent times, this edifice is slipping and these are somewhat trying, if not testing times for the Medical Profession. As new progress happens, but at increasing cost; as aspirations of people rise, more than what they can afford; as attitudes change, and old values disappear; as health expenses soar in the face of a dwindling governmental support; Medical Profession is facing new challenges—challenges of cost, challenges of adhering to old time ethics in a fast-changing world of advertisement and social media, challenges of demands of transparency and accountability in the face of increasing patient autonomy, challenges of meeting the expectations amidst the inevitable fallibility and inconsistency of Medical Science. Doctors need to respond to these challenges and find new, yet ethical ways of practicing their profession and to maintain the highest standards that are expected from them.

Meeting these challenges needs doctors to change and adapt; they need to define new standards in the way they conduct their profession, acquire knowledge of Ethics and Law, adopt and adhere to protocols and guidelines. Doctors need to get educated to do these effectively. It is no longer enough if they practice ethically, they should be seen to practice ethically; not just by peers and patients, but also by Society, Media and at Times law.

It is, therefore, heartening to see a book of this kind, of the first of it's kind meant to explain Legal aspects of Medicine. I am also happy that Senior Doctors from across the country have contributed chapters on different aspects. In particular, the book emphasizes Cosmetic Surgery; different and higher standards are needed in this field, as a Cosmetic Surgery " patient" is not really a sick person, but more a client/consumer—a healthy person-seeking improvement. It is also a reflection of today's scenario, that many chapters in Dermatology are included, formerly regarded as a safe specialty. New issues such as advertisements, social media are also included. Issues of Quackery, socially relevant chapters such as POCSO Act, are included.

I complement the editors, Dr Venkataram Mysore, Dr Subodh Permanand Sirur, and Dr Satish Bhat and all the authors for this effort. I hope the book will succeed in educating doctors to practice safe, but ethical and effective Medicine to ensure safe outcomes both for doctors and patients, for a better society.

Bengaluru (N. Santosh Hegde)

Preface

Medicine is a noble profession. *Vaidyo narayano harihi* (translates to *The doctor is equal to God, Lord Narayan*).

This quote reflected the spirit of practice of medicine—at least, until recently. However, this scenario is changing and changing fast; gone are the days when physicians were regarded healers; now the profession is regarded as trade by the city administration which asks for a trade license by doctors; commercial activity (by the tax official); service (by the service tax official); and a business and enterprise by the banks. Patients, who once implicitly trusted their physicians as healers now view doctors with suspicion. They now question their integrity, their costs, and even their ability to deliver treatments. This changing scenario has resulted in greater medicolegal issues than ever before. Who would have imagined that the highest ever compensation in Indian medicolegal history would happen in a dermatological case? It is now an accepted presumption, a cliché to say that the most doctors will face abuse and legal challenge at some stage in their career. This is a change that physicians will have to adapt if the profession has to continue performing its prime task of healing the patients.

It is not the most intellectual of the species that survives; it is not the strongest that survives; but the species that survives is the one that is able to adapt to and to adjust best to the changing environment in which it finds itself.

—**Charles Darwin**

The medical profession has been slow to respond to these challenges and doctors have generally been ill-equipped to handle the problems. The subject still does not form part of the medical syllabus and it is no wonder that when a doctor faces a legal challenge, he is at a loss and panics. All through medical education aspiring medical practitioners are taught about the human body, drugs and diseases so that one day they can practice medicine; to restore health, to treat and prevent disease, and serve society—staying out of courts or facing courts is not taught at any stage !!!. It is only now that doctors are now slowly learning and adopting to enhanced requirements in documentation, adhering to protocols and guidelines, knowledge of the law, etc. This book is an effort to educate doctors in such medicolegal issues. Ethics and law are about knowing the difference between what you have a right to do and what is right to do.

The book is different from a usual medical book; it is more of a compendium of facts, scenarios, court cases and possible strategies. There is a lot that is based on previous documented case studies, but not everything is written in this fast-changing field. Hence, the book includes much that is based on experience and practice. After all, the law reacts to and follows the practice; courts interpret and judge what is brought before them. The book seeks to inform not just how to face situations, but also how to prevent facing such situations.

Writing a book of this nature has, therefore, its challenges. Finding authors to write the chapters has been one. Fortunately, the editorial board had Dr Subodh Permanand Sirur who is uniquely qualified in dermatology, law, and insurance. Dr Satish Bhat has a keen interest in law and has been assisting doctors in a number of medicolegal situations. We were able to find very experienced physicians who had enough experience in law and practice to write different chapters. We express our sincere thanks to them.

The book has been divided into three principal sections—Section 1; which deals with general medicolegal issues which are relevant to all doctors, such as consent, practice management, malpractice and negligence, civil and criminal liability, social media, clinic regulations, pharmacies and dispensing, consumer courts, advertisement, ethics, quackery, compensation, legal aspects of medical research, photography and confidentiality, and dealing with legal cases. Sections 2 and 3 deal with specific issues of prime relevance to dermatology, viz. cosmetic and aesthetic dermatology, plastic, reconstructive and cosmetic surgery in important diseases, procedures, surgeries and situations.

Our effort has been to keep the book comprehensive, yet simple; to make the book all-inclusive, yet reader-friendly; detailed yet relevant. We hope that we have succeeded in achieving this objective.

The book would not have been possible without the long endeavors of our Associate editors: Dr Madhulika Mhatre, Vivekanshu Verma, and Dr Aniketh Venkataram. In particular, Dr Madhulika has been helpful in coordinating the entire effort amongst authors and with publishers. Dr Vivekanshu has spent hours in putting the right facts and making the book reader-friendly. Dr Aniketh was particularly helpful with the chapters in plastic surgery. Our thanks to them and also to the group of young doctors who helped in proofreading and copyediting.

It is our fond hope that the book will help doctors not just face legal situations, but more importantly, adopt best practices that will help prevent undesirable situations. That will be the apt reward for the effort that has gone into writing the book.

Lastly, any effort at writing a book needs support from the family, who put up with our pre-occupation and the resulting negligence of our family members. Our gratitude to them.

Venkataram Mysore
Satish Bhat
Subodh Permanand Sirur

Acknowledgments

Our sincere thanks to the following doctors who assisted us with proof correction:

Vani Yepuri MBBS DDVL FRGUHS
Consultant Dermatologist
The Venkat Center for Skin and Plastic Surgery
Bengaluru, Karnataka, India

Priyadarshini P Gaddagimath MBBS DDVL FRGUHS
Consultant and Pediatric Dermatologist
The Venkat Center for Skin and Plastic Surgery
Bengaluru, Karnataka, India

Manasa Narayan Kayarkatte MBBS MD(Dermatology)
Senior Resident
Kasturba Medical College
Manipal, Karnataka, India

Hina Jajoria MBBS MD DNB
Fellow
The Venkat Center for Skin and Plastic Surgery
Bengaluru, Karnataka
Guru Gobind Singh Indraprastha University
New Delhi, India

Oliver Clement Lobo MBBS DVD
Fellow
The Venkat Center for Skin and Plastic Surgery
Bengaluru, Karnataka, India

Suman Nepal MD(Dermatology)
Observership Trainee
The Venkat Center for Skin and Plastic Surgery
Bengaluru, Karnataka, India
Helping Hands Hospital
Kathmandu, Nepal

Somodyuti Chandra MBBS MD DNB SCE (UK)
Fellow
The Venkat Center for Skin and Plastic Surgery
Bengaluru, Karnataka, India

M Deepti MBBS MD DVL
Fellow (RGUHS)
The Venkat Center for Skin and Plastic Surgery
Bengaluru, Karnataka, India

M/s Jaypee Brothers Medical Publishers (P) Ltd, New Delhi, India, has done outstanding work in bringing this book out on time. In particular, my thanks to Shri Jitendar P Vij (Group Chairman), Ms Chetna Malhotra Vohra (Associate Director-Content Strategy), Ms Nikita Chauhan (Development Editor), and the production team—our gratitude to them.

Contents

Section 1: General Medical Law

1. **An Overview of Laws and Acts Applicable to Medical Professionals in India** — 3
   Manjunath R

2. **Right to Health; Legal System and Hierarchy of Courts in India** — 15
   Subodh Premanand Sirur

3. **Code of Medical Ethics** — 22
   Putta Srinivas, Nayeem Sadath Haneef

4. **Civil Liability and Civil Negligence including Vicarious Liability** — 38
   Subodh Premanand Sirur

5. **Criminal Medical Negligence and Criminal Liability** — 44
   Subodh Premanand Sirur

6. **Consumer Protect Act-2018 and beyond: What Practicing Doctors need to know?** — 49
   Atul Shah

7. **Defenses in Medical Negligence** — 67
   Neeraj Nagpal

8. **Concept of Compensation** — 78
   Lalit Kapoor

9A. **Informed Consent** — 84
   Satyanarayana Rao KH

9B. **Video Consent in Surgical Procedures** — 88
   Priyadarshini P Gaddagimath, Venkataram Mysore

10. **Right to Confidentiality** — 93
    Santosh Kumar Verma, Vivekanshu Verma, Virender Pal Singh

11. **Legal Implications of Advertising in Medical Practice** — 105
    Lalit Kapoor

12. **Quackery** — 111
    Putta Srinivas, Rajesh Buddhadev

13. **Out-of-Court Settlement: Why, When, and How** — 125
    Venkataram Mysore, Subodh Premanand Sirur, Satish Bhat, KHS Rao

14.	Professional Indemnity Insurance *Subodh Premanand Sirur*	131
15.	Regulations for Starting a Clinic *Dinesh Kumar Devaraj, Sneha Gandhi, Shilpa K*	137
16.	Obligations of a Doctor/Medical Establishment under the POCSO Act *Vivekanshu Verma, Rajesh Verma, Santosh Kumar Verma, Devendra Richhariya*	148
17.	What Ails Medical Laws in India *Chandrashekhar Sohoni*	165
18A.	Self-regulation or State Legislation: An Urgent Choice to Make *Narasimha Rao Kankanala*	173
18B.	Practice Guidelines and Associations: Role in Liability Risk Mitigation *Venkataram Mysore*	180
19.	Legal Aspects of Clinical Research *Manas Chatterjee, Manish Khandare*	184
20.	Role of Social Media in Clinical Practice: Legal Implications *Sidharth Sonthalia, Dharmendra Arora, Aseem Sharma, Madhulika Mhatre*	193
21.	Avenues to Study and Apply Medicolegal Law *Satish Bhat*	223
22.	A Guide for Expert Opinion: Is every Adverse Outcome a Medical Negligence? *Satish Bhat*	232
23.	Who Can Do What? *Putta Srinivas*	245

Section 2: Dermatology

24.	The Changing Face of Dermatology Practice *Venkataram Mysore, Madhulika Mhatre*	253

Part A: General Dermatology

25.	Is Dermatology a Safe Subject? Pitfalls and Safeguards during the Practice of General Dermatology *Rakesh Bharti, Ameesha Mahajan, Vipan Bhasin*	263
26.	Consent for Drug Administration: It is Necessary? *Kiran Godse, Anant Patil*	271
27.	Investigations and Law *Satyanarayana Rao KH*	274

28.	Medicolegal Issues in Cutaneous Adverse Drug Reactions *Lalit Kumar Gupta, Vaishali Masatkar*	277
29.	Legal Issues in HIV and STD Patients *Yogesh S Marfatia, Reema Baxi, Kajal Mehta*	289
30.	Legal Aspects of Leprosy *Nanda B Kishore*	294
31.	Photography and the Law *Feroze Kaliyadan, Karalikkattil T Ashique*	298
32.	Setting up a Pharmacy in a Clinic *DA Satish*	302

Part B: Aesthetic Dermatology

33.	Special Features of an Aesthetic Patient *Namitha Chathra, Venkataram Mysore*	309
34.	Medicolegal Aspects of Hair Practice *Manjot Marwah, Venkataram Mysore*	318
35.	Special Aspects of Dermatosurgery Practice *Savitha AS, Venkataram Mysore*	333
36.	Handling Difficult Patients in Dermatology *Govind S Mittal, Venkataram Mysore*	349
37.	Consent for Injectables in Cosmetic Dermatology *Rasya Dixit*	355
38.	Medicolegal Aspects of Lasers *Sanjeev J Aurangabadkar*	365
39.	Consent in Procedures with Less Evidence and Off-label Indications *Maya Vedamurthy*	384

Section 3: Plastic Surgery

40.	Changing Face of Plastic Surgery: An Overview *Milind S Wagh*	391
41.	How can a Plastic Surgeon Avoid Getting into Trouble or Litigation? *Sanjay Parashar*	400
42.	How to Identify an Unsuitable Patient for Plastic (Aesthetic) Surgery *Lakshyajit D Dhami*	410
43.	Revision Surgery in Aesthetic Plastic Surgery *Shrirang Pandit*	423

44. **Esthetic Procedures and Surgery in Minors** 435
   K Ramachandran, Charan JC

45. **Legal Issues in Medical Tourism** 445
   Rakesh Kalra, Vivekanshu Verma

46. **Delivering Bad News after Plastic Surgery** 453
   Medha A Bhave (Khair)

47. **Photography and the Issue of Patient Confidentiality** 471
   Mukund Jagannathan, Amarnath Munoli

48. **Medicolegal Issues in Burns** 479
   Sunil Keswani, Vivekanshu Verma

49. **Medical Negligence in Plastic, Aesthetic and Reconstructive Surgery** 509
   Rakesh Kumar Khazanchi

50. **Medicolegal Issues in Setting-up a Plastic Surgery Day Care Surgery Set-up** 517
   Milan Doshi, Rani Umul Khair Mulla

51. **Medicolegal Issues in Liposuction** 531
   Shrirang Pandit

52. **Tips and Pearls for Medicolegal Situations** 543
   Bhanuprakash

Index *557*

Plate 1

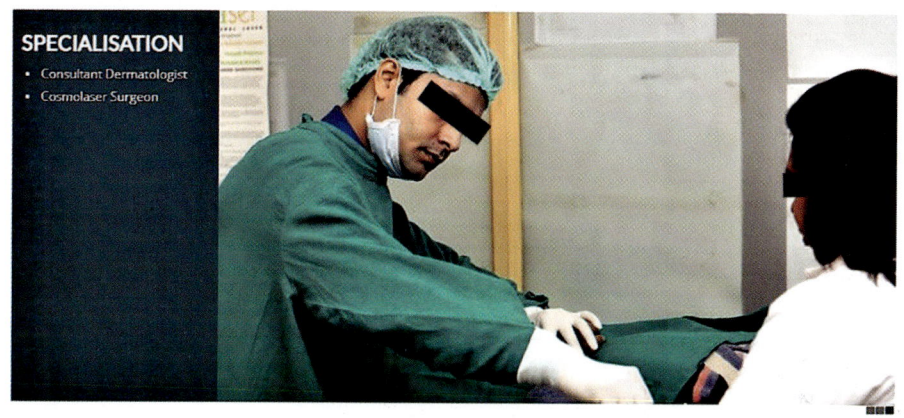

Fig. 4A (Chapter 20): (A) Depicting the value of mere 'web-presence'.

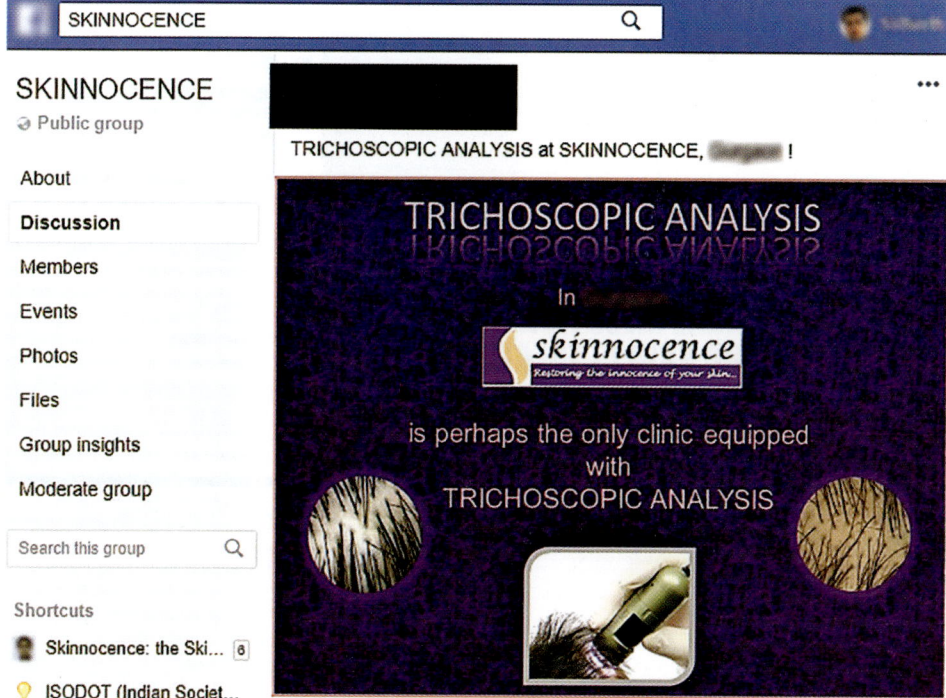

Fig. 4B (Chapter 20): (B) Broadcasting services and facilities available at the clinic.

Plate 2

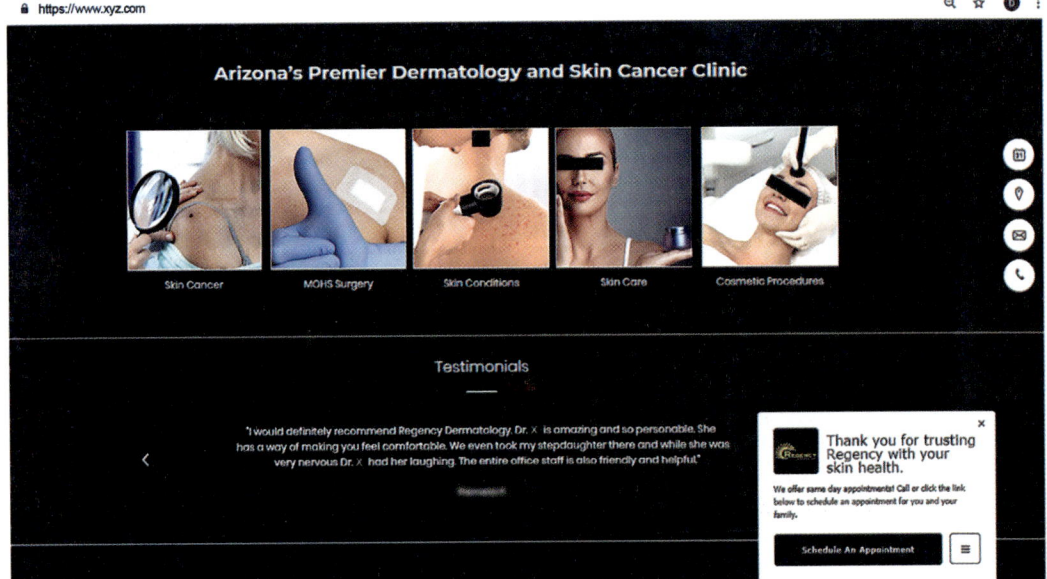

Fig. 4C (Chapter 20): (C) Showcasing the role of an interactive medium to incentivize potential patients.

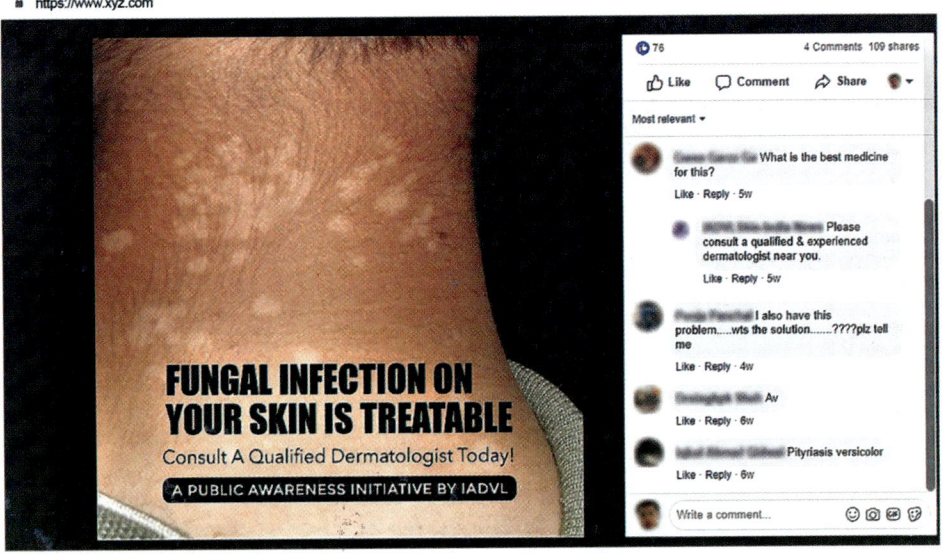

Fig. 5C (Chapter 20): (C) Posting selfless patient awareness information.

Plate 3

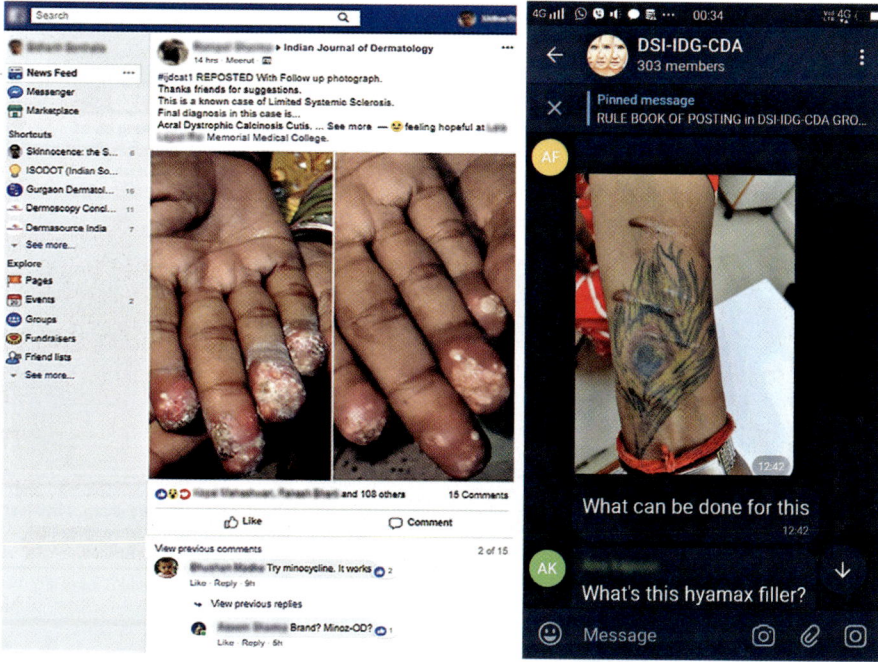

Fig. 7B (Chapter 20): (B) Facebook. **Fig. 7D (Chapter 20):** (C) WhatsApp.

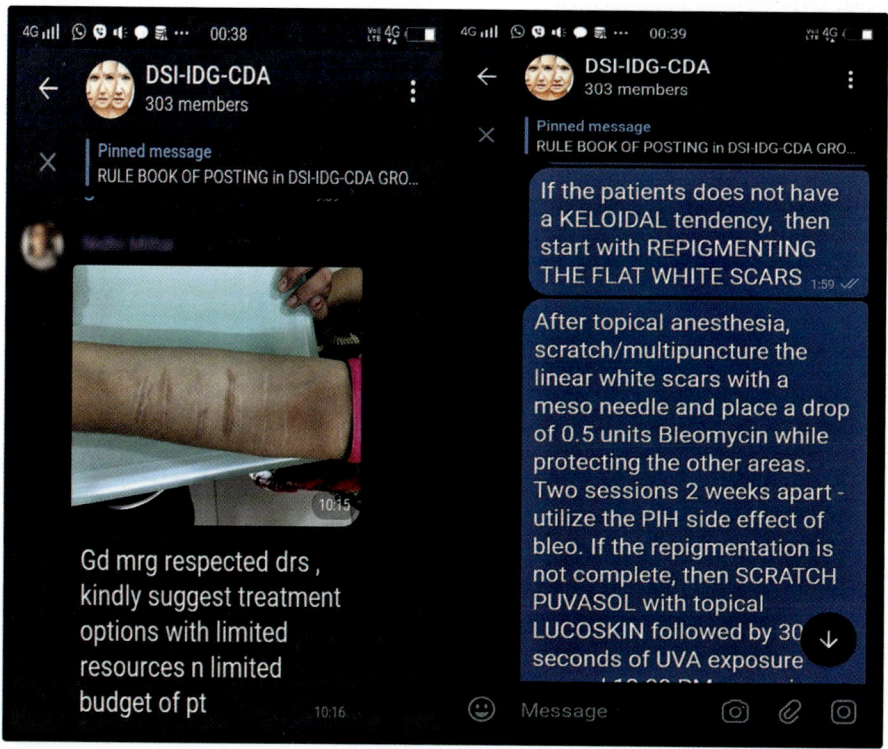

Fig. 8A (Chapter 20): (A) Peers' opinion for managing a case.

Plate 4

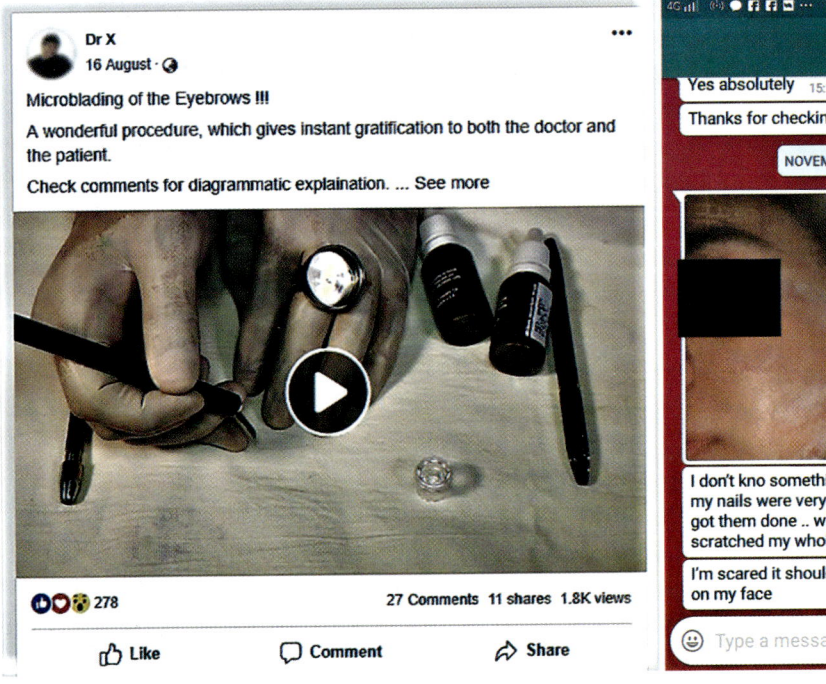

Fig. 8D (Chapter 20): (D) Specific training on a procedure of academic interest.

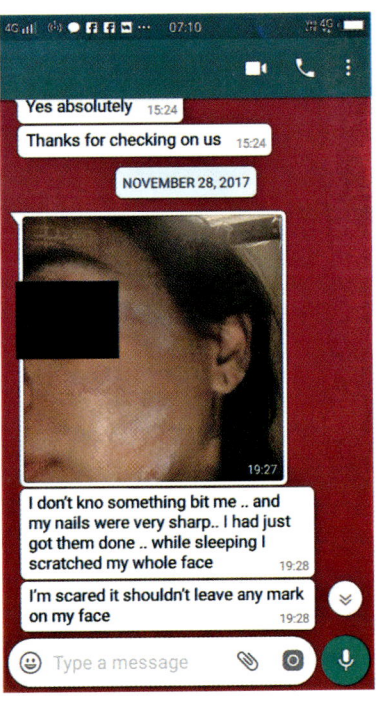

Fig. 9 (Chapter 20): A WhatsApp excerpt showing a patient attempting to gain online consultation to avoid a physical visit to the clinic.

SECTION 1

General Medical Law

- An Overview of Laws and Acts Applicable to Medical Professionals in India
- Right to Health; Legal System and Hierarchy of Courts in India
- Code of Medical Ethics
- Civil Liability and Civil Negligence including Vicarious Liability
- Criminal Medical Negligence and Criminal Liability
- Consumer Protect Act-2018 and beyond: What Practicing Doctors need to know?
- Defenses in Medical Negligence
- Concept of Compensation
- Informed Consent
- Video Consent in Surgical Procedures
- Right to Confidentiality
- Legal Implications of Advertising in Medical Practice
- Quackery
- Out-of-Court Settlement: Why, When, and How
- Professional Indemnity Insurance
- Regulations for Starting a Clinic
- Obligations of a Doctor/Medical Establishment under the POCSO Act
- What Ails Medical Laws in India
- Self-regulation or State Legislation: An Urgent Choice to Make
- Practice Guidelines and Associations: Role in Liability Risk Mitigation
- Legal Aspects of Clinical Research
- Role of Social Media in Clinical Practice: Legal Implications
- Avenues to Study and Apply Medicolegal Law
- A Guide for Expert Opinion: Is every Adverse Outcome a Medical Negligence?
- Who Can Do What?

CHAPTER 1

An Overview of Laws and Acts Applicable to Medical Professionals in India

Manjunath R

INTRODUCTION

Doctors belong to one of the most educated layers of our society. Yet, the legal awareness of doctors in India is surprisingly at a very low level.[1-3] When we hear about "Legal Education and Legal Awareness", we think that it is for law students and lawyers. The truth is that every person in our society needs basic legal education. Doctors are going to need it more than anyone else. Medical professionals in India are facing a multitude of problems. Patients are increasingly becoming aware of their rights and are always ready to take the doctors and hospitals to courts for treatment failures and complications. General public are ready to indulge in physical violence against hospitals and medical professionals for deaths in the hospitals even if they are caused due to road traffic accidents. Statutory bodies and governments are going overboard to please the general public with stringent provisions in the laws even when such provisions violate the fundamental rights of the doctors themselves.

In these testing times, it is essential for doctors and hospitals to have a reasonably good awareness of our laws to—(1) safeguard themselves and their rights, (2) safeguard their patients and the patients' rights, and (3) carry out their duties in accordance with the laws of the land.

The following are a few of the laws which are essential for the clinical establishments and medical professionals in India.

CODE OF MEDICAL ETHICS 2002[4]

The Medical Council of India has laid down certain regulations for modern medical practitioners regarding their professional conduct, etiquette, and ethics.[4] A copy of this is given to all modern medical graduates at the time of their registration at the medical councils, which need to be signed and submitted. Hence, these regulations are binding on all modern medical practitioners. They need to be followed in letter and spirit.

These regulations define—(1) duties and responsibilities of medical professionals to the general public, to their patients, to the paramedical personnel and to one another. (2) Unethical acts, (3) misconduct, (4) punishments and disciplinary actions, and (5) formats for prescription and medical certificates.

FUNDAMENTAL RIGHTS[5]

The Constitution of India has given certain fundamental rights to all citizens of India.[5] They are: right to equality, right to freedom, right against exploitation, right to freedom of religion, cultural, and educational rights, and right to constitutional remedies. Any violation of any of the fundamental rights, even if such violations are committed by governments and statutory bodies, can be successfully challenged in the High Courts and the Supreme Court.

It is surprising that the Indian Medical community have not defended this right as often as they should have been. As a consequence of this apathy, the statutory bodies and the governments have always felt free to ignore the fundamental rights of the doctors while framing the rules and regulations for medical profession.

In 2015, the Government of Karnataka legislated an act making it mandatory for MBBS graduates to undergo 1 year of mandatory rural service after internship to be eligible for registering their MBBS degree at the Karnataka Medical Council.[6] This was challenged at the High Court of Karnataka stating that it violated the rights of the doctors. The High Court of Karnataka has stayed the execution of the above mentioned legislation.[7] As a result, the medical graduates of Karnataka can now register their MBBS degree at the Karnataka medical council by submitting an affidavit, without having to undergo the 1 year rural service that was to be imposed by the Government of Karnataka.[8]

CONCEPT OF MEDICAL NEGLIGENCE AND THE REMEDIES AVAILABLE TO THE ALLEGED VICTIM

Medical professionals in India are in the midst of a highly litiginous atmosphere. The patients are alleging medical negligence for any shortfall in treatments and their outcomes. Under Indian law, the remedies available to a person seeking redress for alleged medical negligence are: (1) suit for damages under the Civil Procedure Code, (2) complaint for negligence under the Criminal Procedure Code, (3) redressal under the Consumer Protection Act, and (4) Medical Council of India for disciplinary action.

However, it is essential for the medical professionals to know that medical negligence is established if and only if the following three criteria are established: (1) existence of legal duty, (2) breach of legal duty, and (3) damage caused directly by the breach of such duty.

Medical professionals should also know that mere complaint alleging medical negligence is not going to form a basis for action against medical professionals. There are legal guidelines for the courts and the police to follow before they can initiate any action against the medical professionals.[9,10]

CONSUMER FORUM

The consumer forum is the most easily accessible forum for the victims of alleged medical negligence. The fees are nominal, there is no need to hire a lawyer and the decisions are faster. Hence, there is a spurt in the number of consumer forum cases against medical professionals. Therefore, it is essential for the medical professionals to know about The Consumer Protection Act, 1986 and Rules, 1987.[11] However, even the consumer courts need to follow the defined criteria and guidelines for establishing medical negligence.

THE KARNATAKA PRIVATE MEDICAL ESTABLISHMENTS ACT, 2007[12] AND THE CLINICAL ESTABLISHMENTS ACT, 2010[13]

For the promotion and monitoring of private medical establishments in the State of Karnataka, the Government of Karnataka has enacted this legislation. All private medical establishments in the state of Karnataka need to register under this act.

A similar act is centrally enacted; The Clinical Establishments (Registration and Regulation) Act, 2010.[13] This Act is applicable to all States, which do not have a Medical Establishments Act of their own.

VIOLENCE AGAINST MEDICAL PROFESSIONALS AND CLINICAL ESTABLISHMENTS

Violence against medical professionals and establishments has become a daily affair in India. There are legislations providing for strict actions against those involved in violence against medical professionals and establishments in many States.[14-16] Karnataka government has issued standard operating procedures to police personnel regarding what is to be done in case of such violence[17] (Appendices 1 and 2). Key aspect of this Act is that any offence committed under section 3 of the Karnataka is that the Act shall be cognizable and nonbailable (Appendix 1). However, despite the Act, incidents of Violence against the Medical Professionals and Medical Establishments are on the rise in the State.

There appears to be a lack of understanding on part of the local police in handling incidents of Violence against Medical Professionals and Medical Establishments. To ensure clarity in this regard, the standard operating procedures (SOPs) were issued (Appendix 2).

However, these laws and SOPs have not been able to deter the perpetrators of such attacks.[18] The situation is so dismal that even the judiciary has indirectly legitimized violence by proclaiming that if doctors can not face violence, they are unfit to work. In such a scenario, all medical professionals need to be well aware of how to identify, prevent, and fight against these violent incidents.[19]

RTI ACT AND CLINICAL ESTABLISHMENTS

Clinical Establishments come under the ambit of Right to Information (RTI) Act of 2005 regarding provision of medical records to patients and their relatives. A decision by the Central Information Commission (CIC) makes it mandatory for all private hospitals to maintain daily reports of medical records of patients and provide them the information.[20] However, medical establishments need to consider the merits of each case with respect to patient confidentiality before giving out medical records under RTI Act.

QUACKERY: RIGHTS AND DUTIES OF MEDICAL PROFESSIONALS

According to the Indian Medical Association (IMA), some 1,000,000 quacks practice in India. These include compounders, assistants to doctors, laboratory technicians, medical store owners, and Vaidyas. Quacks constitute 57% of persons practicing modern medicine in India. Dermatology is one of the most favorite specialties of the quacks. Each and every doctor needs to play an active role in the fight against quackery by identifying quacks, collecting evidence against them, and reporting them to the associations and authorities.

DRUGS AND COSMETICS ACT OF 1940

This Act regulates the manufacture, sale, and distribution of medicines in India. A registered practitioner of modern medicine can dispense medicines to his/her patients without a license under the Drugs and Cosmetics Act, 1940, provided he/she is supplying drugs to his/her own patients, not running an open shop, not selling across the counter, purchasing medicines from a licensed manufacturer or distributor and is maintaining all relevant bills and records.[21]

REFERENCES

1. Varghese AM, Vaswani VR, Kumar BK, et al. Awareness and Attitude of Medical Negligence and Medical Ethics among Interns and Resident Doctors. Int J Curr Microbiol App Sci. 2016;5(11):532-5.
2. Rao GV, Hari N. Medicolegal knowledge assessment of interns and postgraduate students in a medical institution. IAIM. 2016;3(10):105-10.
3. Haripriya A, Haripriya V. Knowledge about Medical Law and its Negligence among Doctors: A Cross-sectional Study. Int J Sci Res Pub. 2014;4(5):1-3.
4. Indian Medical Council. (2002). Indian Medical Council (Professional Conduct, Etiquette and Ethics) Regulations, 2002. [online] Available from https://www.mciindia.org/documents/rulesAndRegulations/Ethics%20Regulations-2002.pdf. [Accessed December, 2018].
5. Know India. The constitution of India, Part III, Fundamental Rights, Articles 12 to 35. [online] Available from http://knowindia.gov.in/profile/fundamental-rights.php. [Accessed December, 2018].
6. Department of Parliamentary Affairs and Legislation. (2015). The Karnataka Compulsory Service Training by Candidates Completed Medical Courses Act, 2012, (Act 26 of 2015). [online] Available from http://dpal.kar.nic.in/ao2015/26%20of%202015%20(E).pdf. [Accessed December, 2018].
7. High Court of Karnataka Daily Orders of the Case Number: WP 25391/2016 for the date of order 28/04/2016.
8. Karnataka Medical Council. (2016). Affidavit for registration. [online] Available from http://karnatakamedicalcouncil.com/userfiles/file/Affidavit%20for%20rural%20service.pdf. [Accessed December, 2018].
9. Wikipedia. (1957). Bolam v Friern Hospital Management Committee. [online] Available from https://en.wikipedia.org/wiki/Bolam_v_Friern_Hospital_Management_Committee. [Accessed December, 2018].
10. Supreme Court of India. (2005). Jacob Mathew vs State of Punjab & Anr on 5 August, 2005. [online] Available from https://indiankanoon.org/doc/871062/. [Accessed December, 2018].
11. Department of Food and Civil Supplies Department (Rajasthan). (1987). The Consumer Protection Act, 1986 & Rules, 1987. [online] Available from http://food.raj.nic.in/Docs/18C.P.Act.pdf. [Accessed December, 2018].
12. Government of Karnataka. (2007). The Karnataka Private Medical Establishments Act, 2007, (Karnataka Act No 21 of 2007). [online] Available from http://dpal.kar.nic.in/pdf_files/21%20of%202007(E).pdf. [Accessed December, 2018].
13. Advocate Khoj. (2010). The Clinical Establishments (Registration and Regulation) Act, 2010. [online] Available from https://www.advocatekhoj.com/library/bareacts/clinical/index.php?Title=Clinical%20Establishments%20(Registration%20and%20Regulation)%20Act,%202010. [Accessed December, 2018].
14. Government of Karnataka. (2009). The Karnataka Prohibition of Violence against Medicare Service Personnel and Damage to

Property in Medicare Service Institutions Act, 2009. [online] Available from http://dpal.kar.nic.in/pdf_files/1of2009(E).pdf. [Accessed December, 2018].
15. The Andhra Pradesh Gazette. (2007). Andhra Pradesh Ordinance against the Violence on Doctors and Medical Establishments. [online] Available from http://medind.nic.in/jal/t08/i1/jalt08i1p54.pdf. [Accessed December, 2018].
16. Government of Maharashtra. (2010). The Maharashtra Medicare Service Persons and Medicare Service Institutions (Prevention of Violence and Damage or Loss to Property) Act, 2010. [online] Available from http://www.lawsofindia.org/pdf/maharashtra/2010/2010MH11.pdf. [Accessed December, 2018].
17. Medical Dialogues. (2017). Standard Operating Procedure to deal with violence against Medical Professionals laid in Karnataka. [online] Available from https://medicaldialogues.in/standard-operating-procedure-to-deal-with-violence-against-medical-professionals-laid-in-karnataka/. [Accessed December, 2018].
18. Kapoor MC. Violence against the medical profession. J Anaesthesiol Clin Pharmacol. 2017;33(2):145-7.
19. Nagpal N. Incidents of violence against doctors in India: can these be prevented? Natl Med J India. 2017;30(2);97-100.
20. Indian Kanoon. (2015). Prabhat Kumar v/s GNCTD, Delhi; CIC/SA/A/2014/000004. [online] Available from https://indiankanoon.org/doc/117751905/. [Accessed December, 2018].
21. Schedule K. (1945) Drugs and cosmetics Rules, 1945. [online] Available from http://www.mogsonline.org/pdfs/shedule_k.pdf. [Accessed December, 2018].

APPENDIX 1: KARNATAKA VIOLENCE ACT

KARNATAKA ACT NO. 1 OF 2009

(First Published in the Karnataka Gazette Extra-ordinary on the Second day of March, 2009)

THE KARNATAKA PROHIBITION OF VIOLENCE AGAINST MEDICARE SERVICE PERSONNEL AND DAMAGE TO PROPERTY IN MEDICARE SERVICE INSTITUTIONS ACT, 2009

Arrangement of Sections

STATEMENT OF OBJECTS AND REASONS
Sections
1. Short title and commencement
2. Definitions
3. Prohibition of violence
4. Penalty
5. Cognizance of offence
6. Recovery of loss for the damage caused to the property
7. The provisions of this Act shall be in addition to other laws.

STATEMENT OF OBJECTS AND REASONS

In order to prevent violence against Medicare Service personnel and damage to property in medicare service, institutions, it is considered necessary to enact a law.

Hence the Bill.
(LA Bill No. 3 of 2009, File No. DPAL 21 Shasana 2008)
(Entry 1 and 6 of List II of the Seventh Schedule to the Constitution of India.)

KARNATAKA ACT NO. 1 OF 2009

(First Published in the Karnataka Gazette Extra-ordinary on the Second day of March, 2009)

THE KARNATAKA PROHIBITION OF VIOLENCE AGAINST MEDICARE SERVICE PERSONNEL AND DAMAGE TO PROPERTY IN MEDICARE SERVICE INSTITUTIONS ACT, 2009

(Received the assent of the Governor on the twenty-sixth day of February, 2009)

An Act to prohibit violence against medicare service personnel and damage to property in medicare service institutions and for matters connected therewith and incidental thereto.

Whereas it is expedient to prohibit violence against medicare service personnel and damage to property in medicare service institutions and for matters connected therewith and incidental thereto;

Be it enacted by the Karnataka State Legislature in the Fifty-ninth year of the Republic of India, as follows:

1. **Short Title and Commencement:** (1) This Act may be called the Karnataka Prohibition of violence against medicare service personnel and damage to property in medicare service institutions Act, 2009.

    (2) It shall come into force at once.

2. **Definitions:** In this Act, unless the context otherwise requires:

    (a) "Medicare Service Institutions" means all institutions, providing medicare services to people, which are under the control of State or Central Government or Local Bodies, etc. including any private hospital having facilities for treatment of the sick and used for their reception or stay, any private maternity home where women are usually received and accommodated for the purpose of confinement and antenatal and postnatal care in connection with child birth or anything connected therewith; and any private nursing home used or intended to be used for the reception and accommodation of persons suffering from any sickness, injury or infirmity whether of body or mind, and providing of treatment for nursing or both of them and includes a maternity home or convalescent home, etc.

    (b) "Medicare service personnel in relation to a medicare service institution" shall include:
    (i) Registered Medical Practitioners, working in Medicare Institutions (including those having provisional registration);
    (ii) Registered nurses;
    (iii) Medical students;
    (iv) Nursing students;
    (v) Paramedical workers employed and working in Medicare Service Institutions;

    (c) 'Offender' means any person who either by himself or as a member or as a leader of a group of persons or organization commits or attempts to commit or abets or incites the commission of violence under this Act;

    (d) 'Violence' means activities of causing any harm, injury or endangering the life or intimidation, obstruction or hindrance to any medicare service personnel in discharge of duty in the medicare service institution or damage to property in medicare service institution;

3. **Prohibition of violence:** Any violence against medicare service personnel or damage to property in a medicare service institution is prohibited.
4. **Penalty:** Any person who commits any act in contravention of section 3, shall be punished with imprisonment for a period of three years with fine which may extend to fifty thousand rupees.
5. **Cognizance of offence:** Any offence committed under section 3 shall be cognizable and non-bailable.
6. **Recovery of loss for the damage caused to the property:** (1) In addition to the punishment specified in section 4, the offender shall also be liable to a penalty of twice the amount of purchase price of medical equipment damaged and loss caused to the property as determined by the Court trying the offender.

   (2) If the offender has not paid the penal amount under sub-section (1), the said sum shall be recovered under the provisions of the Karnataka Land Revenue Act, 1964 (Karnataka Act 12 of 1964) as if it were to be an arrears of land revenue.
7. **The provisions of this Act shall be in addition to other laws:** The provisions of this Act shall be in addition to and not in derogation of the provisions of any other law, for the time being in force.

The above translation of the ಕರ್ನಾಟಕ ವೈದ್ಯೋಪಚಾರ ಸಿಬ್ಬಂದಿಯ ಮೇಲೆ ಹಿಂಸಾಚಾರವನ್ನು ಮತ್ತು ವೈದ್ಯೋಪಚಾರ ಸಂಸ್ಥೆಗಳ ಆಸ್ತಿಗೆ ಹಾನಿ ಮಾಡುವುದನ್ನು ನಿಷೇಧಿಸುವ ಅಧಿನಿಯಮ, 2009 be published in the official Gazette under clause (3) of Article 348 of the Constitution of India.

RAMESHWAR THAKUR
GOVERNOR OF KARNATAKA

By order and in the name of the Governor of Karnataka

G.K. BOREGOWDA
Secretary to Government
Department of Parliamentary Affairs and Legislation.

ಸರ್ಕಾರಿ ಮುದ್ರಣಾಲಯ, ವಿಕಾಸ ಸೌಧ ಘಟಕ, ಬೆಂಗಳೂರು.

APPENDIX 2: STANDARD OPERATING PROCEDURE (SOP)—DIRECTOR GENERAL OF POLICE (DGP) KARNATAKA TO HANDLE VIOLENCE AGAINST MEDICAL PROFESSIONALS AND HOSPITALS.

GOVERNMENT OF KARNATAKA
POLICE DEPARTMENT

Office of the
Director General &
Inspector General of Police
Karnataka State, Bengaluru
Date: 18-05-2017.

No.L&O/MISC-13/2017-18

STANDING ORDER NO. 1018.

Sub: Standard Operating Procedure (SOP) to deal with violence against Medical Professionals and Medical Establishments.

******

Incidents of violence against Medical Professionals and Medical Establishments are on rise in the State, even though 'Karnataka Prohibition of Violence against Medicare Service Personnel and damage to property in Medicare Service Institutions Act' was enacted in 2009 to prevent such violence. There appears to be a lack of understanding on the part of the local police in handling of incidents of violence against Medical Professionals and Medical Care Establishments in the State. To have clarity in this regard this Standard Operating Procedures (SOP) to handle violence against Medical Professionals and Medical Care Establishments is issued.

Karnataka Prohibition of Violence against Medicare Service Personnel and Damage to Property in Medicare Service Institutions Act - 2009:

The Act prohibits violence against Medicare service personnel or damage to property in a medicare service institution. The Act defines a medicare service personnel as any registered medical practitioner, working in medicare institutions (including those having provisional registration, registered nurse, medical student, nursing student and paramedical worker) employed and working in medicare service institution.

The Act defines a Medicare Service Institution as any institution providing medicare services to people, which are under the control of State or Central Government or local bodies, etc. including any private hospital having facilities for treatment of the sick and used for their reception or stay, any private maternity home where women are usually received and accommodated for the purpose of confinement and antenatal and postnatal care in connection with child birth or anything connected therewith; and any private nursing home used or intended to be used for the reception and accommodation of persons suffering from any sickness, injury or infirmity whether of body or mind, and providing of treatment for nursing or both of them and includes a maternity home or convalescent home, etc.

Section 1: General Medical Law

The Act further defines 'violence' as an activity of causing any harm, injury or endangering the life or intimidation, obstruction or hindrance to any medicare service personnel in discharge of duty in the medicare service institution or damage to property in medicare service institution. 'Offender' is defined as any person who either by himself or as a member or as a leader of a group of persons or organization commits or attempts to commit or abets or incites the commission of violence under this Act. Section 3 of the Act prohibits any violence against medicare service personnel or damage to property in a medicare service institution. Offences under the Act are cognizable and non-bailable with imprisonment for a period of three years with fine up to fifty thousand rupees.

Nature of violence against Medical Professionals & Medical Care Establishments:

Violence encountered against Medical Professionals and Medical Care Establishments can broadly be categorized as follows:

1. Verbal abuse by the attendants of the patients.
2. Creating scary situations by the mob.
3. Intimidation
4. Assault on Medical Professionals and Medical Care Establishment staff.
5. Ransacking of the Medical Care Establishment.
6. Preventing Medical professionals from discharging his/her duties.
7. Creating problems/nuisance to the outpatients and inpatients.
8. Entering the restricted areas like Operating theatres, Intensive Care Units, Documentation office and other areas in the Medical Care Establishment.
9. Damaging the property and documents.
10. Refusal to take dead body by the attendants and to pay the bills.
11. Directly or indirectly putting pressure on the Medical Professionals and Medical Care Establishment staff/extortion.
12. Snatching the medical records/documents
13. Forcing the Medical Professionals to treat unrelated treatment.
14. Revengeful act by the patients or their attendees.
15. Unnecessary intervention of media and pressure groups.

Precautionary and Preventive Measures to be taken by the Police:

1. Police personnel at the police station level shall have contact numbers and addresses of all Medical Professionals/Medical Care Establishments in their jurisdiction.
2. Under the new beat system, the Beat Officer shall have such numbers and addresses in his beat area.
3. Police Stations incharge shall form a WhatsApp Group of the Medical Professionals along with beat officers so that there can be regular exchange of information pertaining to any incident of violence.
4. A WhatsApp group at SP/DCP level may also be considered with the Medical Professionals/Medical Care Establishments of the respective jurisdiction.
5. Sensitization of Police personnel about the provisions of the Karnataka Prohibition of Violence against Medicare Service Personnel and Damage to Property in Medicare Service Institutions Act, 2009.

An Overview of Laws and Acts Applicable to Medical Professionals in India

Response by Police:

In case of violence against Medical Professionals and Medical Care Establishments, response of the local police shall be as follows:

1. Once Police Control Room/Mobile Police/Police Station/Higher Authorities receive information of such a violence, responsible police personnel shall immediately reach the place.
2. Immediate protection shall be provided to the Medical professionals/Medical Care Establishment staff/property and other patients.
3. Police personnel on reaching the place, should first disperse the mob from the Medical Care Establishment and control the situation. This is necessary as there are other patients in the Medical Care Establishments as well as doctors attending to them who would be disturbed unless the mob is dispersed. The police should therefore reach the spot with adequate force to do so.
4. In case of death of a patient, the dead body should not be allowed to be kept in the Medical Care Establishment by the agitators as that would instigate further disturbance. The police personnel should talk to the relations/attendants of the concerned patients to shift the body out of the Medical Care Establishments.
5. Immediate steps shall be taken to shift the dead body to mortuary in event of death of a patient.
6. Registration of case under the existing Karnataka Prohibition of Violence against Medicare Service Professional and Damage to Property in Medicare Service Institutions Act 2009 shall be taken up.
7. Protection shall be provided to the Medical Care Establishment till the situation settles.
8. If the attendants of the patient do not have faith on the Medical Care Establishment about their competency in curing of the patient, the attendants of the patients should be asked to shift the patient to any other establishments instead of making a scene in the medical establishment.
9. Any violence at the Medical care establishment shall be brought to the notice of Dy. Commissioner of Police/Superintendent of Police immediately.
10. In case of complaint against doctor by the patient or his relatives, Hon'ble Supreme Court's guidelines shall be followed. In case of deviance, disciplinary action shall be taken against concerned Police Officers.

Relying on Hon'ble Supreme Court Judgments in this connection, the Hon'ble High Court of Madhya Pradesh in its judgment in Dr BC Jain v/s Moulana Saleem on 28-02-2017 has laid down the following guidelines:

I. That, all allegations relating to negligent conduct on the part of a Government Doctor for which a prosecution u/s. 304-A IPC and/or its cognate provisions or under such other law involving penal consequences is sought, the same shall be enquired into by a Medical Board consisting of at least three doctors, constituted by the Dean of any Government Medical College, upon the request of the Police, Administration or the directions of a Court/Tribunal/Commission, within seven days of such requisition.

II. The doctor so selected by the Dean of the Medical College concerned to sit on the Medical Board, shall not be inferior in seniority and experience to that of an Associate Professor.

III. The doctor against whom such negligence is alleged, shall be given an opportunity by the Medical Board to give his reply/explanation in writing and if the doctor so desires to be heard personally, he shall be given such an opportunity by the Medical Board. However, if the Medical Board is of the opinion that the request for personal hearing is with the intent of procrastinating the proceedings before the Board, it may, for reasons to be recorded, waive the opportunity or a personal hearing and proceed to decide the case on the basis of the documents/treatment record and give its finding.
IV. The Medical Board shall endeavor to complete the exercise within sixty days from the date on which it is constituted and upon completion of the enquiry, submit the report to the Police, Administration or the Court/Tribunal/Commission, as the case may be.
V. The police shall not register an FIR against such a doctor in the absence of the report of the Medical Board referred here in above and also, only when the report by the Medical Board has held the doctor prima facie guilty of Gross Negligence and not otherwise.
VI. If a complaint case has been preferred U/s. 200 Cr.P.C, there shall be no order u/s. 156(3) Cr.P.C unless the complaint is accompanied by the report of the Medical Board adverted to in guideline I with prima facie finding of Gross Negligence on the part of the Doctor. However, if the complaint is not accompanied with a report of the Medical Board, the Court may ask the Police to enquire into the case u/s. 202 Cr.P.C. The police, if so directed by the Court, shall approach the Dean of the Medical College for the constitution of the Medical Board and thereafter place the report of the Medical Board before the Court concerned.
VII. If the opinion of the Medical Board is one of Gross Negligence on the part of the doctor, the Court concerned shall direct the police to seek sanction u/s. 197 Cr.P.C from the State Government. The State Government shall, within thirty days from the date of such request for sanction, either grant or refuse the same, which the police shall convey to the Court concerned. Thereafter, the Court concerned shall either dismiss the complaint case against the doctor by exercising jurisdiction u/s. 203 Cr.P.C or issue process u/s. 204 Cr.P.C and try the case in accordance with the law.

All the Commissioners of Police and district Superintendents of Police shall ensure compliance of above instructions.

(RUPAK KUMAR DUTTA, IPS)
Director General &
Inspector General of Police
Karnataka State, Bengaluru

To :
1) All the Addl. DGPs in Karnataka State.
2) All the Commissioners of Police—Bengaluru/Mysore/Belgaum/Hubli-Dharwad/Mangalore cities.
3) All the Inspector-Generals of Police in Karnataka State.
4) All the Dy. Inspector-Generals of Police in Karnataka State.
5) All the Superintendents of Police in Karnataka State.

CHAPTER 2

Right to Health; Legal System and Hierarchy of Courts in India

Subodh Premanand Sirur

INTRODUCTION

The Constitution of India guarantees certain fundamental rights, which includes right to life among others. Article 32 of the Constitution confers the right to move the Supreme Court by appropriate proceedings for enforcement of the fundamental rights and under Article 226 the right to move a High Court for enforcement of the fundamental rights.

Article 21 reads as:

"No person shall be deprived of his life or personal liberty except according to a procedure established by law."

The Supreme Court in a catena of judgment has held that the right to life guaranteed under Article 21 includes the right to healthy life.

PT PARMANAND KATARA VERSUS UNION OF INDIA AND OTHERS

(Decided by the Hon'ble Supreme Court on 28th August, 1989)

"*Article 21 of the Constitution casts the obligation on the State to preserve life. The provision as explained by this Court in scores of decisions has emphasized and reiterated with gradually increasing emphasis that position. A doctor at the Government hospital positioned to meet this State obligation is, therefore, duty-bound to extend medical assistance for preserving life. Every doctor whether at a Government hospital or otherwise has the professional obligation to extend his services with due expertise for protecting life. No law or State action can intervene to avoid/delay the discharge of the paramount obligation cast upon members of the medical profession. The obligation being total, absolute and paramount, laws of procedure whether in statutes or otherwise which would interfere with the discharge of this obligation cannot be sustained and must, therefore, give way.*"

In the case of Paschim Banga Khet Mazdoor Samity versus State of West Bengal, the Supreme Court has reiterated that right to health of a citizen is a fundamental right guaranteed under Article 21 of the Constitution of India. It held as under:

"The Constitution envisages the establishment of a welfare state at the federal level as well as at the state level. In a welfare state, the primary duty of the Government is to secure the welfare of the people. Providing adequate medical facilities for the people is an essential part of the obligations undertaken by the Government in a welfare state. The Government discharges this obligation by running hospitals and health centers, which provide medical care to the person seeking to avail those facilities. Article 21 imposes an obligation on the State to safeguard the right to life of every person. Preservation of human life is thus of paramount importance. The Government hospitals run by the State and the medical officers employed therein are duty-bound to extend medical assistance for preserving human life. Failure on the part of a Government hospital to provide timely medical treatment to a person in need of such treatment results in violation of his right to life guaranteed under Article 21."

LEGAL SYSTEM

There are fundamentally two systems of justice: (1) civil and (2) criminal.

HIERARCHY OF COURTS

In hierarchy, the Supreme Court is the highest Court in India. It is the guardian of the Constitution of India and is also the highest court of appeal. The decisions of the High Courts are challenged before the Supreme Court and the decisions of the Supreme Court under Article 141 of the Constitution are considered to be the law of the land and are binding on all Courts within the territory of India. As noted earlier, the Supreme Court can be approached for enforcement of the fundamental rights guaranteed under the Constitution.

Services that are rendered free of charge fall under the exclusionary clause of service under the provisions of the Consumer Protection Act, 1986. Therefore, if the services are rendered free of charge to everybody availing the said services, there would be no remedy under the Consumer Protection Act. In such a case, regular civil court can be approached seeking compensation or a writ petition can be filed before the High Court or before the Supreme Court. Such a writ petition was filed before the Supreme Court where two petitioners filed the writ on behalf of the affected patients as a public interest litigation.

AS MITTAL AND OTHERS VERSUS STATE OF UP AND OTHERS

(Decided by the Supreme Court of India on 12th May, 1989 under Article 32 of the Constitution of India)

Facts of the Case

An eye camp was conducted in a rural area where ophthalmologists from a city attended the camp conducted the cataract surgery and then returned to the city. Many of the patients developed postoperative infection leading to loss of vision. A writ petition in the nature of public interest litigation was filed.

Decision

The Court directed all States to implement the guidelines and norms issued by the Government of India while holding eye camps and to incorporate the recommendations of an expert sub-committee of the Medical Council of India in these revised guidelines.

The guidelines among others included the following:

"*Staff*: The operations in the camp should only be performed by qualified, experienced Ophthalmic Surgeons registered with Medical

Council of India or any State Medical Council. The camp should not be used as a training ground for postgraduate students, and operative work should not be entrusted to postgraduate students."

Further, it directed payment of compensation to those patients who lost their vision following the cataract surgery at the camp.

Learning Points

1. If a camp is conducted it should be ensured that there is compliance of all local laws, rules and regulations on the conduct of such camp.
2. Sufficient precautions should be taken to prevent infection to the patients. Whatever surgical instruments/materials are required to be used need to be sterilized and medicines to be administered should be of standard quality.
3. The camp should not be used for the purpose of training of postgraduate students. It should be conducted by qualified and skilled specialists.

The highest Court in hierarchy for a State is the High Court of that State. One High Court may have jurisdiction over two or more States. For example, the Bombay High Court has jurisdiction over the States of Maharashtra and Goa. Every High Court has original and appellate jurisdiction, which means it can entertain writ petitions, suits directly filed in the High Courts and such others in original jurisdiction and in appellate jurisdiction it hears appeals from Courts lower to it. The decisions of the High Court are binding on all judicial and quasi-judicial authorities subordinate to that High Court. The High Court in its writ jurisdiction can entertain writ petitions under Article 226 of the Constitution of India for violation of any of the fundamental rights.

CIVIL COURTS

There are Subordinate Civil (District Courts, City Civil Courts, Small Causes Courts) and Criminal Courts in each State. Before the enactment of the Consumer Protection Act, the aggrieved patients or their legal representatives (in the event of the death of the patient) would be required to file a suit before the civil court for seeking compensation for any negligence on the part of the doctor and/or the hospital. However, the regular courts are clogged with pendency of numerous cases leading to a protracted litigation. Further, these Courts have a legalistic approach and have a stricter rule of evidence.

DR TT THOMAS VERSUS SMT ELISA AND OTHERS

(Decided by the Kerala High Court on 11th August, 1986, AIR 1987 Ker 52)

Facts of the Case

The mother, widow and the children of a patient who died due to perforated appendix on 13th July, 1974 filed a suit claiming damages to the tune of ₹ 50,000 from the attending surgeon for failure to perform appendectomy in time and which led to perforation and subsequently death of the patient. The State of Kerala was impleaded as a party to the suit. The lower Court directed the surgeon to pay compensation to the plaintiffs. The challenge came before the Kerala High Court, which gave a decision on 11th August, 1986.

Therefore, the Consumer Disputes Redressal Agencies (commonly referred to as Consumer Courts) established under the provisions of the Consumer Protection Act, 1986 was seen as an alternative and speedier remedy for the patients for seeking compensation in cases of alleged negligence or deficiency of service on the part of the doctor and/or the hospital. In the strictest sense, these agencies are quasi-judicial authorities and not Courts.

There exists a three-tier system under the Consumer Protection Act, 1986.

At the lowest rung, is the Consumer Disputes Redressal Forum or in short District Forum. Every district or one or more districts have one District Forum, which entertains consumer complaints whose value does not extend beyond ₹ 2,000,000. The District Forum is presided by a retired or a sitting District Judge or a person qualified to be a District Judge.

For a consumer complaint whose value exceeds ₹ 2,000,000 but is up to ₹ 10,000,000 can be filed before the State Consumer Disputes Redressal Commission or in short the State Commission. Every State or two or more States may have one State Commission. An appeal from the District Forums subordinate to a particular State Commission will lie before that State Commission. The orders of the State Commission are binding on the District Forums subordinate to that State Commission. The State Commission also has administrative control over these District Forums. The State Commission is presided by a retired or a sitting Judge of the High Court.

An original complaint whose value exceeds ₹ 10,000,000 is required to be filed before the National Consumer Disputes Redressal Commission or in short the National Commission. Appeals or revision applications from the orders of the State Commissions would lie before the National Commission. An appeal from the order of the National Commission lies before the Supreme Court.

A consumer complaint against a doctor or a hospital could be for a negligent act causing loss or injury or death of the patient; deficiency of service (shortcoming in the rendering of service); unfair trade practice (like misleading advertisement) and sale of defective goods (selling of ointments/cosmetics prepared by the doctor or claiming to have been prepared by the doctor).

CRIMINAL COURTS

As per section 6 and 7 of the Criminal Procedure Code (CrPC), 1973, the hierarchy of criminal courts is as follows:

Section 6—Classes of Criminal Courts— Besides the High Courts and the Courts constituted under any law, other than this Code, there shall be, in every State, the following classes of Criminal Courts, namely:

1. Courts of Session;
2. Judicial Magistrates of the first class and, in any metropolitan area, Metropolitan Magistrates;
3. Judicial Magistrates of the second class; and
4. Executive Magistrates.

Section 7—Territorial divisions—(1) Every State shall be a sessions division or shall consist of sessions divisions; and every sessions divisions shall, for the purposes of this Code, be a district or consist of districts:

Provided that every metropolitan area shall, for the said purposes, be a separate sessions division and district. The Chief Metropolitan Magistrate and every Additional Chief Metropolitan Magistrate shall be subordinate to the Sessions Judge; and every other Metropolitan Magistrate shall, subject to the general control of the Sessions Judge, be subordinate to the Chief Metropolitan Magistrate.

As per section 28 of CrPC the sentences which High Courts and Sessions Judges may pass are as follows:

1. A High Court may pass any sentence authorized by law.
2. A Sessions Judge or Additional Sessions Judge may pass any sentence authorized by law; but any sentence of death passed by any such Judge shall be subject to confirmation by the High Court.
3. An Assistant Sessions Judge may pass any sentence authorized by law except a sentence of death or of imprisonment for life or of imprisonment for a term exceeding 10 years.

As per section 29 of CrPC:
Sentences which Magistrates may pass—
1. The Court of a Chief Judicial Magistrate may pass any sentence authorized by law except a sentence of death or of imprisonment for life or of imprisonment for a term exceeding 7 years.
2. The Court of a Magistrate of the first class may pass a sentence of imprisonment for a term not exceeding 3 years, or of fine not exceeding ₹ 10,000, or of both.
3. The Court of Magistrate of the second class may pass a sentence of imprisonment for a term not exceeding 1 year, or of fine not exceeding ₹ 5,000, or of both.
4. The Court of a Chief Metropolitan Magistrate shall have the powers of the Court of a Chief Judicial Magistrate and that of a Metropolitan Magistrate, the powers of the Court of a Magistrate of the first class.

A criminal complaint may be filed by a patient or the patient's legal representative. Generally, the sections of Indian Penal Code (IPC) applied in case of medical negligence include sections 336, 337, 338 (these sections are applied when death has not occurred due to the negligent act of the doctor) and 304-A (when death has occurred due to the rash and negligent act of the doctor).

The Supreme Court in Jacob Mathew versus State of Punjab held as follows with respect to prosecuting medical professionals:

"As we have noticed hereinabove that the cases of doctors (surgeons and physicians) being subjected to criminal prosecution are on an increase. Sometimes such prosecutions are filed by private complainants and sometimes by police on a First Information Report (FIR) being lodged and cognizance taken. The investigating officer and the private complainant cannot always be supposed to have knowledge of medical science so as to determine whether the act of the accused medical professional amounts to rash or negligent act within the domain of criminal law under Section 304-A of IPC. The criminal process once initiated subjects the medical professional to serious embarrassment and sometimes harassment. He has to seek bail to escape arrest, which may or may not be granted to him. At the end, he may be exonerated by acquittal or discharge but the loss which he has suffered in his reputation cannot be compensated by any standards.

The Supreme Court laid down certain guidelines which would govern the prosecution of doctors for offenses of which criminal rashness or criminal negligence is an ingredient. The guidelines are as follows:

"A private complaint may not be entertained unless the complainant has produced prima facie evidence before the Court in the form of a credible opinion given by another competent doctor to support the charge of rashness or negligence on the part of the accused doctor. The investigating officer should, before proceeding against the doctor accused of rash or negligent act or omission, obtain an independent and competent medical opinion preferably from a doctor in Government service qualified in that branch of medical practice who can normally be expected to give an impartial and unbiased

opinion applying Bolam's test to the facts collected in the investigation. A doctor accused of rashness or negligence, may not be arrested in a routine manner (simply because a charge has been leveled against him). Unless his arrest is necessary for furthering the investigation or for collecting evidence or unless the investigation officer feels satisfied that the doctor proceeded against would not make himself available to face the prosecution unless arrested, the arrest may be withheld."

The following case law illustrates the hierarchy of the courts with respect to criminal matters.

In a case of where a patient died of toxic epidermal necrolysis, a relative of the patient filed a Criminal Complaint in the Court of *Chief Judicial Magistrate* against the treating doctors for commission of offense under Section 304-A of IPC. The learned Chief Judicial Magistrate found the two of three doctors (the third doctor was acquitted) guilty of commission of an offense under Section 304-A of IPC and sentenced them to undergo simple imprisonment for 3 months and to pay a fine. The third doctor was acquitted.

Against the order of the learned Magistrate, appeals were filed before the learned *Sessions Judge*, whereas the complainant filed a revision application for enhancement of the punishment imposed on the two doctors. The complainant also filed another revision application before the High Court questioning the legality of the judgment with respect to acquittal of the third doctor. The *High Court* withdrew the appeals preferred by the two doctors before the learned Sessions Judge to itself and heard the criminal appeals and revision petitions together. The High Court held in favor of the doctors and dismissed the applications of the complainant. The said decision of the High Court was challenged before the *Supreme Court* (Criminal Appeal Nos. 1191–1194 of 2005). The Supreme Court dismissed the criminal appeal and acquitted the doctors.

There are often criminal complaints filed and an FIR filed or proceedings commenced against a doctor. There is a remedy available to the doctor if the criminal complaint is false and has been filed to harass the concerned doctor. The remedy is of filing an application under section 482 of CrPC.

Section 482 of CrPC: Saving of Inherent Powers of the High Court

Nothing in this Code shall be deemed to limit or affect the inherent powers of the High Court to make such orders as may be necessary to give effect to any order under this Code, or to prevent abuse of the process of any Court or otherwise to secure the ends of justice.

The Supreme Court laid down the scope of interference by the High Court in the matters of quashing of the FIR or complaint in the State of Haryana and Others versus Bhajanlal and Others, reported in 1992 Supp (1) SCC 335 among others the following:

1. When the allegations made in the FIR or the complaint, even if they are accepted in their entirety do not prima facie constitute any offense against the accused.
2. Where the allegations made in the FIR or complaint are absurd and inherently improbable.
3. Where a criminal proceeding is manifestly attended with mala fide and/or where the proceeding is maliciously instituted with an ulterior motive for wreaking vengeance of the accused.

The Supreme Court, however, cautioned that the power of quashing a criminal proceeding by the High Courts should be exercised very sparingly and with circumspection and that too in the rarest of rare cases.

If an arrest is illegal and an abuse of process of law, the Supreme Court has held in a catena of judgments that it can amount to violation of the fundamental right to life guaranteed Article 21 of the Constitution and compensation can be granted to the victims of such arrest.

POINTS TO REMEMBER

- Right to health is part of right to life enshrined under Article 21 of the Constitution of India.
- Right to health can be enforced against State instrumentalities by filing a writ petition under Article 226 of the Constitution before a High Court or the Supreme Court under Article 32 of the Constitution.
- The disposal of matters pending before the civil courts is tardy as it is clogged with pending matters.
- Consumer Disputes Redressal Agencies (commonly referred to as Consumer Courts) are in strictest sense not Courts but have all the trappings of a Civil Court.
- Criminal liability for doctors (for medical negligence) usually involves filing of criminal complaint before the Magistrate Court and challenge can be made before the Sessions Judge and from there to High Court and from there to the Supreme Court.
- Section 482 of CrPC can be invoked in circumstances such as when an FIR has been filed or criminal proceedings have been commenced against the doctor just for the purpose of harassing the doctor and which is a gross abuse of the process of law.

CHAPTER 3

Code of Medical Ethics

Putta Srinivas, Nayeem Sadath Haneef

KEY OBJECTIVES

- Definition of medical ethics
- Significance of medical ethics
- Technical principles of code of medical ethics
- WMA Declaration of Geneva
- WMA International Code of Medical Ethics
  - Duties of physicians in general
  - Duties of physicians to patients
  - Duties of physicians to colleagues
- American Academy of Dermatology—Code of Ethics for Dermatologists
- IMC Professional Conduct, Etiquette and Ethics Regulations Act 2002
  - Duties and responsibilities of the physicians in general
  - Duties of physicians to their patients
  - Duties of physicians in consultation
  - Responsibilities of physicians to each other
  - Duties of physicians to the public and paramedical profession
  - Unethical acts
  - Misconduct
  - Punishment and disciplinary action
- Relevance of MCI Code of Ethics in today's practice
- Registration of doctors in Indian Medical Register or State Medical Register
- Registration of foreign faculty who perform surgeries or procedures during conferences or CMEs or workshops
- Sign boards and advertisements—need to change in current scenario
- Can a Dermatologist put a board as Cosmetic Dermatologist or Dermato-Surgeon or Cosmetic Surgeon
- Change of nomenclature of PG Course of DVL to that of DVL and Dermato-surgery or Cosmetic Surgery
- Code of ethics: Hospital Industry
- Legal implications of code of medical ethics
- Remedy and prevention of legal implications of code of medical ethics

INTRODUCTION AND HISTORICAL BACKGROUND

Ethics is defined in Oxford English Dictionary as *"moral principles that govern person's behavior or conduct of activities"*.[1] Medical ethics is a *"combination of moral principles and values that are applied to take judgments in medical education, practice and research"*.[2]

Medical ethics is of utmost importance as medical profession is distinguished from other professions by a special moral duty of care to save lives and to relieve suffering. All the great religions of the world have prescribed moral codes of conduct for doctors based on divine instructions as mentioned in their respective holy books, be it the Vedas, Bible, Koran, or others like those of Buddhism.[2] In the ancient recorded history, concerns for the patient's welfare and the appropriate behavior of the physician were noted in the *"Code of Hammurabi"*, a code of ethics dating back to 2000 BC. Ancient Indian scriptures like *"Charaka Samhita"* and *"Sushruta Samhita"* (600 BC) also mention medical ethics in the form of eligibility criteria for being medical students and teachers, counsel on behavior with patients and their relatives and pointers that can be used by us when dealing with such issues as brain death and organ transplantation.[3] Two millennia ago, Greek great Hippocrates gave the *"Hippocratic Oath"*, which established the doctor as a selfless caregiver.

Ethics in modern medicine can be traced back to 1803 when Thomas Percival, a physician based in England, coined the terms medical ethics and medical jurisprudence in his book on medical ethics, which subsequently became widely used reference on medical ethics for quite long.[4] Mass murder of concentration camp prisoners as a result of cruel experimentations by the Nazi Germans during World War II lead to formulation of *"Nuremberg code"* in 1947, mainly dealing with the absolute need for informed consent for human experimentation.[5] Within a month of this development, medical associations of 27 countries founded a global physicians' association, namely, *"World Medical Association (WMA)"* based at Geneva. The WMA, in its second General Assembly in 1948 announced a modernized version of Hippocratic Oath, *"The Declaration of Geneva"*, which binds the physician with the words, "the health of my patient will be my first consideration". In 1949, WMA adopted the *"International Code of Medical Ethics"* urging physicians to act in patients' best interest when providing medical care.[5]

A subject specific *"Code of medical ethics for dermatologists"* was published in 2005 by American Academy of Dermatologists, based on Principles of Medical Ethics and *Current Opinions of the Council on Ethical and Judicial Affairs of the American Medical Association (AMA).*

TECHNICAL PRINCIPLES OF CODE OF MEDICAL ETHICS

Code of medical ethics is based on the following four basic principles:[4]

1. *Respect for autonomy:* Respect the patients' ability to take decisions on behalf of themselves, after being informed thoroughly about the risks and benefits involved in the chosen therapeutic or diagnostic intervention.
2. *Beneficence:* The practitioner should act in "the best interest" of the patient with the intent of doing good to the patient (including constant updating of knowledge and skills).

3. *Justice:* Doctor should treat equitably and distribute scarce resources fairly and wisely.
4. *Nonmaleficence:* Above all *"do no harm".*

Based on these above principles, various codes of medical ethics have been formulated as follows:[5]

WMA Declaration of Geneva[5]

Adopted by the 2nd General Assembly of the WMA, Geneva, Switzerland, September 1948 (amended in 1968, 1983, 1994, 2005, and 2006)

At the time of being admitted as a member of the medical profession:

- *I solemnly pledge* to consecrate my life to the service of humanity;
- *I will give* to my teachers the respect and gratitude that is their due;
- *I will practice* my profession with conscience and dignity;
- *The health of my patient* will be my first consideration;
- *I will respect* the secrets that are confided in me, even after the patient has died;
- *I will maintain* by all the means in my power, the honor and the noble traditions of the medical profession;
- *My colleagues* will be my sisters and brothers;
- *I will not permit* considerations of age, disease or disability, creed, ethnic origin, gender, nationality, political affiliation, race, sexual orientation, social standing, or any other factor to intervene between my duty and my patient;
- *I will maintain* the utmost respect for human life;
- *I will not use* my medical knowledge to violate human rights and civil liberties, even under threat;
- *I make these promises* solemnly, freely and upon my honor.

WMA International Code of Medical Ethics[5]

Adopted by the 3rd General Assembly of the WMA, London, England, October 1949 (amended in 1968, 1983, and 2006)

Duties of Physicians in General

- *A physician shall* always exercise his/her independent professional judgment and maintain the highest standards of professional conduct.
- *A physician shall* respect a competent patient's right to accept or refuse treatment.
- *A physician shall* not allow his/her judgment to be influenced by personal profit or unfair discrimination.
- *A physician shall* be dedicated to providing competent medical service in full professional and moral independence, with compassion and respect for human dignity.
- *A physician shall* deal honestly with patients and colleagues, and report to the appropriate authorities those physicians who practice unethically or incompetently or who engage in fraud or deception.
- *A physician shall* not receive any financial benefits or other incentives solely for referring patients or prescribing specific products.
- *A physician shall* respect the rights and preferences of patients, colleagues, and other health professionals.
- *A physician shall* recognize his/her important role in educating the public but should use due caution in divulging discoveries or new techniques or treatment through nonprofessional channels.
- *A physician shall* certify only that which he/she has personally verified.

- A *physician shall* strive to use healthcare resources in the best way to benefit patients and their community.
- A *physician shall* seek appropriate care and attention if he/she suffers from mental or physical illness.
- A *physician shall* respect the local and national codes of ethics.

Duties of Physicians to Patients

- A *physician shall* always bear in mind the obligation to respect human life.
- A *physician shall* act in the patient's best interest when providing medical care.
- A *physician shall* owe his/her patients complete loyalty and all the scientific resources available to him/her.
- Whenever an examination or treatment is beyond the physician's capacity, he/she should consult with or refer to another physician who has the necessary ability.
- A *physician shall* respect a patient's right to confidentiality. It is ethical to disclose confidential information when the patient consents to it or when there is a real and imminent threat of harm to the patient or to others and this threat can be only removed by a breach of confidentiality.
- A *physician shall* give emergency care as a humanitarian duty unless he/she is assured that others are willing and able to give such care.
- A *physician shall* in situations when he/she is acting for a third party, ensure that the patient has full knowledge of that situation.
- A *physician shall* not enter into a sexual relationship with his/her current patient or into any other abusive or exploitative relationship.

Duties of Physicians to Colleagues

- A *physician shall* behave toward colleagues, as he/she would have them behave toward him/her.
- A *physician shall not* undermine the patient-physician relationship of colleagues in order to attract patients.
- A *physician shall* when medically necessary, communicate with colleagues who are involved in the care of the same patient. This communication should respect patient confidentiality and be confined to necessary information.

American Academy of Dermatology Code of Medical Ethics for Dermatologists (2005)[6]

American Academy of Dermatologists published a specialty specific "code of medical ethics for dermatologists" in 2005, based on Principles of Medical Ethics and *Current Opinions of the Council on Ethical and Judicial Affairs of the AMA*. This code includes various guidelines under nine broad categories, namely, physician-patient relationship, personal conduct, conflicts of interest, maintenance of competence, relationships with dermatologists, nurses, other allied health professionals, relationship with the public, general principles of care, research, and academic responsibilities, and lastly community responsibility.

INDIAN MEDICAL COUNCIL (PROFESSIONAL CONDUCT, ETIQUETTE, AND ETHICS) REGULATIONS, 2002 (AMENDED UP TO 8TH OCTOBER 2016)[7]: EXCERPTS, IMPLICATIONS, AND CONTROVERSIES

The Medical Council of India (MCI) has prescribed regulations relating to the professional conduct, etiquette, and ethics for registered medical practitioners in 2002, under the Indian Medical Council Act, 1956, with approval from the Government of India.

The following are excerpts of the regulations, authors' comments (*in italics*) on their potential implications and controversies surrounding these regulations:

Chapter 1: Code of Medical Ethics

Declaration

At the time of making an application for registration, each applicant is required to submit a signed declaration pledging to serve the humanity with impartial, humane approach while upholding the dignity and nobility of the medical profession.

Duties and Responsibilities of the Physicians in General

- *Character of physician [doctors with qualification of Bachelor of Medicine and Bachelor of Surgery (MBBS) or MBBS with postgraduate degree or diploma or with equivalent qualification in any medical discipline]:*
  - A physician shall uphold the dignity and honor of his profession.
  - The prime object of the medical profession is to render service to humanity; reward or financial gain is a subordinate consideration. Physician shall keep himself pure in character and be diligent in caring for the sick.
  - No person other than a doctor having qualification recognized by MCI and registered with MCI or State Medical Council (s) is allowed to practice.
  - Modern system of Medicine or Surgery. A person obtaining qualification in any other system of, medicine is not allowed to practice Modern system of Medicine in any form.
- *Maintaining good medical practice:*
  - Physicians should serve the patients with devotion and practice methods of healing founded on scientific basis, and continuously improve medical knowledge and skills.
  - Membership in Allopathic Medical Societies for advancement of the profession.
  - A physician should participate in Continuing Medical Education (CME) programs, for at least 30 h every 5 years.

Comment: Many of the State Medical Councils link this requirement of credit hours to renewal of registration once in 5 years. The need for renewal of registration with the State Medical Council once in 5 years or re-registration of doctor belonging to other state in new State Medical Council is itself controversial, as MCI rules indicate that name of any doctor registered with any State Medical Council is automatically entered in Indian Medical Council and hence such doctor can practice anywhere in India lifelong.

- *Maintenance of medical records:*
  - Every physician shall maintain the medical records pertaining to his/her indoor patients for a period of 3 years from the date of commencement of the treatment in a standard proforma.

Comment: The guidelines mention only indoor patients but not outdoor patients' records.

- If any request is made for medical records either by the patients or authorized attendant or legal authorities involved, documents shall be issued within the period of 72 h.
- A Registered medical practitioner shall maintain a Register of Medical Certificates giving full details of certificates issued.
- Efforts shall be made to computerize medical records for quick retrieval.
- *Display of registration numbers:*
  - Every physician shall display the registration number accorded to him

by the State Medical Council or MCI in his clinic and in all his prescriptions, certificates, and money receipts given to his patients.
- Physicians shall display as suffix to their names only recognized medical degrees or such certificates or diplomas and memberships or honors, which confer professional knowledge or recognize any exemplary qualification or achievements.
- *Use of generic names of drugs:* Every physician should prescribe drugs with generic names legibly and preferably in capital letters and he/she shall ensure that there is a rational prescription and use of drugs.

Comment: Prescribing generic names legibly and in capital letters may help in reducing the cost of medicines by curbing recommendation of costly brands by doctors. But in India, there is no guarantee of quality control of such medicines. Also, the pharmacists or salesmen may indulge in profiteering as they can choose a brand or manufacturer to suit their needs. With respect to dermatology, it may be noted that use of irrational combination of topical corticosteroids and antifungal agents has led to outbreak of recalcitrant or resistant dermatophyte infections.

- *Highest quality assurance in patient care:* Every physician should aid in safeguarding the profession against admission to it of those who are deficient in moral character or education. Physician shall not employ in connection with his professional practice any attendant who is neither registered nor enlisted under the Medical Acts in force and shall not permit such persons to attend, treat, or perform operations upon patients wherever professional discretion or skill is required.
- *Exposure of unethical conduct:* A physician should expose, without fear or favor, incompetent or corrupt, and dishonest or unethical conduct on the part of members of the profession.
- *Payment of professional services*: The personal financial interests of a physician should not conflict with the medical interests of patients. A physician should announce his fees before rendering service and not after the operation or treatment is under way.
- *Evasion of legal restrictions:* The physician shall observe the laws of the country in regulating the practice of medicine and shall also not assist others to evade such laws. He should be cooperative in observance and enforcement of sanitary laws and regulations in the interest of public health.

Chapter 2: Duties of Physicians to their Patients

- *Obligations to the sick:*
  - Though a physician is not bound to treat each and every person asking his services, he should be ever ready to respond to the calls of the sick and the injured. A physician advising a patient to seek service of another physician is acceptable; however, in case of emergency a physician must treat the patient. No physician shall arbitrarily refuse treatment to a patient.
  - Medical practitioner having any incapacity detrimental to the patient or which can affect his performance vis-à-vis the patient is not permitted to practice his profession.
- *Patience, delicacy, and secrecy*: Patience and delicacy should characterize the physician. Confidential information about

patient's illness should never be revealed unless their revelation is required by the laws of the State or in order to protect a healthy person against a communicable disease to which he is about to be exposed.
- The physician should neither exaggerate nor minimize the gravity of a patient's condition.
- Once having undertaken a case, the physician should not neglect the patient, nor should he withdraw from the case without giving adequate notice to the patient and his family. Physician shall not willfully commit an act of negligence.
- When a physician who has been engaged to attend an obstetric case is absent and another is sent for and delivery accomplished, the acting physician is entitled to his professional fees, but should secure the patient's consent to resign on the arrival of the physician engaged.

Chapter 3: Duties of Physicians in Consultation

- Unnecessary consultations should be avoided.
- In every consultation, the benefit to the patient is of foremost importance.
- Utmost punctuality should be observed by a physician in consultations.
- All statements to the patient or his representatives should take place in the presence of the consulting physicians, except as otherwise agreed.
- Physician can make subsequent variations in the treatment, if any unexpected change occurs, but reasons for the variations should be discussed or explained.
- When a patient is referred to a specialist by the attending physician, a case summary of the patient should be given to the specialist, who should communicate his opinion in writing to the attending physician.
- A physician shall clearly display his fees and other charges on the board of his chamber and/or the hospitals he is visiting.

Chapter 4: Responsibilities of Physicians to Each Other

- A physician should consider it as a pleasure and privilege to render gratuitous service to all physicians and their immediate family dependents.
- In consultations, no insincerity, rivalry, or envy should be indulged in.
- When a physician has been called for consultation, the consultant should not take charge of the case. The consultant shall not criticize the referring physician. He or she shall discuss the diagnosis treatment plan with the referring physician.
- Whenever a physician requests another physician to attend his patients during his temporary absence from his practice, the other physician should accept only when he has the capacity to discharge the additional responsibility along with his or her other duties.
- The medical officer or physician occupying an official position should avoid remarks upon the diagnosis or the treatment that has been adopted by other physician.

Chapter 5: Duties of Physicians to the Public and to the Paramedical Profession

- Physicians, as good citizens, should advice on public health issues and play their part in enforcing sanitary or public health laws and regulations.
- Physicians should enlighten the public concerning quarantine regulations and measures for the prevention of epidemic and communicable diseases, and also notify public health authorities.

Code of Medical Ethics

- Physicians should recognize and promote the practice of different paramedical services such as, pharmacy and nursing.

Chapter 6: Unethical Acts

A physician shall not aid or abet or commit any of the following acts, which shall be construed as unethical.
- *Advertising:*
  - Soliciting of patients directly or indirectly, by a physician, by a group of physicians, or by institutions or organizations is unethical. A physician shall not make use of him or her (or his or her name) as subject of any form or manner of advertising or publicity through any mode either alone or in conjunction with others, which is of such a character as to invite attention to him or to his professional position, skill, qualification, achievements, attainments, specialties, appointments, associations, affiliations or honors, and/or of such character as would ordinarily result in his self-aggrandizement. A physician shall not give to any person, whether for compensation or otherwise, any approval, recommendation, endorsement, certificate, report or statement with respect of any drug, medicine, nostrum remedy, surgical, or therapeutic article, apparatus or appliance or any commercial product or article with respect of any property, quality or use thereof or any test, demonstration or trial thereof, for use in connection with his name, signature, or photograph in any form or manner of advertising through any mode nor shall he boast of cases, operations, cures or remedies, or permit the publication of report thereof through any mode. A medical practitioner is, however, permitted to make a formal announcement in press regarding the following:
    - On starting practice
    - On change of type of practice
    - On changing address
    - On temporary absence from duty
    - On resumption of another practice
    - On succeeding to another practice
    - Public declaration of charges.
  - Printing of self-photograph, or any such material of publicity in the letter head or on sign board of the consulting room or any such clinical establishment shall be regarded as acts of self-advertisement and unethical conduct on the part of the physician.
- *Patent and copyrights:* A physician may patent surgical instruments, appliances and medicine or copyright applications, methods, and procedures. However, it shall be unethical, if the benefits of such patents or copyrights are not made available in situations where the interest of large population is involved.
- A physician should not run an open shop for sale of medicine for dispensing prescriptions prescribed by doctors other than himself or for sale of medical or surgical appliances. It is not unethical for a physician to prescribe or supply drugs, remedies, or appliances as long as there is no exploitation of the patient. Drugs prescribed by a physician or brought from the market for a patient should explicitly state the proprietary formulae as well as generic name of the drug.
- *Rebates and commission:* A physician shall not give, solicit, or receive nor shall he offer to give solicit or receive, any gift, gratuity, commission or bonus in

consideration of or return for the referring, recommending or procuring of any patient for medical, surgical or other treatment, or for diagnostic tests.
- All the drugs prescribed by a physician should always carry a proprietary formula and clear name. Prescription of secret remedies is prohibited.
- *Human rights:* The physician shall not aid or abet mental or physical trauma or torture in clear violation of human rights.
- Practicing euthanasia shall constitute unethical conduct. However, on specific occasion, the question of withdrawing life-supporting devices even after brain death shall be decided only by a team of doctors and not merely by the treating physician alone.
- *Code of conduct for doctors in their relationship with pharmaceutical and allied health sector industry:*
  - A medical practitioner shall not receive any gift, cash, or monetary grant from any pharmaceutical and allied healthcare industry and their sales representatives. A medical practitioner shall not accept any hospitality or travel facility inside the country or outside, including rail, road, air, ship, cruise tickets, paid vacations, etc. from any pharmaceutical or allied healthcare industry or their representatives for self and family members for vacation or for attending conferences, seminars, workshops, CME program, etc. as a delegate.
  - A medical practitioner may carry out or participate as researchers, treating doctors, or consultants in research projects funded by pharmaceutical and allied healthcare industries, provided all the legal requirements for the medical research, including ethical committee clearing, humane treatment of human volunteers, and experimental animals are fulfilled. Physician should maintain his professional autonomy and patient safety during such participation.
  - A physician shall not indulge in endorsement of any drug or appliance, except in scientific journals for academic purpose only.
  - Any deviation from the above guidelines is punishable with censure, removal of name of the physician from Indian Medical Register or State Medical Register (for a period ranging from 3 months to more than 1 year).

Chapter 7: Misconduct

The following acts of commission or omission on the part of a physician shall constitute professional misconduct rendering him/her liable for disciplinary action:
- If he/she commits any violation of the MCI Regulations.
- Failure to maintain the medical records of indoor patients for a period of 3 years or refusal to provide the same within 72 h when solicited.
- Failure to display registration number in clinic, prescriptions and certificates, etc.
- Abuse of professional position by committing adultery or improper conduct with a patient.
- Conviction by a Court of Law for offences involving moral turpitude or criminal acts.
- Sex determination test undertaken with the intent to terminate the life of a female fetus, unless there are other absolute indications for termination of pregnancy as specified in the Medical Termination of Pregnancy Act, 1971.

- Signing professional certificates, reports, and other documents, which are untrue, misleading, or improper.
- Contravention of provisions of the Drugs and Cosmetics Act and regulations made there under. Accordingly,
  - Prescribing steroids or psychotropic drugs when there is no absolute medical indication;
  - Selling schedule "H" and "L" drugs and poisons to public except to his patient in contravention of the above provisions shall constitute gross professional misconduct by the physician.
- Performing or enabling unqualified person to perform an abortion or any illegal operation for which there is no medical, surgical or psychological indication.
- Issuing certificates of efficiency in modern medicine to unqualified or nonmedical person.

Comment: It is unfortunate that few dermatologists themselves are irresponsibly indulging in providing "certificate courses" for nondermatologist candidates. This is not only unethical, but also creating undue competition for our own fraternity.

- Contributing lay press articles and interviews regarding diseases and treatments for advertising himself or soliciting practices (writing in lay press or delivering public lectures, talks on the radio or TV or internet chat on matters of public health, and hygienic living are allowed).
- An institution run by a physician for a particular purpose such as a maternity home, nursing home, private hospital, rehabilitation center or any type of training institution, etc. may be advertised in the lay press, but such advertisements should not contain anything more than the name of the institution, type of patients admitted, type of training and other facilities offered, and the fees.
- Use of an unusually large signboard and writing anything other than doctor's name, qualifications obtained from a University or a statutory body, titles, and name of specialty, registration number including the name of the State Medical Council under which registered. The same should be the contents of prescription papers. It is improper to affix a signboard on a chemist's shop or in places where the physician does not reside or work.
- *Disclosure the secrets of a patient except:*
  - In a court of law under orders of the presiding judge;
  - In circumstances where there is a serious and identified risk to a specific person and/or community; and
  - Notifiable diseases.
- Refusal on religious grounds alone to give assistance in or conduct of sterility, birth control, circumcision, and medical termination of pregnancy when there is medical indication.
- Failure to obtain written consent before surgery or procedure.

Comment: Not obtaining written informed consent specific to the procedure concerned is the most common mistake, which lands the doctors into medicolegal problems.

- Publishing photographs or case reports of patients without their permission, in any medical or other journal in a manner by which their identity could be made out. If the identity is not to be disclosed, the consent is not needed.
- In the case of running of a nursing home by a physician and employing assistants to help him/her, the ultimate responsibility rests on the physician.

- Use touts or agents for procuring patients.
- Claiming to be specialist unless he has a special qualification in that branch.
- In vitro fertilization or artificial insemination undertaken without the informed consent of the female patient and her spouse as well as the donor.
- *Research*: Clinical drug trials or other research involving patients or volunteers as per the guidelines of Indian Council of Medical Research (ICMR) can be undertaken, provided ethical considerations are borne in mind. Violation of existing ICMR guidelines in this regard shall constitute misconduct. Consent taken from the patient for trial of drug or therapy, which is not as per the guidelines, shall also be construed as misconduct.

Chapter 8: Punishment and Disciplinary Action

Apart from above-mentioned clauses, the MCI and/or State Medical Councils are in no way precluded from considering and dealing with any other form of professional misconduct on the part of a registered practitioner. Upon receipt of any complaint of professional misconduct, the appropriate Medical Council would hold an enquiry within 6 months and give opportunity to the registered medical practitioner to be heard in person or by pleader. During the pendency of the complaint, the appropriate council may restrain the physician from performing the procedure or practice, which is under scrutiny. Professional incompetence shall be judged by peer group as per guidelines prescribed by MCI. If the medical practitioner is found to be guilty of committing professional misconduct, the appropriate Medical Council may award such punishment as deemed necessary. Any person aggrieved by the decision of the State Medical Council on any complaint against a delinquent physician, shall have the right to file an appeal to the MCI within a period of 60 days from the date of receipt of the order passed by the said Medical Council.

RELEVANCE OF MCI CODE OF ETHICS IN TODAY'S PRACTICE

Regulations on MCI code of conduct was issued in 2002 and periodically updated. However, many experts opine that perception of the society, administrators, and policy makers about the medical profession has changed drastically.

Introduction of Consumer Protection Act in 1986, and with bringing of the medical profession within the Consumer Protection Act purview, has dramatically changed the relationship of patient and doctor to that of Consumer and Service Provider. The society generally expects the doctors to be service oriented with humanity, but paradoxically the law deals with doctors as consumer service providers. People when go to a doctor, are expressing that they have full faith and confidence, but when things does not happen as per their expectations, they are treating doctors as villains, without understanding the risk factors and limitations of modern medical science and variations of human response to different treatment methods. Consequently, the patients and their attendants are taking law into their hands and physically assaulting doctors and hospitals. Another aspect is that certain individuals are blackmailing doctors and lodging false complaints or filing cases in consumer courts.

Hence, there is growing feeling among medical profession that Code of Medical Ethics is fixing their responsibilities where as it is silent about protecting their interests. There is an immediate need to make Code of Medical

Ethics more relevant, and shall be updated and shall incorporate changes to protect the interests of doctors also keeping in view the changed circumstances.

REGISTRATION OF DOCTORS: INDIAN MEDICAL REGISTER OR STATE MEDICAL REGISTER

The doctors of modern medicine can register their MBBS, Doctor of Medicine (MD) or Master of Surgery (MS), Doctorate of Medicine (DM), or Master of Chirurgiae (MCh) either with Indian Medical Register maintained at MCI New Delhi or State Medical Register maintained at concerned State Medical Councils. There are certain gray areas where there are elements of ambiguity. When a doctor is registered in Indian Medical Register, it is expected that he should be eligible to practice in any state anywhere in India; however, it is not so. As per the existing regulations, even if a doctor is registered in Indian Medical Register, still he has to register with concerned State Medical Council and state medical register to be eligible to practice in that particular state. This double registration is becoming an area of controversy. There is a need to remove this double registration and ambiguity.

REGISTRATION OF FOREIGN FACULTY WHO PERFORM SURGERIES OR PROCEDURES DURING CONFERENCES OR CME OR WORKSHOPS

It is mandatory that all the foreign doctors to register with concerned State Medical Council, to be eligible to perform on patients surgeries or procedures for live demonstrations during workshops or CME or conferences. The concerned State Medical Council will register them for a minimum period of 3 months during which he can do surgeries or procedures and without such registration, foreign doctors will not be eligible to touch the patients. There is one gray area, that State Medical Council can only register the foreign qualifications, which are recognized by MCI (in reciprocation), but cannot register foreign qualifications, which are not recognized by MCI, and such foreign faculty cannot perform surgeries or procedures. In reality, these rules are not strictly followed by both the organizers and foreign faculty also. However, when an unfortunate incident takes place there will be utter chaos and blaming of each other.

SIGNBOARDS AND ADVERTISEMENTS—NEED TO CHANGE IN CURRENT SCENARIO[7]

The MCI code of ethics 7.13 mentions about the size of signboard and specifies about what matter board should contain. However, there are revolutionary changes in publicity, advertisements, and professional promotion methods, with advent of internet, YouTube, and net-based promotional agencies like Justdial, Practo, etc. These changes in media and advertisements are being used effectively not only by business houses but also by many professional experts. Nowadays, every person looks into these sites for help, guidance as well as opinion generation. With such revolutionary changes, particularly when every professional experts, are using them for their advantage by effective presentation and professional promotion, it is unrealistic to put a bar on doctors from using them.

It is high time that the MCI code of medical ethics should be reviewed and guidelines should be framed for promotion of professional activities of doctors on net-based agencies like Justdial, Practo, and also in print and electronic media, etc. Also there is a need to review regarding the contents of signboards to include facilities that are available and services that are offered. We have to also keep in view the fact that now patient is a consumer and doctor is a service provider and naturally service provider should be allowed to put in signboards, what facilities and services that are available.

Another angle of advertisements is surrogate advertisements by non-Allopathic doctors, chain of clinics of Homeopathic, and Ayurvedic doctors, just to circumvent code of ethics and has become a big menace misleading innocent people and exploiting them just for monitory benefit. Surrogate advertisements by Pharma companies are another problem, as evidenced by recent advertisement by a leading Pharma company of corticosteroid and antifungal combination cream disguised as plain antifungal (miconazole) cream for treatment of tinea infection.

There is an essential and urgent need to curb the menace and represent to Law commission and Government of India to prevent surrogate advertisements.

Can a dermatologist put a board as cosmetic dermatologist or dermatosurgeon or cosmetic surgeon?
Thanks to very rapid advances in science and technology, the scope of dermatology has changed beyond imagination. There were times when one can start dermatology practice with a simple hand lens and a thermal cautery machine. Now one has to have to at least one or two lasers and other dermatosurgical and cosmetic equipment, which may in total need minimum ₹ 1–2 million.

The specialty of dermatology now has developed into subspecialties like dermatosurgery, cosmetic surgery, or medical cosmetology. The curriculum of postgraduate courses and mandatory equipment required as per MCI, includes three types of lasers, cryosurgeries, acne surgeries, vitiligo surgeries, nail surgeries, fillers, dermabrasion, chemical peels, and all dermatosurgical and cosmetic procedures.

However, unfortunately these advances are not reflected in the nomenclature of postgraduate qualifications, which still is by nomenclature of Dermatology, Venereology, and Leprology (DVL). Consequently, people are asking the dermatologists, are you a cosmetologist? are you cosmetic surgeon? are you aesthetic surgeon?, etc. To overcome the nomenclature issues and to counter the propaganda of nonmedical persons claims, many dermatologists are displaying in signboards and letterheads that they are cosmetic dermatologist or cosmetologists or cosmetic surgeon or dermatosurgeon, etc.

As per MCI code of ethics 2002, Regulation 1.4.2, physicians shall display as suffix to their names only recognized medical degrees or *such certificates or diplomas and memberships or honors, which confer professional knowledge* or recognize any exemplary qualification or achievements.

When one has basic postgraduate qualification in dermatology, and subsequently by having hands on training in workshops or CMEs acquiring skills and by getting experience in cosmetic surgery or dermatosurgery or aesthetic surgery, we feel dermatologist can certainly claim and display as member of Association of Cutaneous Surgeons of India (ACSI), Cosmetology Society of India (CSI), etc. and as cosmetic dermatologist or cosmetologists or cosmetic surgeon or dermatosurgeon, etc.

CHANGE OF NOMENCLATURE OF POSTGRADUATE COURSE OF DVL TO DVL AND DERMATOSURGERY/COSMETIC SURGERY

Another aspect is that, after representation of concerned professional associations, basing on scientific advances, MCI has changed the nomenclature of many postgraduate courses. The nomenclature of PG course of TB and CD (Tuberculosis and Chest Diseases) has changed to Pulmonary Medicine or Pulmonology; Similarly nomenclature of PG course of Radiology has changed and separated to Radiodiagnosis and Radiotherapy. It is high time that the professional bodies like Indian Association of Dermatologists, Venereologists, and Leprologists (IADVL), in public interest, to protect the common people from exploitation by unqualified persons, and nonmedical persons, who claim as cosmetic surgeons or cosmetologists, or aesthetic surgeons, and to protect the interests of genuinely qualified dermatologists, should represent to MCI to modify nomenclature of postgraduate course to include cosmetic surgery or dermatosurgery. For example, the nomenclature of MD DVL should be changed to that of MD DVL and Dermato-Surgery or Cosmetic Surgery.

CODE OF ETHICS: HOSPITAL INDUSTRY

All over the world, code of ethics applies to all professions more so to medical profession. However, code of medical ethics applies to individual doctors only but does not apply to nursing homes, hospitals, corporate hospitals, and chain of clinics and cosmetology centers. They all come under the control of local health and municipal administration, who give them permission. But in reality, there is not be much of monitoring on them due factors like huge work load, shortage of staff, administrative bottle necks, and political interference consequently there will be lack of action on erring hospitals or centers.

These days hospitals, particularly corporate hospitals, are established under the category of Health Industry, and by taking huge loans in hundreds of cores of rupees from banks and financial institutions, and they are administered professionally and run as pure business in terms of profit and loss every year. When these hospitals are run as business, naturally ethical values are taking a back seat.

LEGAL IMPLICATIONS OF CODE OF MEDICAL ETHICS

Doctors' behavior in medical education, practice, and research is measured against the above-mentioned code of medical ethics. Any deviation from the same is likely to lead to punitive action against the errant doctors such as removal of name from Indian Medical Council Register. Such deviation may also result in breach of doctor-patient trust leading to litigation by patients, especially in the current era of Consumer Protection Act.[8]

REMEDY AND PREVENTION OF LEGAL IMPLICATIONS OF CODE OF MEDICAL ETHICS

In practice, ethical decision making can be facilitated by adopting the following simple steps:

1. After thorough consideration of technical facts, moral parameters, and legal constraints determines whether the issue at hand is an ethical one.
2. Consult authoritative sources to see how physicians generally deal with such issues.
3. Consider alternative solutions.

4. Discuss your proposed solution with those whom it will affect.
5. Make your decision and act on it.
6. Evaluate your decision and be prepared to act differently in future (in case of objections arising from factual errors, faulty reasoning or conflicting values, etc.).

SUMMARY

Attitude of the society toward medical profession and the outlook of doctors toward their own profession are undergoing tremendous changes with rapid change in socioeconomic status, especially in countries like India. Even then, the medical profession should be viewed differently.

From time to time, various codes of medical ethics have been formulated to uphold the nobility of medical profession. The Indian Medical Council Regulations 2002 are also a step in the same direction, despite some of its fallacies. Following code of medical ethics in letter and spirit is the need of the hour to retain the status of this profession as a noble, fulfilling but yet exciting profession. Doctors should adopt a more humane approach toward patient care. Ethical principles of medical research enshrined in the ethical guidelines of ICMR and *WMA* Declaration of Helsinki should be followed more honestly.[2] The need for a comprehensive overhaul of undergraduate curriculum with regard to ethical and legal medical practices was long felt.[9] Fortunately, this seems to be moving in right direction with the new MCI curriculum for undergraduates, which may hopefully succeed in achieving the highest ethical standards expected out of the doctors of future generations.

SUMMARY WITH KEY MESSAGES AND PEARLS

- Medical ethics is a *"combination of moral principles and values that are applied to take judgements in medical education, practice and research"*.
- Several codes of medical ethics have been prescribed including Code of Hammurabi, Hippocratic Oath, Charaka Samhita, Sushruta Samhita as well as the modern day International Code of Medical Ethics, Indian Medical Council (Professional Conduct, Etiquette and Ethics) Regulations, and AAD code of medical ethics for Dermatologists.
- Code of medical ethics is based on the four basic principles of respect for patient's autonomy, beneficence (patient's best interest), justice and non-maleficence (do no harm).
- Indian Medical Council (Professional Conduct, Etiquette and Ethics) Regulations (2002; amended up to 8th October 2016) deal extensively with duties and responsibilities of physicians towards patients, society, professional colleagues and pharmaceutical companies as well as professional misconduct and its punishment.
- Following the code of medical ethics, such as Indian Medical Council (Professional Conduct, Etiquette and Ethics) Regulations, in letter and spirit is the need of the hour to retain the status of medical profession as a noble and fulfilling profession, devoted to service of humanity.
- However, in the Indian context, there is an urgent need to further amend these regulations to address the modern day concerns such as violence against doctors by patients/attendants, spurious/false consumer forum litigations against doctors/hospitals, double registration/re-registration of degrees in multiple states, surrogate advertisements by non-allopathic medical systems, surrogate advertisements by pharma companies, unnecessarily stringent restrictions on advertisement/display of dermatologists' qualifications (basic and additional) in the modern era of internet and internet based media, competition to dermatologists from unqualified practitioners/beauty clinic chains, etc.

REFERENCES

1. Kamdar BC. Dermatological practice & medical ethics. In: Srinivas P (Ed). A Dermatologists' Perspective of Medical Ethics and Consumer Protection Act: An IADVL Book, 1st edition. Kolkata: IADVL-Printco; 2007. pp. 57-66.
2. Ramana KV, Kandi S, Boinpally PR. Ethics in medical education, practice, and research: An insight. Ann Trop Med Public Health. 2013;6:599-602.
3. Pandya SK. History of medical ethics in India. Eubios J Asian and Int Bioeth. 2000;10:40-4.
4. Boyd KM. Medical ethics: principles, persons, and perspectives: from controversy to conversation. J Med Ethics. 2005;31:481-6.
5. Kuroyonagi T. Historical transition in medical ethics—challenges of the World Medical Association. J Med Assoc J. 2013;56(4):220-6.
6. American Academy of Dermatology. (2014). Code of Medical Ethics For Dermatologists. [online] Available from: https://www.aad.org/Forms/Policies/Uploads/AR/AR%20CODE%20OF%20MEDICAL%20ETHICS%20FOR%20DERMATOLOGISTS.pdf [Accessed December, 2018].
7. MCI Code of Medical Ethics- IMC (Professional conduct, etiquette and ethics) – Regulations 2002; amended upto October 2016.
8. Srinivas P. Consumer Protection Act and dermatological practice. In: Srinivas P (Ed). A Dermatologists' Perspective of Medical Ethics and Consumer Protection Act: An IADVL Book, 1st edition. Kolkata: IADVL-Printco; 2007. pp. 7-14.
9. Eckles ER, Meslin EM, Gaffney M, et al. Medical ethics education: Where are we? Where should we be going? A review. Acad Med. 2005;80:1143-52.

CHAPTER 4

Civil Liability and Civil Negligence including Vicarious Liability

Subodh Premanand Sirur

DANGLING SWORD OF ALLEGATIONS OF NEGLIGENCE

It is indeed distressing for a doctor to be staring at a legal notice or a notice from the Consumer Disputes Redressal Agencies (consumer courts—as they are commonly referred to as) or a civil court or any other judicial or quasi-judicial authority alleging medical negligence on the part of the doctor. The doctor can be caught unaware and respond with disbelief, fear and unfounded apprehensions. Under such circumstances, it is important that the doctors peruse the contents of the notice and verify the facts as also check the nature of allegations contained in the notice. Simply because allegations are made alleging negligence necessarily does not mean that the doctor has been negligent. Before proceeding to take any action, the doctor should assess the matter and the allegations therein. The allegations may be baseless or unsubstantiated and have been made with the sole intention to harass the doctor or to extract money as compensation from the doctor. Even if you have a legal advisor or a lawyer to handle your legal issues a preliminary assessment by the doctor is a good step.

CONCEPT OF NEGLIGENCE

A civil liability can arise as a result of:
1. A contract between two or more parties. If there is breach of the terms and conditions of the contract then a civil liability can arise. Such a liability is termed as "contractual liability".
2. Statutory liability—liability arising out failure to comply with the laws for the time being in force.
3. Tort—negligence is a tort. *Tort is a civil wrong (other than under a contract) which causes loss or harm to the other and for which damages or compensation is payable.* So what does the term "negligence connote"? A doctor is expected to do certain acts as part of his professional commitments and management of patients. If a doctor fails to

do such an act expected of him or her as a prudent or reasonable doctor then such an act would be termed as an act of omission. To illustrate—before injecting a full dose of penicillin one is expected to give a test dose of penicillin to the patient. If the doctor fails to give the test dose, it would be an act of omission.

Likewise, a doctor is not expected to do certain acts, which no prudent and reasonable doctor would do. Such an act is termed as an "act of commission". If a doctor prescribes methotrexate to an elderly patient with known history of chronic kidney disease without adjusting the dose of methotrexate or without considering the safety profile of the drug in chronic kidney disease, it could amount to an act of commission.

Negligence is defined in simple words as doing of an act which no prudent and reasonable doctor would do or not doing an act, which a prudent and reasonable doctor would do under similar circumstances.

PROOF OF NEGLIGENCE

The onus of proving the allegations of negligence is primarily on the person alleging it. Therefore, the burden of proving the allegations is heavily on the patient or the legal representative/s of the patient. But once the patient or the legal representatives prove lack of care on the part of the doctor, the burden shifts on the doctor or the hospital to prove that there has been no negligence.

In *Savita Garg (Smt) versus Director, National Heart Institute*, it has been observed as under:

"*Once an allegation is made that the patient was admitted in a particular hospital and evidence is produced to satisfy that he died because of lack of proper care and negligence, then the burden lies on the hospital to justify that there was no negligence on the part of the treating doctor or hospital. Therefore, in any case, the hospital is in a better position to disclose what care was taken or what medicine was administered to the patient. It is the duty of the hospital to satisfy that there was no lack of care or diligence. The hospitals are institutions, people expect better and efficient service, if the hospital fails to discharge their duties through their doctors, being employed on job basis or employed on contract basis, it is the hospital which has to justify and not impleading a particular doctor will not absolve the hospital of its responsibilities.*"

There are only two exceptions to this rule:

1. *Negligence per se*: In Poonam Verma versus Dr Ashwin Mehta was dealing with a matter alleging medical negligence.

    Facts of the case: The treating doctor was qualified in homeopathic system of medicine but had treated the complainant's husband who was suffering from typhoid by the modern system of medicine. The patient later developed typhoid encephalopathy and died. The complainant alleged negligence on the part of the doctor.

    Decision of the Court: The Supreme Court while holding the doctor negligent observed as below:

    "*Negligence has many manifestations—it may be active negligence, collateral negligence, comparative negligence, concurrent negligence, continued negligence, criminal negligence, gross negligence, hazardous negligence, active and passive negligence, willful or reckless negligence or negligence per se, which is defined in Black's Law Dictionary as under: Negligence per se: Conduct, whether of action or omission, which may be declared and treated as negligence without any* argument or proof as to the particular surrounding circumstances, either because it is in violation of a statute or valid municipal ordinance, or because it is so palpably opposed to the dictates of common prudence that it can be said without hesitation or doubt that no careful person would have been guilty of it. As a general rule, the violation of a public duty, enjoined by law for the protection of person or property, so constitutes."

"A person who does not have knowledge of a particular System of Medicine but practices in that System is a Quack and a mere pretender to medical knowledge or skill, or to put it differently, a Charlatan. Where a person is guilty of negligence per se, no further proof is needed."

Further, it held that a doctor qualified in one system of medicine cannot practice in another system of medicine. Doing so can amount to negligence per se and no further proof of negligence is required.

2. *Res ipsa loquitur (the thing speaks for itself)*: When a gauze piece is left behind in the abdomen after the surgery, the thing speaks for itself, that an event would not happen if the doctor had not been negligent. In such cases, the factum of gauze piece left behind in the abdomen is proved then the onus of proving that there has been no negligence is on the doctor and the patient is not bound to prove negligence.

In *Harjot Ahluwalia (minor) versus Spring Meadows Hospital and another*, the Supreme Court held as under:

"Gross medical mistake will always result in a finding of negligence. Use of wrong drug or wrong gas during the course of anesthetic will frequently lead to the imposition of liability and in some situations even the principle of res ipsa loquitur can be applied."

Essentials of Proof of Negligence

To prove negligence and claim for compensation, the following components are required to be proved:
1. Existence of a legal duty to take care
2. Failure of duty to take care
3. Loss or injury or death of the patient
4. The loss or injury or death is the direct and proximate cause of the failure of duty to take care.

A doctor is legally duty bound to administer a test dose of penicillin before the full dose is administered. Therefore, there exists a duty of care in giving a test dose. If the doctor fails in this duty of care and administers the full dose without giving a test dose and the patient dies of anaphylaxis then there is death due to failure of the duty of care expected of the doctor. The death of the patient due to anaphylaxis is a proximate and direct cause of the failure of the doctor to take care. However, if there is no loss or injury to the patient as a result of the failure on the part of the doctor of the duty to take care then there is no actionable negligence (which means that the claim of compensation will fail).

Duty of Care

While deciding a matter of a medical negligence, the Supreme Court in *Dr Laxman Balakrishna Joshi versus Dr Trimbak Bapu Godbole* held that the three important duties of care of a doctor are the following:

"The duties which a doctor owes to his patient are clear. A person who holds himself out ready to give medical advice and treatment impliedly undertakes that he is possessed of skill and knowledge for the purpose. Such a person when consulted by a patient owes him certain duties, viz. a duty of care in deciding whether to undertake the case, a duty of care in deciding what treatment to give or a duty of care in the administration of that treatment. A breach of any of those, duties gives a right of action for negligence to the patient. The practitioner must bring to his task a reasonable degree of skill and knowledge and must exercise a reasonable degree of care. Neither the very highest nor a very low degree of care and competence judged in the light of the particular circumstances of each case is what the law requires: (cf. Halsbury's Laws of England, 3rd edition. vol. 26, p. 17). The doctor no doubt has discretion in choosing treatment which he proposes to give to the patient and such discretion is relatively ampler in cases of emergency."

CONTRIBUTORY NEGLIGENCE

When the patient is also negligent which results in loss or injury to the patient, it is said to be contributory negligence. While the negligence on the part of the patient does not absolve the doctor of the responsibility to take due care in the management of the patient, the point of contributory negligence is important while assessing the compensation to be paid.

VICARIOUS NEGLIGENCE

Ordinarily the person who commits the negligent act causing loss or injury is liable to pay compensation to the person to whom the loss or injury was caused. However, under certain circumstances, one can be liable for the negligent act of another. For example, the head of the department could be liable for the acts of the junior doctor supervised by him or her; the government running the hospital where the negligent act was committed can be held vicariously for the doctors employed under it and by whom the negligent act was committed.

In a particular case where the gynecologist employed in a State Government hospital left behind a mop in the abdomen, the State Government was held vicariously liable for the negligent act.

In *Kanchanmala Vijay Singh's case* while dealing with a claim for compensation (the matter was not in the realm of medical negligence but the principles of law apply to medical negligence matters also):

"Traditionally, before court directed payment of tort compensation, the claimant had to establish the fault of the person causing injury or damage. But of late, it shall appear from different judicial pronouncements that the fault is being read as because of someone's negligence or carelessness. Same is the approach and attitude of the courts while judging the vicarious liability of the employer for negligence of the employee. Negligence is the omission to do something which a reasonable man is expected to do or a prudent man is expected not to do. Whether in the facts and circumstances of a particular case, the person causing injury to the other was negligent or not has to be examined on the materials produced before the Court. It is the rule that an employer, though guilty of no fault himself, is liable for the damage done by the fault or negligence of his servant acting in the course of his employment. In some case, it can be found that an employee was doing an authorized act in an unauthorized but not a prohibited way. The employer shall be liable for such act, because such employee was acting within the scope of his employment and in so acting done something negligent or wrongful. A master is liable even for acts, which he has not authorized provided they are so connected with acts, which he has been so authorized. On the other hand, if the act of the servant is not even remotely connected within the scope of employment and is an independent act, the master shall not be responsible because the servant is not acting in the course of his employment but has gone outside."

Often, a dermatologist or a plastic surgeon employs juniors for assistance in conducting the outdoor patient department as well for performing certain procedures such as skin biopsy, chemical peels, Botox injection, and filler injections as well for LASER therapy. If the junior fails in his/her duty of care and there is loss or injury to the patient, then the senior doctor will be held vicariously liable for such acts of omission and commission on the part of the junior.

In Harjot Ahluwalia versus Spring Meadows Hospital (referred to earlier in this chapter), the Supreme Court held as below:

Even delegation of responsibility to another may amount to negligence in certain circumstances. A consultant could be negligent where he delegates the responsibility to his junior with the knowledge that the junior was incapable of performing of his duties properly.

Therefore, it is essential that it is ensured that the junior has necessary qualifications and skills before the junior is entrusted with responsibilities. Issuing instructions over the phone on the modality of treatment can prove detrimental to the interests of the dermatologist/plastic surgeon. When a junior requires supervision, physical presence for supervision would be necessary. Further, when a professional indemnity is taken, it is prudent to take a cover for the juniors also, as the ultimate liability may lie with the senior dermatologist/plastic surgeon.

However, it is to be remembered that vicarious liability applies in case of civil liability and not in case of criminal liability for negligence.

CONSUMER PROTECTION ACT AND NEGLIGENCE

The Section 2(g) of the Consumer Protection Act, 1986 defines deficiency of service as under:

"deficiency" means any fault, imperfection, shortcoming or inadequacy in the quality, nature and manner of performance which is required to be maintained by or under any law for the time being in force or has been undertaken to be performed by a person in pursuance of a contract or otherwise in relation to any service.

Thus, in other words, negligence is equivalent to deficiency of service under the Act as negligence is also a shortcoming or imperfection in the quality, nature and manner of performance which is required to be maintained by the doctor. In case of hospitals and other healthcare facilities, failure to keep functional oxygen cylinders, maintain the toilets clean and such others amount to deficiency of service.

For example, if the dermatologist or the plastic surgeon undertakes to perform the hair removal with a promise to completely remove the unwanted hair then lack of removal of complete hair can amount to deficiency of service under the Act as the promise to remove completely the unwanted hair becomes a part of the contract between the dermatologist/plastic surgeon and the patient. Therefore, it is not right to make assurances as sometimes the complete removal may not be possible for reasons beyond the control of the dermatologist and or the plastic surgeon.

Similarly, if there is failure of hair to grow following a hair transplant surgery would by itself not amount to deficiency of service as there are factors beyond the control of operating surgeon.

The Consumer Disputes Redressal Agencies are empowered to award compensation to the patient or his legal representatives (in the event of death of the patient) for any loss or injury suffered by the patient due to the negligence of the doctor.

In a matter decided by the Supreme Court where a dermatologist was also dragged into litigation for alleged negligence.

Facts of the Case

A non-resident Indian (NRI) doctor who visited India along with his wife went out for dinner following which the wife developed some allergic reaction. The physician who saw her diagnosed it to be "allergic vasculitis" and prescribed her injection Depo-Medrol in the dose of 80 mg, which was to be administered twice a day for 3 days. The clinical condition of the patient did not improve and was later hospitalized. The dermatologist diagnosed her to be having toxic epidermal necrolysis and prescribed tablet prednisolone in the dose of 120 mg/day. The patient's condition worsened and the patient was flown from one city to another for "better treatment". The patient later died of septicemia.

Decision

Based on the evidence of experts in the field and extract of standard textbooks on the subjects and articles in the journals, it was held that Depo-Medrol (a depot preparation) should not have been prescribed twice a day for 3 days and that the dose of prednisolone of 120 mg/day was on the higher side and was not recommended for toxic epidermal necrolysis. Further, the patient was certified to be fit to be transferred to another city in another State for "better treatment". This hastened the progression to septicemia and death of the patient. The Court, thus, held the concerned doctors and the hospital liable for negligence.

POINT TO REMEMBER

The line of management should be as per accepted professional practices. As Depo-Medrol is a depot preparation, it was not expected to be prescribed in a frequency of twice a day and that too for 3 consecutive days. While a doctor is expected to treat a patient in accordance to accepted professional practices, the doctor is allowed to make deviation to accepted professional practices depending upon the clinical condition and the clinical judgment of the doctor but should be able to scientifically justify the deviation. If such a deviation is one that no prudent doctor under similar clinical circumstances would do then it may amount to medical negligence.

CIVIL NEGLIGENCE VIS-À-VIS CRIMINAL NEGLIGENCE

1. *Preponderance of evidence*: Whereas in criminal liability the negligence has to be proved beyond a shadow of doubt or beyond reasonable doubt, a liability of civil negligence can be decided on the basis of preponderance of evidence.
2. *Relief sought*: In criminal complaint, the intention is to punish the offender either by way of a fine (as opposed to compensation) and/or imprisonment of the offender whereas in case of civil negligence the objective is to put the patient or his legal representatives in a financial state (by awarding a compensation) in which they would have been in case the adverse consequences of medical negligence would not have occurred.

SUGGESTED READING

1. Supreme Court of India. Civil Appeal No. 1727 of 2007. New Delhi, 2007.
2. Supreme Court of India. Civil Appeal No. 7858 of 1997. New Delhi, 1997.
3. Supreme Court of India. Reported in All India Reporter 1969 at page no. 128. New Delhi, 1969.

CHAPTER 5

Criminal Medical Negligence and Criminal Liability

Subodh Premanand Sirur

INTRODUCTION

It is not uncommon that criminal complaints have been filed against a doctor alleging negligence on the part of the doctor. It is often resorted to extract some amount from the doctor for the alleged negligence. The sections of Indian Penal Code applied for negligence include sections 336, 337, 338 (these sections are applied when death has not occurred due to the negligent act of the doctor) and 304-A (when death has occurred due to the rash and negligent act of the doctor). Rashness has not been defined under the Indian Penal Code; however, rashness means doing an act that has a risk of ensuing adverse consequences but there is indifference on the part of the offender to the risk of such adverse consequences.

SECTION 336: ACT ENDANGERING LIFE OR PERSONAL SAFETY OF OTHERS

Whoever does any act so rashly or negligently as to endanger human life or the personal safety of others shall be punished with imprisonment of either description for a term, which may extend to 3 months, or with fine which may extend to ₹ 250, or with both.

SECTION 337

Whoever causes hurt to any person by doing any act so rashly or negligently as to endanger human life, or the personal safety of others, shall be punished with imprisonment of either description for a term, which may extend to 6 months, or with fine which may extend to ₹ 500, or with both.
(*Hurt:*[1] Whoever causes bodily pain, disease or infirmity to any person is said to cause hurt.)

SECTION 338

Whoever causes grievous hurt to any person by doing any act so rashly or negligently as to endanger human life, or the personal safety of others, shall be punished with imprisonment of either description for a term, which may extend to 2 years, or with fine, which may extend to ₹ 2000, or with both.

(*Grievous hurt:*[2] The following kinds of hurt only are designated as "grievous":

Emasculation, permanent privation of the sight of either eye; permanent privation of the hearing of either ear, privation of any member or joint; destruction or permanent impairing of the powers of any member or joint; permanent disfiguration of the head or face, fracture or dislocation of a bone or tooth, any hurt which endangers life or which causes the sufferer to be during the space of 20 days in severe bodily pain, or unable to follow his ordinary pursuits.)

304-A: CAUSING DEATH BY NEGLIGENCE

"Whoever causes the death of any person by doing any rash or negligent act not amounting to culpable homicide, shall be punished with imprisonment of either description for a term which may extend to 2 years, or with fine, or with both."

It is pertinent to note that the above-mentioned sections are applied commonly in vehicular accidents but have been applied in case of criminal medical negligence also. There were instances when criminal complaints were filed against doctors alleging negligence causing death, following which, the doctor would get arrested. Notably the above-mentioned offenses are bailable offenses. However, the professional reputation of the doctor would be adversely affected following such an arrest.

An important ingredient of criminal liability is presence of "mens rea" or guilty mind of the offender. Rashness or recklessness on the part of the doctor is itself of the "mens rea" of the offending doctor. The doctor ordinarily does not intend to harm the health of the patient but being so rash (reckless or utter disregard to the consequences of his act and knowing fully that the recklessness is most likely to result in adverse consequences for the patient) would indicate the "mens rea" an essential ingredient to prove criminal liability of the offender.

There are extreme instances where the police have applied section 304 II (dealing with culpable homicide not amounting to murder) while dealing with a case of alleged criminal medical negligence. However, such a section would not apply to a doctor unless the criminal intent is proved.

The Supreme Court delivered two landmark judgments on the criminal liability of the doctors in case of alleged negligence and the procedure to be followed in case of such allegations in a criminal complaint.

Jacob Mathew versus State of Punjab[3]

Facts of the Case

The complainant's father diagnosed with terminal cancer had difficulty in breathing while he was in the hospital. The doctors attempted to administer oxygen to the patient. However, the oxygen cylinder was found to be empty. It was alleged that as the oxygen cylinder was unavailable the patient died and that this was due to the negligence on the part of the doctors.

Following the filing of the First Information Report (FIR) an offense under Section 304-A IPC was registered and charges were framed by the Judicial Magistrate First Class, against the two doctors. The revision filed by the doctors in the Court of Sessions Judge was dismissed. A petition was filed by the doctors in the High Court for quashing of the FIR and all the subsequent proceedings. However, the High Court dismissed the petition. A Special Leave Petition was filed before the Supreme Court of India. The matter was placed for hearing before a Bench of two Judges of the Supreme Court, which referred the matter to a Bench of three judges.

The Court referred to its earlier judgment[4] where a young man was treated for nasal deformity. It was shown following investigations that the cause of death was found to be "not introducing a cuffed endotracheal tube of proper size as to prevent aspiration of blood from the wound in the respiratory passage". In that matter, the Supreme Court had held that even if the allegations were to be held to be true such an act though could be an act of negligence (civil) cannot make the doctor criminally liable.

Decision

The three Judge Bench approved the decision in the previous judgment and held that to prove negligence under criminal law, the prosecution must prove:
1. The existence of duty to take care
2. A breach of the duty to take care resulting in death of the patient
3. The breach of the duty must be such so as to amount to gross negligence.

Negligence must be of a gross or a very high degree to amount to criminal negligence unlike in civil negligence. Further, in criminal negligence, the negligence has to be proved beyond a shadow of doubt whereas the civil negligence is decided on preponderance of evidence.

While holding that the doctors in the instant case were not liable under criminal law for negligence, the Supreme Court in *Jacob Mathew versus State of Punjab* laid down certain guidelines in case of a complaint against a doctor alleging criminal negligence.

"A private complaint may not be entertained unless the complainant has produced prima facie evidence before the Court in the form of a credible opinion given by another competent doctor to support the charge of rashness or negligence on the part of the accused doctor."

The investigating officer should, before proceeding against the doctor accused of rash or negligent act or omission, obtain an independent and competent medical opinion preferably from a doctor in government service qualified in that branch of medical practice who can normally be expected to give an impartial and unbiased opinion applying Bolam's test to the facts collected in the investigation.

A doctor accused of rashness or negligence, may not be arrested in a routine manner (simply because a charge has been leveled against him). Unless his arrest is necessary for furthering the investigation or for collecting evidence or unless the investigation officer feels satisfied that the doctor proceeded against would not make himself available to face the prosecution.

Further, it held that—*"Statutory Rules or Executive Instructions incorporating certain guidelines need to be framed and issued by the Government of India and/or the State Governments in consultation with the Medical Council of India. So long as it is not done, we propose to lay down certain guidelines for the future which should govern the prosecution of doctors for offenses of which criminal rashness or criminal negligence is an ingredient."*

In the said judgment, the Supreme Court had directed framing of guidelines by the Government for prosecution of medical professionals. However, such guidelines are yet to be framed and till such time, the guidelines laid by the Supreme Court will govern the prosecution of doctors for alleged criminal negligence.

The complaints against dermatologists alleging negligence is definitely lower than other specialties such as general surgery, gynecology, ophthalmology, anesthesiology and such others. Criminal complaints alleging negligence on the part of the dermatologists are even much lower. The following is an instance where a dermatologist was dragged into a prolonged litigation in a criminal matter.

Facts of the case: In a case where a lady diagnosed to be suffering from Toxic Epidermal Necrolysis[5] was transported from a hospital in one city to another where the condition of the patient worsened and ultimately the patient died of septicemia.

A criminal complaint was filed against three doctors (including a dermatologist) in the Court of Chief Judicial Magistrate for commission of offense under section 304-A of the Indian Penal Code.

The learned Chief Judicial Magistrate found the dermatologist and another doctor criminally liable and sentenced them to undergo simple imprisonment for 3 months and to pay a fine. The appeals of the doctors were allowed by the Hon'ble High Court and the doctors were acquitted. The complainant filed a criminal appeal before the Hon'ble Supreme Court.

Decision: The Supreme Court dismissed the criminal appeal (acquitting the doctors of criminal charges) while holding the doctors liable in civil law for negligence.

It held as follows:

The jurisprudential concept of negligence differs in civil and criminal law. What may be negligence in civil law may not necessarily be negligence in criminal law. For negligence to amount to an offense, the element of mens rea must be shown to exist. For an act to amount to criminal negligence, the degree of negligence should be of a much higher degree. A negligence which is not of such a high degree may provide a ground for action in civil law but cannot form the basis for prosecution. To prosecute a medical professional for negligence under criminal law it must be shown that the accused did something or failed to do something which in the given facts and circumstances no medical professional in his ordinary senses and prudence would have done or failed to do.

It also held as under:

"We may not be understood as holding that doctors can never be prosecuted for an offense of which rashness or negligence is an essential ingredient. All that we are doing is to emphasize the need for care and caution in the interest of society; for, the service which the medical profession renders to human beings is probably the noblest of all, and hence there is a need for protecting doctors from frivolous or unjust prosecutions. Many a complainant prefers recourse to criminal process as a tool for pressurizing the medical professional for extracting uncalled for or unjust compensation. Such malicious proceedings have to be guarded against."

Thus, the Supreme Court has not provided total immunity against criminal liability for doctors but has only protected them from any frivolous or unjust prosecutions.

In case of civil negligence, there is a concept of vicarious liability. This means liability incurred for the wrongdoing of some else than the person on whom the liability is fastened. However, in case of criminal medical negligence, there is no concept of vicarious liability. The wrongdoer is criminally liable for the wrongdoing.

If a dermatologist or a plastic surgeon visits a particular hospital or healthcare facility only for the purpose of performing the aesthetic procedure and serious adverse consequences occur inviting criminal liability then the particular doctor will be held liable for the criminal act. The person who commits the crime is responsible for the crime unless some else has participated in some manner in this crime in which case section 34 of Indian Penal Code may apply if a criminal offense is made out.

SECTION 34 OF THE INDIAN PENAL CODE

Acts done by several persons in furtherance of common intention: When a criminal act is done by several persons in furtherance of the common intention of all, each of such persons is liable for that act in the same manner as if it were done by him alone.

POINTS TO REMEMBER

- Criminal complaints alleging medical negligence on the part of a dermatologist is extremely rare.
- Fastening of criminal liability for negligence on the part of a dermatologist has not been reported so far.
- Sections 336, 337 and 338 of Indian Penal Code are applied in case of criminal complaint alleging medical negligence where death has not occurred and section 304-A when death has occurred following alleged medical negligence.
- A doctor should not be arrested in a routine manner simply because a criminal complaint alleging rashness and negligence has been filed.
- The police officer is bound to seek an independent opinion of an expert in that field before proceeding against the doctor.

REFERENCES

1. Section 319 of the Indian Penal Code.
2. Section 320 of the Indian Penal Code.
3. Supreme Court of India. Criminal Appeal No. 778 of 2004. New Delhi, 2004.
4. Supreme Court of India. Criminal Appeal Nos. 144-145 of 2004. New Delhi, 2004.
5. Supreme Court of India. Criminal Appeal Nos. 1191-1194 of 2005. New Delhi, 2005.

CHAPTER 6

Consumer Protect Act-2018 and beyond: What Practicing Doctors need to know?

Atul Shah

KEY OBJECTIVES
- Medical and healthcare services and consumer protection
- Consumer Protection Law in India
- Instances of complains under the Act
- Precautions by clinicians and healthcare organizations
- Frivolous and vexatious complaints against doctors
- Pearls

MEDICAL AND HEALTHCARE SERVICES AND CONSUMER PROTECTION

Since after the commercialization of plastic surgery and cosmetic dermatology, with introduction of surgical procedures for not only repairing the traumatic/congenital defect, but improving the facial appearance, and beautification of body parts by removing the extra skin and fat, and surgical injections for improving the curves and contours. Thus, the plastic surgeons (along with other doctors in every clinical specialty) have been legally recognized as "Healthcare Providers", since the synthetic materials and technological tools are termed as "Consumables" in Corporate Hospitals, so the person undergoing the surgical correction (who may or may not be suffering for disease) is labeled as "Consumer". Thus, Consumers expect 100% satisfaction even in medical science (unpredictable adverse events have happened in spite of best of care), and if anything goes wrong before, during or even within 24 months after the surgery (plus the age till the consumer becomes major in age, when operated on children), consumers can sues the surgeon for claiming monetary compensation for damages, as per the law of the Land [Consumer

Protection Act (CPA) in India]. The whole legal hassle can be easily recalled as all Ps:
- P—Protection of
- P—Patient (consumer) from
- P—Physical trauma due to wrong surgery, by wrong method, by wrong doctor
- P—Physiological dysfunction of vital organs due to complication of surgery
- P—Psychological trauma due to loss of quality of life after surgery
- P—Personal trauma (loss of spouse due to death that is immediate or late consequence of medical treatment or surgery)
- P—Performance reduction in doing his work, due to unexpected result of surgery. Or P—Paisa (money) excessive expenditure beyond the estimate given before surgery.

But legal hassle can be prevented by:
- P—Paper documentation of Consent, Procedure, and Adverse events during surgery, and steps taken for rectification of expected/unexpected complication
- P—Pursue any consumer complaint in proper manner with guidance of personal lawyer (do not ignore the threats and allegations)
- P—Professional indemnity coverage can be very helpful in saving
- P—Profession of
- P—Plastic surgeons (healthcare P-Provider) by
- P—Paying proposed premium regularly without pendency and
- P—Providing financial support for surgeon to compensate patient with Jackpot amount in Crores awarded by Consumer Courts in India today for
- P—Proven allegation of deficiency in service
- P—Professional training and update with legal bans and sanctions of new Devices/Drugs/Decisions for yourself and your attending junior surgeons, staff, resident doctors (Captain of the ship doctrine)
- P—Pray to almighty God regularly for safe surgical practice.

CONSUMER PROTECTION LAW IN INDIA

The all revamp Consumer Protection Bill 2018 (1 of 2018) was introduced by Minister of Consumer Affairs in Lok Sabha on 5th March, 2018, after it was cleared by standing committee in 2015, many amendments on floor in 2016 and approval was expected by Council of Ministers in 2018. However, when Parliament monsoon session ended on 10th August, 2018, the bill was still pending. In winter session of 2018, Lower house has cleared the bill and sent to Rajya Sabha.

Some salient features of this new bill are:
a. The 2018 Bill provides for fine up to ₹ 5,000,000 and jail up to 5 years for service providers for false and misleading advertisements.
b. The 2018 Bill in chapter III prescribes to set up Central Consumer Protection Authority (CCPA). Chapter II of existing act already refers to such a council naming it as Central Consumer Protection Council (CCPC). CCPA shall have powers to initiate class action enforcing recall, refund and return of products.
c. CCPA shall prevent consumer harassment arising from unfair trade practice. Interestingly the bill has provisions for electronic complaint filing system and mediation as an alternative dispute redressal mechanism.
d. Also in a bid to inhibit patients from registering frivolous complaints, the 2018 bill provides to increase the penalty from ₹ 10,000 to ₹ 50,000.

e. The Consumer Protection Bill, 2018 also proposes some new clauses that will affect health personnel and health organizations. District Forum's limit has now been extended to ₹ 10,000,000, State Forums ₹ 100,000,000, and the National Forums ₹ 100,000,000 and above. The 2018 Bill states that if it appears to the Consumer Forum that there is possibility of a settlement, Forum may direct the parties to give in writing for their dispute to be settled by mediation.[1]

Consumer Protection Act of 1986 (Act 68 of 1986) with two small amendments in 1991 (No. 34 of 1991) and 2002 (No. 62 of 2002)[2] with new sections added is now almost 32 years old.[3] Lot of changes have surfaced in the consumer behaviors since this act was formulated. Here we will prefer to address the Act as CoPrA.

To begin with CoPrA was not explicitly applicable to health and medical care services. In all probability, First State High Court Judgment on this issue can be traced to 1992. Honorable Justice M Rao, writing for two judge bench of himself and Justice VN Rao from Andhra Pradesh High Court in a case of Dr AS Chandra and Others versus Union of India (UoI) and Others[4] wrote on 17th April, 1992.

"...26. The intention of Parliament, in our view, was not and could not be to confine the definition of "service" to what are specifically mentioned in Clause (1)(o) of Section 2 (of CoPrA 1986). The opening words of the clause, "service means service of any description....." clearly bring out the intention of Parliament that service of every description is comprehended by Clause (o); inclusively certain services are mentioned. By no stretch of reasoning can it be said that services mean only what are specified in that clause especially when the opening part comprehends service of any description. Therefore, in the context the expression "includes" enlarges the meaning of word "service" without confining it to what are specifically mentioned in the clause. The Act does not exclude services rendered by professionals. They are too numerous to be specified and that was the reason why inclusive definition was adopted.

27. Two categories are excluded from the definition of service under Section 2(1)(o) of the (CoPrA) Act: (a) Service rendered free of charge; (b) Service rendered under a contract of personal service.

28. In Simmons versus Heath Laundry Company, 1910 (1) KB 543. One of the earliest cases, the Court considered the meaning of the term "contract of service" in the Workmen's Compensation Act. A girl aged 19, employed in a laundry as a skirt machine hand, sustained an injury in the course of her employment which rendered her left hand practically useless; the hand was crushed between two hot rollers. Besides her employment at the laundry she had extra income as a teacher of music lessons and playing accompaniments on the piano. She claimed that her other earnings also should be taken into account in assessing the amount of compensation. Her plea was negatived. The Workmen's Compensation Act comprehended only cases of "contract of service or apprenticeship, with an employer whether by way of manual, labor, clerical work or otherwise". A skilled music teacher who gives lessons to a pupil either in his own house or in the pupil's house could not be regarded as a workman and the pupil as the employer. There was no relationship of master and servant between a music teacher and his pupil. It was a case of contract for services but not a contract of service. The difference between "contract of service" and "contract for services" was explained by Fletcher Moulton, LJ, as follows:

"The greater the amount of direct control exercised over the person rendering the services by the person contracting for them the stronger the grounds for holding it to be a contract of service, and similarly the greater the probability that the services rendered are of the nature of professional services and that the contract is not one of service... Where a person goes to a music and singing master to take lessons it would be absurd to hold that the person giving the lessons is the servant of the person taking them in any sense of the word....

...38. We, therefore, hold that in this batch of cases the complainants before the consumer redressal agencies are consumers within the meaning of Section 2(1)(d) and that the services rendered by private medical practitioners and private medical institutions for consideration fall within the ambit of service under Section 2(1)(o) of the Act."

But it is obvious that the Indian Medical Association, Andhra Pradesh sought a writ of prohibition against the foregoing decision in judgment of Dr AS Chandra, requesting court to direct all the District Forums of Andhra Pradesh not to proceed against members of the medical profession. It was stated that one of the objects of the Indian Medical Association is "to protect the interests of the medical science and medical profession in the State of Andhra Pradesh and it is the duty of the Association to maintain the honor and dignity of the noble profession". Andhra Pradesh high court held that the CoPrA includes Nursing Homes and Private Medical Practitioners within the purview of the Act when they provide service against payment. [Dr AS Chandra versus Union of India (1994) CPJ 509 and (1994) MLJ 438.]

Honorable Justice RM Sahai of Supreme Court of India while delivering judgment from two judge bench of himself and Justice Kuldip Singh in appeal on National Consumer Redressal Forum judgment in case of Lucknow Development Authority versus MK Gupta on 5th November, 1993 had discussed about "services" is and reproduced here.[5] These two judgments can be considered as foundation, which led to inclusion of medical services under CoPrA in a later Supreme Court Judgment of November 1995.

(CoPrA 1986)...Clause (o) of the definition section defines it as under: "service" means service of any description which is made available to potential users and includes the provision of facilities in connection with banking, financing, insurance, transport, processing, supply of electrical or other energy, board or lodging or both, housing construction, entertainment, amusement or the purveying of news or other information, but does not include the rendering of any service free of charge or under a contract of personal service.

It is in three parts. The main part is followed by inclusive clause and ends by exclusionary clause. The main clause itself is very wide. It applies to any service made available to potential users. The words "any" and "potential" are significant. Both are of wide amplitude. The word "any" usually may mean "one or some or all". In Black's Law Dictionary, it is explained thus, "word any" has a diversity of meaning and may be employed to indicate "all" or "every" as well as "some" or "one" and its meaning in a given statute depends upon the context and the subject matter of the statute. The use of the word "any" in the context it has been used in clause (o) indicates that it has been used in wider sense extending from one to all. The other word "potential" is again very wide. In Oxford Dictionary, it is defined as "capable of coming into being, possibility". In Black's Law Dictionary, it is defined as "existing in possibility but not in act.... The legislative intention is thus clear to protect a consumer against services rendered even by statutory bodies. The test, therefore, is not if a person against whom complaint is made is a

Consumer Protect Act-2018 and beyond: What Practicing Doctors need to know?

statutory body but whether the nature of the duty and function performed by it is service or even facility......

The final nail was hammered in the VP Shantha judgment.[6] Interesting to note that Counsels for IMA included Mr Harish Salve and Mr Abhishek Manu Singhvi, and they tried their best to impress upon Apex Court way medical services cannot be brought under CoPrA. It was a three judge Bench and judgment was delivered on 13th November 1995 by Justice SC Agrawal for himself and Justice Kuldip Singh and Justice BL Hansaria. The judgment listed following conclusions:

"...... (1) Service rendered to a patient by a medical practitioner (except where the doctor renders service free of charge to every patient or under a contract of personal service), by way of consultation, diagnosis and treatment, both medicinal and surgical, would fall within the ambit of "service" as defined in Section 2(1)(o) of the Act.

(2) The fact that medical practitioners belong to the medical profession and are subject to the disciplinary control of the Medical Council of India (MCI) and/or State Medical Councils constituted under the provisions of the Indian Medical Council Act would not exclude the services rendered by them from the ambit of the Act.

(3) A "contract of personal service" has to be distinguished from a "contract for personal services". In the absence of a relationship of master and servant between the patient and medical practitioner, the service rendered by a medical practitioner to the patient cannot be regarded as service rendered under a "contract of personal service". Such service is service rendered under a "contract for personal services" and is not covered by exclusionary clause of the definition of "service" contained in Section 2(1)(o) of the Act.

(4) The expression "contract of personal service" in Section 2(1)(o) of the Act cannot be confined to contracts for employment of domestic servants only and the said expression would include the employment of a medical officer for the purpose of rendering medical service to the employer. The service rendered by a medical officer to his employer under the contract of employment would be outside the purview of "service" as defined in Section 2(1)(o) of the Act.

(5) Service rendered free of charge by a medical practitioner attached to a hospital/nursing home or a medical officer employed in a hospital/nursing home where such services are rendered free of charge to everybody, would not be "service" as defined in Section 2(1)(o) of the Act. The payment of a token amount for registration purpose only at the hospital/nursing home would not alter the position.

(6) Service rendered at a non-government hospital/nursing home where no charge whatsoever is made from any person availing the service and all patients (rich and poor) are given free service—is outside the purview of the expression "service" as defined in Section 2(1)(o) of the Act. The payment of a token amount for registration purpose only at the hospital/nursing home would not alter the position.

(7) Service rendered at a non-government hospital/nursing home where charges are required to be paid by the persons availing such services falls within the purview of the expression "service" as defined in Section 2(1)(o) of the Act.

(8) Service rendered at a non-government hospital/nursing home where charges are required to be paid by persons who are in a position to pay and persons who cannot afford to pay are rendered service free of charge would fall within the ambit of the expression "service" as defined in Section 2(1)(o) of the

Act irrespective of the fact that the service is rendered free of charge to persons who are not in a position to pay for such services. Free service would also be "service" and the recipient a "consumer" under the Act.

(9) Service rendered at a Government hospital/health center/dispensary where no charge whatsoever is made from any person availing the services and all patients (rich and poor) are given free service—is outside the purview of the expression "service" as defined in Section 2(1)(o) of the Act. The payment of a token amount for registration purpose only at the hospital/nursing home would not alter the position.

(10) Service rendered at a Government hospital/health center/dispensary where services are rendered on payment of charges and also rendered free of charge to other persons availing such services would fall within the ambit of the expression "service" as defined in Section 2(1)(o) of the Act irrespective of the fact that the service is rendered free of charge to persons who do not pay for such service. Free service would also be "service" and the recipient a "consumer" under the Act.

(11) Service rendered by a medical practitioner or hospital/nursing home cannot be regarded as service rendered free of charge, if the person availing the service has taken an insurance policy for medical care where under the charges for consultation, diagnosis and medical treatment are borne by the insurance company and such service would fall within the ambit of "service" as defined in Section 2(1)(o) of the Act.

(12) Similarly, where, as a part of the conditions of service, the employer bears the expenses of medical treatment of an employee and his family members dependent on him, the service rendered to such an employee and his family members by a medical practitioner or a hospital/nursing home would not be free of charge and would constitute "service" under Section 2(1)(o) of the Act...."

With 2002 amendments, the act became smoother. The negligence of medical professional comes within the expression of deficiency in service. So, when doctors do not perform duties to the best of ability and with proper care and caution it is deficiency as per CoPrA. On the other hand, we do come across faults like removal of the wrong part or surgery on the wrong patient or giving injection of wrong drug is obvious negligence and invokes latin maxim res ipsa loquitur—the wrong speaking for itself. Here it is believed that the complete control of the situation rested with the treating team and there was no contributory negligence of any sort from patient and relatives. Also it is taken for granted that the mishap in question has happened due to negligence. When this maxim is applied, the burden is on the defendant to explain how the incident could have occurred without medical negligence.

Before CoPrA came into existence and even now, medical negligence cases are filed in civil courts under Law of Torts. Quoting English view on Law of Torts and English judgment, Hon'ble Apex Court defined Medical.... "Negligence as a tort is the breach of a duty caused by omission to do something which a reasonable man would do or doing something which a prudent and reasonable man would not do".... The definition involves the following constituents: (1) a legal duty to exercise due care; (2) breach of the duty; and (3) consequential damages.[7] So, Consumer forums and commissions are now given the responsibility to decide what a due care in any circumstances is, and was there deficiency in that due care, and if there was any deficiency, was there any damage. Plastic and Cosmetic surgeons, Dermatologists and Cosmetologists are parading the court rooms of consumer

courts (instead of their operating rooms) in the prime of their career nowadays, due to allegation made by their consumer (patients and relatives) for suffering different types of alleged negligences as mentioned here:
- Wrongful surgical procedure (consent for different procedure and doing another surgery without informed consent)
- On wrong patient (exchange of patient on day of surgery with another)
- On wrongful pair of another limb/finger/eyelid/lip
- Using wrong instruments (corroded scalpel)
- Administering wrong medications/anesthetic during surgery
- Forgetting wrong material inside the surgical part repaired (gauze piece/glass pieces/gravel in RTA)
- At wrong time (high bleeding tendency due to blood thinners in cardiac patients)
- By wrong doctor (vital organs like lung/liver/heart/brain surgery by plastic surgeon)
- In wrong place [Procedure carried outside operation theater (OT) like in office or in emergency room (ER)—consumer hence alleges infected environment]
- For wrong duration (prolonged surgery/repeated surgery).

To avoid litigations under CoPrA or other courts, Dr Chandra Prakash and others in their article stressed on prevention at personal level and at site of medical practice.[8] Their list of personal qualities include Qualification that is approved by MCI, frequent updates, experience, timely and detailed communication with patient and relatives and updated knowledge about medical law and ethics. At site of medical practice, the support staff must be well trained as well as updated. Valid and detailed consent is very important.

Valid consent and proper documentation are two very important aspects of litigation free medical career. Needless to say reasonable care is to be practiced during management of a case. This article stresses on three aspects of skills: (1) medical, (2) social and (3) legal. The stress is also laid on negative consents like refusal for investigation, failure to follow instruction, follow-up failure, etc. Professional Indemnity must be sufficient for all. This can be subscribed from IMA NPPS, State PPS and specialty associations, GIC and private insurance companies.

In spite of all such precautions, litigations may happen. One must actively understand and participate in litigation process because lawyers have limited knowledge about medical processes. There can be several points specified as defense like seniority, expertise in a particular type of management, wrong intention of patient, only to shy away from making payment. Here our documentation and consent will come to our rescue. You must try to ascertain that there was no contributory negligence on part of the patient, and if there was any, the same may be highlighted forthwith. Juthika Debbarma and Others also discuss about defenses, classifying them as technical and factual.[9] Noted Lawyer Mr SV Joga Rao has summarized the CoPrA.[10]

It will be worth the space to briefly specify some judgments of Consumer Forums, Commission and Courts here for further understanding the consumer activism and deficiency in medical services.

INSTANCES OF COMPLAINTS UNDER THE ACT

Case of Nadiya versus Fathima Hospital

Nadiya aged 15 years, with height of 135 cm, got admitted to Fathima Hospital for surgery for increasing her height, for a charge of ₹ 32,000. Ilizarov rings were fixed on legs, which had to be adjusted every 6 hours. However, on her discharge, she found her left leg short by almost 15 cm, could not walk, pain increased, fixators had to be removed and the plaster was applied, skin grafting was required and she remained bedridden. The Commission found negligence and deficiency in service and directed hospital to pay ₹ 500,000 with costs.[11]

Case of Prashant Tamhane versus Hinduja Hospital

In the case of Mr Prashant Tamhane versus the Chief Executive Officer, PD Hinduja Hospital and Intensivist Dr Ashit V Hegde before the Hon'ble State Consumer Disputes Redressal Commission, Maharashtra, at Mumbai, the judgment delivered by President of Commission Justice AP Bhangale and member Mr DR Shirasao has brought out several points.[12] The claimed compensation was ₹ 8,750,000. Judgment reads.... "Compensation cannot be a lottery or jackpot for a Patient who was suffering from ailments...." Also in this judgment only the intensivist has to pay the entire amount of compensation of ₹ 4,125,000 and hospital has been spared looking at circumstances of the case. Reading this judgment shall make reader aware about several other principles of consumer protection aspect of commissions.

In exactly opposite judgment in case of P Manjula versus Global Hospital,[13] "There was agreement of hiring of services of the hospital. There was no privity of contract about hiring (of a particular consultant). Hospital is liable for payment of compensation and not the individual doctor...."

Case of Vikas Arya versus SDM Hospital

In case of Vikas Arya versus Santokba Durlabhji Memorial Hospital while awarding compensation of nearly five million fifty lakh, the Jaipur bench of Rajasthan state commission has made following observation.[14] "It is a common experience that patient and their attendants remain unaware about the diagnosis, treatment and procedure during their stay in the hospital. Attendants are kept away from the patient and they are not even allowed to enter in the room where his patient is kept, in the name of hygiene, cleanliness, individuality and specialty of treatment, etc. This is need of the day that patient and his attendants should be made known the diagnosis, treatment and procedure, etc. and also when and how it was given as the ultimate object of the enactment is not getting or giving compensation but to have flawless service. It is much more essential in the medical field as compared to other types of services, as it is question of life and death and if results are not favorable at the end of procedure, it affects the quality of life. Hospital should not claim immunity by only getting a consent letter signed by the patient or attendant, which is also in many cases blank. Cases like, in hand should not repeat which left the patient and family in life long regret. Hence, we direct the Principal Secretary, Consumer Affairs and Principal Secretary, Medical and Health to formulate a scheme/guideline for keeping transparency in the hospital that patient and their attendants should know exact diagnosis, treatment procedure required and given to the patient from time to time without compromising the quality and urgent nature of the treatment and procedure given or required in the situation. The above scheme/guidelines shall be formulated within 3 months and be placed before this Commission...."

Case of Geeta Rani versus Chandigarh Administration

In case of Geeta Rani Kakkar versus Chandigarh Administration, eye opening judgment is pronounced by state commission of Chandigarh Union territory.[15] It stresses upon proper disinfection of patient bed and cot in managing a burn victim and also about quantum of compensation.

Case of Dipankar versus late Dr Banerjee

"In a tort of medical negligence, the cause of action is personal against the person who has been negligent in discharging his duties and that the cause of action does not survive against his estate or the legal representatives. In this case, the maxim *actio personalis moritur cum persona*, meaning personal right of action dies with the person, a general rule, is applicable to action in torts and, therefore, the cause of action against the party against whom an action in tort is brought is extinguished on his death. It is unfortunate that no relief in the present case can be accorded to the patient on account of Dr Banerjee's death." Thus, wrote the West Bengal state commission judgment when treating doctor died before the conclusion of the matter.[16]

There are variety of such judgments from District Forums, State and National Commissions and State High Courts and Supreme Court. Medical practitioners, health administrators and healthcare organizations have to be watchful at every step of patient care. Individualized cases in relation to dermatologist or plastic surgeon are however limited, but general precautions apply to all alike.

Case of Saurabh Saini versus New Delhi Centre for Sight

It shall be pertinent to conclude the chapter with one more judgment which speaks about casual approach of some patients toward a worthy tool of consumer protection. Decided on 10th May, 2018 while new bill was yet to be debated, the judgment in Saurabh Saini versus New Delhi Centre for Sight delivered by national Commission shows the red light thus.....[17] "We are constrained to note that of late there is an increased tendency on the part of the complainants to overvalue their claim. The reasons why the complainants tend to do this are not difficult to understand. The one reason for doing this may be that a very meager fee as compared to the Court fee payable in civil suit, is payable on complaints filed before the consumer fora. The optimum fee payable for filing original complaint is ₹ 5,000 irrespective of the valuation of the claim made in the complaint. Yet another reason may be is that when it comes to settlement of the claim, the complainant may have an edge and will be in better bargaining position to settle the claim on his own terms. Such a tendency needs to be curbed, lest the complaints of overvalued claim keep on mounting in the National Commission."

Ministry of Consumer affairs publishes judgments of particular period and one such collection can be accessed.[18]

Precautions by Clinicians and Healthcare Organizations

An interesting medicolegal case of minor Facial Trauma will be sufficient to highlight the routine precautins that must be observed. This incidence highlights how medical negligence could be proved from history taking, clinical examination and case notes.

Facts: A 65-year-old male is found by his employer on the floor, unable to speak or get up, lying in a pool of blood from apparent facial injuries. EMS is called and he is brought to the emergency department (ED) for a reported "slip and fall" with associated facial abrasions. He is awake and denies any preceding symptoms, falls or loss of consciousness. EMS report includes concern for cerebrovascular accident (CVA), with variable documentation of face and extremity weakness. Nursing documentation includes the presence of a facial droop. None of this is otherwise communicated to the ED provider and surgeon—only noted in reports. Care is limited to cleaning and dressing the patient's abrasions and he is then discharged. Later that day the patient is found on the front porch of a neighbor's house. He is confused, his wallet and shoes are missing and his pants are around his ankles. Facial trauma is noted but EMS has none of the information from earlier episode in the factory and visit to ED that same day. He is transported to a *different* hospital as possible trauma. There, his initial neurological examination is documented as normal, but a head computed tomography (CT) reveals evidence of a possible acute CVA in the right hemisphere. Patient then develops (*or perhaps is noted to have*) left-sided weakness and neglect. He is eventually diagnosed as having a large right internal carotid artery (ICA) thrombus with downstream embolism and middle cerebral artery (MCA) infarct. He is treated with aspirin and clopidogrel, but infarct and symptoms progress. When discharged, he requires a feeding tube and continuous care at nursing home. A lawsuit is filed against the first hospital, EMS, ED duty doctor, nurse and surgeon.

Plaintiff: Both EMS and the nurse documented the presence of symptoms suggestive of a possible CVA. You either did not read that or ignored it. Your examination was superficial and based on your own presumption that this was nothing more than a "slip and fall". If you had examined my client appropriately, you would have discovered the cause of his "slip and fall". He could then have been treated for his stroke and not have to be in a nursing home for the rest of his life.

Defense: The defense acknowledged that the discrepancies among the EMS, nursing and surgeon documentation were apparent and difficult to defend. They also acknowledged being faced with an involved family and a sympathetic plaintiff with massive damages and the need of high-level lifelong care. Pretrial settlement negotiations ensued.

Result: The hospital agreed to a seven figure settlement during mediation. The surgeon settled for a lesser seven figure amount after refusing to pay the plaintiff's demand for policy limit.

Takeaways:
- Read the nurses notes. Pay attention to their reports. Discrepancies between nursing notes and physician notes are hard to defend.
- Assure that you have good relationships with your nursing staff. Believe it or not, nurses may not talk to a physician for two rare but unfortunate reasons: (1) fear and (2) dislike, i.e. they may consciously or subconsciously want you gone.
- Listen to the history from your EMS providers. They are our eyes and ears in the field.
- Remember that a "slip and fall" is a symptom, not a diagnosis. One must always ascertain the exact cause of the "slip and fall". This is especially true with hip fractures in the elderly. The broken hip may be only the consequence of something much more significant, e.g. a stroke or cardiac event.

There is thin margin between deficiency in service that can be raised as contention in consumer case under CoPrA and claiming medical negligence under tort or the Indian

Penal Code (IPC). Indian judiciary is heavily burdened with cases at all levels.[19]

FRIVOLOUS AND VEXATIOUS COMPLAINTS AGAINST DOCTORS

Section 26 of the CoPrA covers dismissal of false complaints, Where a complaint instituted before the District Forum, the State Commission or, as the case may be, the National Commission is found to be frivolous or vexatious, it shall, for reasons to be recorded in writing, dismiss the complaint and make an order that the complainant shall pay to the opposite party such cost, not exceeding ₹ 10,000, as may be specified in the order. An accusation may be frivolous or vexatious without being wholly false. A "vexatious" charge may be partly true, but the object of the person making the accusation should be primarily to harass the persons accused.

As the numbers of frivolous complaints being filed in the court have increased tremendously, the courts have started taking stringent steps with respect to certain sectors. An example of a recent development is a judgment of the Apex Court given by a bench comprising of Justice Markandey Katju and RM Lodha delivered on 17th February, 2009 which held that police cannot arrest doctors in cases of medical negligence without prima facie evidence. The bench said that frivolous complaints against doctors have increased by leaps and bounds, thus it is necessary to have certain safety measures. The bench also restrained Consumer forums from issuing notices against doctors in cases of medical negligence, without seeking any expert opinion. This is an important decision of the court, as the numbers of frivolous cases against doctors are on the rise, and it is important to protect the doctors who have actually not been negligent in performing their duties.[20]

Similarly, in landmark case of K Jayaraman versus Poona Hospital, National Consumer Disputes Redressal Commission (NCDRC) held that the complaint was mala fide, frivolous and vexatious and was the misuse of the CPA. It caused harassment to the hospital. The case was dismissed and the complainant directed to pay a sum of ₹ 10,000 as costs to the Hospital.[21]

These above cases make it clear that nobody can misuse the act of CPA and harass doctors for extortion of money, to settle the unpaid Hospital bills by greedy and unscrupulous patients. Doctors should get themselves insured under professional indemnity insurance, and fight the false allegations in the court, by maintaining proper documentation of their treatment prescriptions and hospital records in admitted patients.

PEARLS

Best approach to a litigation-free practice would therefore be to be very vigilant with communication, consent and case paper documentation. Added to this shall be good amount of professional indemnity coverage.

REFERENCES

1. http://164.100.47.4/BillsTexts/LSBillTexts/Asintroduced/1_2018_LS_Eng.pdf
2. https://indiankanoon.org/doc/1819218
3. http://ncdrc.nic.in/bare_acts/consumer%20protection%20act-1986.html
4. https://indiankanoon.org/doc/1595175; Equivalent citations: 1992 (1)ALT 713
5. https://indiankanoon.org/doc/1375046; Equivalent citations: 1994 AIR787, 1994 SCC (1) 243
6. https://indiankanoon.org/doc/723973; Citation: 1996 AIR 550, 1995 SCC(6) 651, JT 1995 (8) 119, 1995 SCALE (6)273
7. Poonam Verma versus, Ashwin Patel and Others Judgment delivered on 10th May, 1996; Equivalent citations: 1996 AIR 2111, 1996 SCC (4) 332 https://indiankanoon. org/doc/611474
8. JIAFM. 2007;29(3):39-41; ISSN: 0971-3

9. Delhi Psychiatry J. 2009;12(2):302-5
10. Joga Rao SV. Medical negligence liability under the Consumer Protection Act: a review of judicial perspective. Indian J Urol. 2009;25:361-71. [online] Available from: http://www.indianjurol.com/text.asp?2009/25/3/361/56205. This is in question and answer format and free to download
11. CPJ—Consumer Protection Judgments, Monthly, DLT Publications, 2002; Vol. 1. p. 190
12. https://indiankanoon.org/doc/185407198
13. https://www.deccanchronicle.com/nation/currentaffairs/111116/telangana-global-hospitalstold-to-pay-compensation-to-patients-kin.html
14. https://indiankanoon.org/doc/119567720
15. https://indiankanoon.org/doc/171255602
16. http://www.imlindia.com/blog/Patient-hope-of-compensation-dies-with-the-doctor.htm
17. https://indiankanoon.org/doc/65337646
18. https://consumeraffairs.nic.in/WriteReadData/userfiles/file/Compendium.pdf
19. https://www.ijariit.com/manuscripts/v3i6/V3I6-1360.pdf?872128&872128
20. Martin F D'Souza versus Mohd Ishfaq. 2009 (2) Supreme Court 40
21. 3 (1993) CPJ 70 NCDRC

ANNEXURES*

ANNEXURE 1

Definitions of Various Terms

"Consumer" is defined in Section 2(1)(d) in the Consumer Protection Act, 1986

"Consumer" means any person who: (i) Buys any goods for a consideration which has been paid or promised or partly paid and partly promised, or under any system of deferred payment and includes any user of such goods other than the person who buys such goods for consideration paid or promised or partly paid or partly promised, or under any system of deferred payment, when such use is made with the approval of such person, but does not include a person who obtains such goods for resale or for any commercial purpose; or

(ii) Hires or avails of any services for a consideration which has been paid or promised or partly paid and partly promised, or under any system of deferred payment and includes any beneficiary of such services other than the person who hires or avails of the services for consideration paid or promised, or partly paid and partly promised, or under any system of deferred payment, when such services are availed of with the approval of the first mentioned person but does not include a person who avails of such services for any commercial purpose.

ANNEXURE 2

*In the case of **M/S Spring Meadows Hospital and Anr vs Harjol Ahluwalia Through, KS Ahluwalia** (https://indiankanoon.org/doc/1715546/), Hon Supreme Court considered clause (ii) of Section 2(1)(d). In the said clause a consumer would mean a person who hires or avails of the services and includes any beneficiary of such services other than the person who hires or avails of the services. In the case on hand when a young child was taken to a hospital by his parents and the child was treated by the doctor, the parents would come within the definition of consumer having hired the services and the young child would also become a consumer under the inclusive definition being a beneficiary of such services. The definition clause being wide enough to include not only the person who hires the services but also the beneficiary of such services which beneficiary is other than the person who hires the services, the conclusion is irresistible that both the parents of the child as well as the child would be consumer within the meaning of Section 2(1)(d)(ii) of the Act and as such both can claim compensation under the Act.*

---

* The Consumer Protection Act will see several changes when it is cleared by Rajya Sabha during February 2019 Budget Session and hopefully becomes a law during the 2014-2019 government. The reading of bare act, rules and judgments can always throw more light on the subject.

"Service" is defined in Section 2(1)(o) in the Consumer Protection Act, 1986

"Service" means service of any description which is made available to potential users and includes, but not limited to, the provision of facilities in connection with banking, financing insurance, transport, processing, supply of electrical or other energy, board or lodging or both, housing construction, entertainment, amusement or the purveying of news or other information, but does not include the rendering of any service free of charge or under a contract of personal service.

ANNEXURE 3

Unfair Trade Practices

Unfair Trade Practice' is defined in Section 2(1)(r) of Consumer Protection Act, 1986.

"Unfair trade practice" means a trade practice which, for the purpose of promoting the sale, use or supply of any goods or for the provision of any service, adopts any unfair method or unfair or deceptive practice including any of the following practices, namely:

(1) The practice of making any statement, whether orally or in writing or by visible representation which:
  (i) Falsely represents that the goods are of a particular standard, quality, quantity, grade, composition, style or model.
  (ii) Falsely represents that the services are of a particular standard, quality or grade.
  (iii) Falsely represents any re-built, second-hand, renovated, reconditioned or old goods as new goods.
  (iv) Represents that the goods or services have sponsorship, approval, performance, characteristics, accessories, uses or benefits which such goods or services do not have.
  (v) Represents that the seller or the supplier has a sponsorship or approval or affiliation which such seller or supplier does not have.
  (vi) Makes a false or misleading representation concerning the need for, or the usefulness of, any goods or services.
  (vii) Gives to the public any warranty or guarantee of the performance, efficacy or length of life of a product or of any goods that is not based on an adequate or proper test thereof.
  Provided that where a defense is raised to the effect that such warranty or guarantee is based on adequate or proper test, the burden of proof of such defense shall lie on the person raising such defense.
  (viii) Makes to the public a representation in a form that purports to be:
    (i) A warranty or guarantee of a product or of any goods or services; or
    (ii) A promise to replace, maintain or repair an article or any part thereof or to repeat or continue a service until it has achieved a specified result, if such purported warranty or guarantee or promise is materially misleading or if there is no reasonable prospect that such warranty, guarantee or promise will be carried out.
  (ix) Materially misleads the public concerning the price at which a product or like products or goods or services, have been or are, ordinarily sold or provided, and, for this purpose, a

representation as to price shall be deemed to refer to the price at which the product or goods or services has or have been sold by sellers or provided by suppliers generally in the relevant market unless it is clearly specified to be the price at which the product has been sold or services have been provided by the person by whom or on whose behalf the representation is made.

(x) Gives false or misleading facts disparaging the goods, services or trade of another person.

Explanation—For the purposes of clause (1), a statement that is:

(a) Expressed on an article offered or displayed for sale, or on its wrapper or container; or

(b) Expressed on anything attached to, inserted in, or accompanying, an article offered or displayed for sale, or on anything on which the article is mounted for display or sale; or

(c) Contained in or on anything that is sold, sent, delivered, transmitted or in any other manner whatsoever made available to a member of the public, shall be deemed to be a statement made to the public by, and only by, the person who had caused the statement to be so expressed, made or contained.

(2) Permits the publication of any advertisement whether in any newspaper or otherwise, for the sale or supply at a bargain price, of goods or services that are not intended to be offered for sale or supply at the bargain price, or for a period that is, and in quantities that are, reasonable, having regard to the nature of the market in which the business is carried on, the nature and size of business, and the nature of the advertisement.

Explanation—For the purpose of clause (2), "bargaining price" means:

(a) A price that is stated in any advertisement to be a bargain price, by reference to an ordinary price or otherwise, or

(b) A price that a person who reads, hears or sees the advertisement, would reasonably understand to be a bargain price having regard to the prices at which the product advertised or like products are ordinarily sold.

(3) Permits:

(a) The offering of gifts, prizes or other items with the intention of not providing them as offered or creating impression that something is being given or offered free of charge when it is fully or partly covered by the amount charged in the transaction as a whole.

(b) The conduct of any contest, lottery, game of chance or skill, for the purpose of promoting, directly or indirectly, the sale, use or supply of any product or any business interest.

(3A) Withholding from the participants of any scheme offering gifts, prizes or other items free of charge, on its closure the information about final results of the scheme.

Explanation—For the purposes of this sub-clause, the participants of a scheme shall be deemed to have been informed of the final results of the scheme where such results are within a reasonable time, published, prominently in the same newspapers in which the scheme was originally advertised.

(4) Permits the sale or supply of goods intended to be used, or are of a kind likely to be used, by consumers, knowing or having reason to believe that the goods do not comply with the standards prescribed by competent authority relating to performance,

composition, contents, design, constructions, finishing or packaging as are necessary to prevent or reduce the risk of injury to the person using the goods.

(5) Permits the hoarding or destruction of goods, or refuses to sell the goods or to make them available for sale or to provide any service, if such hoarding or destruction or refusal raises or tends to raise or is intended to raise, the cost of those or other similar goods or services.

(6) Manufacture of spurious goods or offering such goods for sale or adopts deceptive practices in the provision of services.

ANNEXURE 4

Jurisdiction

Territorial jurisdiction for Every District Forum having geographical limits within which it can exercise its jurisdiction. A consumer complaint falls within district forum when at the time of the complaint—(a) The cause of action, arises in that area of district. Or (b) The party against whom the complaint is made, resides or carries on business or has a branch in that area, or (c) for more than one opposite party, each such party carries on business in that area or (d) for more than one opposite party, party working in the area agrees, or the District Forum gives permission in this regard.

Pecuniary jurisdiction: District Forum entertains the cases where the value of claim is upto ₹ 20 Lakh. Where a claim exceed this limit, the matter is beyond the jurisdiction of the Forum. For deciding Pecuniary Jurisdiction, the amount spent for good or service, and the compensation to be claimed are added together. The complainant has a right to reduce value of his claim in order to bring his claim within the jurisdiction of a junior forum.

State Commission entertains the cases where the value of claim exceeds ₹ 20 lakh. But where value of a claim exceed ₹ 100 lakh, the matter is beyond the jurisdiction of the State Commission. In that case the matter foes to national Commission.

Appellate Jurisdiction: State Commission has power to adjudicate upon the appeals made against the order of the District Forums. Any person aggrieved by an order made by the District Forum may prefer an appeal against such order within 30 days from the date of order. However, the State Commission may entertain an appeal after the expiry of 30 days if it is satisfied that there was sufficient cause for delay. 30 days are counted not from the date of order but from the date when the order is communicated to the appellant.

Revisional Jurisdiction: State Commission may call for the records and pass appropriate orders in any consumer dispute which is pending before or has been decided by any District Forum within the State, where State Commission is of the view that the District Forum has exercised jurisdiction which it was not entitled to, or has failed to exercise such jurisdiction which it was entitled to, or has exercised its jurisdiction illegally or with material irregularity. Such revisional jurisdiction may be exercised by the Commission on its own or on the application of a party.

ANNEXURE 5

Enforcing Consumer Forum Order

Compensation awarded by forum can be recovered through legal process as defined in Section 25 in the Consumer Protection Act, 1986.

Enforcement of orders of the District Forum, the State Commission or the National Commission:

(1) Where an interim order made under this Act is not complied with, the District Forum or the State Commission or the National Commission, as the case may be, may order the property of the person, not complying with such order to be attached.

(2) No attachment made under sub-section: (1) Shall remain in force for more than three months at the end of which, if the non-compliance continues, the property attached may be sold and out of the proceeds thereof, the District Forum or the State Commission or the National Commission may award such damages as it thinks fit to the complainant and shall pay the balance, if any, to the party entitled thereto.

(3) Where any amount is due from any person under an order made by a District Forum, State Commission or the National Commission, as the case may be, the person entitled to the amount may make an application to the District Forum, the State Commission or the National Commission, as the case may be, and such District Forum or the State Commission or the National Commission may issue a certificate for the said amount to the Collector of the district (by whatever name called) and the Collector shall proceed to recover the amount in the same manner as arrears of land revenue.

If Forum considers the complain to be frivolous, the procedure is defined in Section 26 in the Consumer Protection Act, 1986.

Dismissal of frivolous or vexatious complaints. Where a complaint instituted before the District Forum, the State Commission or, as the case may be, the National Commission is found to be frivolous or vexatious, it shall, for reasons to be recorded in writing, dismiss the complaint and make an order that the complainant shall pay to the opposite party such cost, not exceeding **ten thousand** rupees, as may be specified in the order.

Failure to comply with order of the forum can lead to **award of penalty** as defined in Section 27 in the Consumer Protection Act, 1986.

(1) Where a trader or a person against whom a complaint is made or the complainant fails or omits to comply with any order made by the District Forum, the State Commission or the National Commission, as the case may be, such trader or person or complainant shall be punishable with imprisonment for a term which shall not be less than one month but which may extend to three years, or with fine which shall not be less than two thousands rupees but which may extend to ten thousand rupees, or with both.

(2) Notwithstanding anything contained in the Code of Criminal Procedure, 1973 (2 of 1974), the District Forum or the State Commission or the National Commission, as the case may be, shall have the power of a Judicial Magistrate of the first class for the trial of offences under this Act, and on such conferment of powers, the District Forum or the State Commission or the National Commission, as the case may be, on whom the powers are so conferred, shall be deemed to be a Judicial Magistrate of the first class for the purpose of the Code of Criminal Procedure, 1973 (2 of 1974).

(3) All offences under this Act may be tried summarily by the District Forum or the State Commission or the National Commission, as the case may be.

ANNEXURE 6

Period of Limitation

For initial application as per Section 24A of the Consumer Protection Act.1986 the District Forum, the State Commission or the National Commission may not admit a complaint unless it is filed within two years from the date on which the cause of action had arisen. But a complaint may be entertained after the period specified above, if the complainant satisfies the District Forum, the State Commission or the National Commission, as the case may be, that he had sufficient cause for not filing the complaint within such period. Hon. Apex Court in this regards has stated that in a dispute concerning a consumer, it is necessary for the courts to take a pragmatic view of the rights of the consumer principally since it is the consumer who is placed at a disadvantage vis-à-vis the supplier of services or goods.

Appeals

Appeal from the order of the District Forum lies to the State Commission, against the order of the State Commission to the National Commission and against the order of the National Commission to the Supreme Court and appeals are to be filed within 30 days of the order appealed against and are to be accompanied by a certified copy of the order.

ANNEXURE 7

Compensation

Usually courts follow a arithmetical equation known as multiplier method to calculate amount of compensation to be awarded. In Dr Balram Prasad Vs Dr Kunal Saha's Case (https://indiankanoon.org/doc/35346928/) The Supreme Court rejected the multiplier method and provided an illustration to show how useless the method can be for medical negligence cases. Hon'ble Justice Mr V Gopala Gowda opined that the multiplier method was provided for convenience and speedy disposal of no fault motor accident cases. Therefore, if a child, housewife or other non-working person fall victim to reckless medical treatment by wayward doctors, the maximum pecuniary damages that the unfortunate victim may collect would be only ₹ 1.8 lakh. It is stated in view of the aforesaid reasons that in today's India, Hospitals, Nursing Homes and doctors make lakhs and crores of rupees on a regular basis. Under such scenario, allowing the multiplier method to be used to determine compensation in medical negligence cases would not have any deterrent effect on them for their medical negligence but in contrast, this would encourage more incidents of medical negligence in India bringing even greater danger for the society at large.

In the case National Insurance Co. Ltd. v. Kusuma, (https://indiankanoon.org/doc/29565/) Hon'ble Supreme Court has held that payment of compensation to parents for the death of a child, including a stillborn, in an accident must be just and not be a pittance. A Bench of Hon'ble Justices DK Jain and RM Lodha said: "The determination of the just amount of compensation is beset with difficulties, more so when the deceased happens to be an infant/child because the future of a child is full of glorious uncertainties." In the case of death of an infant, many imponderables had to be taken into account such as life expectancy and his prospects of earning, saving, spending and distributing. Writing the judgment, Hon'ble Mr Justice DK Jain said, it was quite possible that there would be no actual pecuniary benefit derived by the parents during the lifetime of the child. But that could not be a ground for rejecting their claim of reasonable expectation of pecuniary benefit if the child had lived. The Bench said: "The word 'just' connotes something which is equitable, fair and reasonable, conforming to rectitude and justice, and not arbitrary. It may be true that Section 168 of the Motor Vehicles Act confers a wide discretion on the [Motor Accidents Claims] Tribunal to determine the amount of compensation, but this discretion is also coupled with a duty to see that this exercise is carried out rationally and judiciously by accepted legal standards, and not whimsically and arbitrarily, a concept unknown to public law." The Bench, however, cautioned the tribunals, saying the amount of compensation awarded was not expected to be a windfall or bonanza, nor should it be niggardly or a pittance. "Whether there exists a reasonable expectation of pecuniary benefit" was always a mixed question of fact and law, but a mere speculative possibility of benefit was not sufficient.

In National Consumer Commission Judgement of Dr Mrs Indiu Sharma Vs Apollo Hospital decided on 22th April, 2015, (http://cms.nic.in/ncdrcusersWeb/GetJudgement.do?method=GetJudgement&caseidin=0%2F0%2FOP%2F104%2F2002&dtofhearing=2015-04-22) the compensation awarded for medical negligence in a delayed LSCS and subsequent death of a child that had suffered from cerebral atrophy was ₹ One Crore. Out of these, ₹ Eighty Lakh to be paid by the Hospital.

CHAPTER

7

Defenses in Medical Negligence

Neeraj Nagpal

SUMMARY

This article provides important defenses, which can be used in cases of alleged medical negligence.

ABSTRACT

In recent times, we are witnessing a spurt in litigation involving medical negligence. There is a rising trend wherein huge amounts of compensations are being awarded to litigants for alleged negligence, by the consumer friendly courts of law. The conflict between court-mandated evidence-based medicine and the ground reality of myths, misconceptions, and poor health literacy gives rise to a peculiar situation for doctors of modern scientific medicine in India. On one hand, they are forced to use clinical acumen to keep the costs of treatment down to compete with the omnipresent quackery and crosspathy, while on the other hand in case of an adverse outcome, the courts demand proof that stringent norms have been adhered to. The allegations are unfortunately adjudicated by the judges, who themselves are not from the medical field. All this leads to prolonged and at times frivolous litigations running for a number of years the process of which is in itself a severe punishment for a doctor. All that is required to avoid institution of such unsavory litigation is to always follow the practice guidelines, rules, norms, and regulations that have been prescribed under the law and also take precautionary steps, which may prevent or discourage a prospective litigant. If it makes treatment costly, so be it. It should be made a necessity and not a formality to keep oneself up-to-date and continuing medical education in legal aspects of medicine. This article addresses the preventive steps as well the defenses, which a medical practitioner may use and apply according to the circumstances of a particular case to deal with unwanted litigation. Doing everything listed may still not avoid litigation but if by misfortune, it happens it has to be countered like the first marital skirmish, i.e. stoically, with a resolve not to lose the first fight, and knowing that this was inevitable with or without your fault.

INTRODUCTION

There is no denying that there is a recent spurt in litigation against medical professionals and their establishments. The Consumer Protection Act 1986 and the judgment of VP Shantha and Others versus Indian Medical Association[1] in a way, led to the conversion of a noble service into a purchasable commodity. The policy impact of being included under the purview of the Consumer Protection Act, 1986, is that the treatment provided by a doctor which by all definitions is an inexact and variable science with rapid advancement, changing paradigms, and substantial responsibility, is subject to the same scrutiny as any other service provider, therefore increasing the propensity of the system to solve such matters purely by awarding compensation.[2] Exorbitant compensation awards have given an impetus to increasing demands for compensation for perceived negligence, which is currently going overboard and the occasional prosecution of doctors up to two decades ago, is now turning into ubiquitous persecution for them.

Doctors are usually well-trained in their core subjects in which they practice but what is not taught to them and what they are never adequately prepared for is an allegation of medical negligence made against them. Once an allegation of negligence is made, invariably there is a sinking feeling, fear of the unknown, feeling of hurt and anger at the system, and confusion, which is seen in all of them. Doctors know how to treat a perforation following an unsuccessful Endoscopic Retrograde Cholangiopancreatography (ERCP) but are clueless, when it comes to knowing how to handle the consequences following allegations of medical negligence. There is feeling of guilt, incompetence and inadequacy coupled with fear of ridicule, suspicion of fellow practitioners having instigated the allegations, and unwillingness to openly discuss the issue with colleagues who may be in a better position to guide them.[3]

There is also a universal lament by doctors, who have lost their case that their advocates who defended them could not understand the medical facts or explain them in court. Fact, however, is that doctors do not take adequate interest in their cases, depend heavily on the insurance company to provide them a advocate and then do not spend time and effort with the advocate to prepare the proper defense. They also do not make personal appearance in court and do not provide adequate medical references to their advocates.

ALLEGATIONS AND THE ROLE OF HEALTH LITERACY

Having successfully cured hundreds or more patients prior to the particular incident is no guarantee that outcome will be perfect in the next case. Allegations of medical negligence can, however, occur following a medical accident, a known complication, or even when treatment is proceeding on expected lines. The allegations are dependent more on the perception of the patient or his relative than on the actual acts of omission or commission done by the individual doctor. The perception of the patient or his relatives is based on their health literacy, which anyway in India is very poor[4] as well as the inputs received from various (semiqualified and unqualified) "doctors" who may have earlier treated the patient. Outright cases of negligence where even death has occurred may be ignored or condoned by patients depending on their outlook and the trust and faith they have in their treating physician. On the other hand, use of a dose of medicine outside the recommended range by a senior physician with loads of experience may be construed as negligence sufficient to be prosecuted at multiple levels and finally penalized with heavy compensation by the Honorable Supreme Court.[5] The qualified doctors competing with the omnipresent quacks and crosspaths in the country try and use clinical acumen to keep cost of treatment low, however, in court, they are penalized for not being able to prove the correctness of their clinical decisions in the absence of appropriate investigations or absence of a ventilator, intensive care unit (ICU), neonatal intensive care unit (NICU), or a designated burn unit in hospital.

LITIGIOUS SOCIETY: LEGAL PITFALLS

Though increasing cost of treatment has become one of the factors in increasing number of cases of alleged medical negligence in courts but this not true in entirety. Cases are also filed against Government Hospitals where free treatment is given. Approximately 1.8 million plus 6% interest has been awarded for negligence in treatment given at a Government Hospital in Tamil Nadu by the honorable Supreme Court.[6] Our society is now increasingly litigious and promoted by Government, Press, and so-called civil society, medical profession is now viewed with suspicion and cases of medical negligence are filed at the drop of a hat whenever suboptimal result of medical treatment occurs. The ambulance chasers of the west have now surfaced in our country as well with even for hire protestors available to cut hospital bill.

Though most doctors in India today have either faced such allegations themselves or have knowledge of other doctors having faced such allegations, the desire to update oneself of the legal pitfalls of medical practice is still lacking. Until and unless, one gets embroiled in one such case against his own self the gravity of the problem is not understood in its entirety. Doctors in their naivety at times make blunders on being confronted with such allegations, which becomes difficult to rectify later. To defend oneself against allegations of medical negligence, doctors need to take preventive, remedial, and damage control measures all of which first require knowledge to be attained of the same. The most common mistake is when they give a detailed reply to a legal notice from an advocate hired by the complainant, providing all defense arguments, which then leads the complainant to improve on his complaint when he goes to consumer court. Using the defense arguments, the modified complaint then skirts the easily defendable allegations and concocts or uses those allegations, which the doctor would find difficult to defend. Not giving a reply to a notice from the consumer court within the prescribed 45 days or not informing the insurance company of the incident, which may later result in a claim, and frequent ill thought of attempt to hush up matter by making some monetary out of court settlement are other common mistakes made by doctors which lead to legal problems for them later.

Documentation

Irrespective of the cause of action, nearly all cases of alleged medical negligence are to be contested on basis of documentary evidence and that is where nearly all doctors falter. In their busy schedule and the adrenaline rush of conducting multiple technically complex procedures successfully, they ignore or forget to document the events as they unfold during the treatment process. These documents are what are of prime importance when it comes to defending cases of medical negligence. Indian doctors' common refrain is that we are overloaded with work and if we start documenting the way doctors do in western countries, we will not be able to see more than 10–15 patients per day as against 50–100 plus patients, which is the current norm. On the other hands, courts unrealistically expect minute-to-minute documentation of events as they unfold[7] specially during emergency unmindful of the fact that it is impossible in an emergency for a doctor to focus on anything other than the task at hand. It is also the court's view that documentation done afterwards (after death) is not admissible.[8] With ubiquitous presence of smart phones, patient relatives mostly have photographs of medical records, which they manage to take from time-to-time. It is easy to allege fabrication of records later with such photographs in possession in case when doctors have written notes at a later time or date.

Cutting, overwriting, or discrepancy of medical records between what is written by nurses and what is written by doctors is a problem not easy to defend in court. Sometimes, notes are added in a curved line over the signature to add something. The courts are very expert and sensitive to such tampering of records. Conflicting notes between anesthetist and surgeon are a recipe for disaster as happened in a recent case where anesthetist claimed the patient was fit for giving anesthesia and surgeon claimed she was extremely sick and critical to start with.[9] Using short forms or exceedingly brief notes are frowned upon by courts. In one recent case, the ophthalmologist writing "No ROP seen" was held to be inadequate and negligent by court while awarding ₹ 64 lakhs compensation.

The court demanded that complete procedure of "retinal examination with binocular indirect ophthalmoscope on dilatation of pupil with scleral depression to ascertain avascular zone at periphery of retina" should have been done and documented. The short statement actually written appears a cover up and hence the penalty.[10] Unsigned medical records have no legal validity in courts, including the blank consent form signed by patient but not filled and countersigned by the consultant.[11]

Medical Practitioners' Professional Indemnity Insurance

One of the risk management tools in medical negligence is a professional indemnity insurance. It is surprising that in today's day and age there still are doctors mostly in Government sector (but also some in private sector) who do not take professional indemnity insurance. Resident doctors doing their postgraduation or senior residency are never advised to take indemnity insurance and once dragged into a litigation needs to keep going to court long after finishing their residency and settling in a different city besides having to pay compensation, if awarded, from their own pockets. The indemnity insurance is cheap in India currently and if taken through a Doctors Group or Association for ₹ 50 lakhs can be even cheaper than cost of a dinner eaten in a swank restaurant. At times, this is also due to oversight and failure to renew an ongoing insurance policy but then a policy lapsed is a policy not taken.

Another factor which is unknown to doctors is that these policies are given in different AOA and AOY ratio [Any One Accident (AOA) limit and Any One Year limit ratio]. A ₹ 10 lakhs policy in 1:4 will pay only ₹ 2.5 lakhs for any one case even though the award may be ₹ 10 lakhs. This happens when insurance agents are asked by doctors to reduce the premium quoted and they then clandestinely change the same policy for 10 lakhs from 1:1 to 1:4 with far lower premium making the bargaining doctor happy. This, however, can be very costly in long run.

Frequently changing the policy insurers without understanding the policy terms regarding retroactive cover can also be foolhardy. It is to be understood that the policies being issued to doctors in India are "claim" based policies and not "event or occurrence" based policies which are more expensive worldwide. It is frequently misconstrued by doctors that only when they get a notice from a consumer court that they have to inform the insurance company. As per terms of the policy, if an incident occurs which the doctor feels could result in a claim later he is bound to report the same to the insurer failing which the insurer would be within its rights to deny an liability. This means that one must inform the insurance company of any adverse event like death which could give rise to a claim at a later date specially, if the doctor has been threatened telephonically, verbally, or there has been a complaint made in State Medical Council or to the employer or to the police even when a legal notice has not been received from patient or consumer court.

Some doctors at times take multiple policies from different insurers. This is also not advisable because in case of an award the insurers will then claim to cover only a proportion of the liability. This is especially true in today's era of generous compensation awards made by courts who feel justified in awarding astronomical compensations, given that the doctor is insured for a large amount. Producing only a limited indemnity cover in court may help in restraining the galloping quantum of the compensations being awarded.

It is also important to carefully fill all columns of the proposal form by own self, including where one practices. There is no extra premium to be paid for practicing in more than one establishment but in case, the place of practice is mentioned as only one and later the doctor needs indemnity cover for professional work having done in emergency elsewhere it leaves the insurers a loophole to escape liability. The habit among doctors to sign the proposal form and ask the insurance agent to fill in the columns later is deplorable to say the least.

Legal Cover

It is also important that the indemnity insurance today is taken through a doctors group, or a firm specializing in professional indemnity insurance. Routine insurers may provide legal cover for a consumer case but proper negotiation with insurers by a collective group gets advantages like legal cover for criminal cases, expenses of travel, and stay in case matter goes to National Consumer Disputes Redressal Commission (NCDRC) and overall better quality of advocates. In a recent case, where a firm professing to be an insurance agent specializing in professional indemnity insurance refused to provide legal help to doctor because complaint filed was to Health Minister who marked it to civil surgeon. The company wanted the doctor to appear before the committee formed by the civil surgeon with a self-drafted reply assuring that when the matter goes to consumer court they would provide legal help. Urgent intervention by Medicos Legal Action Group and its advocate salvaged the situation because a negative opinion of this committee formed by the civil surgeon would have weighed heavily later in consumer court and even criminal complaint.

Opinion: Reasonable Degree of Care

Since courts expect a doctor to be qualified as claimed and to have brought reasonable degree of care and caution to his task it is helpful, if doctors support other doctors with affidavits. A statement by a colleague that "under the circumstances I would have done the same" can go a long way to influence the bench favorably. As of now, the courts do not expect doctors to be the best in the field but only as good as another average practicing doctor of same field. Medical literature and references from standard textbooks as defense holds weightage over obscure but latest journals in court.

A medical board constituted by the police or the health authorities on receiving a complaint of alleged medical negligence is made of doctors preferably from Government services and at times give an adverse report suggesting negligence. When this is done by a Board constituted by the police as per the guidelines given in Jacob Mathew versus State of Punjab judgment by the honorable Supreme Court, the police register a first information report (FIR) with alacrity.[12] Most of the defense then comprises of rejection of the opinion given by this Board. Members not being legal experts they do not distinguish "simple" negligence from "gross" negligence leading to erroneous prosecution of the doctor concerned. If no doctor in the medical board is of specialty of the defendant then this opinion is easily rebutted. This frequently occurs when cases of superspecialty doctors are before this board. Not all Government hospitals have doctors of all superspecialties available in its employ and a urologists case may have a surgeon giving an opinion, which would be easily challenged.

Consent

Having taken a proper consent is the biggest defense in cases of alleged medical negligence. As of today in India, we are expected to take "real" consent, which is a British concept as against "informed consent" which is a US Concept. In real consent, a doctor is expected to inform the patient of possible complications, which another average practicing doctor would inform. There is no need to inform about rare complications, which may scare the patient one way or the other. Informed consent on the other hand requires all information to be given to patient and it is left up to him to decide. If the rare complication not mentioned was told to another patient and he would not have agreed to undergo the procedure then it is not informed consent. So, test for real consent is another "reasonable doctor" whereas test for informed consent is another "reasonable patient".

Unfortunately, besides the content of the consent there are other issues, which arise in consent as obtained in India. Ideally, it should be taken in the language that the patient understands, and should be taken and signed by the consultant himself or his junior. Consent should be taken from the patient only in case he is 18 year or older and is conscious with maintained mental faculties without any fraud, force, or coercion. Taking consent from brother, sister, father, mother, and son for a patient who is "compos mentis" is rampant in our country and this is considered as not being valid consent by the courts irrespective of the act of omission or commission which may have been done.

Quality Inputs in a Case

When a medical negligence case is in court, you need both case laws as well as medical literature to buttress your argument. Research to provide reliable medical literature as defense in court cannot be underscored enough. Something, which may seem clear and standard to the medical professionals, will still need evidence in form of a published matter before a court. This is where the advocates are helpless and useless. The doctor needs to spend time personally to find references or take help of other doctors in teaching institutes for the same. Standard textbook references have more evidentiary value than case reports or obscure studies published in some journal.

Role of a medicolegal consultant separates from the advocate also cannot be overemphasized. This new breed of doctors who are also qualified in law provide inputs to the doctor and his advocate and bridge the gaps left by the advocate as well as the accused. At times, their help is crucial as they have more experience of medicolegal problems than an average advocate. Their inputs in drafting of replies and rejoinders are immensely valuable and should be solicited.

Use of Legal Principles in Defense

Besides, the above-mentioned defenses are the actual legal maneuvering in court, which needs a deft legal mind. You can defend yourself in a negligence suit by eliminating one of the four elements:
1. Could argue that you owed no duty to the complainant
2. Could claim that you were as careful as a reasonable person would have been
3. Could state that your actions did not cause the victim's injury
4. Could try to prove that the victim was not really injured in the way that he or she claims.

A doctor may argue that his care was in line with the standards upheld in the medical profession, or that the patient's injuries were not the result of a medical error. Standard of care may be proven using affidavits of other average practicing doctors of same specialty or using medical literature and standard treatment guidelines. Volenti non fit injuria or voluntary assumption of risk is a defense, which can be used if proper real and valid consent has been taken. This legal principle provides protection when a person engages in an event accepting and aware of the risks inherent in that event, then he cannot later complain of, or seek compensation for an injury suffered during the event.

Patient's Duty as Defense

The doctor or patient relationship includes two separate duties. The physician's standard of care duties are well known, but few realize that a patient has a duty in this relationship too. It is this forgotten duty that often becomes the basis for a patient negligence defense in a medical malpractice case.

A prominent duty of the patient occurs in relation to informed consent. Throughout the diagnostic and treatment phases, the doctor and patient communicate and agree upon a course of action. If the doctor breaches this agreement, then there is cause for malpractice. However, a patient can also breach informed consent by not completing his or her part of the agreement. This includes, but is not limited to, failure in attending appointments, taking any tests, and following any instructions for lifestyles changes (dietary, activity restrictions, etc.), and/or taking medicine that might interfere with treatment or not taking diagnosed medication. A breach of informed consent on the patient's behalf is considered patient negligence and can be used as a defense in a malpractice case. Another often-neglected patient responsibility occurs during the very first visit with the doctor: The all-important medical history. The patient must disclose any and all allergies, past and present medical conditions and treatments, as well as any pertinent familial conditions that he or she is aware of. Nondisclosure of this information can seriously jeopardize care, and is cause for patient negligence and can be used in defense against allegations of medical negligence.

The concept of contributory negligence has been used successfully to defend doctors specially ophthalmologists who have been accused of negligence by patients who develop postoperative infection. Lack of proper postoperative care at home has been used as a defense by many doctors in their cases.[13] The most prominent case was the Dr Kunal Saha case, where NCDRC, probably for the first time, imposed contributory negligence penalty on the complainant for interfering with treatment of the patient.[14]

Free Service: Consumer or Not

Many doctors and their legal advisors also use the argument of free service, claiming that no charges were taken hence patient cannot be regarded as a consumer. Though free service was mentioned as an exclusion in Consumer Protection Act but this defense became inherently unacceptable after the[15] and others judgment, which has firmly established that even patients who have not been charged remain consumers, if other patients have been charged. Despite this there have been cases decided by NCDRC,[16] which has given opinion that free treatment in Government Hospitals cannot be dragged to consumer courts.

ERROR OF JUDGMENT

A simple lack of care, an error of judgment or an accident, is not proof of negligence on the part of a medical professional. So long as a doctor follows a practice acceptable to the medical profession of that day, he cannot be held liable for negligence merely because a better alternative course or method of treatment was also available or simply because a more skilled doctor would not have chosen to follow or resort to that practice or procedure, which the accused followed. This concept of "Error of Judgment" though does not provide a blanket immunity to the doctor is sometimes used as a defense successfully but this will vary on a case-to-case basis. Claiming error of judgment which is nonpunishable from negligence can be difficult and requires superior legal assistance. The "Error of Judgment" line of defense works best when there are two or more lines of reasonable management choices all of which are acceptable with their own risks and benefits. The defense of "Error of Judgment" will work better, if the different choices are documented and so is the reason for choosing one of them along with patient's consent regarding this decision.[17]

LIMITATION: DISCOVERY RULE

Another frequently used defense by doctors is that case has been filed more than 2 years from cause of action, which is more than the limitation stipulated by Consumer Protection Act 1986. Being consumer friendly, the consumer fora frequently, however, condone any delay by the complainant especially, if he gives a cogent reason for the delay. Another aspect of this defense of "limitation" is that it is now established case law by honorable Supreme Court that using "Discovery Rule" a complainant has 2 years from the time he discovered that negligence had been committed for him to file a case in consumer courts. The problem for doctors arises from the fact that they need the medical records to defend themselves and as yet in India except for corporate hospitals electronic health record (EHR) is not the norm. Also Indian Medical Council Act Regulations 2002 ask for doctors to maintain inpatient records for 3 years.[18] However, using Discovery rule a patient may file a complaint 15 years or more after cause of action.[19] Most doctors then are left with no option but to defend themselves without the help of medical records, which may have been destroyed long before the case was filed in consumer fora. This defense without medical records is given no weightage in courts. Even detailed affidavits from memory by doctors detailing the sequence of events without medical records have been dismissed by NCDRC in Apollo Hospitals case.[20]

RESEARCH: MEDICAL LITERATURE AND CASE LAWS

However, the argument raised by a cardiologist buttressed with the medical literature he referred to recently had this author transfixed. He actually proved to court that oxygen was not necessary in a patient of acute myocardial infarction. It is a different issue that the court still penalized him for not providing ambulance.[21] The case in point proves that good research both of medical literature and case laws are essential for a good defense. The time invested by a medical practitioner in preparation of his defense is invaluable and the tendency of doctors to depend on the lawyers provided by insurers is mostly the reason for inappropriate defense and hence an adverse outcome.

Good research and information regarding the complainant also at times helps as in a recent case where as on pecuniary damages the complainant sought ₹ 5 lakhs for loss of spouse. The doctor prayed that since the complainant remarried within 1 year of his wife's death his loss could not be calculated so high and court awarded only ₹ 1 lakh.[22] Quantum of compensation calculated and claimed by the complainant is challenged on various grounds and frequently leads to a much reduced compensation that what was demanded. This reduction or elimination of claimed compensation, which may be arbitrarily and unjustifiably inflated, may require some admission of guilt but focus on reduction of liability.

LAW OF TORT: NEGLIGENCE

In some situations, a doctor in his defense may completely skirt the issue whether a mistake was made and focused only on whether patient was harmed. The definition of negligence as given in Law of Torts, Ratanlal and Dhirajlal (edited by Justice GP Singh), holds good. Negligence becomes actionable on account of injury resulting from the act or omission amounting to negligence attributable to the person sued. The essential components of negligence are three—(1) duty, (2) breach, and (3) resulting damage. Even in the presence of breach of duty, if there is no damage then it would not amount to negligence, which warrants to be compensated. This has been stated in Jacob Mathew case by honorable Supreme Court as well as in other judgments.

In case of death, the distinction between causa causans versus causa sine qua non and causa interveniens need to be understood and elaborated not only during criminal trials, but the principle broadly also holds true in consumer and civil courts. All deaths after a procedure may not be because of the procedure. In today's date, when multiple interventions and procedures are needed and patient may need to be in ICU, it is difficult to clearly identify causa causans. A doctor may use "absence of causation" as a defense arguing that any harm that the patient may have experienced was not actually caused by any mistake made by the doctor. For example, a patient might visit a doctor, complaining of severe headaches. The doctor fails to look for ominous signs and diagnoses it as simple migraine giving medication for the same. If this patient now dies within a month from advanced case of brain cancer, in this case, the patient's family might sue the doctor for medical negligence for failure of diagnosis of serious disease leading to death of patient. The doctor could defend by arguing that the negligence did not actually cause any harm. The patient had an incurable form of brain cancer. Even if the doctor had properly diagnosed the patient, the death would have occurred, so the death of the patient was not due to the error in diagnosis. Consumer courts being patient friendly may still award compensation but as a defense, this absence of causa causans stands the test of time in defending doctors during allegations of medical negligence.

CONCLUSION

A medical practitioner must know and follow a reasonable standard of care and caution as expected of them by the public, their profession, and the law of the land. The importance of getting up-to-date information or awareness must never be disregarded.

The doctor should develop good patient relationship, take valid and informed consent, form must be completely filled. All prescribed documentation must be prepared at each stage of the treatment and endorsed by the treating physician. There should be no ambiguity left in the treatment and the procedure followed should be the standard one followed at that time. The litigious society, although there may be fair cases of medical negligence, however, is always on the prowl to somehow implicate the doctor with a view to obtain unfair monetary gains, as is evident from the numerous frivolous medical negligence cases being filed everyday in courts of law. In a news report, a study was published by a leading authority on medical law.[23] According to which there was a 110% rise in the number of medical negligence cases in India every year. That 12% of all cases decided by consumer court are on medical negligence. The main reason for filing cases is attributed to hospitals taking improper consent before performing certain procedures or switching hospitals, or improper documentation throughout the course of diagnosis and treatment. All this is due to lack of awareness among doctors.

The method, too, of calculation of compensation is unpredictable as it varies hugely across different cases, courts, and tribunals, therefore, the medical practitioner should be proactive in every approach touching the treatment of any particular patient. This will not only help in planning professional indemnity insurance but also stress free practice without undue worry about facing litigation for alleged medical negligence.

REFERENCES

1. Agrawal S. Indian Medical Association vs V.P. Shantha, & Ors on 13 November, 1995. Supreme Court of India. 1995;6 SCC 651.
2. Chandra MS, Math SB. Progress in Medicine: Compensation and medical negligence in India: Does the system need a quick fix or an overhaul? Ann Indian Acad Neurol. 2016;19(Suppl 1):S21-7.
3. Scott SD. The Second Victim Phenomenon: (2011). A Harsh Reality of Health Care Professions. [online] Available from: https://psnet.ahrq.gov/perspectives/perspective/102/the-second-victim-phenomenon-a-harsh-reality-of-health-care-professions [Accessed December, 2018].

4. Kaur R, Rajvanshi H. SWOT Analysis of Health Literacy in India. Int J Healthcare Edu Med Inform. 2017;4(2):28-31.
5. Balram Prasad vs Kunal Saha & Ors on 24 October, 2013. Supreme Court of India. 2014;1 SCC 384.
6. V. Krishnakumar vs. State of Tamil Nadu & Ors. Supreme Court of India. 2015;9 SCC 388.
7. D. Uma Devi vs M/S. Yashoda Hospital & 3 Ors. on 11 April, 2016. A.P. National Consumer Disputes Redressal Commission, FA 1169 of 2014.
8. Dr. Rajni Kumari vs. Amar Kant Sharan, NCDRC. 2014 (4) CPR 764.
9. Devendra Kantilal Nayak vs. Dr. Kalyaniben Dhruv Shah. 1996; 3 CPR 56; I (1997) CPJ 103.
10. Master Rishab Sharma & Ors. vs Dr. Rama Sharma & Ors., National Consumer Disputes Redressal Commission, CC/119/2007.
11. A Padmavati vs Dr M Vijayendra & Another. 2016 (2) CPR 662.
12. Jacob Mathew vs State of Punjab & Anr on 5 August, 2005 (2006) 6 SCC 1.
13. Air Commodore Satyanarayan vs LV Prasad Eye Institute. SCDRC, AP, C.D. No. 30 of 1990, DoD Aug-26-1997.
14. Dr Kunal Saha vs Dr Sukumar Mukherjee & Ors. NCDRC. OP No. 240 of 1999, DoD 21-Oct-2011.
15. Indian Medical Association vs V P Shantha, 1(1996) CLT 81 (SC).
16. Major Singh vs State of Punjab & Ors. NCDRC, RP/4734/2012.
17. Dr. Sou Jayshree Ujwal Ingole vs. State of Maharashtra & Anr. SC, Crl Apl No. 636 of 2017.
18. The Indian Medical Council (Professional Conduct, Etiquette and Ethics) Regulations, 2002, 1.3 Maintenance of medical records: 1.3.1 Every physician shall maintain the medical records pertaining to his / her indoor patients for a period of 3 years from the date of commencement of the treatment in a standard proforma laid down by the Medical Council of India and attached as Appendix 3.
19. VN Shrikhande (Dr) vs Anita Sena Fernandes. SC, Cvl Apl No. 8983 of 2010.
20. Apollo Hospitals vs M Sathyanarayana & Others NCDRC, OP 10 of 1998, DoD 28-Apr-2011.
21. Grewal Hospital vs Sher Singh, NCDRC, RP No. 946 of 2013, DoD 11-Nov-2014.
22. Shri Joginder Singh vs. Dr Rajeev Kumar Majumdar, NCDRC, OP No. 289 of 1997, DoD 13-Aug-2009.
23. Medical Times (2016). 110% Rise in number of medical negligence cases in India every year: Study. [online] Available from: http://www.indiamedicaltimes.com/2016/11/20/110-rise-in-number-of-medical-negligence-cases-in-india-every-year-study/ [Accessed December, 2018].

CHAPTER 8

Concept of Compensation

Lalit Kapoor

INTRODUCTION

The Indian Supreme Court recently awarded a record compensation payout for medical negligence that resulted in the death of a patient. In the case known as Dr Balram Prasad versus Dr Kunal Saha and others, the patient who was a US resident, had died following development of drug-induced toxic epidermal necrolysis (TEN). The doctors and the hospital were found to be guilty of negligence and a sum of ₹ 60,800,550 + interest amounting to a total of over ₹ 11 million was awarded. There were also a few other recent cases where huge compensations were awarded by the courts—Krishna Kumar versus State of Tamil Nadu—₹ 13,800,000 + 41.37 lakhs for medical expenses; Nizam Institute of Medical Sciences versus Prasanth Dhanaka—₹ 1 million + interest; Dr Indu Sharma versus Indraprastha Apollo Hospital and Dr Sohini Verma—₹ 1 million.

It may be noted that in motor vehicle accident cases, the compensation is calculated by the multiplier formula. The formula is somewhat like this—70 minus age of patient at the time of death × annual income + 30% inflation minus one-third as personal expenses. In medical negligence cases, the courts have not restricted to this formula and have added other dimensions in calculating the compensation.

The basic concept of awarding compensation lies in the principle of *restitution in integrum,* which a person who suffered some damage due to a wrong committed to him ought to be restored to the position in which he or she would have been had the wrong not been committed. In the medical setting, it would imply that the victim of medical negligence would need to be compensated for the incurred medical expenses, future medical expenses, compensation for mental agony and physical pain, loss of consortium and, even cost of litigation.

The Supreme Court judgment in Harjot Singh Ahluwalia versus Spring Meadows Hospital, laid down another principle that can determine compensation. It answered the following questions:

- In the case of a minor child, being admitted into the hospital for treatment, can the parents of the child be held to be consumers so as to claim compensation under the provisions of the Consumer Protection Act?
- Is the commission under the Act entitled to award compensation to the parents for mental agony in view of the powers of the commission under Section 14 of the Act?
- Even if the child as well as the parents of the child would come under definition of the "Consumer" under Section 2(1) (d) of the Act whether compensation can be awarded in favor of both the consumers or compensation can be awarded only to the beneficiary of the services rendered, who in the present case would be child who was admitted into the hospital?

All the questions were answered in the affirmative and compensation was awarded in favor of the parents in addition to the compensation in favor of the minor child.

In all fairness, it should also be noted that Courts have occasionally come down heavily against plaintiffs making exaggerated claims of compensation and have asked them to revise their claims to reasonable figures or risk their case being dismissed.

NAZIA SULTANA VERSUS DR GULSHANT PANESAR

Facts of the case: *The patient visited the clinic, where laser hair removal was done by the assistant of the doctor, who was not a doctor by himself. It resulted in burns and hyperpigmentation. Following this 50% glycolic acid + Mesoglow was recommended, but it further caused burn at the chin. The whole procedure cost ₹10,000. The patient demanded a compensation of 50 lakhs.*

Verdict—court dismissed the plea as the compensation asked for was very high, giving an option to file a new case again with request for lower compensation.

Thus, compensation in medical negligence cases go beyond the multiplier formula and the Supreme Court has decreed that this is fair and just.

If a 35-year-old patient were to have died due to medical negligence and had a monthly income of ₹ 2 lakhs, the amount payable as compensation would be calculated thus:

70 – 35 = 35 × 24 lakhs = 8.5 million. Add 30% (inflation) = 10.92 million minus one-third for expenses if he was alive = 7.28 million. Add to this mental anguish to the family and litigation costs. Total will amount to ₹ 8–9 million. In the same case, if the income had been ₹ 5 lakhs per month, the compensation amount will be over ₹ 20 million.

These judgments have petrified most doctors and hospital administrators (at least those who read newspapers!) though there are many who are blissfully ignorant of these developments.

Unfortunately, currently, the problem with compensation awards against doctors and hospitals is that there is inconsistency, arbitrariness, and unpredictability in the awards by the various courts. The quantum is entirely dependent on the discretion of the court.

This is especially evident in nonfatal cases where compensation has been demanded not for death of the patient but for complications following treatment wherein permanent damage or disability may have resulted, such as postoperative infection, disfigurement, under or over correction, scarring, asymmetry, etc. Occurrence of serious adverse drug reactions such as Steven-Johnson syndrome is another important cause for demanding compensation. The quantum of compensation demanded could vary in various situations based on individual circumstances. Thus a scarring or disfigurement in a person aspiring to be a model or actor could evoke greater sympathy from the courts and be considered meritorious of a higher compensation. As said earlier, it depends entirely on the discretion of the judge and there is no laid down formula for this.

The Supreme Court has in fact noted the following:

- "The lack of uniformity and consistency in awarding compensation has been a matter of grave concern. If different tribunals calculate compensation differently on the same facts, the claimant, the litigant, and the common man will be confused, perplexed, and bewildered. If there is significant divergence among tribunals in determining the quantum of compensation in similar facts, it will lead to dissatisfaction and distrust in the system."
- In the USA, when multimillion dollar compensation payouts started crippling their healthcare system, a need was felt for "capping" or limiting, the astronomical damages that were being awarded. This restriction was sought to be applied particularly to the noneconomic damages (i.e. for pain, suffering and mental anguish as well as what is called loss of consortium). These are difficult to calculate and there is no formula for it. These were being awarded arbitrarily and were huge and hence the demand for "capping". Some states in USA like California, passed laws capping the compensation to even as low as 25,000 dollars. As a result, the Annual Malpractice Insurance premium in Los Angeles (California) for an obstetrician/gynecologist (Ob/Gyn) specialist is 50,000 dollars. Compared to this the premium for the same specialty is 140,000 dollars in Chicago (Illinois) and 17,500 dollars in Long Island (New York) because these two states do not have capping of compensation.
- A similar thought process has started in India following large compensations awarded by courts, as illustrated above.

What is the justification for huge compensation payouts?

The proponents of large payouts advance the following justification:

Large compensation payouts send out a strong message to negligent or unscrupulous doctors and hospitals and act as an effective deterrent. No other redressal mechanism available to patients does this. A patient activist says—"Large payouts are the only way of improving healthcare in India. Medical Councils have failed to regulate the conduct of doctors".

Will large compensation awards achieve the stated objective and what will be the fallout that can be expected?

The Americans are still reeling under the effects of astronomical awards being handed out by the courts. The fallout is quite apparent and if one was to study it, one would get a pretty good idea of the shape of things to come in our country as well if this trend continues.

It will not be surprising, if this triggers off and replicates the worst aspects of American Healthcare in India. This will be disastrous as (1) governmental healthcare spending is miniscule and the majority of citizens depend heavily on private doctors and hospitals, (2) medical insurance penetration in the population is meager, (3) the judicial system which is already hopelessly clogged, inefficient, and tortuous will be in danger of being choked further.

Will practicing defensive medicine become inevitable for Indian doctors?

Defensive medicine means doctors ordering tests and procedures, making multispecialty references and taking other measures not because the patient need these but in order to protect themselves from any potential malpractice liability.

In the USA, 82 % of physicians order more tests than are necessary, 650 million dollars are lost by American healthcare system because of unnecessary tests and procedures in the process of defensive medicine.

In India, after medical services coming under the purview of the Consumer laws, defensive medicine got legitimacy in view of "consumerization" of the patient. The recent massive compensation awards could only provide a boost for such defensive practice.

- The need for enhanced professional liability insurance cover has already become evident and Association of Medical Consultants (AMC) is presently advising its members to indemnify themselves for at least ₹ 1 million and much more if they practice high-risk specialties. With more number of claims and higher quantum of compensations awarded, the cost of this insurance (which of course will be passed onto the patient or consumer) can only rise.
- High compensations can only further enhance the risky and hazardous nature of pursuing a medical career, as if, fear of physical assaults by patients and relatives was not enough to disincentivize the bright young students from opting for medicine as a profession. This is already evident in coffee table conversations in drawing rooms across the country like in "your daughter wants to take up medicine? Is she mad?"
- It is well known that doctors in the USA are now retiring very early. I am personally aware of my several friends and relatives in US who have opted out of the medical profession at a young age, undoubtedly because of the risk perception of continuing to practice. This is likely to replicate in India and one can well imagine the situation, it will create in a country where the doctor-patient ratio is already hopelessly skewed. The country will lose out on the expertise and experience of thousands of doctors who may even be at the peak of their careers. Almost on a regular basis, I have been receiving enquiries from colleagues, the medicolegal implications of leasing out their nursing home premises to other agencies—whether medical or nonmedical and the common thought process is—it is now getting increasingly hazardous to continue practice—physically, mentally, and financially. The hostility of patients is now quite apparent and perceptible and it is difficult to give your best if you are constrained to look upon every patient as a potential plaintiff!
- Compensation or damages awarded to a patient or relatives should not become a bonanza, largesse or source of profit. But, this is what huge compensations may end up becoming and may be looked forward to as a lottery or jackpot.

Should medical accidents be compared with road traffic accidents?

Injuries arising out of medical accidents are being equated to injuries arising out of road traffic accidents. Is it fair to do so? What are the differences?

- If everyone motorists, pedestrians, and traffic regulators were to be careful on the roads, there should be no accidents at all.
- Victims of road accidents are healthy individuals (or were so until the accident took place).
- In the medical setting, sick and diseased individuals with pre-existing medical risk factors are undergoing attempts to cure them of their infirmities and all actions are being done in good faith for the benefit of the persons presenting themselves. Some are suffering from incurable, even terminal conditions. Many of them may have unsuccessful outcomes of treatment. And even if everyone concerned were to be diligent, accidents, mishaps and complications, unlike in road accidents, will occur. Comparison with road accidents is positively untenable and it would be a travesty of justice to do so.
- One of the objectives of compensating road accident victims, as is sought to be applied to medical accident cases, is deterrence of carelessness of drivers of vehicles. However, in medical cases, it is important to remember that though compensations will deter carelessness by doctors, *it will also deter the desirable risk-taking involved in crucial medical decisions, which may optimize chances of recovery of the patient, especially in life-and-death situations. Fear of being foisted with liability will take away what may be the only chance of recovery of the patient in a given situation.*

If at all, the concept of no-fault compensation, like that existing for road traffic accidents, ought to be looked into. In other words, for a medical accident victim, it should not be necessary for the claimant to prove that someone was negligent and he or she should be compensated irrespective of that fact. An exclusive fund or corpus should be created and a methodology for the same should be devised. Such a system exists in New Zealand, where the compensation for permanent injury arising out medical treatment is paid by a corpus or fund created by the government. However, for the government to fund healthcare injury (error or accident), it needs to initially fund the service (healthcare) itself. Compared with a medical malpractice system, the New Zealand system offers more-timely compensation to a greater number of injured patients and more effective processes for complaint resolution and provider accountability.

Should not courts factor in the woeful lack of healthcare infrastructure in our country while upholding charges of negligence against a doctor? Government spending on healthcare infrastructure is a miserable 1% of the gross domestic product (GDP), lesser than many underdeveloped African countries. Should we implement a first world regulatory structure (large compensations) in a country with pathetic infrastructure (*poor blood banking system, shocking lack of qualified nurses and paramedical personnel, nonexisting emergency response systems and primitive ambulances, and so on*) which leaves doctors hamstrung in exercising their professional skills. Should not Government be penalized for it and made to compensate for being negligent rather than the doctor who is working under difficult conditions not of his making?

It is estimated that there is a shortage in this country of 1 million doctors, 2 million nurses, and 3 million hospital beds.

Another moot point that calls for a debate is the fact that since quantum of compensations is being linked to the earning capacity of the patient, should it not be considered reasonable, if a differential system of charging professional fees by doctors based on the earning capacity of the patient is put in place.

The advisory that is now making the rounds amongst doctors is that whilst taking the medical history of the patient; do not omit to record the income of the patient as it will help you to determine whether or not you can afford the patient in the event of a malpractice claim against you.

This author believes efforts are being made by the national Indian Medical Association (IMA) to get the central government to intervene in the form of an interministerial committee to introduce maximum limits in compensation payouts to medical negligence cases. Hopefully, if this materializes some sanity will return to the system, which is otherwise likely to spin out of control with fatal consequences for the healthcare delivery system. In any case, the fact of the matter is that we are poised at the brink of what the Americans have gone through and call the malpractice crisis situation.

SUGGESTED READING

1. Chandra MS, Math SB. Progress in Medicine: Compensation and medical negligence in India: Does the system need a quick fix or an overhaul? Ann Indian Acad Neurol. 2016;19(Suppl 1):S21-7.
2. Bag RK. Law of Medical Negligence and Compensation. India: Eastern Law House; 1996.
3. Agarwal AK. Medical Negligence and Compensation in India: How Much is Just and Effective? Ahmedabad: Indian Institute of Management; 2014.
4. Bismark M, Paterson R. No-fault compensation in New Zealand: Harmonizing injury compensation, provider accountability, and patient safety. Health Aff (Millwood). 2006;25(1):278-83.

CHAPTER 9A

Informed Consent

Satyanarayana Rao KH

INTRODUCTION

The concept of consent arises from the right to self-determination[1] of each individual with respect to taking decisions affecting his or her well-being. Legally, consent is a contract. Two or more persons are said to consent when they agree upon the same thing in the same sense.

Consent in the medical context involves mutual communication between doctor and patient with an expression of choice, permission, or authorization by the patient for the doctor to act or not act in a particular way. Consent is more important in aesthetic surgery than in conventional medical practice as the intervention is desire or demand based rather than therapeutic.

Treating a patient without permission amounts to physical assault, which is legally called "battery", a punishable offence.[2] Taking consent is also an ethical obligation arising out of the principle of patient's autonomy.[3,4]

Written consent is mandatory even for minor surgery or cosmetic procedure.[5]

LEGAL LIABILITY

Insufficient or lack of informed consent is a frequent cause for medical malpractice litigation.[6,7] In cases of alleged medical negligence, the complainant has to prove that there was medical error or that standard care was not provided or that there was negligence on the part of the doctor. When it is difficult to do so, the easier option for the complainant is to allege improper or inadequate informed consent,[8] in which case it is for the doctor to prove[9] that the patient was adequately informed before taking consent.

Lack of documentation of the informed consent process, incompletely filled printed forms of consent,[5] blanket consents, and consents taken as a ritual in a casual manner are likely to go against the doctor in case of litigation.

Failure to take consent before doing any surgical intervention is a "professional misconduct" and liable for disciplinary action by the State or Indian Medical Council.[10]

> Obtaining patient's signature on a dotted line as a ritual cannot constitute a proper consent and can be contested legally.[11]

Validity of Consent

There are three criteria for consent to be valid:
1. It should be given by an adult. In case of minors, one of the parents or legal guardian can give. In case of persons, aged between 12 and 18 years, the law is not clear. It is preferable to take assent of the teenager as well as consent of a parent.[11]
2. It should be voluntary, i.e. free from compulsion, pressure, inducement, influence, or misrepresentation of facts.
3. Individual giving consent must be of sound mind and must be in the right state of mind at the time of giving consent.

Informed Consent[12-19]

Doctors are legally bound to provide adequate information and disclose all material risks before administering treatment or performing any procedure so that the patient can decide to undergo the procedure or otherwise. It may not be possible or practical to disclose all side effects of drugs or very rare complications of surgery or anesthesia. In fact, such a move may create a sense of scare rather than helping the patient to take a decision.

There is no clear enunciation of the level of disclosure that can be considered adequate. Two standards[20,21] have been mentioned—(1) what a reasonable patient would want in a similar situation; (2) what a reasonable doctor would provide in a similar circumstance.

In case of litigation, there being no clarity of what constitutes a truly informed consent, judicial forums have to decide whether the information provided was adequate based on the circumstances of the particular case. In other words, no doctor can be 100% sure that the informed consent taken is foolproof.

In general, following information has to be provided:
- *Procedure* or treatment details and the benefits thereof.
- *Alternative* options including "no treatment" and its benefits and consequences.
- *Risks* involved in both options, if possible with approximate quantification.[5]
- *Complications* that can arise and their expected frequency.
- *Outcome* expected which should be realistic.
- *Duration* of treatment and *downtime*—including average number of sittings, top-up procedures, etc.
- *Expenditure* involved (approximate).

A mnemonic "*PARCODE*" may be helpful in quickly recalling the components of the information to be discussed with the patient.[11]

Components of a Proper Informed Consent

- Written consent should be signed by both patient and doctor.
- An uninterested third person should sign as witness.
- There is no prescribed fixed format for a consent form. It should be customized for each procedure.
- The contents should be in simple terms without technical jargon and in a language that the patient can understand.
- It should be clearly mentioned that adequate opportunity has been given to seek additional information or clarifications.
- Consent taking should be preceded by adequate disclosure of material information.
- Consent should be taken a few days earlier to the day of procedure, and not on the day of the procedure or weeks prior to it.

- Consent is procedure specific. Consent taken for one procedure does not hold good for doing another or additional procedure.[22]
- Consent is person specific. If consent is taken by Dr A, procedure can only be done by Dr A and not by Dr A's assistant or Dr B.
- Consent is purpose specific. Consent taken for diagnostic procedure cannot hold good for therapeutic procedure.[23]
- If anesthesia is to be used, consent form must mention the type of anesthesia, anesthesiologist's name and his or her endorsement that possible side effects of anesthesia have been explained to the patient. Alternatively, there can be a separate consent.[24]
- Specific consent is necessary for photographing the patient for documentation, scientific, academic or research purpose, or for follow-up. Specific consent must be taken, if the identity of the patient is likely to be revealed while publishing.
- Specific mention in the consent form is a must, if a new procedure or equipment is being tried out along with associated risks.
- In case a printed form is used, all blank spaces must be filled.
- There must not be any cuttings, overwriting but corrections under signature are acceptable.
- Consent form must indicate the place and date.[25]
- Patient retains the right to revoke the consent at any time.
- Denied consent also needs documentation as "informed refusal of consent"
- No kind of surety, guarantee, or money back policy can be a part of the consent.
- *Consent from should mention at the end*: "I have read and understood everything that is stated above. I have been given adequate time to think and decide. I have been given enough opportunity to seek clarifications and all my questions have been addressed satisfactorily. I hereby give my voluntary consent".

Some tips:
- Audio-visual recording of the consent process is not mandatory but may be useful.
- Consent taken well ahead of surgery suggests that time has been given to patient to think.
- If consent taken is several weeks old, it is preferable to take consent again on the day of surgery.
- It is useful that some part of consent is in patients hand writing.
- Witness signature is important. If no one is there from patient's side, a hospital staff can be a witness.
- If consent form is more than one page, patient should sign on all pages.

CONCLUSION

Disclosing adequate information and taking an informed consent before performing any plastic or cosmetic surgery or procedure is mandatory. Insufficient and improper informed consents have resulted in judicial decisions going against doctors. It is important to note that informed consent is not a protective shield against litigations arising out of alleged medical error, negligence, or failure to provide standard medical care.

CONFLICT OF INTEREST

None.

REFERENCES

1. Mallardi V. The origin of informed consent. Acta Otorhinolaryngol Ital. 2005;25(5):312-27.
2. Trehan SP, Sankhari D. Medical Professional, Patient and the Law: The Institute of Law and Ethics in Medicine, 2nd edition. Bangalore: National Law School of India University; 2002.

3. Francis CM. Autonomy and Informed Consent, Medical Ethics, 2nd edition. New Delhi: Jaypee Brothers Medical Publishers (P) Ltd; 2004.
4. Rao KHS. Ethics, Etiquettes and Legal Issues, Management Issues for a Dermatologist, 1st edition. New Delhi: Jaypee Brothers Medical Publishers (P) Ltd; 2009.
5. Kapoor L. Informed consent in aesthetic surgery. J Cutan Aesthet Surg. 2015;8:173-4.
6. Vila-Nova da Silva DB, Nahas FX, Ferreira LM. Factors influencing judicial decisions on medical disputes in plastic surgery. Aesthet Surg J. 2015;35(4):477-83.
7. Therattil PJ, Chung S, Sood A, et al. An analysis of malpractice litigation and expert witnesses in plastic surgery. Eplasty. 2017;17:e30.
8. Park BY, Kwon J, Kang SR, et al. Informed consent as a litigation strategy in the field of aesthetic surgery: an analysis based on court precedents. Arch Plast Surg. 2016;43(5):402-10.
9. Bastia BK, Kuruvilla A, Saralaya KM. Validity of consent—a review of statutes. Indian J Med Sci. 2005;59:74-8.
10. Indian Journal of Medical Ethics. (2002) Indian Medical Council (Professional Conduct, Etiquette and Ethics) Regulations, 2002, published in Gazette of India, No.14, Part III, Section 4 dated 6.4.2002. [online] Available from: http://ijme.in/articles/the-indian-medical-council-professional-conduct-etiquette-and-ethics-regulations-2002/?galley=html [Accessed December, 2018].
11. Rao KHS. Informed Consent: An Ethical Obligation or Legal Compulsion? J Cutan Aesthet Surg. 2008;1(1):33-5.
12. Sacchidanand SA, Bhat S. Safe practice of cosmetic dermatology: Avoiding legal tangles. J Cutan Aesthet Surg. 2012;5(3):170-5.
13. Goldberg DJ. Legal issues in dermatology: Informed consent, complications and medical malpractice. Semin Cutan Med Surg. 2007;26:2-5.
14. Rao KHS. Safer practice of dermatosurgery. Indian J Dermatol Venereol Leprol. 2008;74: S75-7.
15. Goldberg DJ. Cosmetic dermatology: legal issues. Dermatol Clin. 2009;27:501-5.
16. Nejadsarvari N, Ebrahimi A. Different aspects of informed consent in aesthetic surgeries. World J Plast Surg. 2014;3(2):81-6.
17. Srinivas P. Consumer Protection Act and Dermatological Practice, a Dermatologists' Perspective of Medical Ethics and Consumer Protection Act: An IADVL Book, 1st edition. 2007.
18. Goldberg DJ. Medicolegal issues for the dermatologist. Semin Cutan Med Surg. 2000;19:181-8.
19. Sharma A, Arora S. Current Scenario of Informed Consent in India. [online] Available from http://knowledgeisotopes.com/blog/wp-content/uploads/dlm_uploads/2016/02/AS_Whitepaper-Informed-Consent_230216-2-1.pdf [Accessed December, 2018].
20. Reisman NR. Medicolegal issues in plastic surgery. [online] Available from: https://plasticsurgerykey.com/medico-legal-issues-in-plastic-surgery/ [Accessed December, 2018].
21. Weinmeyer R. Lack of standardized informed consent practices and medical malpractice. Virtual Mentor. 2014;16(2):120-3.
22. Shah AK. Newer implications of medicolegal and consent issues in plastic surgery. Indian J Plast Surg. 2014;47:199-202.
23. Nandimath OV. Consent and medical treatment: The legal paradigm in India. Indian J Urol. 2009;25(3):343-7.
24. Kumar A, Mullick P, Prakash S, et al. Consent and the Indian medical practitioner. Indian J Anaesth. 2015;59:695-700.
25. Sharma R. Informed consent in clinical practice and research: ethical and legal perspective. International J Healthcare Biomedical Res. 2014;3(1):144-51.

CHAPTER 9B

Video Consent in Surgical Procedures

Priyadarshini P Gaddagimath, Venkataram Mysore

INTRODUCTION

Informed consent is the process by which the patient learns about the need, benefits, and the risk about the medical or surgical intervention, clinical trial and grants permission in full knowledge. The patient and the concerned relatives normally sign a statement confirming that they understand the same.

Dermatosurgery is one such emerging field in dermatology that specializes in minor surgical procedures and minimal invasive treatments pertaining to skin and its appendages, hair, and nails. It becomes an integral part of dermatology practice over the last decade. With expansion of the surgical skills in this field, patient education about realistic expectation is a need of the hour to be legally errorless. Procuring an informed consent before subjecting a patient to any procedure, surgery, or clinical trial is very essential. Informed consent is an ethical obligation for physicians and required by law prior to any treatment. Consequences of failure to pursue informed consent may be grave not only for the patient but also the physician.[1]

Consent forms are increasingly long and complicated, obscuring important details, and it may not be possible to convey all the information. Also, such written forms may be designed to suit the needs of the institution than the patient. Expression and language in the consent form may also not lead to full understanding of all issues by the patient. On the other hand, the physician may also feel that written consent forms are often inadequate in evolving situations and complex treatment situations. With the advent of newer technologies and their use in the medical field, it is considerably easy to record, copy, or transmit the recording of the patients. Video consent is one of such changing advances in taking the informed consent. This article explains this topic and its relevance to medical practice.

BACKGROUND

The quality of informed consent has been questioned mainly in clinical trials vowing to lack of understanding of the trial by the participants. Thus, Central Drug Standard Control Organization (CDSCO), Ministry of Health and Family Welfare, Government of India, proposed to make draft rule that "an audio–video (AV) recording of the informed consent process of individual subjects, including the procedure of providing information to the subject and his understanding on such consent, shall be maintained by the investigator for record" while conducting clinical trials in India.[2] With this scenario in the country for clinical trials, the same can be used for consents in medical practice, including dermatology mainly dermatosurgery procedures like hair transplantations, scar revisions, and other aesthetic procedures like injection of fillers and botulinum toxins.

TYPES OF CONSENT

Consents are of two types—(1) implied consent and (2) expressed consent.

Implied Consent

The patient seeking a consultation from a doctor and expressing his concerns is taken as implied (or implicit) consent for general physical examination and routine investigations.

Expressed Consent

The expressed consent is either written or oral.[3]

Written consents are useful in procedures involving long-term follow-ups, immunosuppressive drugs, biologics, drugs that cannot be used in pregnancy such as retinoid, methotrexate, etc. high risk interventions, aesthetic procedures such as hair transplantations, rhinoplasties, liposuction, face-lifts, etc. and other similar surgeries. The present scenario expects written consents taken from relatives and the patient for admission in intensive care units also. In dermatology, it is required to take written consents in cases requiring skin biopsy, psoralen with ultraviolet A (PUVA) therapy, intralesional injection, electrocautery, etc.[4]

Dermatology and its allied subjects are mainly involving visible lesions on the skin. Thus, photographs are basic requirement to assess the progress and cure rates. Pre- and post-treatments results are evident. This makes it easier for use of these photographs in promotions, as education material, publications in journals. Consent is required before taking photographs of a patient for such purposes.

Specific consent must be taken, if the identity of the patient is likely to be revealed while publishing.[5] Consent is must for participation in clinical trials and research projects.

CONTENTS OF AN INFORMED CONSENT

The patients' competence to make voluntary decision decides the validity, of the consent. In certain situations, the patient may be unable to give a consent. The declaration of Helsinki addresses this. If a patient is unfit physically or mentally to give a voluntary informed consent for his healthcare needs, a suitable surrogate decision maker is required. Minors, pregnant women, prisoners, human fetuses, or adults that are physically or mentally incapable of giving consent fall in this category. The treating doctor is expected to act in the best interest of the patient, if no appropriate decision maker is not found.[6] The information provided to the patient or client should be in the language best understood by the patient, alternative treatment if any should be informed and patient needs to be given time and space to choose the alternative treatment, if any.

The consent form should be dated and signed by the patient or guardian, the doctor, and an independent witness. A copy of informed consent should be handed over to the patient and the original copy should be preserved for at least 3 years. An aggrieved patient can approach the consumer forum with a complaint of medical negligence within a period of 2 years from the date of cause of action.[7]

What is Video Consent and Why it is Necessary?

- Video recording refers to the use of a camera for the digital recording of meetings.
- Audio recording refers to the use of audio recording using digital recording method.

There has to be regular written consent form taken from the subject and the willingness to agree for the consent process to be taped must be recorded as a separate line on the consent form.

Audio-video (AV) recording of consent can be considered necessary for interventions involving risk, major dermatologic surgeries, and clinical trials. In any case if the purpose of the recording is changed other than for which it was obtained, additional consent has to be acquired. Then specific additional consent must be acquired.

The other purposes of AV recording include the following:[8]
- *Teaching*: Illustration of interviewing techniques
- *Training*: For demonstration purposes to others in the research team
- *Research*: As a defined aspect of a clinical study
- *Educational purpose*: The recorded tape can be used as presentation for the general patient education and awareness about the need and easy understanding of the procedure, which would aid them in taking an appropriate decision. For example, vitiligo surgeries, scar revisions, hair transplantations.

REQUIREMENTS OF AN AUDIO-VIDEO CONSENT

Audio-video recording for consent requires quiet room that can accommodate the patient or client for the procedure or clinical trial, the physician, nurse and a witness (in case of illiterate), and a videographer who despite being able to use small and high-resolution cameras still need to have sufficient distance from those being recorded to record two or three people going through the consent documents, the discussion, and the initials and signatures. In the case of children being recruited, the room also needs to be large enough to accommodate additional family members.[9] The requirement of oral consent for the recording and of the provision of initial information, followed by the discussion and the recording of the process of informed consent, results in multiple sessions for some studies, particularly when the participants need time for discussion with their families.[9]

ADVANTAGES

- Transparency in the treatment and it increases the confidence of the public on the ethical conduct, its safeguards the rights, safety, and well-being of the client/patient, but majorly the treating physician or surgeon.

- It simplifies the process of consent and improves its conduct.
- It helps the physician to understand the areas of the procedures that are poorly grasped by the patients and helps him to improve on the counseling and further simplification the consent.
- It leads to the conformation of the informed decision made by patients that largely helps the physician in case of litigations.

Procedure for Video Recording

Prior starting of the recording, the patient and his family members have to be given an oral and a written information of the recording of the consent stating the voluntary participations of the patient, confidentiality of identity, and location. The patient has to be informed that nonparticipation in the recording will not influence the treatment offered and the patient has a right to withdraw consent at any time, including before, during, or after the recording.

Patient should never be forced and cautioned not to mention third party names (in case of clinical trials). They must be cautioned before the recording to refrain from mentioning names or identifying information about third parties. If done inadvertently, the recording should be stopped and the identifying information erased before resuming taping. After or during the recording, if the patient does not give consent for the recording to be kept, the recording must be stopped and deleted immediately.

Storage and Erasure of Recordings[8,11]

Patient's records, including audio and Digital Versatile Disc (DVDs), must be stored securely in locked cupboards and cataloged. All staff must take responsibility for finding out the procedure for locking AV tapes in their Directorate and comply. Any personal data stored in any form, including electronically, must be completely safe and confidential, in accordance with current legislation. Staff must familiarize themselves with these requirements. One CD per participant will be archived with appropriate labeling in participant binder. The soft copies of the recordings will also be stored in a password protected hard drive. In cases of clinical trials, the original recording in the laptop will be deleted when study is closed out.

A professional tape wiper should be used to erase video tapes. DVD or CD hard copies that cannot be erased must be physically destroyed. The patient should receive a written notification that the recording has been erased.

Copyright of Recordings[8,11]

Audio-video recordings need to be treated in the same way as written medical records with regard to confidentiality. Similar to medical records, they can be subpoenaed by the courts. In ensuring the safe storage of recordings within institutes, it is desirable to create an audit loop to check for adherence to institutional guidelines.

CHALLENGES

- Larger infrastructure and cost implications
- Language barrier, regional and religious hindrances, unwillingness to discuss ailments in camera, interpretation of the behavior on the camera, scare of thefts or misuse of data and identity disclosure.

SUMMARY

Video recording is boon in dermatosurgery. It gives a new meaning to the informed consent making the whole procedure transparent leading to ethical way of conduct of procedures with equal responsibility and involvement of the patient in the procedure. This could reduce the legal litigation burden to a certain extent in the doctors. If the fewer challenges are overcome and protocol is made it becomes an easy tool in day-to-day clinical practice.

REFERENCES

1. Stoff BK, Payne LC, Shih J, et al. What form of informed consent? A nationwide pilot survey. J Clin Exp Dermatol Res. 2012;3:158.
2. Chauhan RC, Purty AJ, Singh N. Consent for audio-video recording of informed consent process in rural South India. Perspect Clin Res. 2015;6(3):159-62.
3. World Medical Association, Inc. (2005). Medical Ethics Manual. [online] Available from: http://www.wma.net/. [Accessed December, 2018].
4. Srinivas P. Consumer Protection Act and Dermatological Practice, a Dermatologists' Perspective of Medical Ethics and Consumer Protection Act: An IADVL Book, 1st edition; 2007. pp. 7–21.
5. Joga Rao SV. Medical Ethics. A Ready Referencer, 1st edition. Bangalore: Legalaxy Publications; 2004. p. 84.
6. Liesegang TJ. The meaning and need for informed consent in research. Indian J Ophthalmol. 2007;55:1-3.
7. Rao KH; IADVL Dermatosurgery Task force. Safer practice of dermatosurgery. Indian J Dermatol Venereol Leprol. 2008;74 Suppl:S75-7.
8. Nirmal B, Sacchidananda SA. Informed consent in dermatology: What's known and What's new? Indian J Dermatol Venereol Leprol. 2014;80(1):58-61.
9. Grady C, Cummings SR, Rowbotham MC, et al. Informed Consent. Review Article: The Changing Face of Clinical Trials. N Engl J Med. 2017;376:856-67.
10. Kulkarni NG, Dalal JJ, Kulkarni TN. Audio-video recording of informed consent process: Boon or bane. Perspect Clin Res. 2014;5(1):6-10.
11. National Health Service. Obtaining consent to record patient sessions procedure. NHS. 2016;3:1-15. Last accessed 30 Dec. 2018.

CHAPTER 10

Right to Confidentiality

Santosh Kumar Verma, Vivekanshu Verma, Virender Pal Singh

INTRODUCTION

The terms "privacy" and "confidentiality" are commonly used interchangeably. However, they are related but not identical concepts. Privacy refers to the right to control access to oneself, and includes physical privacy such as ensuring curtains are closed during physical examinations. Privacy may also relate to information about oneself, and information privacy laws regulate the handling of personal information through enforceable privacy principles. Confidentiality relates to information only. The legal duty of confidentiality obliges healthcare practitioners to protect their patients against inappropriate disclosure of personal health information. There is difference between need to know versus the right to know: as it is related to privacy of patient medical data in an information-based democratic society, although information is the currency of democracy. But the doctors need to be careful in balancing public "Right to Know" versus the Right to Say "No" to release confidential information, to maintain secrecy and privacy of patient medical data in diseases with social stigma like HIV-AIDS, because doctor can be penalized for it.

RIGHT TO INFORMATION

Right to Information Act, 2005[1] has been enacted to ensure effective exercise of right to get information given to citizens by the Parliament to bring about transparency in the functioning of government/public authorities/private body, which can be accessed by a public authority under any other law for the time being in force. It is well known that the doctors are governed by the provisions of Clinical Establishment act, 2010 and Medical code of ethics and regulations under Indian Medical Council Act, 1956 (till National Medical Commission Bill 2018 still pending in Parliament) as well as Consumer Protection Act, 1986. A slight deviation or noncompliance of the applicable provisions at the end of doctor makes them liable for action.

As defined under section 2(f) of the Act—"Information" means any material in any form, including records, documents, memos, e-mails, opinions, advices, press releases, circulars, order, logbooks, contracts, reports, papers, samples, models, date material, held in any electronic form and information relating to any private body, which can be accessed by a public authority under any law for the time being in force.[1]

Referring to an order of Central Information Commission (CIC), said that according to the CIC's July 23 order, a patient has a right to his/her medical record, which is rooted in Article 19 and 21 of the Constitution and the hospital authorities have a duty to provide the same under RTI (Right to Information) Act, Consumer Protection Act, Medical Council Act, and world medical ethics dealt with constitutional rights.[2]

"If there are existing instructions to this effect, the same need to be reiterated and the concerned authorities sensitized about the same, and if there are no existing instructions, the health ministry may consider issuing suitable orders or rules, so that patients get copies of their medical record, including details of treatment, as a matter of right."[2]

The law ministry has stated that "most of the time, the hospital authorities do not provide details of the medical record or the treatment given to a patient".[3]

According to Section 3 of the RTI act, 2005—all citizens shall have the right to access the medical information that is useful for the patient/public benefit without showing any reason.[1]

As per section 4 (1) (a) of the act—every public authority shall maintain all records in proper manner, which facilitates the right to information under this Act while as per subsection-4(1)(b)—shall suo moto publish within 180 days from the enactment of this Act, the particulars of its organization, functions, duties, powers, decision-making process, channels of supervision and accountability, rules, regulations, instructions, manuals, records, arrangements, directory of its officers, and the monthly remuneration received by each of its officers and many more details in most effective method of communication easily accessible to the extent possible in electronic format with the Central Public Information Officer (CPIO) or SPIO as the case may be.[1]

Public Information Officers (PIOs) designated under section 5 (1) of the Act shall deal with requests from persons seeking information and render reasonable assistance to the person seeking information and also provide the required information with the help of any other officer as he or she considers it necessary for proper discharge of his or her duties, on payment of the prescribed fee. In private hospitals, the medical superintendent takes care of RTI applications as PIO, mostly. Large number of requests are received by health authorities under the RTI Act to provide information like copies of postmortem reports (PMR), medicolegal reports (MLR), day-to-day treatment records, test reports/results, etc.[1]

Section 6 of RTI Act 2005[1] gives right to receive information to a person who is a citizen of India from the PIO of the concerned public authority who as per section 7 of the Act shall either provide the information on payment of such fee as may be prescribed within 30 days of receipt of such request or reject for any of the reasons specified in sections 8 or 9:

Provided that where the information sought for concerns the life or liberty of a person, the same shall be provided within 48 hours of the receipt of request.

Section 8 of RTI Act 2005 provides certain conditions, wherein medical information about a patient is exempted from disclosure. However, it has been noticed that different PIOs respond differently to such requests. In this context, it is very important that PIOs are aware of important legal provisions of the RTI Act, especially section 8(1), relevant portion of which is reproduced below:[1] "Notwithstanding anything contained in this Act, there shall be no obligation to give any citizen":

a. *Information*, disclosure of which would prejudicially affect the sovereignty and integrity of India, the security, strategic, scientific or economic interests of the State, relation with foreign State or lead to incitement of an offence.
b. *Information*, which has been expressly forbidden to be published by any court of law or tribunal or the disclosure of which may constitute contempt of court.
c. *Information*, the disclosure of which would cause a breach of privilege of Parliament or the State Legislature.
d. *Information* including commercial confidence, trade secrets, or intellectual property, the disclosure of which would harm the competitive position of a third party, unless the competent authority is satisfied that larger public interest warrants the disclosure of such information.
e. *Information* available to a person in his fiduciary relationship, unless the competent authority is satisfied that the larger public interest warrants the disclosure of such information.
f. *Information* received in confidence from foreign Government.
g. *Information*, the disclosure of which would endanger the life or physical safety of any person or identify the source of information or assistance given in confidence for law enforcement or security purposes
h. *Information*, which would impede the process of investigation or apprehension or prosecution of offenders
i. Cabinet papers including records of deliberations of the council of ministers, secretaries, and other officers
j. *Information*, which relates to personal information the disclosure of which has no relationship to any public activity or interest, or which would cause unwarranted invasion of the privacy of the individual.

Easy recall for "information exempted under RTI— not to be revealed": All S's mnemonic:
- S—Security of the state is affected in revealing information
- S—Secured information by the court of law
- S—Security of patient is affected—endangering life of him
- S—State legislature privileges are breached in revealing information
- S—Secrets of commerce—"information about trade secrets, commercial confidence, intellectual property (IP) rights"
- S—Security of foreign government is affected in revealing information
- S—Safety of life of any person is affected in revealing information
- S—Source of information—affecting confidence of law enforcement agency
- S—Slow the process of investigation in revealing information
- S—Secrets personal—private information of the individual

It may be seen that clause (e) of this section provides for exemption of information, which is available to a person in his "fiduciary relationship". Doctor–patient relationship falls under this category. Therefore, the PIO can claim exemption u/s 8(1) (e) of the RTI Act, if information pertaining to a victim/patient is sought by a 3rd person after following the procedure prescribed u/s 11 of RTI.[1]

Patients and their relatives are entitled to know the treatment details including names and qualifications/experience of doctors.[4]

Further, in doubtful cases where an FIR has been registered and investigation is in progress, the PIO may officially write to the Police and ascertain the status and after obtaining confirmation from the investigation officer, the PIO can claim exemption under clause (h) on the ground that providing copy of PMR or MLR would impede the investigation and/or apprehension or prosecution of offenders.[1]

Similarly, in cases where the disclosure of information may endanger the life and safety of any person (potential witnesses, victim, etc.), exemption can be claimed under Section 8(1)(g) of RTI.[1]

Section 11 of RTI deals with the third party information:

1. Where a CPIO or the SPIO, as the case may be, intends to disclose any information or record, or part thereof on a request made under this Act, which relates to or has been applied by a third party and has been treated as confidential by the third party, the CPIO or the SPIO, as the case may be, shall, within 5 days from the receipt of the request, give a written notice to such third party of the request and of the fact that the CPIO or the SPIO, as the case may be, intends to disclose the information or record, or part thereof, and invite the third party to make a submission in writing or orally, regarding whether the information should be disclosed, and such submission of the third party shall be kept in view while taking a decision about disclosure of information.[1]
   Provided that except in the case of trade or commercial secrets protected by law, disclosure may be allowed, if the public interest in disclosure outweighs in importance any possible harm or injury to the interests of such third party.

2. Where a notice is served by the CPIO or the SPIO, as the case may be, under subsection (1) to a third party in respect of any information or record or part thereof, the third party shall, within 10 days from the date of receipt of such notice, be given the opportunity to make representation against the proposed disclosure.

3. Notwithstanding anything contained in Section 7, the CPIO or SPIO, as the case may be, shall, within 40 days after receipt of the request under section 6, if the third party has been given an opportunity to make representation under subsection (2), make a decision as to whether or not to disclose the information or record or part thereof and give in writing the notice of his decision to the third party.

4. A notice given under section (3) shall include a statement that the third party to whom the notice is given is entitled to prefer an appeal under section 19 against the decision.

It is the discretion of the CPIO or SPIO, as the case may be, to decide whether the disclosure of particular information is in larger public interest or not. If it is not so, the information may be denied.

In a matter relating to marital dispute case, the CIC has held that there is a larger public interest that requires disclosure of medical records of a patient as mandated under section 8(1)(j) of RTI and directed the respondent authority to furnish the information about the medical records of her husband to the extent she needed to establish the disease he was suffering from—its impact, continuity, and incurability or curability, whatever it is along with necessary certified copies to protect her interest/right to secure divorce under the Hindu Marriage Act, 1955 to prevent crime of beating or cruelty against her allegedly being perpetrated by her husband because of mental illness shall be provided.[5]

Section 19 of RTI appeal:
1. Any person, who does not receive a decision within the time specified in subsection (1) or clause (a) of subsection (3) of section 7, or is aggrieved by a decision of the CPIO or SPIO, as the case may be, may within 30 days from the expiry of such period or from the receipt of such a decision prefer an appeal to such officer who is senior in rank to the CPIO or SPIO, as the case may be, in each public authority.[1]
2. Where an appeal is preferred against an order made by a CPIO or an SPIO, as the case may be, under Section 11 to disclose third party information, the appeal by the concerned third party shall be made within 30 days from the date of order.
3. A second appeal against the decision under subsection (1) shall lie within 90 days from the date on which the decision should have been made or was actually received, with the CIC or the SIC.
4. If the decision of the CPIO or SPIO, as the case may be, against which an appeal is preferred relates to information of third party, the CIC or the SIC, as the case may be, shall give an opportunity of being heard to that third party.
5. In an appeal proceedings, the onus to prove that a denial of a request was justified shall lie on the CPIO or SPIO, as the case may be, who denied the request.
6. An appeal under subsection (1) or subsection (2) shall be disposed of within 30 days of receipt of the appeal or within such extended period not exceeding a total of 45 days from the date of filing thereof, as the case may be, for reasons to be recorded in writing.

Besides, under section 20 of the RTI Act dealing with penalties—a complaint can also be filed before the CIC or SIC against the CPIO or SPIO, as the case may be, in case he acts against the prescribed procedure under the Act causing undue inconvenience to the citizen seeking any information.[1]

Q. Can doctors/hospital administrators, as PIO officials, be punished if they do not comply with the RTI?
Public officials who deliberately delay or obstruct an application for information, or who deliberately provide incorrect or misleading information can be punished under the RTI laws. Penalties are an important part of an RTI law because they play a vital role in changing the cultures of secrecy that are common within many of India's bureaucracies. Without the threat of sanction, there is little incentive for bureaucrats to comply with the new terms of the Act. The Central Act allows for the imposition of penalties. Most notably, where a PIO has, without any reasonable cause:
- Refused to receive an application
- Not furnished information within time limits
- Malafidely denied the request
- Knowingly given incorrect, incomplete, or misleading information
- Destroyed information subject to a request, or
- Obstructed the process.

In above findings, the Information Commission can impose a penalty of Rupees 250 per day. The total penalty cannot exceed Rupees 25,000. Section 20(1) of RTI states that "Public Information Officers" can be penalized, but when read with section 5(5) of the RTI Act (which states that any officer whose assistance is sought by a PIO will be treated as a PIO for purposes of the Act's penalty clauses), it is clear that in practice any official can be sanctioned for noncompliance, if they have shirked their duties under the law.

Before a penalty is imposed under section 20(1), an official must be given a reasonably opportunity of being heard. The official is responsible for providing that he/she acted reasonable and diligently. Under the Central RTI Act, where a monetary penalty is imposed, the Information Commission can also recommend disciplinary action against the PIO under the applicable service rules.

Penalties can usually be imposed by appeal bodies, whether or not they are internal appeals bodies or external appeals bodies. Unfortunately, under the Central Act, it is unclear under the law whether the first Appellate Authority can impose penalties, although it is explicit that the Information Commission can. It is not clear, therefore, whether there can be any penalty for noncompliance that is identified during an internal appeal. Information Commissions will need to clarify whether Appellate Authorities can refer cases to the Commission for consideration under section 20. It is possible that Commissions could hear such cases under the broad appeal remit under section 18(1)(f), which empowers Commissions to handle any complaint "in respect of any other matter relating to requesting or obtaining access to records under this Act".

Right of Mentally Ill Patients to Access their Medical Records

As per Section 25 of Mental Healthcare Act, 2017[6]

1. All persons with mental illness shall have the right to access their basic medical records as may be prescribed.
2. The mental health professional in charge of such records may withhold specific information in the medical records, if disclosure would result in:
   a. Serious mental harm to the person with mental illness; or
   b. Likelihood of harm to other persons.
3. When any information in the medical records is withheld from the person, the mental health professional shall inform the person with mental illness of his right to apply to the concerned board for an order to release such information.

RIGHT TO CONFIDENTIALITY

The right to confidentiality of person with illness shall also apply to all information stored in electronic or digital format in real or virtual space.[6]

The Mental Health Act (MHA),[6] in India section 13(1) states that Inspector of psychiatric hospital or nursing home requires to keep confidentiality in relation to personal records of patient. As per section 38 of MHA, even visitors cannot be allowed to inspect records of patients.[6]

As per section 23 of MHA, A person with mental illness shall have the right to confidentiality in respect of his mental health, mental healthcare, treatment, and physical healthcare.[6]

All health professionals providing care or treatment to a person with mental illness shall have a duty to keep all such information confidential, which has been obtained during care or treatment with the following exceptions, namely: (1) release of information to the nominated representative to enable him to fulfill his duties under this Act; (2) release of information to other mental health professionals and other health professionals to enable them to provide care and treatment to the person with mental illness; (3) release of information, if it is necessary to protect any other person from harm or violence; (4) only such information that is necessary to protect against the harm identified shall be released; (5) release only such information as is necessary to prevent threat to life; (6) release of information upon an order by concerned board or the central authority or High Court or Supreme Court or any other statutory authority competent to do so; and (7) release of information in the interests of public safety and security.[6]

Privileged communication of medical professional secrecy:
Easy recall for "Confidential Medical Information of patient to be revealed" in:
All Ps:
- P—Protect patient against further harm/violence in mentally unfit
- P—Patient's own interest in revealing warning signs to legal guardians in minors
- P—Protect other patients from contagious infectious disease
- P—Protect the interests of the community or the state
- P—Prohibit the visit of patients of contagious venereal disease (syphilis) to public swimming pools
- P—Prevent threat to life of patient
- P—Persuade patient suffering from epilepsy to change the high-risk occupation—driver, pilot
- P—Provide further care to patient while referring to another healthcare provider
- P—Public safety and security—suicidal/homicidal tendencies in schizophrenia
- P—Permission of court of law in medicolegal cases
- P—Professional negligence by another healthcare provider
- P—Police enquiry in alleged medical negligence and suspected crimes related to patient
- P—Public health notification—birth and death register, dengue, cholera, tuberculosis (TB)

In Mr Surupsingh Hrya Naik versus State of Maharashtra,[7] a private citizen sought information from the Public Information Officer—of Sir JJ Hospital, Byculla, Mumbai, the medical reports of Mr Naik, legislator who was convicted for contempt of court. Appellant claimed that it was in public interest to know why a convict is allowed to stay in an air conditioned comfort of the hospital and there had been intensive questioning about this aspect in the media and the peoples mind. There is, therefore, a legitimate doubt about the true reasons for a convict being accommodated in air conditioned comfort of the hospital, thereby ensuring that the convict escapes the punishment imposed on him and also denies a scarce facility to the needy.

The medical records of a person are generally confidential, considering the Indian Medical Council (Professional Conduct, Etiquette, and Ethics) Regulations 2002 framed under the provisions of the Indian Medical Council Act, 1956, which hereinafter are referred to as the Regulations. Regulation 2.2, which is relevant, reads as under:

2.2. Patience, Delicacy, and Secrecy: Patience and delicacy should characterize the physician. Confidences concerning individual or domestic life entrusted by patients to a physician and defects in the disposition or character of patients observed during medical attendance should never be revealed unless their revelation is required by the law of the State. Sometimes, however, a physician must determine whether his duty to society requires him to employ knowledge, obtained through confidence as a physician, to protect a healthy person against a communicable disease to which he is about to be exposed. In such instance, the physician should act as he would wish another to act toward one of his own family in like circumstances.[8]

It appears from this Regulation that the information as sought should not be revealed unless the revelation is required by the law of the State.

The next relevant Regulation of Indian Medical Council Act is Regulation 7.14, which reads as under:[8]

The registered medical practitioner shall not disclose the secrets of patient that have been learnt in the exercise of his/her profession, except:
- In a court of law under orders of the Presiding Judge

- In circumstances where there is a serious and identified risk to a specific, person and/or community; and
- *Notifiable diseases*: In case of communicable/notifiable diseases, concerned public health authorities should be informed immediately.[8]

RIGHT TO PRIVACY

Privacy principles governing minimum privacy standards for handling personal information, including:
- The need to gain consent for the collection of health information
- What to tell individuals when information is collected?
- What to consider before passing health information on to others?
- The details that should be included in a health service provider's privacy policy
- Securing and storing information in their health records
- Providing individuals with a right to access their health records.

It is important to maintain privacy and confidentiality because:
- Patients are concerned about the stigma and discrimination associated with their HIV and related conditions.
- Patients want to know that they can choose who has access to information about them.
- Patients are far more likely to seek medical care and give full and honest accounts of their symptoms, if they feel comfortable, respected, and secure.
- A health system with strong privacy mechanisms will promote public confidence and trust in healthcare services generally.

Right to privacy has been culled out of the provisions of Article 21 and other provisions of the Constitution relating to Fundamental Rights read with Directive Principles of State Policy.[9]

"The right to privacy is implicit in the right to life and liberty guaranteed to the citizens of this country by Article 21. It is a "right to be let alone": A citizen has a right to safeguard the privacy of his own, his family, marriage, procreation, motherhood, child-bearing, and education among other matters. None can publish anything concerning the above matters without his consent—whether truthful of otherwise and whether laudatory or critical. If he does so, he would be violating the right to privacy of the person concerned and would be liable in an action for damages. Position may, however, be different, if a person voluntarily thrusts himself into controversy or voluntarily invites or raises a controversy."[9]

"Right to privacy is not absolute": Right of privacy may, apart from contract, also arise out of a particular specific relationship, which may be commercial, matrimonial, or even political. As already discussed above, doctor–patient relationship, though basically commercial, is, professionally, a matter of confidence; and, therefore, doctors are morally and ethically bound to maintain confidentiality. In such a situation, public disclosure of even true private facts may amount to an invasion of the Right of Privacy, which may sometimes lead to the clash of one person's "right to be let alone" with another person's right to be informed. Disclosure of even true private facts has the tenancy to disturb a person's tranquility. It may generate many complexes in him and may even lead to psychological problems. He may, thereafter, have a disturbed life all through. In the face of these potentialities and as already held by this Court in its various decisions referred to above, the Right of Privacy is an essential component of right to life envisaged by Article 21, The right, however, is not absolute and may be lawfully restricted for the prevention of crime, disorder or protection of health or morals or protection of rights and freedom of others.[9]

The declaration of Geneva,[10] in which there is a provision pertaining to right to confidentiality of information about the patient's health status, medical condition, diagnosis, prognosis, and treatment and all other information of a personal kind with the exception, that descendants may have a right of access to information that would inform them of their health risk. A citizen has a right "to safeguard the privacy of his own, his family, marriage, procreation, motherhood, childbearing, and education among other matters".

Supreme Court then observed as under "Right to privacy—by itself—has not been identified under the Constitution. As a concept, it may be too broad and moralistic to define it judicially. Whether right to privacy can be claimed or has been infringed in a given case would depend on the facts of the said case".[9]

In Mr "X" versus Hospital "Z" case, the issue was disclosure of information of a patient affected by HIV. The person, whose information was disclosed, sought an action in damages, by moving the National Consumer Disputes Redressal Commission, which was rejected and then he appealed to the Supreme Court. In considering the duty to maintain confidentially, the Court observed that in doctor–patient relationship, the most important aspect is the doctor's duty of maintaining secrecy and the doctor cannot disclose to a person any information regarding his patient, which he has gathered in the course of treatment nor can the doctor disclose to anyone else the mode of treatment or the advice given by him to the patient. Supreme Court said: The Code of Medical Ethics carves out an exception to the rule of confidentiality and permits the disclosure in the circumstances enumerated in the judgment under which public interest would override the duty of confidentiality particularly where there is an immediate or future health risk to others.[9]

The Human Immunodeficiency Virus and Acquired Immune Deficiency Syndrome (Prevention and Control) Act, 2017 mandates that confidentiality of the medical information of the patient should not be disclosed to any third party.

The "HIV-related information" means any information relating to the HIV status of a person and includes:
- Information relating to the undertaking performing the HIV test or result of an HIV test
- Information relating to the care, support, or treatment of that person
- Information, which may identify that person; and
- Any other information concerning that person, which is collected, received, accessed, or recorded in connection with an HIV test, HIV treatment, or HIV-related research or the HIV status of that person.[11]

As per the HIV and AIDS (Prevention and Control) 2017, every establishment keeping the records of HIV-related information of protected persons shall adopt data protection measures in accordance with the guidelines to ensure that such information is protected from disclosure.

Explanation: For the purpose of this section, data protection measures shall include procedures for protecting information from disclosure, procedures for accessing information, provision for security systems to protect the information stored in any form and mechanisms, to ensure accountability and liability of persons in the establishment.[11]

Q. When is disclosure of HIV status is permitted in law?

(1) Notwithstanding anything contained in any other law for the time being in force:

(i) No person shall be compelled to disclose his HIV status except by an order of the court that the disclosure of such information is necessary in the interest of justice, for the determination of issues in the matter before it.

(ii) No person shall disclose or be compelled to disclose the HIV status or any other private information of other person imparted in confidence or in a relationship of a fiduciary nature, except with the informed consent of that other person or a representative of such another person obtained in the manner as specified in section 5 of the HIV and AIDS (prevention and control) Act, as the case may be, and the fact of such consent has been recorded in writing by the person making such disclosure: provided that, in case of a relationship of a fiduciary nature, informed consent shall be recorded in writing.[11]

(2) The informed consent for disclosure of HIV-related information under clause (ii) of subsection (1) is not required where the disclosure is made:

a. By a healthcare provider to another healthcare provider who is involved in the care, treatment, or counseling of such person, when such disclosure is necessary to provide care or treatment to that person

b. By an order of a court that the disclosure of such information is necessary in the interest of justice for the determination of issues and in the matter before it

c. In suits or legal proceedings between persons, where the disclosure of such information is necessary in filing suits or legal proceedings or for instructing their counsel

d. As required under the provisions of section 9

e. If it relates to statistical or other information of a person that could not reasonably be expected to lead to the identification of that person; and

f. To the officers of the Central Government or the State Government or State AIDS Control Society of the concerned State Government, as the case may be, for the purposes of monitoring, evaluation, or supervision.[11]

Exemptions to HIV-related confidentiality:
When can privileged communications of private medical information related to patient may be disclosed?
All Ws mnemonic for easy recall:
- W—When the person consents to disclosure
- W—When it is necessary to provide care, treatment, or counseling
- W—When patient is referred to another hospital in critical state for advanced care
- W—When the person is receiving particular services in a hospital
- W—When the Director General of Health Services (DGHS) has reasonable grounds to suspect the information is necessary to prevent a risk to public health
- W—When the purposes of legal proceedings arising from the Public Health and accompanying regulations, including reporting those proceedings
- W—When insurance company claims the information for providing mediclaim cover to patient
- W—When public health safety is getting compromised

Q. What are the duties of doctor in disclosure of HIV-positive status to partner of HIV-positive person?

1. No healthcare provider, except a physician or a counselor, shall disclose the HIV-positive status of a person to his or her partner.

2. A healthcare provider, who is a physician or counselor, may disclose the HIV-positive status of a person under his direct care to his or her partner, if such healthcare provider:

a. Reasonably believes that the partner is at the significant risk of transmission of HIV from such person; and
b. Such HIV-positive person has been counseled to inform such partner; and
c. Is satisfied that the HIV-positive person will not inform such partner; and
d. Has informed the HIV-positive person of the intention to disclose the HIV-positive status to such partner:
   i. Provided that disclosure under this subsection to the partner shall be made in person after counseling
   ii. Provided further that such healthcare provider shall have no obligation to identify or locate the partner of an HIV-positive person
   iii. Provided also that such healthcare provider shall not inform the partner of a woman where there is a reasonable apprehension that such information may result in violence, abandonment, or actions, which may have a severe negative effect on the physical or mental health or safety of such woman, her children, her relatives or someone who is close to her.
3. The healthcare provider under subsection (1) shall not be liable for any criminal or civil action for any disclosure or nondisclosure of confidential HIV-related information made to a partner under this section.[11]

The HIV ombudsman shall, upon a complaint made by any person, inquire into the violations of the provisions of this HIV and AIDS (prevention and control) Act, 2017, in relation to acts of discrimination mentioned in section 3 and providing of healthcare services by any person, in such manner as may be prescribed by the State Government. The ombudsman may require any person to furnish information on such points or matters, as he considers necessary, for inquiring into the matter and any person so required shall be deemed to be legally bound to furnish such information and failure to do so shall be punishable under sections 176 and 177 of the Indian Penal Code.[11]

Q. Can journalist be restrained for the publication of the confidential records of HIV-positive doctors? Yes

Case: A journalist obtained confidential records of two HIV-positive doctors who continued their general practice. The doctors sought a permanent injunction to restrain the publication of the information. The Court granted the injunction. It held: "I keep in the forefront of my mind the very important public interest in freedom of the press. And I accept that there is some public interest in knowing that which the defendants seek to publish. But in my judgment, those public interests are substantially outweighed when measured against the public interest in relation to loyalty and confidentiality both generally and with particular reference to AIDS patients' hospital records".[12]

CONCLUSION

Privacy and confidentiality of a patient's medical information create the foundation upon which a patient reposes trust in his or her doctor. While defining the physician–patient privilege, patient's relationship with the modern healthcare delivery system often includes a team of physicians, surgeons, nurses, and other clinical support personnel. This relationship extends beyond direct caregivers and may include healthcare administrators, payor organizations, and persons unfamiliar with a patient's identity, such as researchers and public health officials. Accessing a patient's medical information links these participants to the patient's healthcare delivery relationship. The combination of broad access, individual privacy rights, public's right to information under RTI Act, and computer technology requires a rethinking of measures designed to protect the realities of the modern medical information society.

REFERENCES

1. Ministry of Law and Justice. (2005). Right to Information Act, 2005. [online] Available from: https://rti.gov.in/rti-act.pdf. [Accessed December, 2018].
2. CIC order quoting Union Law Secretary, in a letter to Union Health Secretary. Available from: http://jksic.nic.in/E%20-library/Prabat%20KUmar%20-%20Fortis.pdf [Accessed December, 2018].
3. Central Information Commission. (2014). CIC's decision in File No. CIC/SA/A/2014/000004 dated 03-11-2014/7-4-15-Shri Prabhat Kumar vs Director of Health Services. GNCTD, Delhi. [online] Available from: http://jksic.nic.in/E%20-library/Prabat%20KUmar%20-%20Fortis.pdf. [Accessed December, 2018].
4. Central Information Commission. (2016). Decision of CIC in Appeal No. CIC/SA/A/2015/001894 Anita Singh vs Director of Health Services, GNCTD. [online] Available from: https://indiankanoon.org/doc/138170762/?type=print. [Accessed December, 2018].
5. Central Information Commission. (2015). CIC/KY/A/2014/001348-SA dated 10.04.2015 Mrs Jyoti Jeena vs PIO, Institute of Human Behavior & Allied Science. [online] Available from: https://dtf.in/wp-content/files/CIC_Decision_dated_10.04.2015_on_Appeal_from_Ms._Jyoti_Jeena_Vs._Institue_of_Human_Behaviour__Allied_Sciences_Delhi.pdf. [Accessed December, 2018].
6. Ministry of Law and Justice. (2017). Mental Healthcare Act, 2017. [online] Available from: https://www.prsindia.org/uploads/media/Mental%20Health/Mental%20Healthcare%20Act,%202017.pdf. [Accessed December, 2018].
7. Bombay High Court. (2007). Mr. Surupsingh Hrya Naik vs State Of Maharashtra decided on 23 March, 2007, AIR 2007 Bom 121. [online] Available from: https://indiankanoon.org/doc/570038/. [Accessed December, 2018].
8. Medical Council of India. (2002). Indian Medical Council (Professional Conduct, Etiquette and Ethics) Regulations, 2002. [online] Available from: https://www.mciindia.org/documents/rulesAndRegulations/Ethics%20Regulations-2002.pdf. [Accessed December, 2018].
9. Singh J, Bhushan V. Medical Negligence and Compensation. 4th edition. Bharat Law Publications. Jaipur. 2018. HIV related medicolegal issues. p. 306.
10. World Medical Association. (2005). Declaration of Geneva, adopted by the 2nd General Assembly of the World Medical Association, Geneva, Switzerland, September 1948. [online] Available from: https://www.wma.net/wp-content/uploads/2017/12/Decl-of-Geneva-v2005.pdf. [Accessed December, 2018].
11. Ministry of Law and Justice. (2017). The Human Immunodeficiency Virus and Acquired Immune Deficiency Syndrome (Prevention and Control) Act, 2017. [online] Available from: http://naco.gov.in/sites/default/files/HIV%20AIDS%20Act.pdf. [Accessed December, 2018].
12. Swarb.Co.Uk. (2017). X v Y [1988] 2 All ER 648 UK. [online] Available from: https://swarb.co.uk/x-v-y-1988/. [Accessed December, 2018].

CHAPTER 11

Legal Implications of Advertising in Medical Practice

Lalit Kapoor

INTRODUCTION

If one were to give a short answer to the above question, it would be NIL. The fact of the matter is that there is no law or statute in this country, which makes it illegal for a doctor to advertise his services. But the entire position changes, if the issue is reframed as "ethical implications of advertising in medical practice".

Before we delve into the implications of advertising by doctors, it would be useful to understand the difference between law and ethics.

Since the evolution of mankind, efforts have been to regulate the behavior of individuals and groups of individuals in society by voluntarily enunciating a code of ethics for their respective members. Ethics has been defined as a science of moral principles. It is a code of conduct, a way of behavior, and almost a way of life. The oldest code of ethics for medical practitioners was the Oath of Hippocrates, which formed the basis of a self-inflicted code of conduct.

The link between ethics and law has been neatly summed up thus—law cannot reach where enforcement cannot follow. Hence, ethics begins where the law ends or cannot reach.

Historically, the code of conduct was self-inflicted. However, with the passage of time and the evolution of society along with the tremendous scientific progress and rapid industrialization there was a sea change in the social and cultural behavior of people. Physicians found themselves wedged between several interacting forces like politics, government, law, media, etc. It became necessary to frame statutory measures enforcing the principles laid down in the code of ethics and that is how the Medical Councils were born.

It must be recognized that there may be areas of dissonance and conflict between ethics and law. As a result, an act could be legal yet unethical or vice versa.

Coming to the question of advertising by doctors, the medical profession, which is considered as a liberal profession for example, the legal profession considers advertising as unethical. This is specifically enshrined in the Indian Medical Council (Professional Conduct, Etiquette and Ethics) Regulations, 2002.

ADVERTISING

- Soliciting of patients directly or indirectly, by a physician, by a group of physicians, or by institutions or organizations is unethical. A physician shall not make use of him or her (or his or her name) as subject of any form or manner of advertising or publicity through any mode either alone or in conjunction with others, which is of such a character as to invite attention to him or to his professional position, skill, qualification, achievements, attainments, specialties, appointments, associations, affiliations or honors, and/or of such character as would ordinarily result in his self-aggrandizement. A physician shall not give to any person, whether for compensation or otherwise, any approval, recommendation, endorsement, certificate, report, or statement with respect of any drug, medicine, nostrum remedy, surgical, or therapeutic article, apparatus or appliance or any commercial product, or article with respect of any property, quality or use thereof or any test, demonstration or trial thereof, for use in connection with his name, signature, or photograph in any form or manner of advertising through any mode nor shall he boast of cases, operations, cures or remedies, or permit the publication of report thereof through any mode. A medical practitioner is, however, permitted to make a formal announcement in press regarding the following:
  - On starting practice
  - On change of type of practice
  - On changing address
  - On temporary absence from duty
  - On resumption of another practice
  - On succeeding to another practice
  - Public declaration of charges.
- Printing of self-photograph, or any such material of publicity in the letterhead or on sign board of the consulting room or any such clinical establishment shall be regarded as acts of self-advertisement and unethical conduct on the part of the physician. However, printing of sketches, diagrams, and picture of human system shall not be treated as unethical.

Let us analyze the key issues on this subject.

Why is advertising by doctors considered unethical and should not be allowed?

(1) Conventionally, the medical profession, in particular the medical councils have raised concerns that advertising commercializes the practice of medicine and lowers the dignity of the profession.

(2) It was always felt that a satisfied patient was the best advertisement for a doctor and word of mouth publicity along with referrals from fellow physicians was considered to be good enough. *Advertising by doctors puts them at par with peddlers of commercial goods.*

The real objection to advertising by doctors and healthcare institutions is that unlike as in commercial advertisements, the consequences of misleading or false advertisements could be irreversible and serious or even life-threatening. A person suffering from a medical problem could be easily influenced by claims of cure and would tend to trust any promise easily as is in a vulnerable position and is likely to generate false hopes. While no serious consequences are likely to ensue by believing a false claim of the efficacy of a toothpaste or superiority of a car model or a laptop, believing and acting on a false or misleading medical advertisement could lead to grave, irreversible consequences to the hapless patient. Hence, it is felt by many that permitting doctors to advertise would lead to exploitation of patients.

Why advertising by doctors should be permitted or what are the benefits?

It is argued by many that the thinking that advertising by doctors is unethical is antiquated and no longer compatible with the current scenario. Patients now want to be more and more informed and be able to make informed choices based on truthful advertising and the healthcare professionals should have a right to inform the public of the services they provide information given to patients by doctors about their qualifications, experience, services provided, and cost of treatment can only help patients in making informed choices.

A healthcare consultant had this to say; "consumers are probably being a bit more active in the selection of which hospital they're admitted to and where they seek care, whereas in the past that decision was driven by the physician. Now that consumers are more activated, there's room for other influences in that decision. Advertising can be one of those".

Advertising by Hospitals vis-à-vis Advertising by Individual Doctors

Presently, in our country, though the Medical Council of India (MCI) code of ethics elaborately prohibits advertising by doctors, it appears that hospitals and large healthcare institutions are exempt from this ban on advertising. I have yet to hear of any action by medical councils on such hospitals who indulge in massive and virulent advertising and marketing. It appears that they do not come under the purview of this code of ethics. This has caused a lot of heartburning amongst individual doctors and small healthcare establishments as this obviates "a level playing field". Interestingly, the provision in the relevant clause of the code of ethics says:

- "Soliciting of patients directly or indirectly, by a physician, by *a group of physicians or by institutions or organizations is unethical".*
- It is quite clear that as per the code of ethics, the restriction on advertising was intended to apply to hospitals and organizations as well, there is no evidence of any punitive action being taken to prevent this.
- It is also a fact that the huge amounts being spent on marketing and advertising by these corporate and larger hospitals are further driving up the costs of treatment since these amounts will be eventually passed on to the patient.
- As to the question of taking action against advertising by organizations owned or run by nonmedical owners is concerned, quite clearly Medical Councils are not empowered by the Medical Council Acts to have a jurisdiction over such establishments. Undoubtedly, Acts like Drugs and Magical Remedies Act, etc. can be invoked to take action, but this would come under the jurisdiction of the Police who are generally loathe to pursue such matters.
- One of the solutions would be to amend the Medical Council Acts to bring such healthcare providers in their jurisdiction. Also suitable fresh legislation could be enacted to fill this lacuna.

Advertising by Nonmedical Owners of Clinical Establishments

Another trend recently, particularly in the field of cosmetic surgery, is for beauty clinics, spas, etc. to advertise freely for medical procedures, as they do for beauty treatments. They advertise a laser treatment in the same cavalier way as they treat a facial. This is particularly true of hair transplantation, where advertisements such as "unlimited grafts", nonsurgical transplantation, "stem cells" "no scar surgery", etc. are found routinely in newspapers. Many of these clinics are owned by nonmedical investors who feel they are not under any code. Medical councils have generally been lax in acting against these. While the code covers these organizations as mentioned above, taking action against them may be difficult as no punishment is prescribed in Medical Council Act, which is basically directed against doctors.

Advertising on Social Media

Social media has changed the way advertisement is done—websites, Facebook, Instagram, and YouTube allow people to speak or write what they wish. In general, social media is difficult to control in any field, and laws have generally lagged behind the progress in these fields. However, same yardstick of the code needs to apply to the social media also, though these may be difficult to track.

Advertising on social media, websites, etc. is an entirely new area and there is currently no finality on the legality or ethicality of doing so. There are plenty of gray areas and laws and codes of ethics are appropriately vague and ambiguous on the subject. Apparently, it is extremely difficult to rein in unbridled advertising and self-promotion in the social media. Possibly, a realistic redefining of the code of ethics coupled with assistance from cyber laws, etc. is called for so as to crystallize the issues around advertising and marketing on the social media.

Should the code of ethics be amended in India so as to codify a balanced and contemporary approach on the question of advertising by doctors? What is the current position in the other countries?

There have been several cases of disciplinary action being taken against doctors and nursing homes by medical councils for advertising their services. The names of many of them were struck of the register for varying periods though many were let off with strict warnings. There is no clarity on what constitutes advertising, as no definite guidelines have been laid down and hence judgments by the Councils have been arbitrary and capricious.

Several cases of paid news by doctors in the media are ignored and continued unabated, even though *Suo moto* action by Councils is possible. On the other hand, a complaint against a doctor for giving an interview to a media person on a genuine medical advancement, may be given serious cognizance and an enquiry initiated. The lines between spreading patient awareness on medical matters and self-advertisement are so blurred and liable to being interpreted arbitrarily.

The MCI needs to formulate clear-cut guidelines on this issue so as to dissipate the current ambiguity and doublethink, and delineate the positive and negative aspects of advertising by the medical profession. It needs to clarify its position on use of social media, personal websites, and online announcements.

It will be useful to study the situation in other countries and integrate features appropriate to the Indian milieu.

Back in 1847, the first code of ethics was released by the American Medical Association. It expressly prohibited all advertising as unethical.

This "No Advertising" rule was the standard until 1980. That year, the Federal Trade Commission (FTC) ruled that the Australian Medical Association's (AMA's) ethical restriction of ALL advertising by physicians was actually a restriction of trade. Although the FTC completely agreed with the ethical concerns, they felt that physicians had the right to let people know who they were, what certifications they held, and where their office was located. And this created the current guidelines followed by pretty much every physicians' society, which has then been adopted as a general ethical standard for medical institutions, groups, and clinics around the world. Here they are in a nutshell:

- *Appropriate forms of communication*: The medium must allow for complete, objectively true explanations. Sound bites, billboards, bus ads, etc. are discouraged since they lend themselves to misleading and vague statements.
- *Objectively true, inarguable statements:* The most common examples of this would be the provider's name, certification, and services they provide, pricing structure, and contact information.
- *No claims promising results*: Most medical results are uncertain so claims like "we'll make your knee feel better," are considered misleading and therefore unethical. Most testimonials are also discouraged since they imply guaranteed results. A testimonial like "I appreciate that every patient gets 30 minutes with the therapist" is fine if that is objectively true.
- *No use of superlatives*: Cannot use terms like "best", "world-famous", "pioneer", etc. because they are considered misleading and designed to attract vulnerable patients.
- *No disparaging other providers*: Stating that your profession is "the best" (see above) at something, implies that the other professions are inadequate for that service. This is unethical unless you have objective, inarguable evidence to support such a claim. You actually do not know what is best for a patient that you have not evaluated. You also cannot say that you are a better physical therapist than another.
- *Other stuff:* There are also other limitations that are self-evident like being a paid spokesperson, using actors to represent patients, use of an agency for traditional advertising campaigns that typically exaggerate the truth, being discriminatory against specific groups in your advertising, etc.

Today, so long as the advertisement does not contain any false or deceptive information, an American physician is free to advertise her or himself through any commercial or other form of public communication. However, certain restrictions still apply. To the extent that testimonials regarding a physician's skill or quality of professional services from patients who do not have a comprehensive access to the physician's practice are often misleading, such endorsements are not permitted. Ethical obligations to share medical knowledge and skills make it improbable that a physician is likely to have unique skills or equipment. An advertisement that makes such a claim would be questioned. However, such a claim may be justifiable in a restricted geographic area. Claims regarding competence and quality of care supported by objective data are permissible.

Information about doctors, their qualifications, fees, and services, they provide is of obvious value to the community. The AMA's guidelines underscore this point:

- The AMA believes that a doctor's reputation and capacity to increase their practice should be based on good medical practice and appropriate provision of information about the medical services they offer. The AMA believes that all such information should (1) be demonstrably true in all respects; (2) not be misleading, vulgar, or sensational; (3) seek to maintain the decorum and dignity of the profession; (4) not contain any testimonial or endorsement of clinical skills; (5) not claim that one doctor is superior to others nor contain endorsements for any particular doctor; and (6) avoid aggressive forms of competitive persuasion, such as those that prevail in commerce and industry.
- *In accordance with the general guidelines detailed above, the chief purpose of any advertisement for a doctor's services should be to present information that is reasonably needed by any patient to make an informed decision about the appropriateness and availability of the medical services offered.*

In summary, undoubtedly advertising by doctors has been traditionally considered to be derogatory to the medical profession. However, times have changed and we need to discard outdated concepts and revise our statutes and guidelines in sync with modern times. With the runaway advances in information technology, we need to redefine ethicality pertaining to advertising and marketing in the healthcare setting.

Instead of "no advertisements allowed" (which in any case is being flouted with immunity), it should be "only ethical advertising allowed". Ethical advertising should be unambiguously defined, an Ethical Advertising Board should be created and quick, visible, and strict action should be taken against those violating the guidelines.

Vague and unclear directions on the issue can do no good as they are followed more in the breach.

SUGGESTED READING

1. Harlow AD. 7 Dangerous Legal Issues to avoid in Doctor Advertising. [online] Available from: https://www.healthcaresuccess.com/blog/doctor-marketing/dangerous-legal-issues.html [Accessed December, 2018].
2. Jones JW, McCullough LB. Is medical advertising always unethical, or does it just seem to be? J Vasc Surg. 2015;61(6):1635-6.
3. Medical Council of India. INDIAN MEDICAL COUNCIL (Professional Conduct, Etiquette and Ethics) Regulations, 2002 (AMENDED UP TO 8th OCTOBER 2016). [online] Available from: https://www.mciindia.org/documents/rulesAndRegulations/Ethics%20Regulations-2002.pdf [Accessed December, 2018].
4. Meira E. (20017). The ethics of healthcare advertising. [online] Available from: https://thesciencept.com/ethics-of-healthcare-advertising/ [Accessed December, 2018].
5. PANDYA, Sunil K. Advertising remains unethical even in the digital age. Indian Journal of Medical Ethics, [S.l.], v. 9, n. 1, p. 15, nov. 2016. ISSN 0975-5691.
6. Schenker Y, Arnold RM, London AJ. The ethics of advertising for healthcare services, Am J Bioeth. 2014;14(3):34-43.

CHAPTER 12

Quackery

Putta Srinivas*, Rajesh Buddhadev*

"Quackery is the legitimate offspring of ignorance and can only be abridged by elevating the standards of medicine and disseminating a correct public statement."
—**Charles K Winston and Paul E Eve (1851)**

KEY OBJECTIVES

- Definition of Quackery
- Brief history
- Types of quacks
- Charlatans
- Cranks
- Health hucksters
- Medical quackery
- Nutritional quackery
- Device quackery
- Why quacks are succeeding and flourishing?
- Health quackery hazards
  - Direct health hazard:
  - Indirect health hazards
  - Economic hazards
- Dermatology and quackery
- Present legal status of dealing with quackery
- Legal references
- Fighting against quackery
  - Prevention of quackery
  - law enforcement
- Unauthorized and unqualified hair and cosmetology centers
- Unauthorized and illegal diplomas/degrees
- Factories awarding unauthorized and illegal diplomas in India
- Quackery—in hair transplantation
- Google, facebook, and YouTube medical quackery
- Amazon medical quackery

---

* Members of IADVL Taskforce against Quackery (ITAQ)

DEFINITION

Health quackery is defined as the promotion and commercialization of unproven and often dangerous health products and procedures.[1]

BRIEF HISTORY

Quackery refers to unproven or fraudulent medical practices, often through the sale or application of "quack medicines". The word "quack" derives from the archaic Dutch word "quacksalver", meaning "boaster who applies a salve". A closely associated German word, "Quacksalver", means "questionable salesperson". In the middle ages the word quack meant "shouting". The quacksalvers sold their wares on the market shouting in a loud voice.[2]

Quack medicines were especially prevalent in the British Empire for centuries, including in the American colonies. Following the American Revolution and the War of 1812, American products began to dominate the domestic market. The American term for quack medicine was "snake oil", a reference to sales pitches in which the sometimes outrageous claims of medicinal successes.

The snake oil was used for inflammation. Original Chinese snake was made with the fat from Chinese water snakes. However, the snake oil marketed in US in nearly contains mineral oil, beef fat, red pepper, and turpentine but no snake oil. Cocaine was used as local anesthetic agent, during dental surgeries. Opiates were used for crying babies to put them to sleep.[2]

In 1800, the quackery at its best of exploitation was prescribing tapeworm eggs for reduction of obesity, with the claim that one can eat whatever they like and then consume tapeworm eggs and tapeworms, will eat away whatever one has eaten. But the results were not as promised, as the tapeworm eggs supplied through mail were often dead on arrival. US government has enacted Pure Food and Drug Act of 1906 and sale snake oil was banned. With the introduction of in 1914 the Harrison Narcotics Act, the sale of cocaine drops and opiates was banned.

TYPES OF QUACKS

Quacks can be categorized in to three types: (1) charlatans, (2) cranks, and (3) health hucksters.[3]

Charlatans

"One who is not what he or she claims to be."[4] Charlatans are deliberate fakers and they exploit people without feeling guilty. They want and do whatever they like, and they are blind to the conscience and totally indifferent to feelings of others. They are health predators, who charm, manipulate ruthlessly go ahead with their deception leaving a trail of broken hearts, shattered expectations, and empty wallets.[3]

Cranks

They are delusional individuals who sincerely believe in themselves and their nostrums. However, they likely to be honest and they exhibit generosity and selflessness. They defend themselves blindly and vehemently and they are often paranoid and counter scientific criticism as persecution done with vengeance. Usually charlatans are cautious and limit their claims and they try to escape from law and regulations, on the contrary cranks do not accept their limitations and are more dangerous to society.[3]

Health Hucksters

They are business persons and use marketing techniques to promote their secret remedies without any scientific evidence of efficacy and safety, which any responsible business person or health professional will do. They idealize entrepreneurialism and exploit the potential offered by public interest in areas which modern science provides slow and long-term and sometimes limited solutions for which general public feel difficult to follow, like reducing obesity, improving color and complexion, etc.

They do not have any ethics and on the other hand they expect buyers to be aware "caveat emptor" (meaning thereby "without a warranty, the buyer must take the risk"). *"They operate with a principle that if people are not aware and intelligent enough to identify useless health remedies they are foolish enough to survive in modern economic society which is called as social Darwinism"*. Vigorous business promotion and showmanship are hallmarks of health hucksters and they continuously use celebrities like movie stars, models, sportsman, and women who are usually worshipped by common people to promote their health remedies/drugs. Presently, it is there in almost all sectors of life, but unfortunately more so in dermatology field![3]

Quackery can be also classified as medical quackery, nutrition quackery, and device quackery.

Medical Quackery

It pertains to the malpractice in the medical profession where pseudo doctors, claim to be experts and competent in treating diseases. Their intention is always to make profit at the expense of deceiving people; they capitalize on the hope, ignorance, and fear of people.

Nutritional Quackery

Any form of fake or unclassified claims of nutritional value or impact. Some of the most popular and profitable hoaxes that goes in the form of dietary supplements, herbal remedies, weight loss products, energy boosters, and which do not have any scientific evidence. More often than not, these products become detrimental to one's health, ironic from what its label tells.

Device Quackery

It pertains to the claims or information about the products that are "too good to be true". They deceive the customers by exaggerating about the quality, efficiency, and try to justify the cost or lower its price along with quality.

WHY QUACKS ARE SUCCEEDING AND FLOURISHING?

It was expected that as the medical sciences progressed, as many diseases became curable and quality of health of people improved remarkably as reflected by increase of life expectancy, decrease of infant mortality rate (IMR) and maternal mortality ratio (MMR), will lead to gradual elimination of quackery. But surprisingly it is not so and on the contrary, quackery is booming!

In spite of advanced state of medical science, many people with health problems turn to dubious methods. Faced with the prospect of chronic suffering, deformity, or death, many individuals are tempted to try anything that offers relief or hope. The terminally ill, the elderly, and various cultural minorities are especially vulnerable to health frauds and quackery. Many intelligent and well-educated individuals resort to worthless methods procedures with the belief that anything is better than nothing.[5]

The success and survival of quackery has multiple reasons and composite in nature. There are psychological, sociocultural, educational, and economic factors.[6]

- Quacks listens, spare more time, show concerns with sympathy, take care and establish, rapport and cordial relationship which is their trump card, however, it may not be true every time and many a times they show rigid attitude also when asked a question or querry.[7]
- Various studies have raveled that whenever humans are not able to get benefits of science and technology, they revert and look towards quacks. Quacks exploit the dimension that science and modern medicine cannot.
- Appeal of the quack is not unlike that of gambler, the quack offers a *"get well quick"* temptation akin to the gamblers inducement to *"get rich quick"*.[6]
- *Lack of suspicion*: Many a times people believe that if something is printed or broadcast, it must be true or otherwise its publication or broadcast would not be allowed and are attracted by promises of quick, painless, or drugless solutions to their problems.[5] The mass media both print and electronic media provide much false and misleading information in advertisements, news reports, feature articles, and books, and on radio and television programs. News reports are often sensationalized, stimulating false hopes, and by creating fear psychosis by misleading and false propaganda. The most unfortunate aspect is that the producers of print and electronic media escape from responsibility by putting a disclaimer and also claim that they are providing entertainment and have no ethical duty to check the claims. In India there is a need of more stringent advertisement rules and regulations and strict penalty, which is not there unfortunately.
- *Desperation*: Whenever people faced with a serious health problem or beauty-related issues that doctors cannot solve, become desperate enough to try almost anything that arouses hope. Many victims of cancer, arthritis, multiple sclerosis, and acquired immunodeficiency syndrome (AIDS) are vulnerable in this way. Some squander their life's savings searching for a "cure". Many people suffer from chronic aches, pains, or other discomforts for which medicine cannot offer clear-cut diagnoses or effective treatment. The more persistent the condition, the more susceptible the sufferer may be to promises of a "cure". Fears of social unacceptability or growing old wrinkles, loss of hair and sensory acuity, and decreased sexual potency can also lead people astray.
- *Alienation*: Some people have deep antagonism toward scientific medicine, but are attracted to methods represented as "natural" or otherwise unconventional. They may also harbor extreme distrust of the medical profession, the food industry, drug companies, and Government agencies.[5]

HEALTH QUACKERY HAZARDS

There are three categories:
1. *Direct health hazard*: These are harmful effects of using unsafe and unscientific medicines.
2. *Indirect health hazards*: These are not directly due to the medicines, as they have no proven clinically proven therapeutic value, but they cause severe and sometimes irreparable indirect damage, like stoppage modern medicines by patients suffering from diabetes, hypertension or cancer patients. "Penelope Dingle" incident in Australia *is classical example of indirect health hazard.*

"Penelope Dingle Incident in Australia"
Penelope Dingle was an Australian woman, 45 years old, died of colorectal cancer on 25th August 2005. She was treated by homeopath Francine Scrayen with homeopathy alone and forbade Penelope to take even pain killers for her extremely painful condition. Penelope at last sought medical help, but by then it was far too late.

3. *Economic hazards*: Usage of ineffective and useless medicines or procedures may not cause any direct damage, however, in the process it will have wastage of hard earned of the individuals but also overall public expenditure on health related issues.

DERMATOLOGY AND QUACKERY

Quackery in treatment of skin diseases is not new and quackery has no boundaries. The quackery of treatment of skin diseases became that much easier as it is accessible directly and anything and everything can be blindly applied basing on assumptions and imaginations.

With advances in medical science and technology, lasers, acne scar/cosmetic surgeries, chemical peels, hair transplant surgeries led to development of different subspecialty, especially dermatosurgery, aesthetic medicine, and medical cosmetology. There is an enormous increase in awareness about beauty, appearance, and to look young in all sections of society and among all age groups. Unfortunately there are many grey areas in statutory regulations which are not updated this has led to mushrooming of many chain of cosmetology centers, aesthetic centers, and hair transplant centers.

Quacks and quackery in relation to dermatology can be divided in to six basic categories as follows:

1. *Quacks with no qualification whatsoever*: Who sees, prescribes allopathic medicines, and performs procedures which only a qualified dermatologist can do it.
   - Beauty parlors/salons/who are not qualified as per laws to treat any medical skin conditions without knowledge of any skin path physiology which can cause certain skin changes and still they treat it with various peels/lasers, etc. and may end up with short- or long-term complications.
   - In many institution or so called skin clinics under the name of a doctor unqualified staff/technicians who performs certain aesthetic procedures without direct supervision of a qualified dermatologist is another form of quackery.

2. Practitioners of Indian medicine Ayurveda, Yoga and Naturopathy Unani, Siddha Homeopathy, commonly called AYUSH, who are not qualified to practice modern medicine (allopathy), but are practicing modern medicine in dermatology.

3. Practitioners of so called integrated medicine, alternative system of medicine, electrohomeopathy, indo allopathy, etc. terms which do not exist in any act.

4. *Those dermatologists themselves, who trains*: Practitioners of Indian medicine (*Ayurveda, Siddha, Tibb,* and *Unani*), Homeopathy, Naturopathy, commonly called AYUSH, who are not qualified to practice modern medicine (allopathy), beauticians and salon workers and provides them certificate of training. These type of practice, in turn produces more quacks and they use these certificates as their qualifications.

5. *Training of quacks by eminent dermatologists and certain training institutions—those dermatologists themselves, who trains*: Dentists, gynecologists, and other specialists (with PG diploma/degree)

provides them certificate of training. These type of practice, in turn produces more quacks and they use these certificates as their qualifications.
6. *Pharmacist and chemist-based quackery*: A big issue in India today: Why? As they:
   - Dispense by themselves: Schedule H/H1 medicines without a genuine prescription by a qualified allopathic practitioners
   - Redispense by themselves without a fresh prescription, which in long run harms the skin and produces harmful adverse/side effects also.
   - Remember, a prescription is not only advice for patient's recovery, but it also is a legitimate order for the sale of controlled drugs and pharmaceutical product; thereby functions as a regulatory tool for consumption of pharmaceutical products at retail level.

There is acute lack of awareness amongst state governments, the legislature(s), judiciary, and even doctors themselves regarding threat to nation's health from quackery and about nonentitlement of practitioners of Indian medicine who are practicing modern medicine.

Having *not* succeeded to take advantage of ambiguity in State Medical Acts and Drugs and Cosmetics Act and rules some practitioners of *Ayurveda, Siddha, Unani* and *Tibb*, commonly called AYUSH, have concocted a fake name like integrated medicine and practice modern medicine (allopathy) under its grab. The Government has clarified that they have not recognized integrated system of medicine and currently there is no proposal to develop integrated system of medicine by Government of India. Even Central Council of Indian Medicine (CCIM) in their letter dated 5-12-2008 has announced that the term "Integrated System of Medicine" has not been defined in their Act and it is not one of the approved systems of medicine in India. The practitioners of Integrated System of Medicine are quacks and should be treated alike them.

Then there is a variety of fake medical degrees like electrohomeopathy, indo allopathy, etc. who call themselves alternative system of medicine and under this guise practice modern medicine. Alternative system of medicine is not recognized by law. Since they are a danger to the nation, there is a need to take action against such quacks wherever we find them. In fact, practitioners of *Ayurveda, Siddha, Unani,* and *Tibb* keep jumping from their original system of medicine to integrated or alternative system of medicine just to keep practicing modern medicine under different façade. If required, they are not averse to concoct new system of medicine just to avoid detection.

PRESENT LEGAL STATUS OF DEALING WITH QUACKERY

- *Beauty clinics*: Quack is an unqualified person. He/she cannot practice modern scientific medicine. As per section 15(2) of Indian Medical Council (IMC) Act, 1956, and clause 1.1.3 of IMC, (Professional Conduct, Etiquette, and Ethics) Regulations 2002, an unqualified person, i.e. quack cannot practice modern medicine.
- Doctors with BHMS-homeopathy BAMS-ayurvedic, and BUMS-Unani.

Nowadays, it is very common that many homeopathic doctors with BHMS, ayurvedic doctors with BAMS and Unani doctors with BUMS, claiming as skin specialists' and dermatologists, treating and prescribing allopathic drugs for skin diseases. Some of them are getting trained by bogus illegal institutions and with fake certificates are claiming themselves as dermatologists, cosmetologists and aestheticians, trichologists, etc.

Now it is well settled in law that prescribing allopathic medicines by homeopaths, ayurvedic, and Unani doctors are unlawful and amounts negligent act.[8-22]

Legal References

Honorable Supreme Court of India, in the case of Poonam Verma versus Ashwin Patel and also in case of Dr Mukhtiar Chand versus State of Punjab, held that:

"The right to practice modern scientific medicine (allopathic medicine) or Indian system of medicine cannot be based on the provisions of drug rules and declarations made there under by State Governments. Indeed the right to practice a system of medicine is derived from the Act under which a medical practitioner is registered."

In pursuance of the above judgments "a person having obtained qualification in particular system of medicine can practice medicine in that system of medicine only. If a person having qualification in alternative medicine or ayurvedic medicine or homeopathy or Unani and found practicing modern medicine, he/she is liable for disciplinary action by the authorities of AYUSH. If a person having qualification in other system of medicine and prescribing drugs of modern medicine, he/she is liable for prosecution as per the provisions contained in Drugs Act/Drugs Rules.

Government of India has issued Government Notification vide Memo No. 8914/L2/97-1 dated, 17-3-1997, implementing the Supreme Court judgment in Poonam Verma versus Dr Ashwin Patel, the judgment of Honorable Supreme Court in Dr Mukhtiar Chand and Others versus State of Punjab and others.

Quack

Quack is an unqualified person. He/she cannot practice modern scientific medicine. As per Section 15(2) of IMC Act, 1956 read with clause 1.1.3 of IMC Regulations, an unqualified person, i.e. quack cannot practice modern medicine. In case a quack is found practicing modern medicine, police complaint shall be given and the procedure laid down in police manual shall be followed. An aggrieved/affected person may file a criminal complaint before competent magistrate. The procedure laid down in section 200 Criminal Procedure Code (CrPC) shall be followed.

- The State Government's authorities have the power to control or abolish or eradicate the quackery/unethical/unregistered/unauthorized modern medicine practice. The concerned state authorities are: (1) The District Collector, being the District Magistrate. (2) The Superintendent of Police/Deputy Superintendents of Police of the concerned district/subdivision. In the case of cities, the Commissioners of Police. (3) The District Medical and Health Officers of the district concerned as per the provisions contained.
- There are several Central/State Acts, like Indian Medical Degrees Act, 1916, IMC Act, 1956, several notifications of Medical Council of India (MCI) and Notification of State Government in the year 1997.
- State Medical Councils have to take appropriate action against quacks/unqualified persons, whenever complaints have been received. State Medical Council Law has to address letters to the police authorities and District Medical and Health Officers to take action as per law.
- The authorities concerned in the districts to eradicate or control quackery are concerned police authorities or the District Medical and Health Officers.

FIGHTING AGAINST QUACKERY[1]

Professional bodies like concerned associations, e.g. IADVL (Indian Association of Dermatologists, Venereologists and Leprologists) shall actively oppose quackery and fraudulent medical practices. Dermatologists should educate patients and their attendants. They should also disseminate this information by educating the people and through print and electronic media.

Prevention of quackery—to deal with quackery, we have to focus attention on multiple factors responsible for its existence.

- First is to educate the people about the accurate factual information about the health and specific conditions, including the areas where people are more concerned like, beauty, color improvement, hair fall, baldness, lasers, chemical peels, aesthetics, etc. Quacks are always agile, they sense quickly and rush to exploit the people's real concerns. We shall also make aware the real facts about the false and extravagant claims of quacks. These educational and awareness programs will tackle the aspect of "ignorance" which is one of the major factor for survival of quackery.
- Second factor is emotional aspect, which makes the patient feels that "something is better than nothing" and gets attracted towards quacks. These types of patients with emotional immaturities and variations, need, extra degree of support, care, sparing extra time, and thorough and meaning full discussion with patients and attendants will go a long way in preventing them from getting attracted by quackery.
- Dermatology and all subspecialty services should reach all the areas particularly semi-urban and rural and tribal areas to meet the needs of people and very crucial to reduce the public receptivity to quackery.[6] There are about ten thousand dermatologists in our country for a population of 1.3 crores. There is a dire need to interact and conduct awareness programs not only to general practitioners but also to sister medical organizations, Indian Medical Association (IMA), associations of other specialties and super specialties, nurses, and paramedical associations.
- *Law enforcement*: Vigilance and proactive approach of medical associations and creation of special task force groups to tackle the menace of quackery and approach statutory authorities for effective law enforcement.

Unauthorized and Unqualified Hair and Cosmetology Centers

In the last two decades innumerable numbers of cosmetic clinics/centers have come up in all major metros and cities, just to exploit the people's desires, expectations particularly with regard to "beauty and appearance". If we go through, especially Sunday edition of any newspaper of any language we will find innumerable advertisements of these cosmetology or beauty centers with attractive catchy titles. But if we check carefully, they will not mention about the names and qualifications of experts who are doing the cosmetic/aesthetic procedures. They do not engage the services of either dermatologists or plastic surgeons, who are the actual, qualified to perform all these procedures.

Typically they offer discounts and festival offers and sometimes bumper offers of cars, two-wheelers, and TV's total worth of ₹ 1,000,000–1,500,000 for booking and making initial payments.

Most of them take permission from municipal authorities for running a salon, but later gradually start doing cosmetic procedures and sometimes surgeries, without obtaining any permission or license from health authorities.

Court Orders "Cosmetic Clinic" to Pay ₹ 100,000 Compensation plus Refund of ₹ 95,000 and Additional ₹ 20,000 toward Cost of Litigation

Brief facts of the case: In 2015 one consumer resident of Pernem in the state of Goa, known diabetic, approached a cosmetic clinic for transplantation of 6,000 strands of hair for ₹ 140,000. He developed, after first session of transplant of 500 hair, headache, giddiness, and diarrhea and having paid the full amount, he underwent second session but subsequently developed boils in the head and unsteadiness of his legs.

He approached the consumer forum and forum held that there was complete negligence and gross deficiency of service. The entire conduct of the clinic in the matter so far has been *totally unethical, unprofessional, highly casual and unconcerned*, and regardless towards complaint and his health the quorum stated, in its order.

The forum has directed looks cosmetics clinical in Calangute to pay a compensation of ₹ 100,000 for harming a consumer with "illegal activities of hair transplant".

The quorum also observed that the opposite parties *did not have a license to operate the Looks Health Services. The directorate of health services informed that the clinic has not taken any license to operate under the Goa Medical Practitioner's Act, 2004 and Rules 2011, as a health clinic.*

"Based on the above three letters from the Food and Drug Administration (FDA), directorate of health services from Panaji, Campla, and from the letter of the primary health center, Candolim, it is clear that the *Opposite Party No. 2 Mrs Leema George, who is the incharge of Opposite Party No. 1, that is the Looks Cosmetic Clinic, is doing illegal business and cheating people and making wrongful gains for herself at the cost of the clients who come to her Looks Cosmetic Clinic also known as Looks Health Services,*" the order stated.[23]

Unauthorized and Illegal Diplomas/Degrees

We find many MBBS, BDS, and other doctors claiming as dermatologists, cosmetologist, aesthetician, etc. by obtaining attending a course of few days to few months and being awarded by these diplomas and degrees.

Examples:
- PGDCC: Postgraduate Diploma in Clinical Cosmetology given by ILAMED
- PGMT: Postgraduate Diploma in Medical Trichology given by ILAMED
- PGDCC: Postgraduate Diploma in Clinical Cosmetology given—Germany
- Diploma in Practical Dermatology
- MSc Clinical Dermatology
- MSc Dermatology Skills and Treatment, University of Hertfordshire
- Masters in Clinical Dermatology
- Diploma in Clinical Dermatology (UK).

Fellowships:
1. Advanced Fellowship in Cosmetic Dermatology, Mahatma Gandhi University, Jaipur

Unfortunately sometimes reputed medical journals also print advertisements endorsing unrecognized postgraduate diplomas, fellowship, and certificate courses of dermatology, cosmetology, and aesthetics conducted by private institutions and hospitals for MBBS/BDS and other ineligible doctors.

Various judgments of Indian Courts, make it amply clear that any postgraduate medical course conducted under any title (diploma, postgraduate diploma, certificate, fellowship, etc.) become illegal unless it is recognized by MCI and/or the central government.

According to the MCI ethics code regulation 7.20, a physician should not claim to be a specialist unless he/she has a special qualification in that branch. Practicing a specialty, without having a qualification in that branch, amounts to flouting regulation 7.20 of the ethics code.

In 2008, the Madras High Court quashed *a State Government Order (GO) which had allowed a certificate course in diabetology without the prior permission of MCI.*

The judges reasoned that the executive power of every state should be exercised ensuring compliance with the laws made by parliament and any existing law applied in the state. *Therefore, the GO was ruled unconstitutional and preventable in view of Entry 66 of List I of the constitution. The judges clearly stated that no course in medical education by any name could be started without the permission of MCI and the Central Government.*

Factories Awarding Unauthorized and Illegal Diplomas in India

There are many unauthorized and illegal certificates of diploma, degree or fellowship awarded by private and non-MCI recognized institutions like, ILAMED, LEMED, Cosmetica India Academy, and Facial Aesthetics in Rajasthan.

Legal Status

In 2011, the Madras High Court declared 11 postgraduate diploma courses conducted by Tamil Nadu, Dr MGR University as illegal since they were being conducted without the prior approval of MCI or the central government. Justice N Paul Vasantkumar said *"The University is not empowered to grant permission to any institution or medical college to conduct any PG diploma course in medical science without prior approval of the MCI Act, 1956".* The judge also pointed out that according to the MCI ethics code regulations, 2002, a physician is supposed to suffix only recognized qualifications. *The Honorable Judge said that "Without such recognition, if any person is allowed to suffix PG diploma in medical sciences along with MBBS degree, the general public will definitely get an impression that the physician is a specialist. Special status can be claimed by any physician only after getting an approved PG diploma and not half-baked diploma courses offered by the university".*

So, the legal status of these unauthorized institutions, ILAMED, LEMED, etc. is crystal clear and well-settled in law that they are not only completely unauthorized but also illegal.

Quackery—In Hair Transplantation

Throughout India there are multiple hair transplantation centers established and some have chain of centers and in majority of them hair transplantation is not done by dermatologists or plastic surgeons, who are the actual eligible experts, but unfortunately by MBBS, BDS, nonallopathic doctors, and sometimes by so called technicians. They take permission from municipal authorities for hair saloon services, but gradually start doing hair transplantation surgeries also, for which permission from health authorities is mandatory.

Death of a Final-year Medico in Chennai in June 2016 after Hair Transplantation

A final year medical student in Chennai, 22-year-old Santosh was shy of his slight baldness and decided to go for a hair transplant procedure last month. But 2 days after the surgery, he was dead. The MBBS doctor, the doctor at Advanced Robotic Hair Transplantation Center who performed the procedure, was not a surgeon equipped with either a dermatology or plastic surgery degree—a basic qualification in the field. Moreover, the Dr Hariprasad Kasturi, the anesthetist was not present throughout the procedure after administering anesthesia—another basic requirement ignored. Later, when the parents lodged complaint and on verification by authorities, it was found that, the hair transplant center Advanced Robotic Hair Transplantation Center had *obtained a license only to run a hair salon which too expired two months* before. Although they had qualified doctors one of who was trained in China, there was no infrastructure to tackle any complication. The center has no sterile place or an operation theatre. The authorities have sealed the center. The drug controller has recovered a huge stock of medicines kept without license.

The health department is recommended using a tough law to regulate such centers dealing with surgical procedures including hair and wart removal, often masquerading as beauty parlors, spas, and hair treatment centers.

Later Tamil Nadu Medical Council has acted firmly and an anesthetist, has been barred from practice for 6 months. an MBBS doctor, an MBBS graduate from a Chinese university, has been barred for a year.

Google, Facebook, and YouTube Medical Quackery

The new dimension of medical quackery is spread of inaccurate, unscientific, and deliberately false content at high speed and making even educated to believe them, unsuspectingly (Goebbels' propaganda). If one goes into YouTube and searches for treatment of melasma, one gets the wide range of suggestions from lemon face pack, turmeric, tomato, papaya face packs to lasers, and promoted and recommenced by self-styled experts from nonmedical individuals to all varieties of nonallopathic doctors. The most shocking is, for dog bite it is well-established scientifically that active and passive immunization as well as wound treatment are gold standards throughout the world, but treatment recommendations in YouTube consists of a range of treatments from banana, garlic, homeopathy, ayurvedic to lasers also.

The consequences of such treatments will be disastrous to the individuals and society. In South Africa, the country's President in the late 1990s and 2000, came to believe that AIDS is nonexistent and a hoax and Government policies were framed accordingly, which has led to an estimated, more than 330,000 deaths as per the researchers.[24]

Amazon Medical Quackery

Quacks are always agile and take advantage of patient's eagerness.[25] Amazon websites are hawking a universe of dangerous, pseudoscience health products—to cure human immunodeficiency virus (HIV) infection to bleach enemas for autism.

That is according to an investigation by *UK's Sun newspaper*, which accuses, the main internet giant of profiting off people's desperation and illness by selling unproven, snake-oil products.

If one looks for treatment of acne and melasma in Amazon, you will find a range of products including unscientific and unproven products from attractive cosmetic products to "do yourself" physical modalities and instruments.

The main reason why Amazon sells such products is that though these products are recommended and promoted for medical purpose, but technically fall in the category of "dietary supplements" or "cosmetics" which are very loosely regulated by FDA or our Indian regulatory authorities.[26]

SUMMARY WITH KEY MESSAGES AND PEARLS

- Medical Quackery is malpractice in the medical profession where pseudo doctors, claim to be experts and competent in treating diseases.
- Quacks always try to make profit at the expense of deceiving people; they capitalize on the hope, ignorance, and fear of people.
- Health quackery hazards are direct health hazards, Indirect health hazards and Economic hazards.
- Quackery in Dermatology became much easier as skin is accessible directly and anything and everything can be blindly applied basing on assumptions and imaginations.
- In a Land mark judgments, Honorable Supreme Court of India, in the case of Poonam Verma versus Ashwin Patel and also in case of Dr Mukhtiar Chand versus State of Punjab, has given judgment that "A person having obtained qualification in particular system of medicine can practice medicine in that system of medicine only. If a person having qualification in alternative medicine or ayurvedic medicine or homeopathy or Unani and found practicing modern medicine, he/she is liable for disciplinary action
- Government of India has issued Government Notification vide Memo No. 8914/L2/97-1 dated, 17-3-1997, implementing the Supreme Court judgment in Poonam Verma versus Dr Ashwin Patel.
- As per Section 15(2) of IMC Act, 1956 read with clause 1.1.3 of IMC Regulations, an unqualified person, i.e. quack cannot practice modern medicine.
- The State Government's authorities have the power to control or abolish or eradicate the quackery/ unethical/unregistered/ unauthorized modern medicine practice. The concerned state authorities are: (1) The District Collector, being the District Magistrate. (2) The Superintendent of Police/Deputy Superintendents of Police of the concerned district/subdivision. In the case of cities, the Commissioners of Police. (3) The District Medical and Health Officers of the district concerned as per the provisions contained.
- Types of Quacks and quackery
  - Quacks with no qualification whatsoever
  - Practitioners of India medicine Ayurveda, Yoga, Naturopathy, Unani, Siddha and Homeopathy, commonly called AYUSH, who are not qualified to practice modern medicine (allopathy), but are practicing modern medicine in dermatology.
  - Certain dermatologists themselves, are training practitioners of Indian medicine with qualifications of BHMS, BAMS, BUMS.BYNS which is not only un-ethical but illegal.
  - Training of quacks by certain unauthorized, unrecognized and illegal training institutions training Dentists, gynecologists, and other specialists in dermatosurgical procedures.
- **Prevention of quackery**
- Educate the people about the accurate factual information about the health and specific conditions
- Patients with emotional immaturities and variations, need extra degree of support, care, sparing extra time and thorough and meaningful discussion with patients and attendants
- Dermatology and all subspecialty services should reach all the areas particularly semiurban and rural and tribal areas to meet the needs of people and very crucial to reduce the public receptivity to quackery
- Law enforcement-Vigilance and proactive approach of medical associations and creation of special task force groups to tackle the menace of quackery and approach statutory authorities for effective law enforcement.

- **Legal status of Unauthorized and unqualified hair and Cosmetology centers.** The Consumer forum of Goa state has given judgment that Hair and Cosmetology centers are doing illegal business and cheating people and making wrongful gains for herself at the cost of the clients
- **Legal status of Unauthorized and illegal Diplomas/Degrees.** Various Judgments of Indian Courts, make it amply clear that any postgraduate medical course conducted under any title (diploma, postgraduate diploma, certificate, fellowship, etc.) become illegal unless it is recognized by MCI and/or the Central Government
- **Legal status of centers awarding Unauthorized and illegal Diplomas in India.** There are many unauthorized and illegal certificates of diploma, degree or Fellowship are awarded by private and Non-MCI recognized institutions like, ILAMED, LEMED, Cosmetic India Academy, Facial Aesthetics in Rajasthan. In 2011, the Madras High Court declared 11 postgraduate diploma courses conducted by Tamil Nadu Dr. MGR University as illegal since they were being conducted without the prior approval of MCI or the central government. Justice N Paul Vasantkumar said "The University is not empowered to grant permission to any institution or medical college to conduct any PG diploma course in medical science without prior approval of the Medical Council of India Act, 1956."
- **Legal status—Hair Transplantation**
Death of a final year medico in Chennai in June 2016 after Hair transplantation and the doctor at ARHT Transplant center who performed the procedure, was not a surgeon equipped with either a dermatology or plastic surgery degree—a basic qualification in the field and later Tamil Nadu Medical Council has acted firmly and, Dr Hariprasad Kasturi, an anesthetist, has been barred from practice for six months. An MBBS graduate from a Chinese university, has been barred for a year".

REFERENCES

1. American College of Physicians. Health quackery. Philadelphia, PA: American College of Physicians; 1989.
2. Quackery, Workman Publishing. Credit: available from https://www.sciencefriday.com/segments/medical-cures-that-did-more-harm-than-good/ [Accessed December 2018].
3. NCAHF (2001). Some notes on Quackery. [online] Available from: https://www.ncahf.org/articles/o-r/quackery.html [Accessed December 2018].
4. Stanford Libraries. Webster's II New Riverside University Dictionary. Boston, MA: Riverside Pub. Co.; 1984.
5. Quackwatch (2005). Vulnerability to Quackery. [online] Available from: https://www.quackwatch.org/01QuackeryRelatedTopics/quackvul.html [Accessed December 2018].
6. Bernard NW. Why people become the victims of medical quackery. Am J Public Health Nations Health. 1965;55(8):1142-7.
7. Datta R. The World of Quacks: A parallel Health Care system in Rural West Bengal. IOSR J Human Soc Sci. 2013;14(2):44-53.
8. Poonam verma vs. Ashwin Patel & Ors. 1996 AIR 2111, 1996 SCC (4) 332.
9. Dr Mukhtiar Chand & Ors vs. The State of Punjab & Ors. 1998
10. Martin F D' Souza vs. Mohd. Ishfaq. 2009
11. Shiva Kumar Gautham (Dr) vs Alima. 2006
12. Kanaiyalal Ramanlal Trivedi vs Dr Satyanarayan Vishwakarma. 1997
13. Jalaluddin Khan (Dr) vs. India Sen Verma 2009 (4) CPJ 89: 2009 (3) CPR 208 NCDRC
14. SN Namboodri (Dr) vs Haneeefa, 1998 CPJ 389 (Ker.SCDRC)
15. Khairaiti Lal vs Kewal Krishna,1998 (1) CPJ 181: 1998 (1) CLT 637: 1998 (1) CPC 153 (Punj. SCDRC).
16. 16. Manpreet Kaur vs Veena Ghumber (Dr) 2005 (2) CPJ 63: 2005 (1) CPR 656 (Punj SCDRC).
17. Sher Singh (Dr) vs Billu Khan, 2007 (4) CPJ 295: 2008 (1) CPR 45 (NCDRC).
18. Arun Dewangan (Dr) vs Madhu (Preti Chandei) 2009 (2) CPJ 315: 2009 (2) CPR 389 (NCDRC).
19. RR Singh AVV (Bom) vs Pratibha P Gamre, 2012 (2) CPJ 534 (NCDRC).
20. Alok Kumar (Dr) vs Devlal, 2013 (4) CPJ 31 (NCDRC).
21. PN Thakur (Prof) vs Hans Charitable Hospital, 2007 (3) CPJ 340: 2007 (3) CPR 157 (NCDRC).

22. Azizul Haq Khan (Dr @ Lallan) vs Shyamapati 2009 (2) CPR 61: 2009 (2) CPJ 49 (NCDRC).
23. The Times of India 5th August 2017.
24. UNDARK (2018). Social media algorithms help charlatans spread autism cures, vaccine disinformation, and AIDS denialism through online videos. Who's really to blame? [online] Available from https://undark.org/article/aids-denialism-quackery-facebook-youtube/ [Accessed December 2018].
25. Yuong JH. American Health Quackery: Collected Essays of James Harvey Young. Princeton, United States: Princeton University Press; 1972.
26. Julia Belluz@juliaoftorontojulia.belluz@voxmedia.com

CHAPTER 13

Out-of-Court Settlement: Why, When, and How

Venkataram Mysore, Subodh Premanand Sirur, Satish Bhat, KHS Rao

INTRODUCTION

It is generally accepted that medicolegal cases have increased several folds over the last few years. Generally, a medical practitioner is taken by surprise and does not know how to react, when the notice hits him/her. Every practitioner should expect a medicolegal case at some point and be prepared, if it indeed happens. This is particularly so in the prevailing situation in India, where healers are often treated as predators. It can be said that, in the authors' opinion, situation changed drastically, after a TV reality show made an issue out of an exaggerated of a renal transplant recipient, and after a huge compensation of several crores in a case of toxic epidermal necrolysis leading to death of a therapist practicing abroad who was a doctor's wife.

WARNING SIGNS OF A MEDICOLEGAL SITUATION

The most important part of being prepared is to recognize a potential medicolegal case early.

Here are some tips to recognize a potential legal situation:
- When something has gone adverse in a case, results are not as anticipated or a complication has happened.
- Patient is unhappy either for above reasons or over payment issues.
- Relatives argue in reception over different issues.
- Request for a patient's records. This should not be ignored; patient records cannot be refused, but should be handed over only to a patient or an authorized person. An acknowledgement is to be taken for having received the documents. Whatever documents are requested should be handed over, without any modification.
- Doctor bashing happens in the media: whether conventional (print/online) or social media.

It should be noted that in cosmetic surgeries, such issues can arise months or even years after surgery as results are often delayed and doctor may not remember all facts of the case. Hence, proper documentation is vital.

PROCESS OF LAW IN NEGLIGENCE

At this stage, it is important to understand the process of law for medical negligence. An outline is presented here as this is dealt in detail in other chapters:

- *Step 1*: Patient sends a notice. The claim officially begins with the issuance of a legal notice. The legal notice outlines what the claimant wants, and gives a time frame for reply. The letter also serves as a warning that you will be taken to court, if you do not comply with the demands in the legal notice within the said time frame.
- *Step 2*: Doctor decides whether to defend or settle.
- *Step 3*: If doctor decides to defend, he responds to notice.
- *Step 4*: If patient is unsatisfied with the reply, and is convinced there is a deficiency of service and negligence, the patient files a case and court serves a summons. Even at this stage, doctor can choose to settle if he/she wishes or to respond to summons and defend.
  On the occasions where the reply by doctor answers the queries/allegations satisfactorily, with facts and information that the patient may not have revealed to their advocate, the patient's advocate may advise the patient to drop the matter there itself.
- *Step 5*: Once matter is in court/consumer forum, a notice is sent to the doctor, who responds to the same and the proceeding starts. The process is usually long, with arguments and counterarguments by the two parties. The onus is on the patient to prove negligence. Evidence is presented and witnesses are called and they can be cross-examined. The ensuing judgment can then be followed by a review or appeal.

Out-of-court settlement is possible at this stage also.

If both the parties agree on an out of court settlement, the memorandum of settlement detailing the terms of settlement and the settlement is executed with formal approval of the Court.

Respond or to defend?

There are two choices in every claim on how to respond, settle the case out of court, or defend to trial. This is not a decision to be taken lightly; if doctor settles too easily, it is a sign of panic, and he will be regarded as a soft target; if he defends then he has to follow the long process and pay for the costs. *This decision needs a proper consultation with a lawyer, with all the factual information, which will include a copy of the patient's records, preferably in consultation with another medical expert. The medical expert is consulted to give an impartial opinion as to whether there is any deviation from accepted guidelines of care.*

However, in India, doctors tend to be secretive and often do not wish to consult another doctor, which is not recommended.

Why out-of-court settlement?

Not all cases reach judicial and quasi-judicial authorities but there is no data available on the number of matters that get settled out of court. Some cases do get settled after a legal notice is issued or even after a threat of legal notice or a threat of filing of a consumer complaint or a criminal complaint. No doctor wants to get entangled in litigation. There are certain factors, which would favor an out-of-court settlement whereas there would be factors, which would not favor such recourse. A balanced decision should be taken based on the facts and circumstances of the matter after consultation of the defense team and the medical experts in that field.

There are several concerns about the process of adjudication that cross the minds of the affected Doctors, as well as their immediate well-wishers, which may make them initially inclined to think of a settlement:

- The whole trial process is stressful—time consuming, may drag on for years. *The author is aware of a case where in a case of death after angioplasty dragged on for several years, as patient who was a judge took the case right up to the Supreme Court. The anesthetist and cardiac surgeons in the case came under immense stress, with a possible adverse judgment dangling over them.*
- Prohibitive costs of defense.
- Frequent visits to the court affect practice; this may involve travelling to another place where court is located. Though it is not mandatory that the doctor attends each hearing after having appointed a duly authorized representative or a lawyer, it is in the interests of the doctor to do so.

Some examples for this are:
  - *In a case, the patient, in a claim for compensation for poor results after hair transplantation, said he bought a laser machine for hair growth on doctor's advice, and included the cost of the machine in compensation claim. The doctor had not advised the machine, but what had happened was that patient had sought advice on the machine and doctor on the back of prescription, wrote the name of the website of the machine for patient to study and get more information. Doctor could claim that this was just for education of the patient and not a prescription and hence escaped any adverse outcome in court.*

- Even if facts are in favor of the doctor, the lawyer has to present them properly—often the lawyer may not be fully aware of medical aspects, and hence close coordination is essential between the two. This consumes considerable time and expense.
- Often media gets into the issue, and adverse publicity affects the reputation and the practice of the doctor.
- Lastly, a doctor does not basically like the idea of standing in trial.
- Often patient complains in several agencies; Civil Court, Criminal Court, Medical Council, Women's Commission, Human Rights Commission, etc. It is difficult to fight in so many different agencies for an individual doctor.

A decision regarding "Out-of-court settlement" should preferably be taken after involving the local medical fraternity—whether the Indian Medical Association (IMA) or any other medical association or an expert group related to the Doctor's area of and after due consideration of all facts as outlined above. The decision should not be taken as a reaction to the pressure created by the impending proceedings, as this is the very impression that the patient's lawyer wants to create, to have an upper hand in the negotiations that would inevitably happen, if the matter does proceed for a settlement. The approval for a settlement should be seen as an option agreed to by the doctor and his/her lawyer, out of compassion for the patient more than anything else. It should be emphatically conveyed in no uncertain terms, that the doctor is more than willing to fight the case, else most of the benefits that the doctor gets from a settlement may be lost.

A Peer Group, which gives the accused doctor moral support, and ensures the decision for settlement is not taken out of pressure, but rather on genuine grounds is of great help to the doctor. In the personal experience of one of the authors as the convener of the Medicolegal Cell of an Association of Specialist Doctors (AMC Mangalore), a group of 10 odd doctors committed to the cause have been meeting at least one evening a week, for the last 6–7 years. This gives a strong sense of support to all members of the association that their colleagues are available in the event of any matter, any time during the progress of their matter with the authorities.

The most accepted scenario in which an out-of-court settlement is recommended by all experts is when there is an "indefensible case". Classic examples include:
- Mop in the abdomen
- Operating on the wrong side of the body
- Injury to an organ/structure during the course of the surgery—ureter during a gynecological procedure.

There is no way such cases can be defended in court, by even the most brilliant lawyer. By having an out-of-court settlement, there is an additional benefit for the medical fraternity, besides the benefits to the patient and the doctor involved. Only a case that goes for trial, and is adjudicated finally, makes its way to law books, literature, and Journals, and can be used as a "Case Law" or a precedent. By having an out-of-court settlement, the fraternity is avoiding a Case Law with a higher compensation amount, which the judgment may have.

WAYS OF SETTLING

- The most common way, which is not often realized, is in the clinic, before patient serves a notice, when there is a warning sign as mentioned above. As soon as patient is noticed to be unhappy, the physician identifies the potential of the situation and takes preventive action. This may be in the form of free treatment, procedures to correct the problem, or even refund of the cost of treatment.

In aesthetic dermatology, there can be several examples:
- In cases of laser hair removal, additional sessions can be offered in cases of lack of response.
- In case of hair transplantation, additional touch up sessions can be done to correct lack of density.
- In some cases, refund or partial refund of treatment cost may be done. For example, in one case, patient said, doctor, I have got only 50% of result, so please refund 50% of costs, I do not want to go to court.
- A patient who underwent Botulinum toxin treatment was unhappy over lack of results. Since he was from another country, he could not come for a touch up session. He threatened the doctor to complain to medical council, to take him to court and report media. Doctor counseled him about need for touch up session, and arranged a treatment with a doctor whom he knew. The condition improved and the case was settled.

Note: Offering free treatment or refund of fees carries the risk of being taken as an admission of guilt on the part of the doctor. Such allegations have been the grounds for claims for compensation in some cases. If such a course is found to be desirable then it is essential that the patient is counseled and explained that the refund of fees or free treatment is way of good will and in no way indicates admission of negligence or deficiency of service. It is preferable to have this in the written form. Refund of fees or free treatment can be part of the terms of the settlement.

It is advisable to ensure proper documentation in all such cases, as to why refund or additional sessions are being done with the consent signed by patient, in presence of a witness. All guidelines of care are to be followed thoroughly.

- This can also be done after a notice is issued, with involvement of the lawyer as mentioned above. At this stage, it is preferable to involve a lawyer or a mutual friend and ensure proper documentation.

Documentation of settlement: The document should state the details of settlement, compensation provided, with specific confirmation that the patient will not pursue the case in any court, and will not indulge in any action on social media or visual or print media adverse to the doctor. It should also mention among other points that the doctor does not admit any lack of duty of care in the management of the patient or any deficiency of service on the part of the doctor or his staff, nurses, and others.

MAKING THE DECISION TO FIGHT

When not to settle?

Just as there are reasons to settle, there are also reasons to fight.

1. *The doctor believes there is no negligence, and hence no liability, patient is being unreasonable.*

   For example, the first author successfully fought a case in consumer court, where he believed he was fully correct in every way and decided to fight just to get the experience of a trial. The attitude was, "if I cannot fight this case, how will I fight case which may be difficult". Of course, he was aided by the fact that documentation was perfect with signatures by patient about 10 places for every aspect in hair transplantation. The patient had claimed lack of results after hair transplantation and blamed the doctor for poor outcome. The author produced an informed consent document in which the patient mentioned that he does not want to take any drug after hair transplantation to prevent future baldness, and the court agreed that "patient was negligent, not the doctor".

2. *The doctor is of the opinion that there is a liability on his part, but the demands of the patient are unreasonable.*

   In the personal experience of one of the authors, a lawyer sent a legal notice to his treating dermatologist for a side effect of a drug. The financial compensation sought was not in commensurate with the alleged loss or injury suffered by the lawyer. Three rounds of discussion did not yield any fruitful outcomes. It was suggested not to settle the matter, if the demand for compensation was unreasonable and excessive and that no further negotiations were possible under such circumstances. Few days later, the lawyer voluntarily agreed to the initially offered compensation as settlement of the matter.

   It is always preferable that the discussion on settlement is initiated by the complainant or his lawyer. Very often, when the discussion is initiated by the doctor or his defense team, it is presumed that the doctor has been negligent and is therefore willing to settle the matter. The negotiating power of the doctor and his team could then be compromised. A statement for settlement can also be made before the Court where the matter is being heard. However, it should be made abundantly clear that the defending doctor does not admit any negligence or deficiency of service.

   There are occasions where criminal complaints have been filed or verbal threats of filing complaints before different judicial and quasi-judicial authorities are made and the doctor is intimidated into make a payment as compensation. Compensation should not be paid unless there is a memorandum of settlement.

For example, the first author is aware of a case where a chemical peel resulted in pigmentation. The patient behaved aggressively in the clinic with a group of four well-built individuals. The doctor panicked and went to the nearby police station. The concerned inspector offered to mediate the case, and the case was settled with a payment of ₹ 25,000 to the patient, even though the pigmentation was temporary and could have been easily treated and hence the doctor was not at fault. This was clearly a case of intimidation.

Further, if the doctor has a professional indemnity insurance, payment of amount of settlement should not be made without the concurrence of the insurance company in writing. If a promise is made or money is paid as compensation as an out of court settlement without the written concurrence of the insurance company then the insurance company will not entertain a claim under the policy for reimbursement of such amount.

It is notable that cases of "out-of-court settlement" do not get reported and the information regarding such settlement or the terms of settlement does not come in public domain.

POINTS TO REMEMBER

- Out-of-court settlement is an option, which should be exercised in appropriate cases.
- It can help a doctor to avoid the protracted trial process.
- It should not be pursued in an overenthusiastic manner by the doctor, as it may be interpreted as an admission of guilt/negligence/deficiency of service.
- It should be done only after proper consultation with experts, both in law and medicine.
- A memorandum of settlement should be entered into between the doctor and the patient/legal representative of the patient as the case may be. Such a memorandum of settlement can be filed before the court/forum where the matter is pending following which the court/forum will close the matter.
- Inform the insurance company, if one has a professional indemnity policy about the possibility of having an "out-of-court settlement" and take their written concurrence for such a course.

CHAPTER 14

Professional Indemnity Insurance

Subodh Premanand Sirur

INTRODUCTION

A medical professional is subjected to numerous risks in the discharge of professional commitments. Such risks include the risk of litigation. It is essential that every doctor (whether having own practice or is attached to a nursing home or to a hospital or employed in a government hospital) has a risk management strategy in place. In simple words, risk management includes measures adopted to minimize the risk (particularly the risk of litigation) in the course of professional commitments. Risk management is not something to be done only by management experts. While it is prudent to have a professional managing the risks in case of larger health facilities, the individual doctor for want of human and financial resources would be constrained to deal with risks himself or herself.

COMPONENTS OF RISK MANAGEMENT

- *Risk identification:* This step involves identification of risks or pitfalls. For example, having unqualified nurses handling some of the esthetic procedures or delegation of responsibilities to an incompetent junior can be pitfalls for litigation.
- *Risk assessment:* This step follows identification of the risks and involves assessment of the possible impact of such risks. In a particular case decided by the Supreme Court on 25 March, 1998 (M/S Spring Meadows Hospital and another versus Harjot Ahluwalia) a child with pyrexia of unknown origin suffered cardiac arrest and slipped into coma due to administration of chloroquine instead of chloramphenicol. The consultant had recommended chloramphenicol whereas the junior doctor asked the unqualified nurse to give a prescription who wrote chloroquine instead of chloramphenicol. An amount of 17.5 lakhs rupees (12.5 lakhs rupees as also 5 lakhs rupees as compensation to the parents of the minor child for the acute mental agony that has been caused to the parents by reason

of their only son having been reduced to a vegetative state requiring lifelong care and attention) was directed to be paid as compensation. This would have certainly had an adverse financial impact on the hospital. The insurance company challenged the decision of the National Commission which directed the insurance company to pay the compensation for the negligent act of the unqualified nurse as the negligent act of the unqualified nurse would not be covered under the terms and conditions of the insurance policy. Most policies do not cover acts done by unqualified staff. A doctor may be vicariously liable for the acts of omission and commission of his unqualified staff. The policy may not cover in case of a claim. The Supreme Court while deciding a matter of medical negligence had left this question open as to whether the insurance companies can deny claim where the act of omission or commission has been caused by an unqualified "nurse."

Notably the insurance policies exclude the following:
- Any criminal act or any act committed in violation of any law or ordinance
- Deliberate, willful or intentional non-compliance of any statutory provision.
- Non-compliance with technical standards commonly observed in professional practice, laid down by law, or regulated by official bodies
- Any dishonest, fraudulent criminal or malicious act or omission
- Deliberate conscious or intentional disregard of the insured's technical or administrative management of the need to take all reasonable steps to prevent claims.

- *Risk handling:* Once the risks have been identified and the possible impact of such risks is assessed then the next step is handling of such risks. This can be aimed at handling litigation as and when they hit. It also aims at prevention of risks such as regular audit systems to ensure that structured operating procedures are being diligently followed. Professional indemnity insurance is one of the risk mitigation tools as part of risk management.

Need for a Professional Indemnity Insurance

A professional indemnity insurance policy essentially covers two events-payment of defense costs in the event of litigation and payment of compensation for legal liability due to bodily injury or death caused by breach of professional duty by the doctor in the event that a Court directs payment of compensation.

There are doctors who believe that spending on a professional indemnity is a waste of financial resources. This is especially when the doctor feels that he or she has taken adequate precautions to avoid litigation and is practicing as per accepted professional practices. It is important to note that the policy covers defense costs (costs of lawyers) which can be prohibitive and a huge drain on financial resources. Further, that the doctor may be held not negligent and that compensation is not payable. However, there will be costs towards payment of fees to lawyers even if the doctor is finally discharged of any liability in the matter. In such a case the professional indemnity insurance will protect the doctor from financial losses.

Cover under the Policy

It is a common practice for the doctors to sign on the dotted line on the proposal form and expect the insurance agent to do the rest. Further, when the policy document is received the terms and conditions are occasionally glanced through. Only a few doctors are known to have really read the terms and conditions. Every doctor needs to read the terms and conditions of the policy to know what all is covered under the policy and what is not.

This author was chatting with a senior dermatologist over a cup of coffee when the dermatologist mentioned that she feels safe with coverage of 1 crore rupees under her professional indemnity insurance policy. This author casually asked her if she had read the contents of the policy. Not surprisingly she had not. Quite aware the dermatologist was more into esthetic medicine she was asked if she was aware that her policy may not be covering cosmetic procedures as a number of policies exclude such a cover unless it is specifically sought and that too for a loading of premium. The dermatologist quipped that she would check with her agent and of course read the policy terms herself. It is better to be safe than sorry.

So, it would be necessary to negotiate with the insurance company to cover the esthetic procedures too and have an endorsement on the policy.

The associations have an important role to play in this matter. The association has numbers and can negotiate for better and reasonable premium to cover esthetic procedures. It can also facilitate better handling and settlement of claims. Indian Association of Dermatologists, Venereologists and Leprologists (IADVL) has started an insurance scheme called Dermatologists, Venereologists and Leprologist (DVL) trust.

It is advisable to be conversant with some basic concepts in insurance. Most of the indemnity policies sold in India are "claims made" basis as opposed to "occurrence" basis. This means that the policy should be in force without a break as on the date when the claim is made. So if the adverse event or the alleged negligent act occurred a year prior and the policy was in force at that time but not renewed later or renewed without a break when the claim was made then the insurance company will not cover the claim. Notably, the limitation for filing a complaint under the Consumer Protection Act, 1986 is 2 years from the date of cause of action and under general law for 3 years. Therefore, if there is a break in renewal or if the policy has not been renewed the insurance company is not bound to settle the claim even if the policy was in force at the time the negligent act is alleged to have occurred. Therefore, it is imperative that the process of renewal is started well before the date of expiry of the term of the policy to avoid any break in the policy.

Therefore, one must always check the retroactive date on the policy. The retroactive date is the date on which the policy incepted for the first time. So if a policy has been purchased on 1/8/2000 for the first time and has been renewed annually without a break then the retroactive date would be 1/8/2000 though the tenure of the current policy would be 1/8/2018 to 31/7/2019.

A doctor should play a participative role in deciding the level of indemnity (erroneously referred to commonly as sum insured). It is impossible to estimate with certainty the level of indemnity as compensation payable will differ from case to case and the level of damage caused to the patient. As compensation includes loss of wages also technically speaking loss or damage to a patient with high income may result in a higher pay out. The risk of litigation would be higher when esthetic procedures are being done (when the expectation of the patient is to improve one's looks and at least not to worsen it or have complications. There can be unrealistic expectations too). Mortality and morbidity can also be a cause for litigation. A doctor has to decide the level of indemnity based on these considerations. No straight jacket formula can be applied. The premium paying capacity of the doctor is also an important determinant. Higher the limit of the indemnity chosen by the doctor, higher will be the premium.

The level of indemnity can be decided by the proposer (doctor proposing to purchase the policy) under two headings. For example, if a doctor has decided to have the limit of indemnity of 20 lakhs rupees for the insurance policy. This can be broken into Any One Accident (event) and Any One Year. So for the year the overall limit of indemnity will be 20 lakhs rupees but if it is expected that there could be three or four adverse events per year and possibly the claim could be in the range of 5 lakhs rupees per adverse event then the limit of indemnity for a single event (termed as accident) can be fixed to 5 lakhs rupees only for each of the 4 events with an overall limit of 20 lakhs rupees.

It is expected of a doctor to inform the insurance company whenever a legal notice is received or even a threat of legal action. Such information forwarded to your insurance company (in written form with acknowledgement for future use) will help in case a court case ensues and there has been a break in the renewal of the policy or has not been renewed at all. The insurance company will consider a claim arising out of such a court case. The insurance company may refuse to settle the claim if no information is forwarded to them.

There are instances when a case is indefensible and an out of court settlement is the best way to go ahead rather than going through the protracted legal battle and its accompanying mental agony. However, it is important to bear in mind not to promise or to go in for an out of court settlement without having the concurrence of the insurance company. If there is no such concurrence the insurance company can refuse to settle the claim. In a matter in Dr T versus New India Assurance Company Limited decided by the National Consumer Disputes Redressal Commission on 2nd April, 2013.

Facts of the Case

A doctor filed a complaint against the insurance company for deficiency of service in not settling the claim under the Professional Indemnity Policy for Doctors and Medical Practitioners which was purchased by the doctor and was validly in force at the time of the making the claim.

A compensation of 267,750 rupees was directed to be paid for medical negligence on the part of the doctor. The doctor immediately informed the insurance company to pay the awarded amount and to indemnify the claim but the insurance company failed to take any steps to indemnify the policy.

The insurance company relied upon the following terms and conditions of the policy:
- The insured shall give written notice to the company as soon as reasonably practicable of any claims made against the insured or any specific event or circumstances that may give rise to a claim being made against the insured and which forms the subject of indemnity under this policy and shall give all such additional information as the company may require.
- Every claim, writ, summons or process and all documents relating to the event shall be forwarded to the company immediately they are received by the insured.

- As the doctor had failed to inform the insurance company as per the terms and conditions of the policy and informed them only after the matter was decided by the Forum and the compensation was awarded against the doctor, the insurance company refused to settle the claim of the doctor and pay the compensation. The doctor paid the compensation to the complainant in compliance of the order and to avoid proceedings under Section 27 of the Consumer Protection Act, 1986. The doctor then filed a complaint against the insurance company for nonsettlement of the claim and to pay the compensation to the complainant.

Decision

The State Commission had dismissed the appeal of the doctor against the insurance company. The doctor filed a revision petition before the National Commission. The National Commission observed that "The State Commission opined that the question is required to be decided as to whether there is any deficiency in service of the insurer. If the insurer has refused to indemnify the claim for nonsatisfaction of the policy condition by the insured, it cannot be held that the action of the insurance company was deficient in service. The condition which has been violated is not a mere procedural redundant requirement. Apparently the said condition gave opportunity to the insurer to have not only notice but also an opportunity to control if possible, any claim or proceeding against the insured."

The National Commission referred to a decision of the Supreme Court *in Oriental Insurance Co. Ltd., versus Sony Cheriyan* (Supreme Court Cases page no. 455, paragraph 17) wherein it was held that—"The insurance policy between the insurer and the insured represents a contract between the parties. Since the insurer undertakes to compensate the loss suffered by the insured on account of risks covered by the insurance policy, the terms of the agreement have to be strictly construed to determine the extent of liability of the insurer. The insured cannot claim anything more than what is covered by the insurance policy. That being so, the insured has also to act strictly in accordance with the statutory limitations or terms of the policy expressly set out therein.

The endeavor of the court must always be to interpret the words in which the contract is expressed by the parties. The court while construing the terms of the policy is not expected to venture into extra liberalism that may result in rewriting the contract or substituting the terms which are not intended by the parties. The insured cannot claim anything more than what is covered by the insurance policy."

The National Commission referred to the clauses 8.1 to 8.3 of the Professional Indemnity Policy for Doctors and Medical Practitioners:
- 8.1 The insured shall give written notice to the Company as soon as reasonably practicable of any claims made against the insured (or any specific event or circumstances that may give to a claim being made against the insured) and which forms the subject of indemnity under this policy and shall give all such additional information as the Company may require. Every claim, writ, summons or process and all documents relating to the event shall be forwarded to the company immediately they are received by the insured.
- 8.2 No admission, offer, promise or payment shall be made or given by or on behalf of the insured without the written consent of the company.

- 8.3 The company will have the right but in no case the obligation, to take over and conduct in the name of the insured the defense of any claims and will have full discretion in the conduct of any proceedings and the settlement of any claim and having taken over the defense of any claim may relinquish the same. All amounts expended by the Company in the defense, settlement or payment of any claim will reduce the limits of indemnity specified in the schedule of the policy.

As the doctor has not complied with the clause 8.1 requiring the doctor to give a written notice to the insurance company of any claims made against the insured (or any specific event or circumstances that may give to a claim being made against the insured) it was held that there is no deficiency of service on the part of the insurance company in not settling the claim.

POINTS TO REMEMBER

- A professional indemnity policy for doctors serves the purpose of covering the compensation payable in case it is held that the doctor was negligent and it also serves the purpose of covering the defense costs (even when there is no finding of medical negligence by the courts).
- It is essential for a doctor to peruse the terms and conditions of the policy and verify if they would cover his needs in case of a legal liability.
- Purchase of a professional indemnity policy through an association has certain advantages as associations have better bargaining powers.
- There is no straight jacket method to determine the limit of liability.
- Factors helping determine the limit of liability include the area of practice (likely pitfalls are use of drugs, such as biological and performance of esthetic procedures); the economic status of the patients and the premium paying capacity of the doctor (more the limit of indemnity chosen higher will the premium be).
- Ensure that the policy is renewed well before the expiry of the term of the policy.
- Inform the insurance company of any claim or any threat of a claim under the insurance policy.

CHAPTER 15

Regulations for Starting a Clinic

Dinesh Kumar Devaraj, Sneha Gandhi, Shilpa K

SUMMARY

Most dermatologists in India practice in independent skin clinics and offer basic dermatosurgery services. As such, skin clinics are regarded as a taxable commercial enterprise by the government. Thus, applying for various approval such as registration of clinic with regional government health authority, trade license from the local city/town corporation and pollution control board for safe biomedical waste disposal are few of the crucial steps in starting and running a skin clinic in a hassle-free manner. In addition, a dermatologist should be sensitized regarding the rules of running a pharmacy, various labor laws to manage staff efficiently as well as should have a sound knowledge about income tax and goods and services tax.

KEY MESSAGES

- Adherence to legal frame-work is a must, in every aspect of clinic establishment.
- Acquaint yourself well with your specialty colleagues, also with lawyers and auditors.
- Adhere to staff regulations pertaining to duties, obligations and privileges.
- Awareness on the legal aspects and significant court judgments pertaining to health care setups is desirable.
- Awareness of various regulations and complying with them is crucial for smooth running of skin clinics.

INTRODUCTION

Dermatology is primarily a non-emergency, outpatient-based specialty with most dermatologists opting to have a private practice, with the exception of a few government and institutional doctors bounded by a non-practice agreement with their institutions. A skin clinic (as indeed all medical clinics) is essentially regarded as a business or commercial or a trade enterprise by the government authorities and as a service provider under Consumer Protection Act, 1986. Further, the expanding forays of dermatology in the last decade have evolved the skin clinics from a primarily prescription-based practice into centers that also offer procedural dermatology including minor surgical and aesthetic procedures at the least and hair transplantation and other major cosmetic services at the best. The impact of these changes has led to an increase in size of the clinic as well as the number of staff on board. This recent paradigm shift in dermatology practice, brings with it, several new practice management issues for the dermatologists as traditionally, doctors have little knowledge or training in business/hospital management. These issues are neither taught in medical curriculum nor addressed in any conferences. This chapter addresses this need and reviews the various licenses and other obligatory regulatory requirements that are required by law to be followed by a dermatologist. However, it is essential to note that the regulations discussed here are of a general nature and the reader is encouraged to consult the local agencies for the precise regulations of his/her state. This chapter also focuses on the rules and regulations regarding the patient records, liability toward the income tax and GST.

TERMINOLOGIES RELEVANT TO THE CHAPTER

"Skin and Hair Clinic" refers to any center which offers treatment for various dermatological conditions (skin, hair, nail, aesthetic treatments, STIs, leprosy) with or without injections, minor operations, dressing, etc. to the patients.

"Consultation Room" means a place where consultation, which includes examination of the patients is carried out and relevant prescription, advice and education pertaining the patient's condition is provided by the dermatologist.

"Dermatologist" refers to a registered medical practitioner (RMP) who is registered with the State Medical Council or Medical Council of India holding a recognized degree/diploma in Dermatology, Venereology, and Leprosy (MD, Diploma or DNB holder), offering consultations and treatment under modern system of medicine (Allopathy).

"Registered Medical Practitioner" includes any person who possesses any of the Government recognized medical qualification and who has been enrolled in the register of the respective State Medical Council.

"Patient" implies a person who reports himself/herself or is brought to a clinic/hospital for the purpose of consultation or treatment or to seek any other services rendered by the clinic/hospital.

"Clinical Establishment" means a hospital, maternity home, nursing home, dispensary, clinic, sanatorium, or any other institution that offers services, facilities requiring diagnosis, treatment or care for illness, injury, deformity, abnormality or pregnancy in any recognized system of medicine. It also includes laboratory and diagnostic center or any other place where pathological, bacteriological, genetic, radiological, chemical, biological investigations or other services with aid of laboratory or other medical equipment are carried out.

"Hospital" (WHO) means healthcare institutions that have an organized medical and other professional staff, and inpatient facilities, and deliver medical, nursing and related services 24 hours per day, 7 days per week. Hospitals offer a varying range of acute, convalescent and terminal care using diagnostic and curative services in response to acute and chronic conditions arising from diseases as well as injuries and genetic anomalies. In doing so, they generate essential information for research, education, and management.

"Clinical/Medical Diagnostic Laboratory" means a laboratory with one or more of the following where microbiological, serological, chemical, hematological, immunohematological, immunological, toxicological, cytogenetic, exfoliative cytogenetic, histological, pathological or other examinations are performed of materials/fluids derived from the human body for the purpose of providing information on diagnosis, prognosis, prevention, or treatment of disease.

"Polyclinic" means a clinic where more than one doctor offers consultation with or without treatment for illness in any recognized system of medicine.

"Staff Nurse" means a person who possess the required qualification from any of the Nursing Teaching Institutions, recognized by the respective State Government and that person must have enrolled in the respective State's Nurses and Midwives Council under the Indian Nursing Council Act, 1947 (Central Act XLVIII of 1947) or any of the State Nursing Council in India recognized by the Indian Nursing Council.

"Dermatology Assistant/Technician" refers to the qualified staff, who supports in-patient care services provided in a clinical establishment and may be involved in assisting the minor surgical/cosmetic procedures offered at the establishment (if any).

MINIMUM STANDARDS FOR A "SKIN AND HAIR" CLINIC

A dermatologist running a skin and hair clinic is required to abide by several regulations and acquire various licenses as prescribed by different local/state authorities.

The Clinical Establishments Act (CEA) provides for registration and regulation of clinical establishments in the country with a view to prescribe basic minimum standards of facilities and services of particular type being provided by the clinical establishment. It is however, important to note that the CEA is currently applicable only in 16 states and union territories while a few states are bound by a separate legislature and are in the process of repealing the current legislature in favor of the CEA. The reader is encouraged to access the website http://www.clinicalestablishments.gov.in to access the various regulations prescribed for his/her particular state. According to these proposals, a clinic offering LASER and cosmetology services must have a dermatologist who has certified laser training of atleast 6 months duration. These guidelines are being reviewed by the Ministry of Health and will be finalized after feedback from all parties concerned. Indian Association of Dermatologists, Venereologists, and Leprologists (IADVL) has already recommended modifications to these on the grounds that these guidelines are too strict and need modification. However, it is important that all members obtain proper hands-on certificates for training. The basic amenities and facilities to be offered at the clinic as per the CEA guidelines have been discussed below.

Infrastructure

A clinic shall have a consultation room and a separate space (waiting area/reception) for the patients awaiting consultation. The consultation room should preferably have a space of not less than 100 ft^2 and be provided with sufficient light and ventilation. The minimum area prescribed under the clinical establishments act is not less than 35 ft^2 carpet area for the reception cum waiting area and a minimum of 70 ft^2 carpet area for consultation room including storage. A minimum of 40 ft^2 area shall be allotted to the pharmacy if present. If the center functions as a polyclinic, then, separate cubicles shall be made available to each specialist/specialties, if they attend simultaneously. Names of the various practicing consultants with their consultation fees, timing and the services offered (if any) shall be exhibited in the waiting room.

Human Resource

There should be a minimum of one qualified dermatologist and one paramedical staff to meet the treatment and service needs of the patient. However, this number may increase depending upon the workload and scope of the service being provided by the clinical establishment. The examination of the patient and prescription of the treatment shall be done only by a registered medical practitioner (qualified dermatologist) as required under the Indian Medical Council Act.

Equipment

The following equipment and furniture/fixtures should be available in the dermatologist's consulting room:
- Examination couch with chairs
- Magnifying lens
- Wood's lamp
- Torch light
- Tongue depressor
- Thermometer
- Weighing machine
- Blood pressure apparatus
- A screen for adequate privacy
- Foot stools
- Storage cabinets for records, etc.
- Autoclave equipment.

Other preferable clinic equipment to be made available in a dermatological setup would be:
- Sterilizer or autoclave.
- Dermatoscope, trichoscope

- Cheatle forceps, sterile scissors, sterile forceps, glucometer, other essential dermatosurgical equipment, sterile gloves, etc.
- Ablative radiofrequency equipment, chemical peel, and lasers.
- Emergency drugs and resuscitation kit.

Other miscellaneous equipment such as those required for biopsy procedures, microscope, dark ground microscope, narrow band or phototherapy chamber are considered mandatory if the establishment comes under the purview of "hospital" but are desirable if the establishment comes under the purview of "dermatology clinic/cosmetic center". The Clinical Establishments Act mandates that all of the equipment should be of adequate capacity and should be functional at all times with periodic inspection, cleaning, maintenance of equipment as per the manufacturer's guidelines.

Licenses

The various licenses needed for a skin clinic are mentioned in Box 1. Box 1A lists all the registrations that need to be done.

BOX 1: Various licenses needed for a skin clinic/establishment.
- Registration under respective Clinical Establishments Act or local municipal rules and regulations
- Pharmacy license (if pharmacy is attached)

BOX 1A: Various registrations needed for a skin clinic/establishment.
- Agreement/MOU with biomedical waste disposal agency
- GST registration (if cosmetic surgeries are done)
- Medical indemnity insurance

> **BOX 2:** Documents needed for clinic registration.*
> - Covering letter to district health officer from doctor/manager of clinic
> - Two passport size photos of proprietor/ doctor
> - State Medical Council Registration Certificate (photocopy)
> - Degree certificate of medical degree/diploma (photocopy)
> - Copy of agreement/MOU with local biomedical waste disposal agency
> - Authorization from pollution control board
> - Price list of services provided—including the consultation fees and the list of procedures. The minimum price/range/precise fees of surgery may be mentioned depending on time taken and complexity of surgery
> - Certificates of concerned paramedical staff—pharmacist, nurse/laboratory technician, etc.
> - Either the ownership documents of the building (if owned by the doctor) or rental agreement with landlord (photocopy or original)
> - Declaration from dermatologist stating that he/she is aware of clinical establishments act and will comply with its rules
>
> *May vary from State-to-State in India, check your respective State.

Registration under Respective Clinical Establishments Act

The registration of the skin clinic is done at a committed cell for registering clinical establishments at the district health office. The requisite documents needed for the registration are mentioned under Box 2.

Agreement/Memorandum of Understanding with Biomedical Waste Disposal Agency

The clinics are required by law to enter into an agreement or memorandum of understanding (MOU) with a government recognized local biomedical waste disposal agency. The clinician is also required to keep a copy of the said agreement at the clinic. Failure to adhere to the biomedical waste disposal system may lead to penalty, license cancellation and even imprisonment. The responsibilities of the dermatologist toward biomedical waste management have been described below.

Pharmacy License (If Pharmacy is Attached)

A dermatologist may run a pharmacy within the clinic premises after he/she appoints a qualified pharmacist and procures a license from local drug inspector in the name of the pharmacist. The practitioner must also inform the local private medical establishment regarding the said pharmacy and submit a photocopy of the degree/diploma certificate of the pharmacist. The law mandates an area of 120 ft^2 for the pharmacy, a separate Taxpayer Identification Number (TIN) and storage of the drugs as per the manufacturer's instructions (temperature, shielding from sunlight, etc.), a refrigerator and an air-conditioner of minimum 1 ton. Further, the sale of medicines comes under the purview of the GST tax and the tax is generally inclusive of the maximum retail price (MRP). If dermatologist intends to manufacture and dispense certain topical or oral medicines—a separate license from the drug inspector has to be procured. However, these licenses do not authorize a dermatologist to either stock or sell medicines in bulk to other chemists (like a stockist) nor is he authorized to dispense/sell medicines without a label and maximum retail price.

A doctor is within the legal framework to dispense medications without a license within his/her clinic; however, certain conditions have to be adhered to the same. As per item 5 of Schedule K of the Drugs and Cosmetics Act and Rules [The Drugs and Cosmetics Act, 1940 (23 of 1940) (amended up to the 30th June, 2005) and the Drugs and Cosmetics Rules, 1945 (amended up to the 30th June, 2005) which states that "Drugs supplied by a registered medical practitioner to his own patient or any drug specified in Schedule C supplied by a registered medical practitioner at the request of another such practitioner if it is specially prepared with reference to the condition and for the use of an individual patient provided the registered medical practitioner is not (a) keeping an open shop or (b) selling across the counter or (c) engaged in the importation, manufacture, distribution or sale of drugs in the provision of Chapter IV of the Act and the rules there under."

Lending credence to the above is clause 6.3, Chapter 6 of MCI regulations, Indian Medical Council (Professional conduct, Etiquette and Ethics) Regulations, 2002 published in Part III, Section 4 of the Gazette of India, dated 6th April, 2002 (amended up to December, 2010), the following is the regulation regarding dispensing of drugs by doctors.

Running an open shop (dispensing of drugs and appliances by physicians): A physician should not run an open shop for sale of medicine for dispensing prescriptions prescribed by doctors other than him or for sale of medical or surgical appliances. It is not unethical for a physician to prescribe or supply drugs, remedies or appliances as long as there is no exploitation of the patient. Drugs prescribed by a physician or brought from the market for a patient should explicitly state the proprietary formulae as well as generic name of the drug.

Further, item 5 of schedule-K of the Drugs and Cosmetics Rules allow a single doctor to stock, prescribe or dispense medicines without having a license. Hence a single medical practitioner can dispense his/her own prescribed medication but when medicine is dispensed to the prescriptions of more than a one doctor in the clinic, a pharmacy license is needed to dispense medicines.

A case verdict in the above context can be accessed from http://www.indiamedicaltimes.com/wp-content/uploads/2014/09/Dr-Kamalasanan-Verdict-Aug-2014.pdf.

GST Registration (If Cosmetic Surgeries are Done)

Goods and Services Tax or simply GST has replaced several indirect taxes in India and is applicable on both goods and services. Good refers to any kind of movable property while services include anything that does not come under the purview of goods including transactions in money. The exemption limit under GST is 20 lakhs above which the person is liable to pay the tax and should register himself within a period of 30 days. Further details have been mentioned below.

Medical Indemnity Insurance

A practitioner may procure medical indemnity insurance with appropriate cover at the initiation of his/her practice. The cover may further depend on the type of practice; for instance, a dermatologist performing frequent surgeries will need a higher cover. This insurance may be procured from private insurance companies, IMA (which also offers legal help through IMA office bearers), and through IADVL. However, the policies under IMA categorize dermatologists under category A (low risk) and hence do not cover procedural dermatology. Indian Association of Dermatologists, Venereologists, and Leprologists has a medical indemnity scheme called DVL trust which covers cosmetic procedures. It is therefore strongly recommended that all dermatologists avail this facility.

Maintenance of Patient Medical Records

Regulations have been set forward with regards to maintenance of the registers as well as the format of patient prescription. Every clinical establishment is required to maintain a "daily case register" replete with

FORM NO. 3C
[See rule 6f{3}]
Form of daily case register

[TO BE MAINTAINED BY PRACTITIONERS OF ANY SYSTEM OF MEDICINE IE, PHYSICIANS, SURGEONS, DENTISTS, PATHOLOGISTS, RADIOLOGISTS, VAIDS, HAKIMS, ETC.]

Date	Sl. No.	Patient's name	Nature of the professional services rendered, i.e. general consultation, surgery, injection, visit, etc.	Fees received	Date of receipt
(1)	(2)	(3)	(4)	(5)	(6)

Fig. 1: Form no. 3C—Format of the daily case register to be maintained by the practitioner.

the following details of the patients such as the name, age, sex, address of the patient and the date of examination in compliance with Form no. 3C prescribed by the IT Act (Fig. 1). Form no. 3C can be downloaded from www.incometaxindia.gov.in. A dermatologist is also required by law to maintain the details of patients, their treatment and procedures for at least a period of 3 years. The prescription given to the patient should contain name, age, sex of the patient, the date of consultation, diagnosis (either provisional or final) and treatment advised, the investigation and its result (if it was undertaken). The dermatologist shall sign the prescription slip with date and seal. This data has to be maintained in an organized manner—preferably computerized. In absentia of a computerized storage facility, an outpatient register and a carbon—copy type of prescription pad is a minimum requirement. However, the author recommends installation of suitable clinic management software with storage of preoperative and postoperative digital photographs as a medicolegal protective measure. Most clinic management software are designed to maintain records in the format of Form no. 3C, but the dermatologist can also record the necessary details manually if he/she so wishes.

Medical Waste Disposal

The Government of India and the State Pollution Control Board have issued directives regarding the facilities necessary to segregate the waste, dressings, etc. generated by a clinic. Pollution control rules mandate that clinics enter into an agreement/MOU with local biomedical waste disposal agency. The clinician is also required to keep a copy of the said agreement at the clinic. Failure to adhere to the biomedical waste disposal system may lead to penalty, license cancellation and even imprisonment. The clinician has the following responsibilities:

- Segregate the solid waste at the source into the respective color-coded bags.
- Hire a government approved agency to collect the waste which then collects it from the clinic on a regular/daily basis (about once to twice a week in smaller cities/taluks) and dispose it in a scientific manner at a common treatment plant.
- It is also crucial to keep the receipts of payment made to the biomedical waste disposal agency, as a proof of the dermatologist's compliance with pollution control laws.
- The clinician may install an incinerator at the center to manage the waste. However,

this needs a special license from, and quarterly reports about its emission to the state pollution board. The incinerator is also required to be robust enough to handle the diverse nature of biomedical waste such as bloody dressings, plastic syringes and excised body parts.
- Needles and sharp waste shall be stored in puncture proof container.
- Liquid waste (not managed by the disposal agency) should be treated with 1% sodium hypochlorite for 1 hour before letting it out into the sewage. This can be easily achieved with a few plumbing alterations. In the operating theater wash basins, a plastic can (25 L capacity) with tap may be connected below the sink. Bleaching powder may be added from the top end and the treated water may be let out through the tap—after 1 hour or even overnight (Fig. 2).

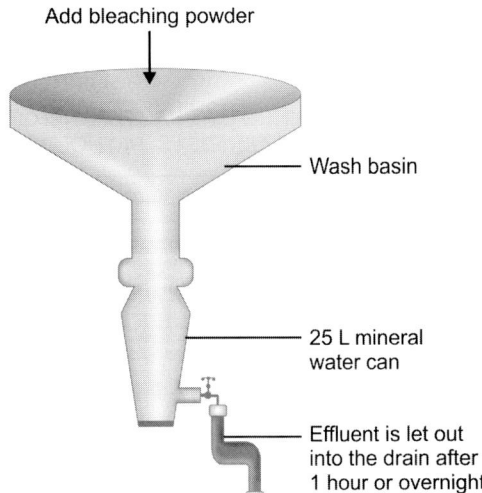

Fig. 2: A wash basin connected to a 25 L mineral water can below. Bleaching powder is added through the wash basin. After 1 hour or overnight immersion the tap of the can may be opened to release the effluent to the drain.

Laboratory in a Clinic

In response to a query by NABL to the Medical Council of India (MCI), the Ethics Committee and Executive Committee of MCI put forth in April 2017 that "All laboratory reports to be signed/countersigned by persons registered with MCI/State Medical Council."*

The Supreme Court of India in December 2017 passed an order that mentioned "We dispose of all these special leave petitions and other pending applications, if any, by taking a view that the stand of the Medical Council of India that Laboratory Report can be countersigned only by a registered medical practitioner with a postgraduate qualification in pathology is correct." **

If the skin clinic is providing laboratory services, the laboratory work shall be done by a qualified laboratory technician who holds a diploma in Medical Laboratory Technician/Certificate in Medical Laboratory Technician course approved by the Government or alternately the dermatologist can get the tests done by trained personnel under his/her direct supervision. However, the dermatologists can only sign for reports pertaining to KOH mount, a slit skin smear (SSS), and fungal cultures. For other investigations it is advisable to get it countersigned by a registered medical

---

*https://medicaldialogues.in/only-mbbs-can-sign-lab-reports-msc-cannot-mci/
https://www.hindustantimes.com/health/only-doctors-registered-with-mci-or-state-council-can-sign-lab-reports-mci/story-PJaD6PXKXWSRIo8wsHlS6J.html
**http://www.livelaw.in/laboratory-report-can-counter-signed-registered-medical-practitioner-post-graduate-qualification-sc-read-order/
https://indiankanoon.org/doc/1170686/

practitioner with a postgraduate qualification in pathology.

Mandatory Holidays for Clinic Staff

As per the labor rules, it is mandatory to declare holidays on 15th August, 26th January, 1st May, 2nd October, although additional mandatory holidays may be added by the respective state. The law upholds that if the clinic staff is made to work on these days, they must be paid double the wages for the day. Alternatively, an additional day-off must be given within a week's time.

TAXES FOR THE DERMATOLOGIST

Income Tax Act for a Dermatologist

The income generated by a dermatologist comes under the purview of professional income and hence is liable to Income tax and the practitioner is expected to abide its various rules and regulations. The practitioner is required to maintain "books of accounts" on the basis of financial year from 1st of April of current year to 31st of March of the following year and should file his/her IT returns by July 31st. Original bills for various expenses of clinic, such as stationery, equipment purchase and consumables must also be preserved. All these books or computerized records and bills are required to be maintained at the premises. This is mandatory when the annual income exceeds ₹ 1.2 lakhs per annum and the practitioner must employ the services of a chartered accountant when the turnover/income exceeds 25 lakhs. Recent income tax act amendments (from the financial year 2014-15*) have raised the standard deduction limit from ₹ 2 lakhs per annum to ₹ 2.5 lakhs per annum up to the age of 60 years. Other than the standard deduction limit, several other expenditure heads come under the purview of legal deductions and exemptions (as mentioned under Section 80C of the Income Tax Act)

Professional Tax Payment

As professionals, dermatologists are required under the law to register themselves with local professional tax officer and pay tax annually in accordance with the slab and location. This tax may also be paid online through government run websites. For instance, the professional tax website for Karnataka state is www.pt.kar.nic.in.

Goods and Services Tax

As professionals, dermatologists are required under the law to pay tax annually in accordance with the relevant slab and location. In addition of the professional taxes the dermatologist should also register for GST if cosmetic procedures are being done. The main entry No. 82 of exemption list of services from GST covers the area of medical sector for medical practitioners. The entry excludes any service provided by a clinical establishment, authorized medical practitioner, paramedics including transportation in an ambulance from GST, but does not define the terms of clinical establishment or authorized medical practitioner. If we consider the same definition for these terms as under the service tax, we can conclude that GST excludes any curative service but applies to beautification procedures. Table 1 provides a comprehensive view of the services included/exempted from GST. The reader is also encouraged to go through the exhaustive

---

*https://www.indiabudget.gov.in/budget2014-2015/ub2014-15/fb/bill1.pdf

TABLE 1: Services included and exempted from GST.

Exempted from GST	Included under GST
Consultation (including regular check-ups) and medical management under OPD basis	Medications sold either directly by a practitioner or via a self-owned shop will be charged GST which will be inclusive in the MRP
All surgeries, rent for OT, bed, patient room, beverages, equipment charges, doctor's consultation/surgery charges	Any service or surgery in relation to plastic/cosmetic surgery for a condition that has not arisen from congenital defects, developmental anomalies, degenerative diseases, injury or trauma
Various tests done in a hospital	
Services used/provided in biomedical waste management	
Services provided/needed by blood bank	

list of procedures complied by the IADVL which apply to GST taxation.

FIRE SAFETY GUIDELINES

The clinics/hospitals which occupy less than 1000 m² and are less than 15 meters in height do not require a license from the fire safety department. The fire safety compliance required in such a scenario is the presence of an alternate exit (other than the main exit) which may be also be a ramp. However, it is advisable to keep chemical fire extinguishers where LASERs are being used. Larger buildings need to obtain a special license from the fire safety license and the center may also apply for NABH accreditation to standardize the clinic operations and gain confidence of the general public. The criteria for accreditation may be accessed on www.nabh.co/.

CONCLUSION

Various licenses and approvals are needed for smooth running of skin clinics. Awareness of these laws and complying with them, through proper documentation is essential.

KEY POINTS

- Check with your state's CEA and follow it regarding the guidelines, licenses, etc.
- Electronic medical records are helpful and are the order of the day; it is advisable to switch over to them.
- Proper and adequate documentation of every procedure/guideline followed is must.
- A dermatologist can dispense medicines only for his prescription by following the framework.
- Biomedical waste segregation and disposal to be followed.
- Always take advice of a qualified auditor, lawyer for any doubts, clarifications.

SUGGESTED READING

1. Bothara RA. Goods and Services Tax: Effect on Health Care. Dermapractice. 2017;02-07.
2. Central Pollution Control Board (2018). [online]. Available from: http://www.cpcb.nic.in/ [Accessed December, 2018].
3. Clinical Establishment Act Standards for Clinic/Poly Clinic only Consultation (2010). List of emergency drugs. [online]. Available from: <http://clinicalestablishments.gov.in/WriteReadData/9361.pdf [Accessed December, 2018].

4. Clinical Establishments (2010). [online]. Available from: http://clinicalestablishments.gov.in/WriteReadData/969.pdf [Accessed December, 2018].
5. Clinical Establishments (2010). Registration of Skin clinics. [online]. Available from: http://www.clinicalestablishments.gov.in [Accessed December, 2018].
6. Clinical Establishments (2012). Guidelines from CEA specialty wise. [online]. Available from: http://clinicalestablishments.gov.in/WriteReadData/311.pdf [Accessed December, 2018].
7. Dhepe N. Minimum standard guidelines of care on requirements for setting up a laser room. Indian J Dermatol Venereol Leprol. 2009;75(Suppl S2):101-10.
8. Guidelines from CEA http://clinicalestablishments.gov.in/WriteReadData/2591.pdf.
9. Income Tax Department (2018). Income tax Form no 3C for maintaining patient records. [online]. Available from: http://www.incometaxindia.gov.in/ [Accessed December, 2018].
10. Indian Association of Dermatologists, Venereologists and Leprologists (2016). Dermapractice 1,2,3,4. [online]. Available from: <http://www.iadvl.org/newsletter.php> [Accessed December, 2018].
11. Jayanth DP, Mysore V. For the Dermatological Entrepreneur: Regulations for setting up a clinic. Dermapractice. 2015;1:15-27.
12. Ministry of Environment and Forests (1998). Biomedical waste management and handling rules 2011. [online]. Available from: http://www.moef.nic.in/downloads/public.../salient-features-draft-bmwmh.pdf [Accessed December, 2018].
13. National Accreditation Board for Hospitals and Health Care Providers (2018). [online]. Available from: http://www.nabh.co/ [Accessed December, 2018].
14. Pharmacy Council of India (2018). Pharmacy council of India guidelines. [online]. Available from: http://www.pci.nic.in/ [Accessed December, 2018].
15. Sathish DA. Setting up a pharmacy in the clinic. Dermapractice. 2016;(1):17-8.
16. Tamil Nadu Government Gazette Extraordinary (2018). Tamil Nadu Clinical Establishments (Regulation) Rules, 2018. [online]. Available from: http://www.stationeryprinting.tn.gov.in/extraordinary/2018/102_Ex_IV_1_E.pdf [Accessed December, 2018].

CHAPTER 16

Obligations of a Doctor/Medical Establishment under the POCSO Act

Vivekanshu Verma, Rajesh Verma, Santosh Kumar Verma, Devendra Richhariya

INTRODUCTION

Doctors have a dual role to play in terms of the Protection of Children from Sexual Offences (POCSO) Act, 2012. They are in a position to detect that a child has been or is being abused [for example, if they come across a child with a sexually transmitted disease (STD)]; they are also often the first point of reference in confirming that a child has indeed been the victim of sexual abuse.

To deal with child sexual abuse cases, the Government has brought in a special law, namely, The POCSO Act, 2012.[1] The Act has come into force with effect from 14th November, 2012 along with the rules framed thereunder.

The POCSO Act, 2012 is a comprehensive law to provide for the protection of children from the offences of sexual assault, sexual harassment, and pornography, while safeguarding the interests of the child at every stage of the judicial process by incorporating child-friendly mechanisms for reporting, recording of evidence, investigation, and speedy trial of offences through designated special courts.

The said Act defines a child as any person below 18 years of age, and defines different forms of sexual abuse, including penetrative and nonpenetrative assault, as well as sexual harassment and pornography, and deems a sexual assault to be "aggravated" under certain circumstances, such as when the abused child is mentally ill or when the abuse is committed by a person in a position of trust or authority vis-à-vis the child, like a family member, police officer, teacher, or doctor.

The role of the doctor in POCSO Act[2] may include:
- Having an in-depth understanding of sexual victimization
- Obtaining a medical history of the child's experience in a facilitating, nonjudgmental, and empathetic manner
- Meticulously documenting historical details

- Conducting a detailed examination to diagnose acute and chronic residual trauma and STDs, and to collect forensic evidence
- Considering a differential diagnosis of behavioral complaints and physical signs that may mimic sexual abuse
- Obtaining photographic/video documentation of all diagnostic findings that appear to be residual to abuse
- Formulating a complete and thorough medical report with diagnosis and recommendations for treatment
- Testifying in court when required.

There are at least three different circumstances when there is no direct allegation, but when the doctor may consider the diagnosis of sexual abuse and have to ask questions of the parent and child. These include but are not limited to:

- When a child has a complaint that might be directly related to the possibility of sexual abuse, such as a girl with a vaginal discharge
- When a child has a complaint that is not directly related to the possibility of sexual abuse, such as abdominal pain or encopresis (soiling)
- When a child has no complaint but an incidental finding, such as an enlarged hymenal ring, makes the doctor suspicious.

MANDATORY REPORTING[3]

When a doctor has reason to suspect that a child has been or is being sexually abused, he/she is required to report this to the appropriate authorities (i.e. the police or the relevant person within his/her organization who will then have to report it to the police). Failure to do this would result in imprisonment of up to 6 months, with or without fine. (Section 21, POCSO Act, 2012).[1]

ROLE OF CONSENT[3]

Where a child is brought to a doctor for a medical examination to confirm sexual abuse, the doctor must:

- Take the written consent of the child. The three main elements of consent are information, comprehension, and voluntariness. The child and his/her family should be given information about the medical examination process and what is involved therein, so that they can choose whether or not to participate. Secondly, they should be allowed enough time to understand the information and to ask questions so that they can clarify their doubts. Lastly, the child and/or his or her parent/guardian should agree to the examination voluntarily, without feeling pressurized to do so. In some situations it may be appropriate to spend time with the child/adolescent alone, without the parent/guardian present. This may make it easier for the child to ask questions and not feel coerced by a parent/guardian.
- Where the child is too young or otherwise incapable of giving consent, consent should be obtained from the child's parent, guardian or other person in whom the child has trust and confidence.
- The right to informed consent implies the right to informed refusal.
- To be able to give informed consent, the child and his/her parents/guardian need to understand that healthcare professionals may have a legal obligation to report the case and to disclose information received during the course of the consultation to the authorities even in the absence of consent.
- Document who was present during the conversation with the child.
- Document questions asked and child's answers in the child's own words.

- Conduct the examination in a sensitive manner. It is important that the exam is never painful. The exam should be done in a manner that is least disturbing to the child.
- Focus on asking simply worded, open-ended, nonleading questions, such as the "what, when, where, and how" questions, which are important to the medical evaluation of suspected child sexual abuse.
- Reliance should be placed as far as possible on such questioning as "tell me more" followed by "and then what happened?"
- Do not ask uncomfortable questions related to details of the abuse, but try to find out more about the medical and family history of the child.
- Using the child's words for body parts may make the child more comfortable with difficult conversations about sexual activities.
- Using drawings may also help children describe where they may have been touched and with what they were touched.
- Ensure that the child has adequate privacy while the examination is being conducted.
- Do not conduct the examination in a labor room or other place that may cause additional trauma to the child.
- Always ensure patient privacy. Be sensitive to the child's feelings of vulnerability and embarrassment and stop the examination if the child indicates discomfort or withdraws permission to continue.
- Always prepare the child by explaining the examination and showing equipment; this has been shown to diminish fears and anxiety. Encourage the child to ask questions about the examination.
- If the child is old enough, and it is deemed appropriate, ask whom they would like in the room for support during the examination. Some older children may choose a trusted adult to be present. Sexual abuse of children is usually not physically violent. In the large majority of children the physical exam is normal. A normal or nonspecific exam does not rule out sexual abuse.
- As a minimum, the medical history should cover any known health problems (including allergies), immunization status, and medications. In terms of obtaining information about the child's general health status, useful questions to ask would be:
  - Tell me about your general health.
  - Have you seen a nurse or doctor lately?
  - Have you been diagnosed with any illnesses?
  - Have you had any operations?
  - Do you suffer from any infectious diseases?
- Carefully collect and preserve forensic evidence.
- Clothing collection is critical when evidence is collected. Clothing, especially underwear, is the most likely positive site for evidentiary deoxyribonucleic acid (DNA).
- Scene investigation, including collection of linens and clothing should be done early. Evidence from clothing and other objects is more likely to be positive than evidence from the patient's body.
- Children often report weeks or months after the abuse event, and physical injuries to the genital or anal regions usually heal within a few days. This is why the medical provider should always consider differential diagnosis and alternative explanations for physical signs and symptoms.
- In the case of a child with special needs, ensure that the procedures are explained

to the child in a manner which he/she understands and that he/she is asked what help he/she requires, if any (e.g. a child with physical disabilities may need help to get on and off the medical examination table or to assume positions necessary for the examination). However, do not assume that the child will need special aid. Also, ask for permission before proceeding to help the child.
- Recognize that it may be the first time the child is having an internal examination. The child may have very limited knowledge of reproductive health issues and not be able to describe what happened to them. He/she may not know how he/she feels about the incident or even identify that a crime was committed against him/her.
- Wherever necessary, refer the child for counseling.
- Wherever applicable, refer the child for testing for human immunodeficiency virus (HIV) and other STDs.

If the Child Resists the Examination

- If a child of any age refuses the genital-anal examination, it is a clinical judgment of how to proceed. A rule of thumb is that the physical exam should not cause any trauma to the child. It may be wise to defer the examination under these circumstances.
- It may be possible to address some of the child's fears and anxieties (e.g. a fear of needles) or potential sources of unease (e.g. the sex of the examining health worker).

Further, utmost comfort and care for the child should be provided, e.g. examining very small children while on their mother's (or caregiver's) lap or lying with her on a couch (POCSO—Model Guidelines).

- If the child still refuses, the examination may need to be deferred or even abandoned. Never force the examination, especially if there are no reported symptoms or injuries, because findings will be minimal and this coercion may represent yet another assault to the child.
- The child should not be held down or restrained for the examination (exception for infants or very young toddlers).

POCSO—MODEL GUIDELINES

Doctors may be faced with some of these questions from children as well as parents and caregivers.

Q. Why is the medical examination necessary?

The medical exam is a very important tool in evaluating sexual abuse. The physical examination can identify both new and old injuries, detect STDs, and provide evidence of sexual contact. If done in a sensitive manner, the examination can answer any questions or concerns the child may have and reassure the child about their well-being and that their body is private. The exam also has evidentiary value in a court of law.

Q. The last time my child was touched in a sexually inappropriate manner was over a year ago. Is the medical exam still necessary?

Yes. Most children reveal their experience of abuse after a long time has passed, for example, when they are older or feel that they are no longer in danger of being abused again. Some even reveal it accidentally. In such cases, the medical examination can reassure the child about their well-being and address any worried the child may have about the injuries they suffered due to the abuse. Some children may have injuries that healed a long time ago, but can be seen with the help of special equipment.

Q. Is the examination uncomfortable for the child?
No. The examination itself is rarely physically uncomfortable for the child; however, what may cause discomfort is the attitude of the person conducting the examination. For this reason, it is important that all medical healthcare professionals be trained in conducting medical examinations of children in a sensitive manner. The doctor is expected to explain the procedure to the child and his/her parents and obtain their consent prior to conducting the examination, as well as answer any questions they may have.

Q. Can the parent(s) be present while the examination is being conducted?
Yes. Section 27 of the new POCSO Act, 2012[1] specifically requires that the examination be conducted in the presence of the child's parents/guardian or other person in whom the child has trust and confidence.

Q. Is the medical examination of the child conducted in the same manner as an adult female gynecological examination?
Unlike routine per speculum examination in adult females. No speculum examination in prepubescent children. During examination of the external genitalia– do not use traction in children under the age of 1 year.

Q. Will the doctor/nurse be able to tell if there was penetration?
Yes, if their are signs and symptoms of penetrative trauma in genitalia of the child, such as bleeding, bruise or swelling, lacerated/incised wound, than it is suggestive of penetration.

Q. How is the examination of a boy different from that of a girl?
Male victims tend to be less willing to report rape than females. Forensic evidence from oral or anal penetration collected within 24–36 hours (72 hours in infants). Additional sterile saline swabs from mouth, penis, scrotum, perineum and anus/rectum in male victims. Pharyngeal gonorrhea is not uncommon after forced oral penetration.

Q. Why cannot a family doctor or another doctor known to the child do the examination?
Code of Medical Ethics states that physicians generally should not treat themselves or members of their immediate families. Obviously, emotions play a role when it comes to family.

Q. What are obligations of a doctor/medical establishment under the POSCO Act?
All medical professionals and nurses providing the first aid and advanced medical care to the survivor child are bound to abide by these principles:
- *Right to life and survival:*[3] Every child has the right to life and survival and to be shielded from any form of further physical, psychological, and mental abuse or neglect during treatment.
- *The best interests of the child:*[3] Protecting the child's best interests means not only protecting the child from secondary victimization and hardship while involved in the justice process as victim or witness, but also enhancing the child's capacity to contribute to that process. Secondary victimization refers to the victimization that occurs not as a direct result of the Criminal Act, but through the response of hospitals and doctors to the victim.
- *The right to be treated with dignity and compassion:*[3] Child victims should be treated in a caring and sensitive manner throughout the treatment process, taking into account their personal situation and immediate needs, age, gender, disability

and level of maturity, and fully respecting their physical, mental and moral integrity. Efforts should also be made to reduce the number of doctors interviewing the child. At the same time, however, it is important that high standards of evidence collection are maintained in order to ensure fair and equitable outcomes of the justice process. In order to avoid further hardship to the child, interviews, examination, and other forms of investigation should be conducted by trained professionals who proceed in a sensitive, respectful, and thorough manner in a child-friendly environment. All interactions should also take place in a language that the child uses and understands. Medical examination should be ordered only where it is necessary for the investigation of the case and is in the best interests of the child and it should be minimally intrusive.

- *The right to be informed*:[3] The important aspects of child victims' right to be informed about the process of medical examination, and informed consent to be taken in age more than 12 years along with guardian's consent.
- *The right to privacy*:[3] The child's privacy and identity must be protected at all stages of the hospital stay. The release of information about a child victim, in particular in the media, may endanger the child's safety, cause the child intense shame and humiliation, discourage him from telling what happened, and cause him severe emotional harm. There are two essential ways of protecting the privacy of child victims: firstly, by restricting the disclosure of information on child victims and secondly, by restricting the attendance of the general public or nonessential persons in hospital wards.
- *The right to safety*:[3] Where the safety of a child victim may be at risk, appropriate measures should be taken to require the reporting of those safety risks to appropriate authorities (security guards) and to protect the child from such risk before, during, and after the surgical treatment in hospital.
- *The right to free medical treatment to the child victim, in case of absence of any financial support by the guardian. Emergency medical care*: The child may be brought to the hospital for emergency medical care as soon as the police receive a report of the commission of an offence against the child. In such cases, the rules under the POCSO Act, 2012 prescribe that the child is to be taken to the nearest hospital or medical care facility. This may be a government facility or a private one. This is reiterated by Section 23 of the Criminal Law Amendment Act,[4] which inserts Section 357C into the Code of Criminal Procedure (CrPC), 1973. This Section provides that all hospitals are required to provide first aid or medical treatment, free of cost, to the victims of a sexual offence.

SECTION 27 OF POCSO ACT—MEDICAL EXAMINATION[1]

- The medical examination of a child in respect of whom any offence has been committed under this Act, shall, notwithstanding that a first information report (FIR) or complaint has not been registered for the offences under this Act, be conducted in accordance with Section 164A of the Code of CrPC, 1973.
- In case the victim is a girl child, the medical examination shall be conducted by a woman doctor.

- The medical examination shall be conducted in the presence of the parent of the child or any other person in whom the child reposes trust or confidence.
- Where, in case the parent of the child or other person referred to in subsection 3 of POCSO Act cannot be present, for any reason, during the medical examination of the child, the medical examination shall be conducted in the presence of a woman nominated by the head of the medical institution.

RULE 5 OF POCSO ACT— EMERGENCY MEDICAL CARE[1]

1. Where an officer of the Special Juvenile Police Unit (SJPU) or the local police receives information under Section 19 of the Act that an offence under the Act has been committed, and is satisfied that the child against whom an offence has been committed is in need of urgent medical care and protection, he shall, as soon as possible, but not later than 24 hours of receiving such information, arrange to take such child to the nearest hospital or medical care facility center for emergency medical care. Provided that where an offence has been committed under Sections 3, 5, 7 or 9 of the Act, the victim shall be referred to emergency medical care.
2. Emergency medical care shall be rendered in such a manner as to protect the privacy of the child, and in the presence of the parent or guardian or any other person in whom the child has trust and confidence.
3. No medical practitioner, hospital or other medical facility center rendering emergency medical care to a child shall demand any legal or magisterial requisition or other documentation as a prerequisite to rendering such care.
4. The registered medical practitioner rendering emergency medical care shall attend to the needs of the child, including:
   - Treatment for cuts, bruises, and other injuries including genital injuries, if any;
   - Treatment for exposure to STDs including prophylaxis for identified STDs;
   - Treatment for exposure to HIV, including prophylaxis for HIV after necessary consultation with infectious disease experts;
   - Possible pregnancy and emergency contraceptives should be discussed with the pubertal child and her parent or any other person in whom the child has trust and confidence; and,
   - Wherever necessary, a referral or consultation for mental or psychological health or other counseling should be made.
5. Any forensic evidence collected in the course of rendering emergency medical care must be collected in accordance with Section 27 of the Act.

Q. Does a doctor have a legal duty to inform the authorities if a minor girl is pregnant?
Yes. Section 19(1) of the POCSO Act[1] requires anyone who knows that a sexual offence has been committed to report the case to the appropriate authorities (the local police or SJPU or child protection committee) or to the relevant person in the organization who could report the pregnancy to the appropriate authorities (for example, the Chief Medical Officer). Anyone who knowingly fails to make this report can be punished with up to 6 months in prison and a fine. However, the doctor does not need to wait till the authorities take action and may proceed with the termination of pregnancy in line with the provisions of the Medical Termination

of Pregnancy (MTP) Act after maintaining complete and detailed records of the case.

Q. Does a doctor have a legal duty to inform the authorities if a minor girl is married and is pregnant by her husband with her will and consent?

Marital status makes no difference to the reporting requirement under the POCSO Act. Anyone who knowingly fails to make this report can be punished with up to 6 months in prison and a fine. As per Section 164(A) of the Criminal Procedure Code, any Registered Medical Practitioner can conduct a medico-legal examination for injuries and abuse.

Q. What to do if there is no proof of age and the victim seems to be a minor?

If the girl's age is uncertain, it is advised to report the pregnancy as per the legal requirement under the POCSO Act and to allow the authorities to decide what actions to take. Not knowing the girl's exact age may bring up the question of reporting requirement under the POCSO Act, but these details should not impact the legality of the termination under the MTP Act. The provider does not need to wait for the authorities to take action and may proceed with the termination of pregnancy in line with the provisions of the MTP Act after maintaining complete and detailed records of the case.

Q. What conduct is sufficient to satisfy a doctor's duty to report under the POCSO Act while offering MTP services to a minor?

Providing a medicolegal certificate to the authorities is sufficient to comply with the reporting requirements of the POCSO Act. A doctor is not obligated to file an FIR or to conduct an investigation; the doctor's duty is only to inform the authorities when providing safe abortion service under the MTP Act.

Q. Under the MTP Act, a minor girl needs written permission from her guardian to get an abortion. Who counts as a "guardian"?

The MTP Act defines guardian as a person "having the care" of the minor person. This is a fairly broad definition and includes anyone who has the care of a minor girl. Thus, an adult, i.e. someone over 18 years of age who accompanies a minor girl to a clinic could be a de-facto guardian and could consent to an abortion on the girl's behalf.

Q. Does a medical provider have to wait for any medicolegal procedure before performing the abortion?

Rule no. 5(3) of the POCSO Rules state that "No medical practitioner, hospital or other medical facility center rendering emergency medical care to a child shall demand any legal or magisterial requisition or other documentation as a prerequisite to rendering" emergency medical care.

Similarly, the 2013 Ministry of Health and Family Welfare Guidelines and Protocols: Medico-legal Care for Survivors/Victims of Sexual Violence[3] state: "Providing treatment and necessary medical investigations is the prime responsibility of the examining doctor" and that "admission, evidence collection or filing a police complaint is not mandatory for providing treatment." This means that providers can even inform the authorities about the pregnant minor after performing the abortion. Rape is a legal ground for terminating a pregnancy under Section 3 of the MTP Act and given the 20-week limit in the Act, it is important to provide medical care at the earliest while legal proceeding can continue simultaneously.

Q. Does the doctor have a legal obligation to preserve the products of conception (POC) for abortion services for minor girls?

Section 201 of the Indian Penal Code (IPC)[5] prohibits causing "any evidence of the commission" of an offence to disappear with the intention of screening the offender from legal punishment. Crucially, this includes an important intent component. It would be considered a violation only if a provider destroys evidence with the intent to protect the accused from legal action. Therefore, doctors who dispose of the POC for a good faith reason (for example, inadequate preservation facilities or following standard operating procedures), should be shielded from prosecution. However, since a minor girl who is pregnant is considered a rape victim under the law, the POC might be evidence of an offence that the medical provider must preserve under Section 201 if possible.

Section 8 of the MTP Act[6] guarantees protection for doctors, who act in good faith. This recognizes that above all else, it is imperative that girls and women receive the highest standard of medical care available. Accordingly, all doctors should fulfill their reporting requirements and legal obligations under the MTP Act and the POCSO Act after ensuring essential services. A doctor is not obligated to file an FIR or to conduct an investigation; the provider's duty is only to inform the authorities when providing safe abortion service under the MTP Act.

THE POCSO ACT AND THE MTP ACT

The MTP Act, 1971[6] governs induced abortion service delivery in India. It very clearly defines by who, where, and when abortion services may be provided. The Government of India enacted the POCSO Act, 2012 to prevent and address child sexual abuse. These Acts overlap where the POCSO Act requires medical providers to report sexual abuse among minors and the MTP Act allows registered providers to terminate pregnancies resulting from rape. The intersection between the MTP Act and the POCSO Act creates confusion, delays, and sometimes denial of abortion services for young girls.

MEDICOLEGAL REPORTING OF CHILD SURVIVOR OF SEXUAL VIOLENCE

Medicolegal reports (MLRs) are documents prepared by a government and private doctors, pertaining to injury, sexual offence, suspected poisoning or unexplained death (Box 1). It contains all the facts observed by the doctor and his opinion drawn therefrom. Doctor's opinion must be based upon the clinical observations made by him, and not on hearsay evidence.

Doctor's Dilemma: What to do First—MLR Documentation or Treatment?

In the hospital, while attending to an emergency, the doctor should understand that his first priority is to save the life of the patient. He

> **BOX 1:** Mnemonics for easy recall for medicolegal report (MLR) for unconscious patient with suspected drug overdose, poisoning and intoxication in survivors of sexual violence: All W's.
> - W: Who is victim (name, age, gender, and address)
> - W: Which occupation of child (school student, farmer, household worker, room cleaner, and sweeper)
> - W: What poison consumed (than call poison control center)
> - W: What quantity consumed (fatal dose)
> - W: When consumed (fatal period)
> - W: What is route of poisoning (ingestion/inhalation/injection—subcutaneous, intramuscular, and intravenous)
> - W: Where consumed (place of crime)—to collect evidence by police
> - W: What number of victims (mass casualty)
> - W: Who gave poison—only in dying declaration (suicidal/homicidal/accidental)
> - W: Why (intentional, nonintentional, suicidal, homicidal, and accidental)

should do everything possible to resuscitate the patient and ensure that he is out of danger. All legal formalities stand suspended till this is achieved. This has been clearly exemplified by the Honorable Supreme Court of India in Parmanand Katara versus Union of India.[7]

Sampling in a Case of Suspected Poisoning with Sexual Violence

- Blood, urine, clothes or gastric lavage are preserved for chemical analysis.
- Three swabs from genitalia, nail clippings, and loose hair on the body/clothes are preserved for DNA study to identify the accused, based on Locard's principle of exchange.
- Containers with forensic and toxicology samples must be well-labeled, the name of suspected poisoning and assault communicated in form of copy of MLR and all sample packets are signed by the doctor, after sealing the sample.
- *Chain of custody*: Samples should be carefully handed over to police investigating officer, to be sent to Forensic Science Laboratory (FSL), and receiving should be taken on MLR, from the police officer.

Do's and Don'ts of MLR Writing for Doctors

- Always intimate the police about medicolegal case (MLC) promptly—not informing police to screen offender—Section 201 IPC—punishable 3 years.
- Medicolegal case reports should be prepared in duplicate preferably with ball pen.
- No overwriting in MLR, if any word corrected, it should be initiated by signature of doctor, any tempering or altercation in entries—Fabricating false evidence—Section 191 IPC—punishable 7 years.
- Medicolegal reports are confidential legal documents, do not issue to anyone in right to information, except the patient.
- Do not miss the court date on summons—arrest warrant will be issued—contempt of court—Section 228 IPC—punishable 6 months.

Query: How to interpret summon of witness?[8]

- I happened to observe that mostly odd numbers of last digit, with regard to IPC Sections are safer in law and bailable than even numbers, which are nonbailable.
- It is helpful in interpreting summon of witness/warrant received by doctors, to appear after making MLR.
- In even numbers IPC in summon (Box 2), Doctors need to be ready to answer in court to defense lawyer and judge, whether the injuries were dangerous to life or not?

In Case of Death due to Sexual Violence on a Child

- Recording date and time of death
- Information to the police
- Death certificate not to be issued
- Body to be sent for medicolegal autopsy
- Postmortem (PM) certificate issued after autopsy may be issued in place of death certificate towards registration of death.

Q. When can a copy of the MLC report be issued by the hospital to the accused?
If an accused wants attested copy of the MLR, he should apply for such a copy to the holder of the original. The original is supposed to be with the police. However, if the original is with the hospital/doctor, a copy can be supplied as per court orders or on production of a No Objection Certificate from the police.[8]

> **BOX 2:** Even numbers Indian Penal Code (IPC) and nonbailable offences in IPC.
> - 124-A IPC: Sedition
> - 148 IPC: Riot by dangerous weapon
> - 232 IPC: Counterfeiting coin and currency notes
> - 274 IPC: Adulteration of drugs
> - 302 IPC: Murder
> - 304 IPC: Culpable homicide
> - 304B: Dowry death
> - 306 IPC: Abetment of suicide
> - 308 IPC: Attempt to commit culpable homicide
> - 314: Causing death by Act with intent of miscarriage
> - 316: Causing death of a quick unborn child
> - 324: Dangerous weapon causing hurt
> - 326: Dangerous weapon/means causing grievous hurt
> - 326A: Grievous hurt by use of acid
> - 326B: Voluntarily throwing acid or attempting to throw
> - 328: Criminal poisoning
> - 332: Voluntarily causing hurt to deter public servant from duty
> - 354: Outrage modesty of woman
> - 354B: Intent to disrobe woman
> - 364: Kidnapping for murder/ransom
> - 370: Human trafficking
> - 372: Selling/hiring minor for prostitution
> - 376 A, B, C, and D: Rape, gang rape, custodial rape, and rape-murder
> - 384: Extortion.
> - 386: Extortion by threat of death/grievous hurt
> - 392: Robbery
> - 406: Criminal breach of trust
> - 420: Cheating
> - 436: Mischief by fire/explosive
> - 466: Forgery of a record of—court/birth and death register/MLR/PMR
> - 498A: Cruelty to married woman for demand of dowry.
> - Section 4 of the POCSO Act: Penetrative sexual assault
> - Section 6 of the POCSO Act: Aggravated penetrative sexual assault
> - Section 8 of the POCSO Act: Sexual assault
> - Section 10 of the POCSO Act: Aggravated sexual assault
> - Section 12 of the POCSO Act: Sexual harassment
> - Section 14 of the POCSO Act: Using child for pornographic purposes
> - Section 18 of the POCSO Act: Attempt to commit an offence[8]
>
> (MLR: medicolegal report; PMR: postmortem report; POCSO: Protection of Children from Sexual Offences)

RECENT UPDATES IN LAWS REGULATING SEXUAL ASSAULT ON CHILDREN: CRIMINAL LAW AMENDMENT ORDINANCE, 2018[9]

An ordinance providing the death penalty for rapists of girls below 12 years of age and other stringent penal provisions for rape.

Salient Features of the Ordinance

- Minimum punishment for rape made 10 years.
- Minimum punishment of 20 years to a person committing rape on a woman aged below 16 years.
- Minimum punishment of 20 years rigorous imprisonment and maximum death penalty/life imprisonment for committing rape on a girl aged below 12 years.
- Fine imposed shall be just and reasonable to meet the medical expenses and rehabilitation of the victim.
- Police officer/doctor/warden committing custodial rape shall be awarded rigorous imprisonment of minimum 10 years.
- Investigation in rape cases to be completed within 2 months.
- No anticipatory bail can be granted to a person accused of rape of girls of age less than 16 years.
- Appeals in rape cases to be disposed within 6 months.
- Section 376DA and 376DB provide minimum punishment of life imprisonment for persons involved in gang rape of woman aged less than 16 years and 12 years, respectively.
- Death penalty is also prescribed for persons involved in gang rape of a girl of age less than 12 years.
- It is also provided in these sections, that such fine shall be imposed which shall be just and reasonable to meet the medical

expenses and rehabilitation of the victim and the fine imposed is to be paid to the victim.

- New subsection has been added to Section 439 which mandates presence of informant or any person authorized by him at the time of hearing application for bail to a person accused of rape of girls of age less than 16 years.

2018 AMENDMENT TO POCSO ACT AND EVIDENCE ACT[9]

Section 42 of the POCSO Act has been also amended to include newly inserted IPC provisions Section 376AB, Section 376DA, and Section 376DB. Section 53A of the Evidence Act that deals with evidence of character or previous sexual experience not relevant in certain cases and Section 146 of the Act that deals with evidence of character or previous sexual experience not relevant in certain cases, has also been amended to include newly inserted IPC provisions Section 376AB, Section 376DA, and Section 376DB.

Q: What are the legal guidelines for hospitals for free treatment of victims of sexual assault in emergency?

All cases coming to emergency services should be registered and stabilized before retransfer to other hospital. As per Clinical Establishment Act (CEA), emergency treatment is free and cannot be charged, CEA has been notified in many states.[8]

The Honorable Supreme Court in their judgment dated 06-05-1996 in SLP (C) No. 796/92—Paschim Banga Khet Mazdoor Samity and Others versus State of West Bengal; suggested remedial measures to ensure immediate medical attention and treatment to persons in real need.

The following guidelines may be kept in view while dealing with emergency cases in addition to the existing guidelines:

- In the hospital, the Medical Officer in the emergency/casualty services should admit a patient whose condition is morbid/serious in consultation with the specialist concerned on duty in the emergency department.
- In case the vacant beds are not available in the concerned department to accommodate such patient, the patient has to be given all necessary attention.
- Subsequently, the Medical Officer will make necessary arrangement to get the patient transferred to another hospital in the ambulance. The position as to whether there is vacant bed in the concerned department has to be ascertained before transferring the patient. The patient will be accompanied by the resident Medical Officer in the ambulance.
- In no case the patient will be left unattended for want of vacant beds in the emergency/casualty department.
- The services of Centralised Accident and Trauma Services (CATS) should be utilized to the extent possible in Delhi.
- The efforts may be made to monitor the functioning of the emergency department periodically by the Heads of the institution.
- The medical record of patient attending the emergency services should be preserved in the medical record department.
- The Medical Superintendent may coordinate with each other for providing better emergency services.[8]

Q: Is consent of the patient/relatives is required for labeling the case as MLC in child victims of rape?

Consent of the patient/relatives is not required for labeling the case as MLC. In fact, even if the patient is stressing that he does not want an MLC, it should still be made.[8]

Q: Can private practitioners (PPs) make an MLC in child victims of rape?
Private practitioners can make an MLC. The practice by PPs of sending patients to government hospitals for getting registered as MLC cases are wrong. If the patient is serious, and dies on the way to government hospital, the PP can be sued under Section 304A IPC. Treatment in serious cases must take precedence over completion of the injury report. Injury report can be completed after patient has stabilized.

Referral to a second hospital: If a case has been labeled as medicolegal and has been referred to another hospital, it is in second doctor's interest to make a fresh MLC (second MLC), so as to record meticulously his own findings. It is because when he is summoned in the court, he has to go by his own findings.

Dead on arrival ("brought dead" cases): All cases which are pronounced dead on arrival at hospital must be labeled as MLC and police be informed.[8]

Q: Who can waive off PM in MLCs, e.g. child dies after rape?
Please remember that police officer of cadre Superintendent of Police (SP) has power to waive off any PM. Doctor conducts PM only on request of police/magistrate. Doctor cannot do PM on its own. Even for pathological autopsy, he needs consent from relatives of deceased.[8]

Q: Can a male doctor examine a female breast of minor or a vaginal exam in survivors of sexual assault under POCSO Act?
Female doctor should do the examination of female minors, if no female doctor is available in nearby center, chaperone female nurse should be present, while managing the victim in emergency, whose signature should be taken on MLR as witness of medicolegal examination. In minor male victims of sexual assault under POCSO, both male/female doctors can examine, with consent of legal guardian of the patient.

Q: Can an AYUSH doctor prepare a MLR or perform an autopsy in child victims under POCSO Act?
No. This can be done only by an MBBS doctor. This is supported by the following legal provisions:
- Indian Medical Council Act, 1956—Clauses (c) and (d) of Section 15(2) of the Indian Medical Council Act, 1956, read as follows:
  - "No person other than a medical practitioner enrolled on a State Medical Register.
  - (c) shall be entitled to sign or authenticate a medical or fitness certificate or any other certificate required by any law to be signed or authenticated by a duly qualified medical practitioner.
  - (d) shall be entitled to give evidence at any inquest or in any court of law as an expert under Section 45 of the Indian Evidence Act (IEA), 1872 on any matter relating to medicine.

IMPORTANT POINTS

- Section 45 of the IEA, 1872 reads—When the Court has to form an opinion upon a point of foreign law or of science, or art, or as to identity of handwriting, or finger impressions, the opinions upon that point of persons especially skilled in such foreign law, science or art, or in questions as to identity of handwriting or finger impressions are relevant facts. Such persons are called experts.

Obligations of a Doctor/Medical Establishment under the POCSO Act

- Code of CrPC, 1973—Section 53 of the Code of CrPC, 1973, reads—"Examination of accused by medical practitioner at the request of police officer:
  - When a person is arrested on a charge of committing an offence of such a nature and alleged to have been committed under such circumstances that there are reasonable grounds for believing that an examination of his person will afford evidence as to the commission of an offence, it shall be lawful for a registered medical practitioner, acting, at the request of a police officer not below the rank of Sub-Inspector, and for—any person acting in good faith in his aid and—under his direction, to make such all examination of the person arrested as is reasonably necessary in order to ascertain the facts which may afford such evidence, and to use such force as is reasonably necessary for that purpose.
  - Whenever the person of a female is to be examined under this Section, the examination shall be made only by, or under the supervision of, a female registered medical practitioner.
  Explanation—In this Section and in Sections 53A and 54:
    - "Examination" shall include the examination of blood, blood stains, semen, swabs in case of sexual offences, sputum and sweat, hair samples and finger nail clippings by the use of modern and scientific techniques including DNA profiling, and such other tests which the registered medical practitioner thinks necessary in a particular case;
    - "Registered medical practitioner" means a medical practitioner who possesses any medical qualification as defined in clause (h) of Section 2 of the Indian Medical Council Act, 1956 and whose name has been entered in a State Medical Register."[8]

RECENT CASE LAWS RELATED TO OBLIGATIONS OF A DOCTOR/MEDICAL ESTABLISHMENT RELATED TO VIOLATION THE POCSO ACT

Case Law 1: Describe a Case Law Resolving Conflict between 375 IPC and POCSO Act in Marital Rape by Husband on his Wife, Who is Minor

The Supreme Court held that a man will be punished for rape if he is found to be guilty of having sexual intercourse with his minor wife. With this verdict, the Supreme Court has ended the disparity between this exception to Section 375, which allows a husband to have sexual relationship with his 15-year-old wife, and the definition of "child" in recent laws such as the POCSO Act, 2012, which includes any person below the age of 18 years.[10]

Case Law 2: Describe a Case Law of Perjury against a Minor Victim of Rape under POCSO Act, for Misusing Law during False Complaint against her Accused Father

The case before the court related to the rape of the girl allegedly done by her father. Though victim testified against her father in the examination-in-chief (a process where the victim is examined by the prosecution), she turned hostile at the end of the cross-examination conducted by the defense counsel. The trial strategy on part of the defense was similar to rape trials involving adult women victims, where attempts are made to devalue the credibility of the victim by questioning her sexual history. Despite the amendment to Section 146(3) of the IEA 1871, where the defense is prohibited from questioning the sexual history of the rape victim; and the repealing of Section 155(4) of the IEA which permitted the defense to argue that the victim was of "immoral character" in the course of the trial, these practices continue. The defense counsel in the case posed questions relating to her association with boys and her father's disapproval of it. It was alleged that she filed a false complaint at the instance of a family feud between her father and maternal relatives. The victim turned hostile towards the end of the cross-examination by stating that the complaint was filed due to a fight with her father. On 22 December 2016, Special Court in Thane, Maharashtra issued a perjury notice to a 16-year-old minor girl in a case under the POCSO Act. But the agonizing aspect of the case is a perjury notice issued against her and her transfer to the Juvenile Justice Board (JJB), under the provisions of the Juvenile Justice Act, 2000.[11]

Case Law 3: Describe a Case Law in Refusing to Extend POCSO to Adults with Mental Retardation

The case before the court related to the rape of a 38-year-old woman with cerebral palsy. Her mother was concerned about the absence of a friendly and congenial atmosphere before the trial court. She approached the courts for a direction to transfer the case to a Special Court under POCSO, a law that mandates child-friendly procedures and features during the trial, taking into account her daughter's mental age, which she said was that of a 6-year-old. In a fateful turn of events, the lone accused died during these proceedings, bringing the criminal case to an end. The implication of the Supreme Court ruling is that the onus is always on trial judges to keep in mind the degree of retardation of victims and their level of understanding while appreciating their evidence. It would be unfortunate if cases get derailed because of either the victims' inability to communicate effectively or because of the court's difficulty in understanding their words or gestures. It is now up to the legislature to consider the introduction of legal provisions to determine mental competence so victims with inadequate mental development may effectively testify against sexual offenders. The Supreme Court has shown due restraint in declining to apply the provisions of the POCSO Act to mentally retarded adults whose mental age may be that of a child. It would have been tempting to give a purposive interpretation to the term "child" under POCSO, which refers to those below 18 years of age, and rule that it encompasses those with a "mental age" of a person below 18 years. It would have been compelling to acknowledge how similarly a child and an adult with inadequate intellectual growth are placed when it comes to sexual assault: both may show the same lack of understanding about the situation they are in and incapacity to protest. No doubt, any expanded definition to encompass both biological and mental age within the POCSO framework would have helped extend its beneficial features to another section of vulnerable persons. The court has chosen the challenging path of analyzing the import of such judicial interpretation, along with the question whether expanding the notion of age is within its remit. It has ruled that it is outside its domain. POCSO is meant to protect children from sexual offences. To extend it to adult victims based on mental age would require determination of their mental competence. This would need statutory provisions and rules; the legislature alone is competent to enact them. Judicial conferment of power to trial courts to treat some adults as children-based on mental capacity would, in the Bench's opinion, do violence to the existing law protecting children from sexual offences.[12]

Case Law 4: Describe a Latest Case Law of Supreme Court, Quashing FIR against Doctor/Medical Establishment Treating Rape Victim, on Failing to Inform the Police, after Knowledge of the Crime of Rape, thus Violating the POCSO Act

In this case, Church priest had raped the victim when she was a minor in the year 2016. As a result, she became pregnant. When the victim started complaining about pain in her abdomen, her mother brought her to the doctor/medical establishment, on 7th February, 2017. It was found by the gynecologist that the victim was in advance stage of pregnancy. In fact, soon after she was brought to the hospital, she went into labor. She delivered the child. When the victim was brought to the hospital, her mother informed the treating doctor that she had been raped by the accused when she was a minor. Doctor/medical establishment did not inform the police about the raped victim. Later, victim filed complaint against doctor/medical establishment, accusing them in FIR, for not informing police under Section 19(1) of the POCSO Act—a person who had an apprehension that an offence under the said Act is likely to be committed or has knowledge that such an offence had been committed would be required to provide such information to the police. The provisions of Section 19(1), reproduced above, put a legal obligation on treating doctor to inform the police, inter alia, when he/she has knowledge that an offence under the Act had been committed. Thus, what is alleged against the treating doctors is that they had the knowledge that an offence under the Act had been committed and, therefore, they were required to provide this information to the relevant authorities which they failed to do. Doctor's defense lawyer argued that they did not knew that the victim was a minor when she had sexual intercourse, the medical records of the victim state that she was 18 years' old as on 7th February, 2017. In these circumstances, it was the professional duty of gynecologist to attend to her and conduct the delivery, which she did dutifully. Likewise, after the baby was born, the pediatrician performed her professional duty. Being the administrator of the hospital it was not possible for her to be aware of the details of each patient. The expression used is "knowledge" which means that some information received by such a person gives him/her knowledge about the commission of the crime. There is no obligation on doctors to investigate and gather knowledge. If at all, the doctors were not careful enough to find the cause of pregnancy as the victim was only 18 years of age at the time of delivery. But that would not be translated into criminality. The entire case set up against the doctors is on the basis that when the victim was brought to the hospital her age was recorded as 18 years. On that basis doctors could have gathered that at the time of conception she was less than 18 years and was, thus, a minor and, therefore, the doctors should have taken due care in finding as to how the victim became pregnant.

Fastening the criminal liability on the basis of the aforesaid allegation is too far-fetched. After going through the record and hearing the counsel for the both parties, Supreme Court was of the opinion that no such case is made out even as per the material collected by the prosecution. Thus the Supreme Court quashed the complaint against the doctors and hospital administrator and discharged the gynecologist, pediatrician, and the hospital administrator from charges of POCSO Act violation.[13]

Case Law 5: Describe a Case Law Related to Male Victim in POCSO Act, in which Accused Attempted to Lure the Minor into Sexual Act, and POCSO Case was Quashed in Victim's Interest

In this case, the accused, an auto-rickshaw driver, had not even touched the boy and that only an attempt had been made to lure the minor into sexual Acts by showing sex videos and his private parts. FIR was registered by the victim, and underwent medicolegal examination by duty doctor, no injuries noted on the body of victim. During police investigation, it was noted that only an attempt was made to lure the boy. Later in court, petition was filed by the accused to quash the case booked against him on the basis of a compromise reached between him and the victim's family. During an in-camera interaction, the boy told the judge that his family had decided to bury the hatchet in the interest of his studies. The Madras High Court has quashed a case booked under the POCSO Act, because the victim, a boy who was hardly a few days away from attaining majority, did not want to pursue the case as it would affect his studies and his future career.[14]

REFERENCES

1. Protection of Children from Sexual Offences Act, 2012. Available from: wcd.nic.in/sites/default/files/POCSO-ModelGuidelines.pdf
2. Moirangthem S, Kumar NC, Math SB. Child sexual abuse: Issues & concerns. Indian J Med Res. 2015;142(1):1-3.
3. Ministry of Health and Family Welfare Guidelines and Protocols: Medico-legal care for survivors/victims of sexual violence. Available from: https://mohfw.gov.in/reports/guidelines-and-protocols-medico-legal-care-survivors-victims-sexual-violence
4. Criminal Law Amendment Act, 2013.
5. Indian Penal Code, 1860.
6. Medical Termination of Pregnancy Act, 1971.
7. Parmanand Katara vs Union of India (1989) 4 SCC 286.
8. Richhariya D. Textbook of Emergency & Trauma Care, 1st edition. New Delhi: Jaypee Brothers Medical Publishers (P) Ltd.; 2018. pp. 35-71.
9. Criminal Law Amendment Ordinance, 2018.
10. The Hindu (2017). What is the Conflict between IPC 375 and POCSO Act? [online] Available from: https://www.thehindu.com/news/national/what-is-the-conflict-between-ipc-375-and-pocso-act/article19839944.ece [Accessed December 2018].
11. Livelaw (2018). A Case of Perjury Against a Minor: The POCSO Act and its Implementation. [online] Available from https://www.livelaw.in/case-perjury-minor-pocso-act-implementation/ [Accessed December 2018].
12. The Hindu. (2017). Questions of Age—On SC's Ruling on POCSO Act. [online] Available from: https://www.thehindu.com/opinion/editorial/questions-of-age/article19365965.ece [Accessed December 2018].
13. Supreme Court quashing Complaint against Doctors in Dr. SR. Tessy Jose and Others vs State of Kerala. SLP(CRL.) No. 3712 of 2018.
14. The Hindu (2018). POCSO Case quashed in 'Victim's Interest'. [online] Available from: https://www.thehindu.com/news/national/tamil-nadu/pocso-case-quashed-in-victims-interest/article23543678.ece [Accessed December 2018].

CHAPTER 17

What Ails Medical Laws in India

Chandrashekhar Sohoni

INTRODUCTION

Over the last two decades or so, a paradigm shift has happened in the way medicine is practiced in India. For a long time after independence, medicine was only subject to the rule of science and judgment of physicians. But over the last 2–3 decades, there has been a rapid influx of legal regulations in medical practice, the seed of which lies in the changing demographic and socioeconomic landscape of India. Liberalization of economy, rapid urbanization, better education, accessibility to internet and technology and consumer rights movement superimposed over deep-rooted traditional beliefs have been largely responsible for this shift.

Unfortunately, physicians in India are struggling to adapt to this shift, and for good reasons. In this chapter, we examine the palpable anomalies, which are primarily responsible for an average Indian doctor feeling unwanted in his own house.

OVER-REGULATION

In 1912, the late Louis D Brandeis, former Supreme Court Justice, United States of America, had remarked: "If we desire respect for the law, we must first make the law respectable". Today, this statement resonates with Indian physicians. The Central Clinical Establishment Act, which was introduced in 2010 with an aim to regulate clinical establishments, has gradually turned into a threat for the survival of small healthcare establishments. The primary reason for the same is the impractical infrastructure and human resource demands that some of the State Clinical Establishment Acts are imposing upon small healthcare establishments.

The West Bengal Clinical Establishment Act (WB CEA), 2017 is a prime example of such over-regulation. As if the infrastructure and human resource requirements were not enough, the WB CEA provides for criminal prosecution of doctors for alleged medical negligence, financial penalty up to ₹ 50 lac for death due to negligence and substantial penalty even for minor rectifiable deficiencies in the clinical establishment that do not pose any imminent danger to the health and safety of any patient. The Act gives unbridled powers to the authorities, enabling them to close down the clinical establishment and even forfeit the property in case of grievous injury or death of a patient. The Act establishes a separate Commission for prosecution of doctors and clinical establishments for medical negligence, deficiency in service or other deviations from the norms. The Commission has the powers of a civil court and it is a remedy in addition to the already existing remedy of Consumer Forums and Consumer Commissions. The Act has a unique provision for the authority to publish the name and place of residence of the negligent doctor, along with the offence and penalty imposed, in case of grievous injury or death of a patient. The Act also provides for regulation of the pricing of various healthcare services. Conveniently, the Act is only applicable to private clinical establishments, leaving government-run clinical establishments out of its ambit.

The Central Clinical Establishment Act provides for mandatory stabilization of a patient brought in emergency to a clinical establishment, without any provision for reimbursement of the cost of such treatment. Healthcare is considered a fundamental right under Article 21 of the Constitution of India and the Directive Principles of State Policy put the onus for providing the same on the State. However, an inadequate public healthcare system, largely a result of abysmal government spending on healthcare (slightly more than 1% of the GDP as of date), is looking to shift the onus of this fundamental duty of State to private healthcare establishments via the way of over-regulation.[1]

As a largely resource-restricted country where a significant percentage of population still lives in poverty, such over-regulation of healthcare is disastrous. An insecure healthcare system gives rise to an unnecessary compliance industry, the costs of which are ultimately borne by the end-user, i.e. the patient. And if over-regulation does not allow the costs to be passed on to the patient, private healthcare system becomes nonviable and ultimately collapses.

OVERCRIMINALIZATION

The Preconception and Prenatal Diagnostic Techniques (PCPNDT) Act, 1994 equates any deficiency or inaccuracy in record-keeping with the offence of sex-determination, and also prescribes the same degree of punishment for errors in record-keeping as for sex-determination. This is a unique piece of legislation, which criminalizes a human error like any deficiency or inaccuracy of record-keeping.

The aims of labeling a particular action or inaction as criminal offence and prescribing punishment for the same are as follows:
- Furthering the greater good of the society
- Creating a deterrent
- Reformation of the criminal.

Criminalizing human error by legislatively removing the need for the element of *mens rea* makes the accused completely defenseless and therefore such a legislative provision should strictly be applied only and only where there is a very high likelihood of the provision directly achieving the desired aims (as stated above). When the mere presence of any deficiency or inaccuracy in record-keeping is criminalized, which of the above aims is achieved? There is no plausible explanation as to how prosecuting someone for errors in record-keeping can prevent the crime of sex-determination.

The terror unleashed by this penal provision has surely created highly-qualified medical clerks efficient in filling forms. But is the severity of the provision primarily aimed at elimination of unintentional documentation errors or prevention of sex-determination. The question of reformation of the criminal does not arise since there is nothing to reform in the first place. You cannot reform human inadvertence, just like you cannot reform human happiness or human sadness.

There are significant downsides of such severe provisions. Firstly, they terrorize physicians to the extent where documentation takes precedence over the interests of the patient. The patients in this case being the pregnant lady and the fetus, it is ironical that a piece of legislation which, in a way, aims at woman empowerment ends up harming the interests of this most vulnerable section of the society.[2] Secondly, it discourages physicians from reporting genuine errors and encourages cover-ups. Thirdly, it perpetrates the culture of inspector-raj, which is the last thing any developing country needs. Upon being thoroughly terrorized by the penal provisions of PCPNDT Act, some doctors even stop practicing ultrasound altogether.[3] This again is a great loss to the nation which is already facing a dearth of qualified modern medicine practitioners. Added to this, the fact that it is easily possible for the real perpetrators of sex-determination and female feticide to go completely undetected by keeping the most accurate records makes this legislative provision severely counterproductive. That the social evil of female feticide stems from the morbid dislike for the girl child for reasons such as dowry and the archaic belief in the son being the torch-bearer of the family name, in addition to being socially believed to be parents' support in their old age, is systematically ignored. The entire focus of the administrative and legal machinery is on prosecuting doctors for errors in record-keeping.[3,4] No wonder then that the child sex ratio has gradually worsened in some states over the past two decades of implementation of PCPNDT Act.[5]

Keeping-up with the tradition of overcriminalization and ignoring the ground realities, the Protection of Children from Sexual Offences (POCSO) Act, 2012 criminalizes an act of omission, i.e. failure to report such information to police if a person has apprehension or knowledge of an offence being committed under this Act. For physicians, this situation usually arises when they come across a pregnancy in a minor girl. That child sexual abuse is a grave problem in our society and needs to be addressed by strong legislative means is beyond argument. At the same time, it is also a fact that pregnancy in unmarried minor girls in an average Indian family is a highly sensitive issue. The social stigma associated with pregnancy in a minor ensures that the family tries its best to keep it under wraps. Social estrangement and honor-killings are a reality in India, and so is frequent violence against doctors.[6] The fact that the mention of the word "police" does not inspire confidence in an average citizen of our country does not help either. In such a scenario, a doctor faces grave predicament while dealing with a pregnancy in a minor. What if the family is aggressively against involving the police? What are the possible consequences if the doctor informs the police against the wishes of the family? What if the physician is willing to inform the police but is afraid to do so for the fear of harassment? Such fears of the physician are not unfounded. Unfortunately, these socially relevant practical problems do not find any consideration in the POCSO Act.

Since it is practically very difficult to prosecute any other ordinary person for non-furnishing of information, the physician, who documents facts in the form of medical records, is the easy target for prosecution under section POCSO Act.[7] This is a classic example of how a perfectly well-meaning professional can be turned into a criminal for not being a whistle-blower in a hostile environment bereft of any safeguards.

The prosecution of physicians under Indian Penal Code for alleged criminal negligence is also on a rise. Despite the honorable Supreme Court in *Jacob Mathew Vs State of Punjab and Anr* making it mandatory for the police to obtain an independent medical opinion before registering an FIR against a doctor upon receipt of a complaint of criminal negligence, innovative ways are used to bypass the directives of SC and register FIRs.[8-10] Despite the honorable Supreme Court in *Lalita Kumari Vs Govt. of UP and Ors* clearly stating that even for cognizable offences, an arrest is not mandatory after registration of FIR in every single case, doctors continue to be arrested and detained.[9,11] The Supreme Court has also held that unnecessary arrest of the accused is in violation of his fundamental right granted under Article 21 of the Constitution.[11] The basic logic behind arrest is to prevent the accused from tampering of evidence, induce threat to the witness and absconding. This is perfectly understandable in case of heinous crimes, but to put white-collared professionals like doctors on the same pedestal as hard-core criminals is completely unjustified. Considering additionally the fact that most of the doctors accused of criminal negligence are ultimately acquitted by the court for want of guilt, the permanent mental and social handicap left behind by the stigma of criminal prosecution is irreparable.[12] When such a treatment is meted out to a highly intellectual class, it has devastating long-term consequences, one of which is repulsion among young intelligent students toward medicine as a career. The ultimate loser is the society, which will be gradually devoid of good physicians.

RETRIBUTIVE JUSTICE

Since the honorable Supreme Court has firmly established the liability of medical professionals under Consumer Protection Act (CPA), the fact that the honorable Supreme Court also holds practice of medicine by qualified professionals as a non-commercial activity does not make the patient any less a "consumer".[13,14] Be that as it may, the "accountability" of doctors under CPA seems largely a victim of outcome bias, i.e. the tendency of people to attribute blame more easily if the outcome is serious than they would if the outcome was comparatively minor. When clinical outcomes primarily determine the attribution of blame and resultant penalties, the process of scientific reasoning becomes a mere side-show. Since compensations are now being liberally awarded under CPA for non-quantifiable damages like "mental agony" and "harassment" even in the absence of medical negligence, one is left wondering whether we are back to the primitive days of retributive justice based primarily on emotions rather than scientific facts.[15]

While delivering a landmark judgment, the honorable Supreme Court in *Balram Prasad vs Kunal Saha and ors* awarded a total compensation of Rs. 11.41 crore (inclusive of 6% interest) to the kin of the deceased patient while holding the concerned hospital and treating physicians guilty of medical negligence. The court used the *restitutio ad integrum* method instead of the multiplier method while assessing the pecuniary damages arising from medical negligence. Simply put, a patient with higher earnings power has a claim to a higher compensation than a patient with lower earnings power, even if the damages and degree of medical negligence suffered are identical.[16] Curiously, the Ethics Code Regulations, 2002 of Medical Council of India do not permit a physician to discriminate between patients based on their earnings profile. Neither does human physiology or disease processes make such discrimination. Such a divergent situation puts physicians in an extremely precarious position and forces them to espouse a guarded attitude. A forced defensive outlook is ultimately deleterious for the society. In 2017, the Delhi government suspended the license of a prominent corporate hospital in Shalimar Bagh, New Delhi following an incident wherein the doctor on-duty missed signs of life in a premature baby and erroneously declared it dead.[17] Such anachronistic ways of delivering justice may temporarily appease the masses but end-up creating morbid fear among healthcare professionals. No professional can do justice to his job acting under morbid fear.

A serious profession like medicine needs a very balanced mix of accountability and responsibility. If accountability is primarily based on *you err, we punish* motto, the responsibility will suffer from demotivation, pathological stress and defensive attitude. When accountability is perceived as being intrusive, insulting and unscientific by the decision-maker, it becomes counter-productive. The problem is compounded by the fact that decision-making in medicine though ideally should be purely scientific, is largely influenced by social, cultural and economic factors which are outside the control of the physician. As Wilkinson stated: "A lot of lip service is paid to the myth of command residing in the cockpit, to the fantasy of the captain as ultimate decision-maker. But today the commander must first consult the accountant."[18]

In case of a mishap, our society constantly looks for someone or something to fix the blame upon while decidedly ignoring the fact that in complex systems, accidents and deaths can happen despite nobody's fault. Selecting a scapegoat provides us with the psychological relief of not having to acknowledge the hard fact that we do not have absolute control over systems and outcomes. Practicing a non-exact science like medicine in such an environment is similar to walking on a minefield. Punishment-oriented accountability greatly hinders learning process because it results in under-reporting of errors, obscuration of facts and defensive posturing. Nothing can be more unfortunate for the future of medicine.

PRESUMPTION OF GUILT

The PCPNDT Act presumes that any deficiency or inaccuracy in record-keeping amounts to the offence of sex-determination, unless the contrary is proven. And even if contrary is proven, error in record-keeping itself is an independent offence carrying the same punishment as sex-determination! The PCPNDT Act presumes the accused physician as guilty and puts the heavy burden of proof on his shoulders, that too under criminal charges! The concept of "reverse burden" is not unique to PCPNDT Act. However, the fact that the PCPNDT Act has applied it while equating *any* deficiency or inaccuracy in record-keeping with the offence of sex-determination is flabbergasting. It appears even more counterintuitive against the backdrop of Article 14(2) of the International Covenant on Civil and Political Rights, 1966 and Article 11(1) of Universal Declaration of Human

Rights, 1948, which recognize presumption of innocence as a human right. The Protection of Human Rights Act, 1993 derives its definition of "human rights" from the International Covenant on Civil and Political Rights, 1966, in addition to Constitution of India. To say that it is unreasonable to deprive a person of his human right for any deficiency or inaccuracy in record-keeping will be a severe understatement.

The Prevention of Cut Practices in Healthcare Bill, an antigraft law proposed to be introduced in the state of Maharashtra, criminalizes the referral of a patient by a healthcare provider if there is an "intention' to indulge in cut-practice.[19] How easy or difficult it will be to suspect such an intention, especially in a world where the element of trust in doctor-patient relationship is rapidly diminishing, is anybody's guess. Will a subjective element like "intention" be a separate offence in the absence of actual reception of kick-backs? Like the PCPNDT Act, will a mere preponderance of probability be enough to initiate criminal proceedings against the accused? Only a constitutional court will be able to tell us that as and when the law takes force. Meanwhile, one can only hope that well-meaning doctors do not become a victim of vague definitions, as has happened under the PCPNDT Act. Even if a substantive law is aimed at achieving important social objectives, the means to achieve them should not be violative of the fundamental rights of people.

DISPROPORTIONATE PUNISHMENT

As highlighted earlier, the PCPNDT Act prescribes the same punishment for deficiency or inaccuracy in record-keeping as for the offence of sex-determination. In the absence of an alternative, the court of law is forced to award imprisonment even for minor deficiencies in record-keeping which may have no material impact on the accuracy or completeness of the desired information. Under the WB CEA, any person violating conditions of registration and license shall be liable for imprisonment up to 3 years, without any alternative penalty like a monetary fine, etc. The rules under the Transplantation of Human Organs Act (THOA), 1994 put the onus upon the registered medical practitioner of establishing the fact that the donor is a near relative of the recipient by verifying the prescribed documents. Failure to do so attracts nothing less than criminal prosecution and imprisonment under THOA. The fact that the registered medical practitioner himself may become a victim of a fraud perpetrated by the donor and recipient acting in collusion has not been addressed explicitly. In 2016, five prominent doctors from a reputed corporate hospital were charge-sheeted under THOA.[20] The provisions under the various Acts mentioned above do not leave any flexibility for courts while awarding penalties. If one examines the provisions of Narcotic Drugs and Psychotropic Substances Act, 1985, a system of graded punishment has been prescribed, depending upon whether the quantity of substance in possession is small, more than small or commercial, thus leaving enough scope for the court to award punishment proportionate to the offence. However, no such flexibility has been granted particularly under the PCPNDT Act, thus making the Act decidedly draconian.

CONCLUSION

The prime objective of making laws is to further the interest of the nation and its people. In a country like India where public healthcare system is found wanting, small and medium private healthcare establishments shoulder the burden of providing affordable healthcare to the masses. The reasonability of legal provisions is usually, though not always, determined by the social setting in which they are implemented. In a resource-constrained country like India, some of the legal provisions cited above are threatening to paralyze the primary saviors of health care, i.e. the physicians running the small and medium healthcare establishments. The society in general and policy-makers in particular need to urgently take cognizance of this fact, lest the nation's health care may land-up in a coma.

REFERENCES

1. Yadavar S. (2018) Rs. 3: here's what the government spends every day on each Indian's health. [online]. Available from: https://www.indiaspend.com/rs-3-amount-india-spends-every-day-on-each-indians-health-53127/ [Accessed December, 2018]
2. Phutke G, Laux TS, Jain P, et al. (2018) Ultrasound in rural India: a failure of the best intentions. Indian J Med Ethics. [online]. Available from: https://ijme.in/articles/ultrasound-in-rural-india-a-failure-of-the-best-intentions/?galley=html [Accessed December, 2018].
3. Tripathi A. (2018). Sex determination in India: doctors tell their side of the story. Scroll. [online]. Available from: https://scroll.in/article/805064/sex-determination-in-india-doctors-tell-their-side-of-the-story [Accessed December, 2018].
4. Yadav A. (2017). Medical association wants doctors to be protected from punishment under sex determination laws. Scroll [online]. Available from: https://scroll.in/pulse/839838/medical-association-wants-doctors-to-be-protected-from-punishment-under-sex-determination-laws [Accessed December, 2018].
5. Tabaie S. Stopping female feticide in India: the failure and unintended consequence of ultrasound restriction. J Glob Health. 2017;7(1):010304.
6. Sharma K. Understanding the concept of honour killing within the social paradigm: theoretical perspectives. IOSR J Human Soc Sci. 2016;9(8),26-32.
7. Live Law News Network. (2018). This is what SC held when it quashed charges under POCSO Act against doctors in Kottiyoor rape case [read judgment]. [online]. Available from: https://www.livelaw.in/this-is-what-sc-held-when-it-quashed-charges-under-pocso-act-against-doctors-in-kottiyoor-rape-case-read-judgment/ [Accessed December, 2018].
8. Jacob Mathew vs State of Punjab and another—(2005) SCCL.COM 456. Criminal Appeal No. 144-145 of 2004 decided by the Supreme Court on 2005.
9. Cross Town News. (2018). Without enquiry arrest of doctors is violation of Supreme Court orders: DAJ. [online]. Available from: https://www.magzter.com/news/887/2390/062018/3g6uk [Accessed December, 2018].
10. Deshpande S. (2018). SC restrains Ratnagiri police from arresting doctor couple in patient death case. The Times of India. [online]. Available from: https://timesofindia.indiatimes.com/city/mumbai/sc-restrains-ratnagiri-police-from-arresting-doctor-couple-in-patient-death-case/articleshow/65242066.cms [Accessed December, 2018].
11. Lalita Kumari vs Govt of U.P. and others—(2014) 2 SCC 1. Writ Petition (Criminal) No. 68 of 2008.
12. Singhal A. Veracity of laws relating to medical malpractice in India. Int J Sci Res Pub. 2015. [online]. Available from: http://www.ijsrp.org/monograph/Veracity_of_laws_relating_to_medical_malpractice_in_India.pdf [Accessed December, 2018].
13. Chairman and Chief Executive Officer, Noida and another vs Mange Ram Sharma and another and Dr. Anupama Bisara and others—(2012) 12 SCC 717. Civil Appeal No. 10535 of 2011.
14. Indian Medical Association v. V. P. Shantha and others—1996 AIR 550, 1995 (6) SCC 651.
15. Anoop Awasthi v. Dr. T. Kataria. National Consumer Disputes Redressal Commission. Consumer Case no. 84 of 2002.

16. Balram Prasad v. Kunal Saha and others—(2014) 1 SCC 384. Civil Appeal No. 2867 of 2012.
17. Jha DN. (2017). Hospital declares live baby dead, gives it to parents in plastic bag. Times of India [online]. Available from: https://timesofindia.indiatimes.com/city/delhi/hospital-declares-live-baby-dead-gives-it-to-parents-in-plastic-bag/articleshow/61887252.cms [Accessed December, 2018].
18. Wilkinson S. The November Oscar incident. Pilot. 1994;32. [online]. Available from: http://forum.aeforum.net/index.php?showtopic=384754 [Accessed December, 2018].
19. The Prevention of Cut Practices in Healthcare Services Act, 2017. [online]. Available from: https://www.dmer.org/new/Prevention%20Healthcare%20Services%20Act%202017.html {Accessed December, 2018].
20. Narayan V. Kidney racket: Five Hiranandani doctors charge sheeted for criminal conspiracy. The Times of India. (2016). [online]. Available from: https://timesofindia.indiatimes.com/city/mumbai/Kidney-racket-Five-Hiranandani-doctors-chargesheeted-for-criminal-conspiracy/articleshow/54789249.cms [accessed December, 2018].

CHAPTER 18A

Self-regulation or State Legislation: An Urgent Choice to Make

Narasimha Rao Kankanala

"If you would take, you must first give, this is the beginning of intelligence"
— ***Lao Tzu***

QUID AGIS–QUO VADIS

[Latin: "What are (we) doing – Where are (we) headed"]

Award of an unprecedented *60 million-plus rupees' compensation* for medical negligence—this landmark judgment's[1] lesser-known parts are:

- "Doctors and senior doctors of high repute —made every *attempt to shift the blame to the other Doctors thereby tainting the medical profession.. unbecoming of a doctor* as renowned and revered as he is.."
- "It is pertinent for us to note the shifting of blames....which is a *shameful act on the dignity of medical profession*..."
- "...*Abhor the shifting of blames* by the senior doctor on the attending physician the appellant Dr... even though the Court held him guilty of negligence..."
- "...had *conducted with utmost callousness*... which led to her unfortunate demise".

While we all have debated at length on the decree's fairness and quantum of compensation, let us look at this decree from a Judge's perspective, who goes by a principle of "Preponderance of Probability"[2] in order to adjudicate civil matters. When doctors blame each other, especially in a court of law, the tone is set for the balance of probabilities tilting against the doctors and the resulting damages awarded include punitive damages (in addition to the pecuniary and non-pecuniary damages) also, which is awarded as a punishment in order to act as a deterrent in future, not only for the accused, but the fraternity at large, which is evident from this part of the same judgment:

"...we, therefore, hope and trust that this decision acts as a *deterrent and a reminder to those doctors, hospitals,* the nursing homes and other connected establishments who do not take their responsibility seriously..."

"...the *Central and the State Governments may consider enacting laws wherever there is absence of one* for effective functioning of the private Hospitals and Nursing Homes..."[1]

Consequentially, when the State or Judiciary, legislate or decree in their respective capacity, the unrest triggered within the medical fraternity results in instant reactions which may not exactly concur with the proposed intent of the State/Judiciary. On reacting to such legislations or decrees, as a fraternity (medical), we tend to get misled into inconclusive/conflictory discussions on the 'Letter of the Law,'[3] not realizing that focusing on the Spirit of the Law, would eventually dictate its Letter, in the best interests of all the stakeholders, doctors included!

BASIC UNDERSTANDING

Let's get to the basics.

What is a Self-regulatory Organization?

The dictionary meaning is: A professional organization, unaffiliated with a Government, having certain, limited regulatory authority over members. An example is the American Dental Association, which has the ability to set standards and enforce discipline over dentists in the United States.[4]

The Regulatory Bodies

- *Statutory*: Medical Council of India (MCI) and the respective State Medical Councils.
- *Nonstatutory*: Associations like the Indian Medical Association (IMA), other specialty Associations like the API (Association of Physicians of India), IOA (Indian Orthopaedic Association), Indian Association of Dermatologists, Venereologists, and Leprologists (IADVL), Associations of Plastic Surgeons of India (APSI), etc.

While the nonstatutory bodies are free to have their own regulations, the statutory body, MCI is governed by the MCI Act, 1956.[5] Under this Act, we have the Indian Medical Council (Professional Conduct, Etiquette and Ethics) Regulations, 2002;[6] with the latest amendment in October, 2016.[7]

Self-regulation: As an Individual

For an individual, while the Statutory Code of Ethics details systematic self-regulation, it is very simple to Self-regulate—a basic outline could be:

- Smile and greet
- Speech—Soft and clear and document
- Stickler for basic protocols
- Sincere and professional approach
- Seek second opinion as needed
- Solve potential problems early—grievance redressal onsite
- Shun professional jousting
- Shun self-promotion
- Shun sponsorships, (e.g. Pharma)

Such self-regulatory norms of ethics and etiquette would be evident to the patient in practice—spoken (communication) and written (documentation). The relationship of Trust (*Fiduciary!*) thus built-up would be an effective way to avert a future Litigation (*Judiciary!*) or at least, mitigate it. In the event of a patient seeking to litigate frivolously, the etiquette and ethical conduct would be written all over the available records, be it, written, circumstantial or audiovisual, which would decide the course of litigation equitably.

While the articulated ethical conduct is important, it is the "unarticulated premise"[8] of a physician's diligent time spent with the patient (which arises naturally when considering the patient as a kin) which determines the standard of care in the patient's mind and also in the adjudicator's mind, should the patient litigate. One such example is the case[9] (Kamalesh versus Dr Ajit Roy, State Commission of West Bengal, 2000) where a doctor shifted a patient with respiratory distress (who eventually expired) by his car and not by an ambulance, was held not guilty; because the Judge felt that "all possible treatment was given to the patient," apparently biased by the diligent time he spent with the patient.

This apparent "**unarticulated premise**" of time with the patient, possibly helped in acquitting the doctors in another case[10] (Ganga Ram Hospital versus DP Bhandari), where the allegation of negligence was that the patient died for not shifting the patient to the intensive care unit (ICU), higher/scan center.

More specifically, it is interesting to note that the *four - Judge* bench of the *High Court* that adjudicated this case, took cognizance of the fact that "*as many as 140 visits were made by the paramedical staff and 25 visits by the doctors to the patient's room during 57 hours, the period when his condition required to be kept under constant watch and there was regular monitoring of his pulse, urine, blood pressure, respiratory functions, etc. Taking into account all the facts and circumstances disclosed by the materials available on record, we find ourselves unable to uphold the finding recorded by the State Commission that there was negligence on the part of the hospital in not transferring the patient to the ICU,*" rather than the details of technicalities of treatment or delay.

"*A mind all logic is like a knife all blade. It makes the hand bleed that uses it.*"

—**Rabindranath Tagore**

Applying Tagore's wisdom to this aforementioned scenario, self-regulatory norms like **diligent time** with the patient could provide a **humane "handle"** to the "**mind all logic**", thus **protecting** the **patient (during treatment)** and the **doctor (during litigation)** from the "knife all blade" (of only logic and letter of law). Due diligence taking precedence over shifting to an ICU—not only helped overrule the order by the State Commission, but could provide the insight to answer the contemporary question of relevance of physical presence of an ICU/ventilator, when adjudicating on alleged negligence.

Self-regulation: As a Fraternity

Sustained violation of ethical practices and failure of the Statutory Regulatory body to impose deterrent disciplinary action on the violators, forces the State/Judiciary to step in and impose Legislative and Judicial restrictions on the accused. Thereafter, violation of ethics would be viewed as violation of law with floodgates open and an exponential rise of litigation follows; to the tune of 400% in a decade, according to a legal resource, Manupatra.[11]

This is when, as a fraternity, we need to stand up to the challenge and strategize, to seek a solution, rather than blaming the State/Judiciary. In this context, it is worth recalling Justice DK Jain, retired Supreme Court Judge and the then President, NCDRC (National Consumer Disputes Redressal Commission), quoting at a National Medicolegal Conclave, Chennai, September, 2017: "I have a lurking fear in my mind that I might give a wrong judgment against doctors, going by western standards. I want you (doctors) to help me with what is appropriate for our set-up and infrastructure."

We need to believe that we are the best at seeking a rational solution going by our training at medical school. A similar understanding on the lines on Etiology/Pathophysiology/Management/Prophylaxis, could help us show the way.

Such an understanding on the lines on Management Studies is the well-known SWOT (*Strengths, Weaknesses, Opportunities,* and *Threats*) analysis.[12]

As a fraternity, a *sample* of our listing could be:
- *Strengths*: Ability for hard work, empathy, knowledge, analytical thinking to conquer disease.
- *Weaknesses*: Lack of uniformity/consensus on consent/treatment/grievance redressal, silence of the ethical majority, unethical practices with absence of structured deterrents, deficient knowledge of medical jurisprudence.
- *Opportunities*: Digital Revolution, vacuum in the areas of Clinical Practice Guidelines (CPG), costing of treatment—our forte, quick redressal, Government's inability to handle the rising cost of healthcare, Judiciary's burden of huge pendency of cases.[13]
- *Threats*: Rise in Patient-Doctor trust deficit, "Draconian" state legislations,[14] insurance companies dictating protocols and pricing,[15] unprofessional advertisements by both 'professionals' and nonprofessionals ('quacks'), corporate culture with entrepreneurs imposing 'targets',[16] Violence against healthcare staff/establishments.

The general approach would be to capitalize on our strengths, using the opportunities and *thus,* progressively strengthening the weaknesses and neutralizing the threats, the nitty-gritty of which can be handled in purposefully structured brain-storming workshops/think-tanks. If we opt to be more advanced/positive in our approach, we could seek to apply the management concept of Appreciative Inquiry,[17] rather than SWOT.

While an in-depth analysis/solution for each of the issues is beyond the scope of this chapter, it suffices to mention here, that solutions are being sought using certain principles like:
- Seeking 'Win-all' solutions
- Employing digital tools like Aadhaar, etc
- Arriving at consensus on CPG, *for practice*
- Structuring protocols for imposing disciplinary action, *upon breach*

In this manner, we are in the process of proposing/implementing solutions/mechanisms like:
- Medical Tribunal to supplant 'Consumer Forum'
- "Beti-Aadhaar" to supplant PC-PNDT Act
- Aadhaar in helping Emergent care
- ABCDE of formulation of CPG (Clinical Practice Guidelines) – **A**pproval-consent/**B**asic Protocols/**C**linical Pathways/**D**uties of Doctor-Patient/**E**thical Guidelines
- Constituting a Patient Grievance Redressal Cell.[18]

Rather than resisting change, we could *propose better change,* in keeping with the aforementioned principles, and, *"make an offer that cannot be refused"!!*

On this note, it would be pertinent to acknowledge MCI's to-be-notified Guidelines on Constitution of peer group which would judge the professional as medical incompetence of a doctor which would be applicable at the medical trial jurisdiction.[19] This could be the foundation for a Medical Tribunal! It would be commendable if the MCI could act positively on the Parliamentary Standing Committee[20] report too, which could possibly deter the State from imposing the proposed National Medical Commission Bill and also the Judiciary from acting *suo moto,* such as, appointing an Oversight Committee[21] and lambasting the MCI: "In March 2016, a

Parliamentary Standing Committee (PSC) on health and family planning tabled its report in Parliament suggesting restructuring Medical Council of India in order to improve healthcare and medical education in our country. Shortly thereafter, endorsing the said PSC report, the Supreme Court has used its rare and extraordinary powers under the constitution (under Article 142) to set-up three members committee, headed by a former Chief Justice of India, to oversee the functioning of the Medical Council of India (MCI) for at least a year. In the Judgment the Supreme Court said "Unethical practices Medical professionals indulge in unethical practices conducting unnecessary diagnostics tests and surgical procedures in order to extract money from hapless patients, the judgment said. The challenges facing medical education of the 21st Century are truly gigantic...Game changer reforms of transformational nature are therefore the need of the hour and they need to be carried out urgently and immediately".

CONCLUSION

While it is relatively easy to self-regulate and be safe at an individual level, we could seek to pitch in collectively to self-regulate as a fraternity in the little capacity that we can, so as to mitigate the trust-deficit and thus practice in peace and counteract objectively, should the patient litigate. Ethical Practice, even if it is in contravention of the Law in a given instance, the Law (its Letter) would amend itself to suit its Spirit.

How Portia successfully invoked the Spirit of the Law to fight its Letter to save Antonio from Shylock's wicked demand for 'the pound of flesh', is worth recalling from Shakespeare's *Merchant of Venice!*

Likewise, we could replicate the unmatched success, we, as a fraternity have hitherto achieved (as evidenced by the rise in life expectancy from 32 years in 1947[22] to 69.09 years in 2018),[23] in the process of Self-regulation too, particularly, way beyond mitigating litigation.

Self-regulation could revive the *Dream* of the traditional/ancestral image of the Indian Physician—

"Vaidyo Narayano Harihi" (translating as, Doctor is equal to God)!

To 'dare to' dream of such a possibility, we could invoke *Dr APJ Abdul Kalam sir's* wisdom

"Dream is not that which you see in sleep, but something that does not let you sleep!"

ACKNOWLEDGMENTS

For teaching the values of life: *My parents, Sri K Nageswara Rao and Smt K Visalakshmi and my teachers of Campion H.S. School, Trichy.*

For teaching Medical Ethics: *All my teachers, especially Prof Benjamin Joseph & Prof Sharath K Rao, KMC, Manipal, Dr K Srinivasan and Dr RD Chakravarthy, Manipal Hospital, Bengaluru and Dr Jacob Varghese, Amrita IMS, Kochi.*

For teaching Medical Jurisprudence: *All my teachers, especially, Prof (Dr) OV Nandimath and Prof (Dr) SV Joga Rao, NLSIU, Bengaluru, Honorable Justice M Sathyanarayanan, Madras High Court.*

For teaching the value of trust and the responsibility imposed by trust: *My Patients over 25 years – to whom I dedicate this chapter, with the hope that we can take this further in the best interests of the health care of our nation.*

REFERENCES

1. Balram Prasad vs Kunal Saha & Ors on 24 October, 2013, Supreme Court of India.

2. "Burden of Proof (Law)", Available at https://en.wikipedia.org/wiki/Burden_of_proof_(law). (Last visited on 24.05.2018).
3. "Letter and Spirit of the Law", Available at https://en.wikipedia.org/wiki/Letter_and_spirit_of_the_law. (Last visited on 29.07.2018).
4. "Self-regulatory Organization"Available at https://financial-dictionary.thefreedictionary.com/Self+Regulatory+Organization. (Last Visited on 24.05.2018).
5. The Indian Medical Council Act, 1956, (102 of 1956) 30th December, 1956, (As amended by the Indian Medical Council (Amendment) Acts, 1964, 1993 & 2001) Available at https://mciindia.org/ActivitiWebClient/actnamendments/theMedicalCouncilAct1956. (Last visited on 11.08.2018).
6. Medical Council of India, Notification, (Published in Part III, Section 4 of the Gazette of India, dated 6th April, 2002), Available at https://old.mciindia.org/RulesandRegulations/CodeofMedicalEthicsRegulations2002.aspx. (Last visited on 11.08.2018).
7. Indian Medical Council, (Professional Conduct, Etiquette and Ethics), Regulations, 2002. Available at https://old.mciindia.org/Rules-and-Regulation/Ethics%20Regulations-2002.pdf. (Last visited on 11.08.2018).
8. A contextual personal communication with Prof Dr OV Nandimath, Professor of Law & Registrar, National Law School of India University, Bengaluru.
9. Shivakumar Kumbar, "Transportation of the patient: Legal binding of anaesthesiologist". Indian Journal of Anaesthesia. 2010;54(4): 367-8.
10. Ganga Ram Hospital vs D.P. Bhandari Ors. on 23 April, 1992, Delhi High Court.
11. Damayanthi Datta, Doctors in the Dock, Doctors are in fear as a storm of litigation hits hospitals. Fuzzy laws and frivolous cases are taking a toll on the profession. Will it change the way medicine is practiced in India?, October 9, 2014. Available at http://indiatoday.intoday.in/story/litigation-doctors-medicine-law-national-accreditation-board-for-hospitals/1/394983.html. (Last visited on 16.04.2016).
12. "SWOT Analysis". Available at https://en.wikipedia.org/wiki/SWOT_analysis. (Last visited on 11.08.2018).
13. Tilak Marg, "National judicial data grid made available online for public access with case pendency statistics, Published data, September 19, 2015. Available at http://tilakmarg.com/news/national-judicial-data-grid-made-available-online-for-public-access-with-case-pendency-statistics. (Last visited on 16.04.2016).
14. Tabassum Barnagarwala, "First of its kind: Maharashtra Bill to stop doctor's commissions cuts both ways", Updated date, October 26, 2017. Available at https://indianexpress.com/article/explained/first-of-its-kind-maharashtra-bill-to-stop-doctors-commissions-cuts-both-ways-4906625. (Last visited on 9.08.2018).
15. Ravi Duggal, "Private Health Insurance and Access to Healthcare", Published Indian Jounal of Med Ethics, Vol 8 No.1, 2011. Available at http://ijme.in/articles/private-health-insurance-and-access-to-healthcare/?galley=html. (Last visited on 9.08.2018).
16. Anne Lowe, "The BMJ reveals 'unethical' targets in India's private hospitals", Public Domain, September 3, 2015.
17. "Appreciative Inquiry". Available at https://en.wikipedia.org/wiki/Appreciative_inquiry (Last visited on 2.09.2018).
18. Inspired by Prof Dr SV Joga Rao's'M/s LegalExcel Healthcare, Solicitors and Advocates, Bengaluru'–run "Patient Grievance Redressal Cell", which witnessed about 40% drop in litigation in the given chain of hospitals – personal communication.
19. Meghna, "MCI defines Professional Incompetence, issues Guidelines", Published date, September 22, 2017. Available at https://medicaldialogues.in/mci-defines-professional-incompetence-issues-guidelines. (Last visited on 11.08.2018).
20. "Parliamentary Panel Pulls up MCI Over Corruption". Available at http://www.livemint.com/Politics/X8cYK9Wdw72XmkLReY2BNK/Parliamentary-panel-pulls-up-MCI-over-corruption.html. (Last visited on 17.04.2016).

21. Dr Sonia Kukreja Pandy, "Supreme Court Clips MCI Wings, Appoints Panel to Monitor", Publised on May 04, 2016. Available at https://www.docplexus.in/#/app/posts/800d3a22-1064-4fbb-8055-fa76dd5bcacc?utm_term=Email-Digest-0-eve&utm_campaign=Email-Digest&utm_medium=Email&utm_source=Docplexus.in&utm_content=CTA. (Last visited on 07.05.2016).
22. Preetika Rana and Joanna Sugden, "India's Record Since Independence, Published date, August 15, 2013, Available at https://blogs.wsj.com/indiarealtime/2013/08/15/indias-record-since-independence/(Last visited on 11.08.2018).
23. The World: Life Expectancy (2018) Top 100+ Available at http://www.geoba.se/population.php?pc=world&page=1&type=15&st=rank&asde=&year=2018. (Last visited on 11.08.2018).

CHAPTER 18B

Practice Guidelines and Associations: Role in Liability Risk Mitigation

Venkataram Mysore

INTRODUCTION

Medical profession has been in the line of fire by the society for different reasons, the most prominent being that the profession at large has failed to regulate itself. There is some truth in this accusation—this profession hitherto regarded as noble and given an exalted position has generally chosen to remain silent and look the other way in all matters of corruption, negligence, and response to societal needs. It has even failed at times, in maintenance and setting up of academic standards. It could not mount an effective resistance even when the profession was threatened, as in the case of inclusion in consumer forum or in the face of mounting violence against hospitals and doctors. If it cannot defend itself, it can hardly be expected to fight on behalf of others. Importantly from the point of view of public, doctors have failed to tackle corruption in health care, such as unethical practices, industry sponsorships, commissions, unnecessary investigations, overpricing by hospitals, spurious drugs and devices, etc.

The main reasons for this are perhaps as follows:
- Medical profession is not one entity and is a diverse group—each specialty looks after itself. The Indian Medical Association (IMA) which is the mother organization, is not the area of active participation for most specialists in the cities. IMA is more representative of the profession in the smaller towns.
- There are divergent areas of interest in the medical profession—each group looking after its own interests. It is not easy to find one common area of interest, except when the profession is threatened, as has happened recently when an act was thrust was on the profession in Karnataka and other States.
- The individual doctor is mostly a "frog in the pond", living happily in the clinic or his department, of which he is the king! Except

- occasional academic interactions, doctors hardly get together for a social cause.
- Ego and a sense of superiority are perhaps prevalent in most specialists and hence they do not relate to the problems of others.
- Doctors are generally poor administrators and find solace mostly in their clinical work.
- A sense of respect for the senior and subservience to the head is prevalent across the profession and this prevents them from protesting adequately when needed.
- Young doctors who would otherwise be expected to be flag bearers of change, have a long tiring education course and are busy in settling down.
- Associations are primarily meant for welfare of its members, and in that sense are self-centered.

The result is a general lack of interest in any issue other than clinical care.

However, associations can contribute in a significant way in number of areas:
- Policy making—trying to influence the government and other agencies
- Setting standards of practice
- Setting up grievance cells for handling patient complaints
- Fighting corruption in health care
- Vigilance cells to help doctors in the face of violence
- Tackling quackery
- Stopping unethical advertisements.

It is somewhat heartening to note that there are many instances wherein associations have taken an active role in at least some of the above issues. Some examples are as follows:
- *Influencing policy*:
  - The IMA has acted forcefully in airing its views on the proposed National Medical Commission Bill and has forced the government to make significant changes.
  - The IMA Karnataka successfully forced the Government of Karnataka to change significant portions of the Karnataka Private Medical Establishment (KPME) Act.
  - Indian Association of Dermatologists, Venereologists and Leprologists (IADVL) has successfully interacted with Drug Controller General of India to initiate a ban on topical steroid drug combinations.
- *Setting standards of practice*: While several associations have made significant contributions, certainly this is an area where more can be done. Some examples:
  - The IADVL published standard guidelines of care in 18 different dermatosurgical procedures. These have been helpful in setting standards of practice and also in helping its members in medicolegal situations (Refer to case example at the end of the chapter).[1]
  - The IADVL has authored guidelines of care in Stevens–Johnson syndrome, after the well-known Saha case where a huge amount of compensation was ordered by the Supreme Court.[2] It has also published guidelines for other diseases and drugs.[3,4]
  - AHRS (Association of Hair Restoration Surgeons) and ISHRS (International Society of Hair Restorations Surgeons) have published a number of position papers on different aspects of hair transplantation practice (www.ahrsindia.org).
- *Tackling corruption in health care*: There has been a lot of attention paid recently to several practices perceived as corruption

in health care, such as unethical practices, commissions, unnecessary investigations, overpricing by hospitals, clinical research on behalf of industry, spurious drugs and devices, etc. There have been instances of associations endorsing companies such as vaccines, toothpaste, water purifiers, etc. The society expects doctors to be whistle blowers in these situations and also in fighting for better health care to patients. It has to be recognized that the role of associations in these situations has not been satisfactory. Most associations have not tackled this issue, beyond issuing statements. More needs to be done in order to enhance the confidence of society in doctors.

- *Establishing grievance cells for patients*: This is again true that associations have been lax in addressing complaints by patients. Most associations do not even have a grievance cell to address complaints by patients.
- *Violence against doctors*: The associations were slow in addressing this new assault on the medical profession initially, but of late they have started uniting and addressing this issue. Their stand has forced most states into enacting acts against violence against doctors. Many local associations have made local vigilance cells to protect doctors.
- *Fight against quackery*: Quackery is a menace and pervades all parts of India. While there are laws against quackery, they have been poorly implemented. Associations have generally been ineffective in launching a fight against this menace.
- *Advertisements*: Hyped, exaggerated advertisements affect health care. These are indulged by companies, corporate hospitals, and quacks. Associations have generally been silent in voicing their opinion against such advertisements, except occasional instances such as the advertisement by a corporate hospital enticing patients for a second consultation in Mumbai, action by IADVL against the company, which marketed a steroid containing cream as a fairness and anti-scar cream.

How to initiate/implement changes on various issues identified by the association:

- *Have an administrative officer*:
  - Can be called CEO or similar
  - Needs to be a non-medical person, who works as a full-time employee of the association
  - Will manage the basic administrative work, with inputs from the association EC, through the secretary
  - This will ensure that the secretary is not pushed to take time out from their clinical work
  - Additional office staff will support the manager in administrative tasks.
- *Have a medicolegal cell*:
  - Practicing doctors with a legal bent of mind, with/without formal training in law, can analyze a given clinical scenario from the legal perspective, and plan the strategy to respond, with inputs from the qualified lawyers
  - If left to lawyers alone to plan the legal strategy in case of a medicolegal situation, the clinical perspective may get totally missed.
- *Have a panel of lawyers*:
  - A qualified lawyer is needed to analyze situations legally and suggest the legal path for executing decisions
  - They ensure that letters sent by the association do not have any legal shortcomings

- Having a panel lawyer ensures legal advice is available without delay, and makes him/her committed to the welfare of the association. Engaging a lawyer only when the need arises, may entail the risk of delayed or suboptimal response.
- Having a media cell to deal with adverse publicity, either on social or visual or print media: Doctors are not media experts and often handle media poorly. It is also difficult for an individual doctor or a small hospital to afford media agents.
- *Role in expert opinion:* It has been repeatedly stressed in several judgments that when in doubt, expert opinion should be sought by the consumer courts. This is an area where associations have a major role to play by forming a peer group of experts to help younger colleagues. An expert group also helps in voicing opinion about incidents, as medical science is highly specialized and complicated. It is also important for a young doctor to have a mentor to consult, and refer when problems arise.

SUMMARY

While associations have started in asserting their role in some areas, a lot more needs to be done in addressing issues of relevance to patients and societies.

CASE EXAMPLE

Tin Anusha versus Dr Brahmaramba Sav.

Complaint

The patient approached the doctor for LASER hair removal of the upper lip. The patient developed two to three blisters, following which she developed keloids. Test patch for LASER was not done and also higher fluence was used.

Verdict: Doctor was Acquitted

The doctor was sued in lower court. An appeal in the higher court was made, wherein the defense (doctor) argued that a long pulsed LASER was used for better safety with 100 J, according to the standard protocols. IADVL guidelines of care mention that test spot is not mandatory and recommended in beginners only; the doctor had 9 years experience as a cosmetologist. Also, the patient had not shown any keloidal tendency previously (https://indiankanoon.org/doc/193268809/).

REFERENCES

1. Patwardhan N, Mysore V; IADVL Dermatosurgery Task Force. Hair transplantation: standard guidelines of care. Indian J Dermatol Venereol Leprol. 2008;74 (Suppl):S46-53.
2. Mysore V, BM Shashikumar. Therapeutic guidelines—IADVL. Indian J Dermatol Venereol Leprol. 2016;82(1):1-6.
3. Mysore V, Mahadevappa OH, Barua S, et al. Standard guidelines of care: Performing procedures in patients on or recently administered with isotretinoin. J Cutan Aesthet Surg. 2017;10:186-94.
4. Mysore V, Shashikumar BM. Guidelines for use of finasteride in androgenetic alopecia. Indian J Dermatol Venereol Leprol. 2016;82:128-34.

CHAPTER 19

Legal Aspects of Clinical Research

Manas Chatterjee, Manish Khandare

INTRODUCTION

There are a number of laws representing clinical research in India. Despite the fact that we have a number of enactments, the vital one for clinical trials is the Indian Council of Medical Research (ICMR)—1947 guidelines (amended in the year 2002). Clinical trials are directed through a controlled approach following certain rules set around the International Conference on Harmonization (ICH), which is led by USA, Europe, and Japan. The Drugs and Cosmetics Act, The Medical Council of India (MCI) Act express that every single clinical trial in India ought to take after the ICMR rules of 2000.[1]

There are number of laws governing clinical research in India. Indian Acts/Orders related to clinical trials are:
- Drugs and Cosmetics Act—1940
- Medical Council of India Act—1956, (amended in the year 2002)
- Central Council for Indian Medicine Act—1970
- Guidelines for Exchange of Biological Material (MOH order, 1997)
- Right to Information Act—2005.

APPROVALS AND ETHICS COMMITTEES

The Drugs Controller General of India (DCGI) is in charge of administrative endorsements of clinical trials in India. The DCGI office relies upon outer specialists and other government organizations for exhortation. Extra consents are required for blood tests to remote focal research centers. The ICMR has a Central Ethics Committee (EC) on Human Research (CECHR). Academic Institutes should ensure that their Institutional Ethics Committees (IECs) are registered with the central licensing authority and the registration renewed at the end of 3 years. This is mandatory for their approval of Regulatory Clinical Trials. All clinical trials need to have approval from IEC. If IEC finds potential overlap between the academic and regulatory purposes of the trial, they should notify DCGI. If the IEC does not hear from the DCGI within 30 days, it should be presumed that no permission is needed. This board of trustees reviews the working of the IEC. The as of late revised Schedule Y of Drugs and Cosmetic Rules arranged the creation of the IEC according to ICMR rules. The DCGI's office in a joint effort with WHO, ICMR, and many experts, has been directing preparation of programs for individuals from the ECs the nation over.

Schedule Y of the Drugs and Cosmetics Rules controls clinical trials in India. The Rules are authorized by the DCGI which is likewise in charge of observing every single clinical trial submitted to that office for endorsement. For new medications being produced in India, clinical trials must be directed in India from stage 1. For advertising endorsement of medications effectively affirmed in different nations, a stage 3 clinical trial is required on around 100 patients in at least three focuses, with a specific end goal to set up the medication's effect on the Indian ethnic populace. Till January 2005, clinical trials of new medications being created outside India were allowed just with a "stage slack": a stage 2 trial could be led in India simply after stage 3 trials were finished somewhere else. Stage 1 trials of outside medications were not permitted, except for medications of exceptional pertinence to India. This proviso empowered, for instance, stage 1 trials of HIV immunizations in India. Stage 2 and stage 3 trials of medications found abroad may now be led in India in a similar stage and in the meantime as they are directed in different parts of the world.

In 2000, the ICMR first distributed point by point rules for biomedical research. In 2006, modified rules distributed, express that the morals survey board of trustees is likewise in charge of observing trials. A draft bill to make the rules legitimately restricting is pending. Once passed, the law will require that all ECs enroll with a Biomedical Research Authority.[2]

It is important to classify clinical trials that are regulated by DCGI and those which are not. Investigator initiated studies on drugs that are not sponsored for commercial exploit may be conducted on approved drugs in an unapproved indication without prior DCGI approval. If an approved drug is being tested for a new route of administration or different dose and is being tested for purely academic purpose without an intention to commercially exploit the results of the trial, then no DCGI approval may be required but an undertaking from the investigator needs to be taken. However, sponsored trials on even approved drugs in an unapproved indication would require DCGI approval prior to EC approval. In clinical studies not involving drug trials, approval of DCGI can be commenced after approval by the EC.

REGISTRATION OF THE CLINICAL TRIAL (CLINICAL TRIALS REGISTRY OF INDIA)

The Clinical Trials Registry of India (CTRI), hosted at the ICMR National Institute of Medical Statistics (NIMS) site, is a free and online public record system for registration of clinical trials being conducted in India that was launched on 20th July 2007. Initiated as a voluntary measure, since 15th June 2009, trial registration in the CTRI website has been made mandatory by the Drugs Controller General (India) (DCGI). Moreover, Editors of Biomedical Journals of 11 major journals of India declared that only registered trials would be considered for publication.[3,4]

Trial registration involves public declaration and identification of trial investigators, sponsors, interventions, patient population, etc. before the enrollment of the first patient. Submission of Ethics Committee approval and DCGI approval (if applicable) are essential for trial registration in the CTRI. Indian entities participating in multi-country trials which have been registered in an international registry are also expected to be registered in the CTRI. In the CTRI, details of Indian investigators, trial sites, Indian target sample size and date of enrollment are captured. After a trial is registered, trialists are expected to regularly update the trial status or other aspects as the case may be. After a trial is registered, all updates and changes will be recorded and available for public display.

INFORMED CONSENT FROM PARTICIPANTS

As per schedule Y, in all clinical trials, investigators must ensure that freely given, written, informed consent is obtained from all participants. Patient information sheet and consent form should be approved by IEC. "Informed Consent Form" is to be written in the form. If a subject is not able to give consent (unconscious/minor), a LAR (legally acceptable representative) can give the same. If LAR is not able to write, then an impartial witness should be present all the time during consent and signature.

Audiovisual Recording of Consent

The Gazette notification dated 19th November 2013, after the approval of the Ministry of Health and Family welfare, has decided that in all clinical trials, in addition to the requirement of obtaining written informed consent, audio-visual recording of the informed consent process of each trial subject, including the procedure of providing information to the subject and his/her understanding on such consent with good quality images, without background noise or disturbances, is required to be done while adhering to the principles of confidentiality and should be preserved for at least 5 years if not possible for lifetime.[2]

Conditions for Granting Waiver of Consent

The EC may grant consent waiver in the following situations:
- Research cannot practically be carried out without the waiver and the waiver is scientifically justified
- Retrospective studies, where the participants are de-identified or cannot be contacted
- Research on anonymized biological samples/data
- Certain types of public health studies/surveillance programs/program evaluation studies
- Research on data available in the public domain; or research during humanitarian emergencies and disasters, when the participant may not be in a position to give consent.

Attempt should be made to obtain the participant's consent at the earliest if at all possible.[5]

RESPONSIBILITY OF INVESTIGATOR

The investigator(s) shall be responsible for the conduct of the trial according to the protocol and Guidelines for Good Clinical Practice (GCP). Standard operating procedures are required to be documented by the investigators for the tasks performed by them. During and following a subject's participation in a trial, the investigator should ensure that adequate medical care is provided to the participant for any adverse events. Investigator(s) shall report all serious and unexpected adverse events to the Licensing Authority within 24 hours of their occurrence. Reporting of Serious Adverse Events (SAEs) may be done through email or fax communication (including on nonworking days). In case, the investigator fails to report any serious adverse event within the stipulated period, he/she shall have to furnish the reason for the delay to the satisfaction of the Licensing Authority along with the report of the serious adverse event. The report of the serious adverse event, after due analysis, shall be forwarded by the investigator to the Licensing Authority as well as the chairman of the EC and the head of the institution where the trial has been conducted, within 14 days of the occurrence of the serious adverse event.[6,7] All research participants who suffer harm, whether related to the trial or not, should be offered appropriate medical care, psychosocial support, referrals, clinical facilities, etc. Medical management should be free if the harm is related to the research.

For sponsored research, it is the responsibility of the sponsor (whether a pharmaceutical company, government or nongovernmental organization (NGO), national or international/bilateral/multilateral donor agency/institution) to include insurance coverage or provision for possible compensation for research related injury or harm within the budget.

In investigator initiated research/student research, the investigator/institution where the research is conducted becomes the sponsor. It is the responsibility of the host institution to provide compensation and/or cover for insurance for research-related injury or harm to be paid as decided by the EC. The institution should create in-built mechanism to be able to provide for compensation, such as a corpus fund in the institution.

ANCILLARY CARE

Participants may be offered free medical care for nonresearch-related conditions or incidental findings if these occur during the course of participation in the research, provided such compensation does not amount to undue inducement as determined by the EC.[5]

RESEARCH CONDUCTED AT THE COST OF SOMEONE'S LIFE

Doctors in India were questioned the ethics of a study which observed the natural course of precancerous uterine cervical lesions without treatment in women who had not given written consent to take part. In at least nine women, the lesions progressed to invasive cancer, and 62 women developed carcinoma in situ of the cervix before they were treated. There were serious flaws in the design of the trial, issues with consent and consent forms, absence of insurance cover, unstated conflict of interest (COI) on the part of a member of the institutional review board and so on.[8]

CONFLICT OF INTEREST

Conflict of Interest (COI) is a set of conditions where professional judgment concerning a primary interest such as participants' welfare or the validity of research tends to be unduly influenced by a secondary interest, financial or nonfinancial (personal, academic or political). COI can be at the level of researchers, EC members, institutions or sponsors. If COI is inherent in the research, it is important to declare this at the outset and establish appropriate mechanisms to manage it. ECs must evaluate each study in light of any disclosed interests and ensure that appropriate means of mitigation are taken.

The broad responsibilities of those involved in research, with respect to COI, are given below:

- *Research institutions must:*
  - Develop policies and SOPs to address COI issues that are dynamic, transparent and actively communicated
  - Implement policies and procedures to address COI and conflicts of commitment, and educate their staff about such policies
  - Monitor the research or check research results for accuracy and objectivity
  - Not interfere in the functioning and decision making of the EC.
- *Researchers must:*
  - Ensure that documents submitted to the EC include disclosure of COI (financial or nonfinancial) that may affect their research
  - Guard against conflicts of commitment that may arise from situations that place competing demands on researchers' time and loyalties
  - Prevent intellectual and personal conflicts by ensuring they do not serve as reviewers for grants and publications submitted by close colleagues, relatives and/or students.
- *Ethics committees must:*
  - Evaluate each study in light of any disclosed COI and ensure appropriate action is taken to mitigate this
  - Require their members to disclose their own COI and take appropriate measures to recuse themselves from reviewing or decision-making on protocols related to their COI
  - Make appropriate suggestions for management, if COI is detected at the institutional or researchers' level.[5]

CLINICAL TRIALS IN SPECIAL POPULATION

Information supporting the use of the drug in children, pregnant women, nursing women, elderly patients, patients with renal or other organ systems failure, and those on specific concomitant medications, is required to be submitted, if relevant to the clinical profile of the drug and its anticipated usage pattern.

Geriatrics

Geriatric patients should be included in Phase III clinical trials (and in Phase II trials, at the Sponsor's option) if:

- The disease intended to be treated is characteristically a disease of aging
- The population to be treated is known to include substantial numbers of geriatric patient
- When there is specific reason to expect that conditions common in the elderly are likely to be encountered
- When the new drug is likely to alter the geriatric patient's response (with regard to safety or efficacy) compared with that of the non-geriatric patient.

Pediatrics

Study in the pediatric age group for a new drug development program will depend on the medicinal product, the type of disease being treated, safety considerations, and the efficacy and safety of available treatments. For a drug expected to be used in children, evaluations should be made in the appropriate age group. It is usually appropriate to begin with older children before extending the trial to younger children and then infants. If the new drug is intended to treat serious or life-threatening diseases occurring in both adults and pediatric patients, for which there are

currently no or limited therapeutic options, pediatric population should be included in the clinical trials early, following assessment of initial safety data and reasonable evidence of potential benefit. The pediatric studies should include:
- Clinical trials
- Relative bioequivalence comparisons of the pediatric formulation with the adult formulation performed in adults
- Definitive pharmacokinetic studies for dose selection across the age ranges of pediatric patients in whom the drug is likely to be used.

Written informed consent should be obtained from the parent/legal guardian. However, all pediatric participants should be informed to the fullest extent possible about the study in a language and in terms that they are able to understand.

Pregnant or Nursing Women

For new drugs intended for use during pregnancy, follow-up data (pertaining to a period appropriate for that drug) on the pregnancy, fetus and child will be required. Where applicable, excretion of the drug or its metabolites into human milk should be examined and the infant should be monitored for predicted pharmacological effects of the drug.[2]

CRITERIA FOR RESEARCH INVOLVING PREGNANT WOMEN AND FETUS

- Appropriate studies on animals and nonpregnant individuals should have been completed (if applicable).
- The risk to the fetus must be the least possible risk for achieving the objectives of the trial, including when the purpose of the trial is to meet the health needs of the mother or the fetus.
- Researchers should not participate in decision-making regarding any termination of a pregnancy.
- No procedural changes, which will cause greater than minimal risk to the woman or fetus, will be introduced into the procedure for terminating the pregnancy solely in the interest of the trial.[5]

STUDIES WITH MEDICAL DEVICES

Investigational medical devices need both IEC and DCGI approval as per draft notification (Medical Devices Rules, 2016) dated 17th October 2016, issued for medical devices by the Ministry of Health and Family Welfare, Department of Health and Family Welfare, Government of India [GSR 983 (E)].

ANIMAL EXPERIMENTATION

Those involved in experimentation on animals must follow all the existing regulations and guidelines including the Prevention of Cruelty to Animals Act, 1960, amended in 1982, the Breeding and Experimentation Rules, 1998, amended in 2001 and 2006, the Guidelines for Care and Use of Animals in Scientific Research (Indian National Science Academy, 1982, amended in 2000), ICMR Guidelines on Humane Care and Use of Laboratory Animals, 2006, Committee for the Purpose of Control and Supervision of Experiments on Animals (CPCSEA) Guidelines for Laboratory Animal Facilities, 2003 to 2018 and Guidelines for Rehabilitation of Animals used in Research, 2010.

SOURCES OF FUNDING FOR ACADEMIC INVESTIGATOR INITIATED RESEARCH

Several governmental and NGOs in India like ICMR, Department of Biotechnology,

Department of Science and Technology and the Council for Scientific and Industrial Research, fund academic research. Several pharmaceutical companies in the country also fund investigator initiated research. The funding from the industry could be provision of drug supplies or monetary support or both.[9]

WORKING WITH A COLLABORATOR OUTSIDE THE COUNTRY

Studies that involve a collaborator from outside India need an additional approval from the Health Ministry Screening Committee, a committee that works out of ICMR and meets quarterly to assess these projects for collaborative merit.[10]

COMPENSATION IN THE CASES OF CLINICAL TRIAL-RELATED SERIOUS ADVERSE EVENTS OCCURRING DURING CLINICAL TRIALS

The Drugs and Cosmetics Rules have been amended vide GSR 53(E) dated 30-01-2013 inserting a Rule 122DAB in Schedule "Y". This includes the procedure for processing of reports to arrive at the cause of injury/death to the subject during clinical trial, and to determine the quantum of compensation, if any, to be paid by the sponsor or his representatives. An Independent Expert Committee shall examine the report and give its recommendation to the Licensing Authority within 30 days of receiving the report from the concerned EC. The Quantum of Compensation to be paid by the sponsor will be decided by the DCG(I) and it shall pass order as deemed necessary within 3 months of receiving the report on the Serious Adverse Event (SAE) or death. Then the sponsor or his representative shall pay the compensation as per the order of the DCG(I) within 30 days of the receipt of such order.

Considering minimum wages as on date as ₹ 7,722.00/month, accordingly, a base amount (rounded) of ₹ 8.0 lakhs was assessed. It was also decided that this base amount should refer to the age of 65 years which corresponds to the factor of 99.37 of the table of Worksmen Compensation Act (Annexure 1). It is evident that the base amount will increase/change with the revision of minimum wage.

Computing the three factors, viz. (1) age, (2) risk, and (3) base amount, following formula emerged for deciding the quantum of compensation in case of SAE (death) related to clinical trial:

Compensation = $B \times F \times R\ A/99.37$

Where, B = Base amount (i.e. 8 lakhs)

F = Factor depending on the age of the subject as per Annexure 1 (based on Workmen Compensation Act)

R = Risk factor depending on the seriousness and severity of the disease, presence of comorbidity and duration of disease of the subject at the time of enrolment in the clinical trial between a scale of 0.5 and 4 as under:

- 0.5 terminally ill patient [expected survival not more than (NMT) 6 months]
- 1.0 patient with high risk (expected survival between 6 and 24 months)
- 2.0 patient with moderate risk
- 3.0 patient with mild risk
- 4.0 healthy volunteers or subject of no risk.

Thus, it will be seen that the compensation amount will vary from a minimum of ₹ 4 lakhs to a maximum of ₹ 73.60 lakhs depending on the age of the deceased and the risk factor. However, in case of patients whose expected mortality is 90% or more within 30 days, a fixed amount of ₹ 2 lakhs should be given.

CONCLUSION

There is increased need for laws relating to clinical research as India had become a hub for clinical trials and the rights of the participants were being violated. The Supreme Court also gave directions to protect the rights of participants including the need to have audio-visual recording of informed consent in clinical trials. In this scenario, it is essential that the various legal aspects of clinical trials and research are known to those who are involved in the design and carrying out of these studies. In this manner, we would be better equipped to get trials approved as well as to carry out trials without legal and ethical issues. Publication of clinical trial data would also be helped by the knowledge of the registration process of clinical trials and studies prior to their commencement. This would go a long way in improving the environment for the conduct of clinical research in India.

REFERENCES

1. Pandey A (2018). Legal issues in conducting clinical trials in India—iPleaders. [online]. iPleaders. Available from: https://blog.ipleaders.in/legal-issues-conducting-clinical-trials-india. {Accessed December, 2018].
2. Cdsco.nic.in. (2018). [online]. Available from: http://cdsco.nic.in/html/D&C_Rules_Schedule_Y.pdf [Accessed December, 2018].
3. Pandey A, Aggarwal AR, Seth SD, et al. Clinical Trials Registry – India: Redefining the conduct of clinical trials. Indian J Cancer. 2008;45(3):79-82.
4. Pandey A, Aggarwal A, Maulik, M, et al. Clinical trial registration gains momentum in India. Indian J Med Res [Letter to Editor]. 2009;130:85-86.
5. Icmr.nic.in. (2017). [online]. Available from: https://www.icmr.nic.in/sites/default/files/guidelines/ICMR_Ethical_Guidelines_2017.pdf [Accessed December, 2018].
6. Cdsco.nic.in. (2018). [online]. Available from: http://www.cdsco.nic.in/writereaddata/Office%20Order%20dated%2019.11.2013.pdf [Accessed December, 2018].
7. Cdsco.nic.in. (2018). [online]. Available from: http://www.cdsco.nic.in/writereaddata/GSR%20313%20(E)%20dated%2016_03_2016.pdf [Accessed December, 2018].
8. Madur G. Indian Study of women with cervical lesions called Unethical. BMJ. 1997;314(7087):1065.
9. Cdsco.nic.in. (2018). [online]. Available from: http://www.cdsco.nic.in/writereaddata/1Draft%20Rules%20on%20compensation.pdf [Accessed December, 2018].
10. Icmr.nic.in. (2018). Indian Council of Medical Research. [online]. Available from: http://www.icmr.nic.in [Accessed December, 2018].

ANNEXURE 1

Factors (F) for calculating the amount of compensation

Age	Factors
<16	228.54
17	227.49
18	226.38
19	225.22
20	224.00
21	222.71
22	221.37
23	219.95
24	218.47
25	216.91
26	215.28
27	213.57
28	211.79
29	209.92
30	207.98
31	205.95
32	203.85
33	201.66
34	199.40
35	197.06
36	194.64
37	192.14
38	189.56
39	186.90
40	184.17
41	181.37
42	178.49
43	175.54
44	172.52
45	169.44
46	166.29
47	163.07
48	159.80
49	156.47
50	153.09
51	149.67
52	146.20
53	142.68
54	139.13
55	135.56
56	131.95
57	128.33
58	124.70
59	121.05
60	117.41
61	113.77
62	110.14
63	106.52
64	102.93
65 or more	99.37

CHAPTER

20

Role of Social Media in Clinical Practice: Legal Implications

Sidharth Sonthalia, Dharmendra Arora, Aseem Sharma, Madhulika Mhatre

INTRODUCTION

There have been four innovations in the history of communication: the printing press, the telephone and telegraph, television and radio, and social media. The transition of a general surgeon from open laparotomy to laparoscopic surgery to robot-assisted minimally invasive surgery; a logical outcome of decades of systematic advancements in the healthcare sector can now considered be too gradual a change in contrast with the transformation of patients from "simple quintessential patients" to "*e-patients*" to "instant messenger (IM)-patients" to "difficult patients" to "clients and customers" and the "litigational patients," an unregulated phenomenon that occurred within years and expected to become the chief determinant of delivery of healthcare services in India and abroad.

Notwithstanding the plethora of problems that a huge section of dermatologists and other medical professionals are facing today following skewed "patient empowerment" through the internet and social media portals, the internet revolution has also rendered a huge peace quotient to everybody's life, both personal and professional. From buying a product from the comfort of our home to selling products online; from instant acquisition and sharing of latest knowledge and skills through discussions on academically-committed mailer groups, Facebook discussion forum and academic groups on instant messaging (IM) service portals such as and Telegram; to exploring the option of widening your outreach to patients through online clinic software– the World Wide Web or WWW seems to rule the roost now. And the independence of social media from need of bulky hardware, strict proprietary regulations and other directives due to sheer lack of them or their enforcement adds on to its desirability for use by patients in varied realms of healthcare. The year 2004 established "Web 2.0" as a term designating an entire range of interactive and collaborative aspects of the Internet, including new ways of approaching and exploiting the organizational possibilities of the Web.[1] Therefore, digital content and information is no longer made available to Internet surfers only by the mass media, but also by private individuals, interconnected through online networks, who use the web for active dissemination of information across the globe.

DEFINING SOCIAL MEDIA

The Merriam-Webster dictionary defines Social Media as *"the forms of electronic communication (such as websites for social networking and microblogging) through which users create online communities to share information, ideas, personal messages, and other content (such as videos)."* It is worth noting that the definition of Social Media ranked amongst the top 1% of the Merriam-Webster pool of words whose definitions are searched on the internet.[2]

This relatively heuristic description can be enhanced with inputs from Wikipedia that states—*"Social media are interactive computer-mediated technologies that facilitate the creation and sharing of information, ideas, career interests and other forms of expression via virtual communities and networks. The variety of stand-alone and built-in social media services currently available introduces challenges of definition; however, there are some common features"* (Box 1).

Social media can be categorized into six broad groups:
- Collaborative projects (e.g. Wikipedia)
- Blogs or microblogs (e.g. Blogger, Twitter)
- Content communities (e.g. YouTube)
- Social networking sites (e.g. Facebook)
- Virtual gaming or social worlds (e.g. Second Life)[3]
- Instant messenger (IM) portals (e.g. WhatsApp, Telegram).

BOX 1: Characteristic features of social media.
- Social media are interactive Web 2.0 Internet-based applications; thus can be accessed through any device that supports these (computer, laptop, I-pad, smartphone, etc.).
- The hardcore content of social media include user-generated content, such as text posts or comments, digital photos or videos, and data generated through all online interactions.
- The engagement of the users involved creation of service-specific profiles for the website or available apps. The job of the social media organization is to design, maintain, update, and periodically upgrade these websites and apps.
- The essential working theme of social media is to facilitate the development of online social networks by interconnecting profiles of users, whether individuals or groups.

IMPACT OF SOCIAL MEDIA ON PRACTICE OF MEDICINE: FACTS, EVIDENCE AND CONTROVERSIES

Social media has literally performed a surgical transformation in healthcare related communication and practice. Prior to the era of the *world wide web (WWW) boom*, the physician-patient relationship was predicated on an asymmetry of medical knowledge; physicians had sequestered all of sequestered all of it and patients were and patients were practically entirely dependent on them. Now, electronic tools empowered with the force of social media have allowed for medical knowledge parity. This has changed the overall approach of patients to physicians resulting in a balancing change in the attitude and carefulness of doctors. Our neolexicon now consists of *e-patients* and *e-doctors, shared decision making, health care tweet chats,* and *online reputation.*[3]

In a nationwide survey of 3,014 adults living in the United States (US) through telephonic (landline or mobile phone) interviews conducted by Princeton Survey

TABLE 1: Important statistical information from the nationwide survey of 3014 adult residents of the US conducted by Princeton Survey Research Associates International from August 7 to September 6, 2012.

Phenomenon	Statistics
Adults who had have gone online at one time or another to try to figure out what medical condition they or someone else might have.	>35%
Respondents/online *diagnosers* who said that the information found online led them to think:	
• They needed the attention of a medical professional	46%
• It was something they could take care of at home	38%
• Both or in-between.	11%
On accuracy of initial self-diagnosis made online: After initial online diagnosis, the respondents who said that:	
• The medical professional confirmed the same diagnosis completely or partially	43%
• The medical professional either did not agree or offered a different opinion about the condition	18%
• Conversation with the clinician was inconclusive	1%
• They did not go to a medical professional.	35%
Online payment to seek information—of those who looked online for health information:	
• Those who were asked to pay for access to the information they sought	26%
• Of those who have been asked to pay:	
– Users who actually paid	2%
– Users who tried to find the same information free of cost somewhere else.	83%
Peer-to-peer sharing attempt—in the past 12 months:	
• Users who read or watched someone else's experience about health or medical issues	26%
• Users who went online find others who might share the same health concerns.	16%
Smart phone users who used their phone to search for health information.	52%
Smartphone owners who downloaded an app specifically to track or manage health-related issues.	19%

Research Associates International from August 7 to September 6, 2012, 72% of Internet users admitted to having searched for health information online within the last year.[4] Other important statistics of this survey are given in Table 1.[4,5] Those who were more likely to seek medical information online included those with net access, younger individuals (18–49 years), women, individuals privileged with higher level of education, and/or residence in higher-income group households, people suffering with chronic or serious health concerns themselves or those with loved ones suffering from such issues.

As per the Bupa Health Pulse 2010 survey conducted by Max Bupa, out of the total number of Indians who access information online, more than one-third (39%) used the net for health information.[6] The primary use of the internet for health purposes as per this 2010 survey was finding information about medicines (68% of respondents) in all countries. Other uses in India included searching for information to make a self-diagnosis (46%), seeking for other patients' experiences (39%), and looking for information on medical professionals (36%). More people in India (e-mail: 36%, text: 35%) and Mexico (e-mail: 38%, text: 35%) report being able to text and e-mail their doctor than elsewhere in the world.[6]

SOCIAL NETWORK PENETRATION IN INDIA

Figure 1 presents the social network penetration in India in 16-64 year age group (*Source*: www.statista.com).[7] In the third quarter of 2017, the most popular social network were YouTube and Facebook (30% penetration rate each), closely followed by WhatsApp (28% reach). Although India ranks among the top three countries with the most Facebook users, accounting for 11% of global Facebook audiences in April 2017, the overall active social networking in India as per January 2017 data was only 14% of the population–one of the lowest rates worldwide.[7]

Even if you are not using social media, your patients are!

It is imperative for dermatologists to be cognizant of the fact that Facebook alone has more than 800 million active users worldwide, with more than 200 million added in 2011. More than 80% of American adults use an online social network, with Facebook grabbing the maximum time of those on social media. With almost 23% of the entire time an average user spends online being spent on social networking, professionals including dermatologists are left with little choice other than harnessing the immense power of social media to their marketing advantage.[8] The three major marketing benefits attainable through social media are:

- High visibility to a large number of people
- Personalized connectivity with potential clients
- Personal image enhancement and self-promotion.

A common question that is often asked by dermatologist unsavvy with social media marketing is–"*I have a very attractive and interactive website; then why do I still need to engage with social media to increase my patient/client number?*"

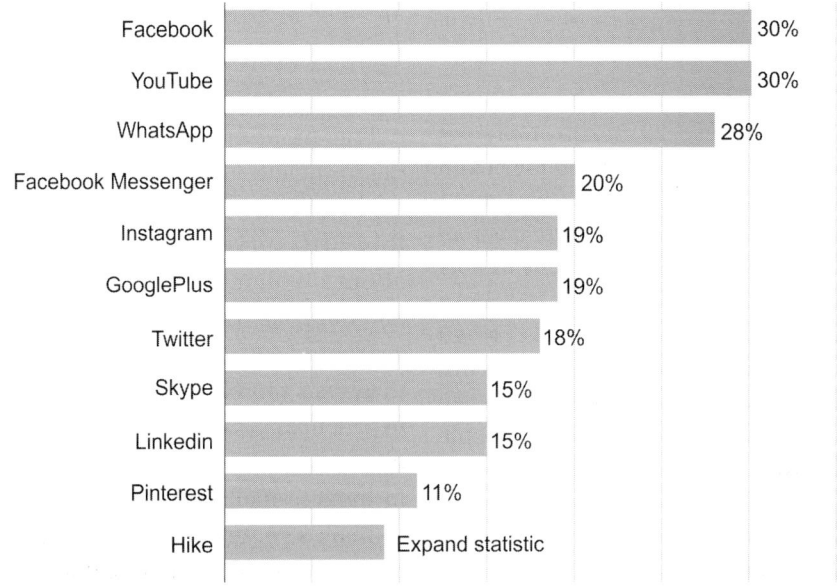

Fig. 1: Bar diagram showing the penetrance of common social media platforms in India.

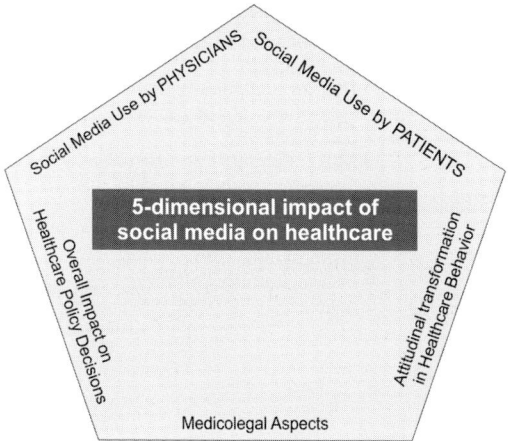

Fig. 2: The 5-dimensional impact of social media on healthcare.

> **BOX 2:** Major uses of social media portals for dermatologists and other healthcare givers.
>
> - To enhance and expand the scope of one's practice
> - Mutual exchange of knowledge, updates and skills
> - Showcasing one's major accomplishments in the field such as Awards, Conference Faculty invitations, Special recognitions, etc.
> - Fostering collegiality with colleagues from other specialties
> - Promoting the principle of patient benefaction, e.g. by posting useful patient awareness information
> - Raising contentious healthcare issues to trigger meaningful discussions, (e.g. the current epidemic of recalcitrant dermatophytic infections, violence against doctors).

Well, the answer is pretty straightforward. Any good or great website including that of a dermatologist needs targeted visibility in an organic search for maximum output. Websites integrated with active social networking tend to receive higher importance by leading search engines such as Google. In fact, social media activities associated with a website have become one of the most reliable forms of evidence to determine the website's worthiness from the point of view of online readers.[8] Every link or mention of the website on a social media platform is sensed by search engines as an endorsement of the content by the internet readers; improving the page rankings with more readers endorsing that socially networked website.

The paradox of great enthusiasm surrounding the use of social media in healthcare versus the paucity of evidence of its outcome and the medicolegal impact is unfortunate. Given the rapid expansion and adoption of social media by doctors and patients alike, confounded by the visual nature of dermatologic diagnosis, evaluation of the ill-defined realms of this issue becomes imperative. The five essential dimensions of this issue that warrant deliberation have been depicted in Figure 2.

SOCIAL MEDIA USE BY DOCTORS: REASONS, MERITS, AND DANGERS (BOX 2)

We have classified the current popular uses of social media portals by dermatologists into three main categories (Fig. 3). The debate on the uses of social networking mediablogs and microblogs (Twitter), social networking sites (Facebook, Myspace, Instagram), IM portals (WhatsApp, Telegram), and content sharing sites (YouTube, Flickr) by medical professionals is now a favorite topic of conversation amongst doctors and ancillary personnel. The primal question is *"What all reasons can/should a doctor use these networking portals for;"* answer to which would further need evidence backing and critical analysis. Social media is being used by doctors for variety of reasons the most common being to enhance and expand the scope of their practice. This is being achieved by elementary indulgences such as ensuring mere web-presence (Fig. 4A), posting information with or without

Section 1: General Medical Law

Knowledge and skill enhancement	Practice enhancement	Deliverance of medical benefaction
• Trouble-shooting • Direct tutorial learning • Dedicated educational forums • Planned learning through conferences and workshops	• Website promotion with social media linking • Projection of special skills and services of the dermatologists and clinic/centre • Sharing of pre-and post-results and patient testimonials • Declaration of special achievements, medals, honors, faculty invites at reputed conferences • Announcements of creation of special interest groups, societies and conducting relevant conferences	• Patient and community awareness about specific conditions • Making patients and community beware of malafide healthcare practices • Specific campaigns against discriminatory yet popular sociocultural/government policies

Fig. 3: Utility of social media by doctors in three tiers.

pictures and videos about "services" including "special facilities" available at one's clinic or center (Fig. 4B), creation of interactive webpages to sensitize and incentivize online patients to seek consultation, (Fig. 4C), sharing testimonials taken from happy patients (Fig. 4D), maintaining a systematic communication channel (tweets, blogs, Facebook posts, etc.) discussing conditions and therapies that people often surf for, regular sloganeering with posting of "words of wisdom" akin to health awareness posts (Fig. 5A), and showcasing one's major accomplishments in the field such as awards, invitations as faculty to conferences, special recognitions (Fig. 5B), etc. Fostering collegiality with colleagues from other specialties to present a perception of providing multispecialty care is a new addendum to this end. The other major reason of some doctors' stint with social media is to advance the pristine principle of benefaction by either posting selfless patient awareness information (Fig. 5C), bringing contentious healthcare issues on the table to trigger meaningful discussions (Fig. 5D), and creating and/or responding in specially created professional groups for mutual exchange of knowledge, updates and skills (*vide infra*). The phenomenon of posting information and/or visual minutia reflecting self-admiration for nonmonetary benefit of ego-boost also seems to be catching up, possibly stemming from peer pressure.

Exchange of Knowledge, Updates and Skills

Social media has become the source for exchange of specialty-relevant as well as interspecialty exchange of medical know-how, updates and skills. An overview with specific mention of few popular community groups catering to this concept has been outlined in Figure 6. It is essential to mention that the preference for a particular social media platform to host such academic-cum-practical exchange is also shifting from relatively "slow response" portals like the Yahoo groups (Fig. 7A) or FB pages (Fig. 7B) to "instant response" portals like WhatsApp (Fig. 7C) and Telegram (Fig. 7D); notwithstanding the fact that this shift is likely to be temporary owing to the rapid availability of smart phone-enabled apps and messenger services of the erstwhile website-predominant social media platforms.

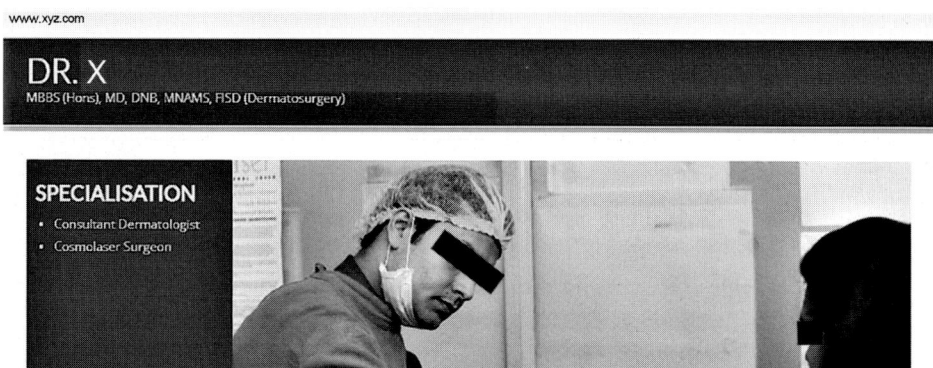

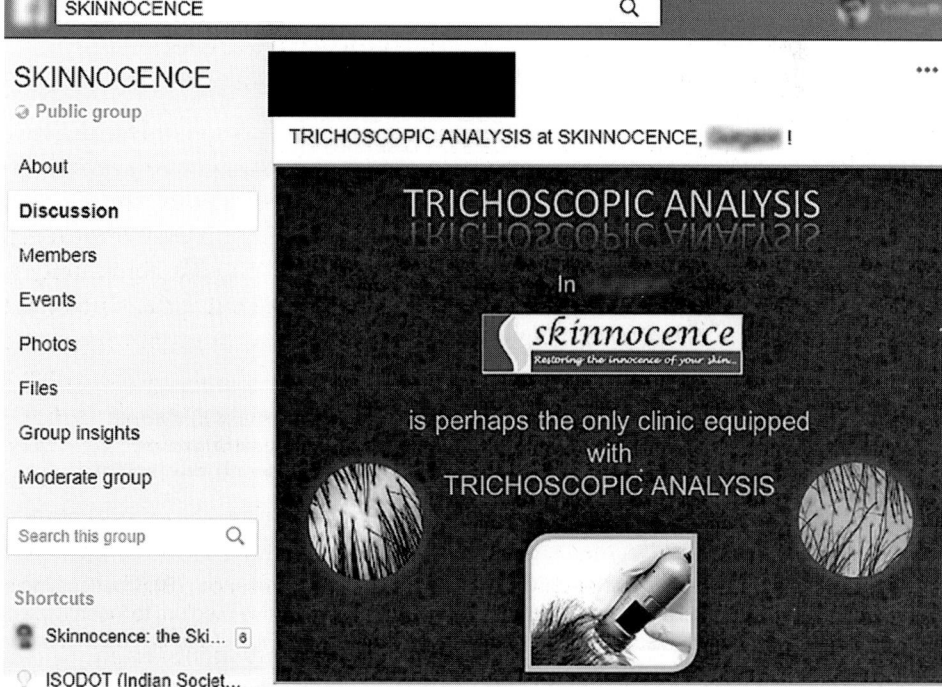

Figs. 4A and B

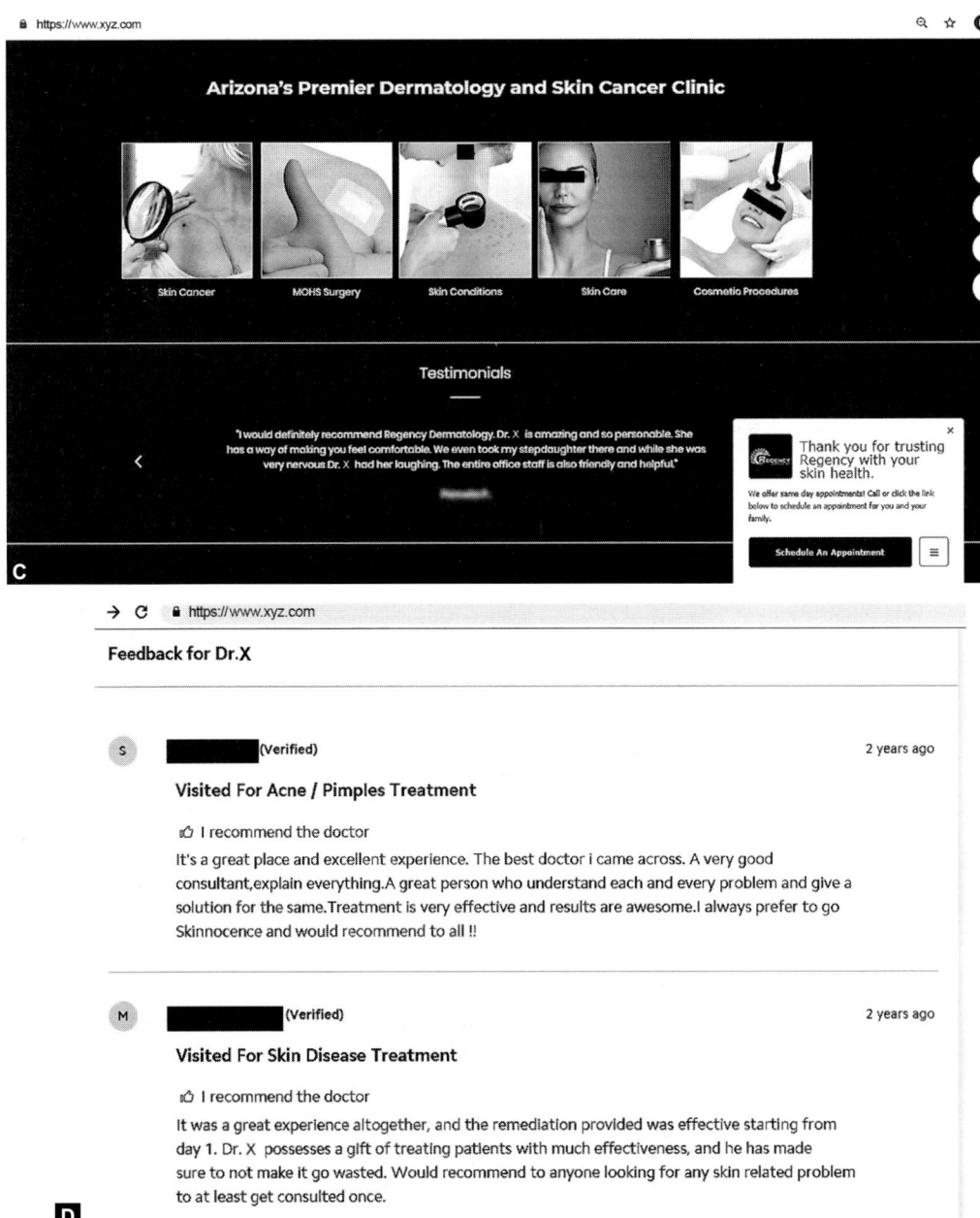

Figs. 4C and D

Figs. 4A to D: A doctor's website: (A) Depicting the value of mere 'web-presence'; (B) Broadcasting services and facilities available at the clinic; (C) Showcasing the role of an interactive medium to incentivize potential patients; (D) Testimonials received from patients. (*For color version of Figs. 4A to C, see Plates 1 and 2*).

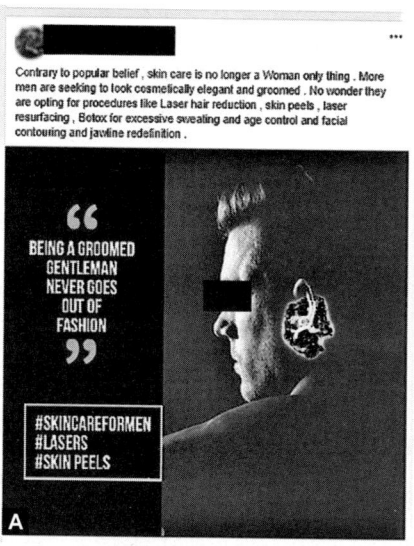

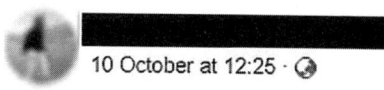

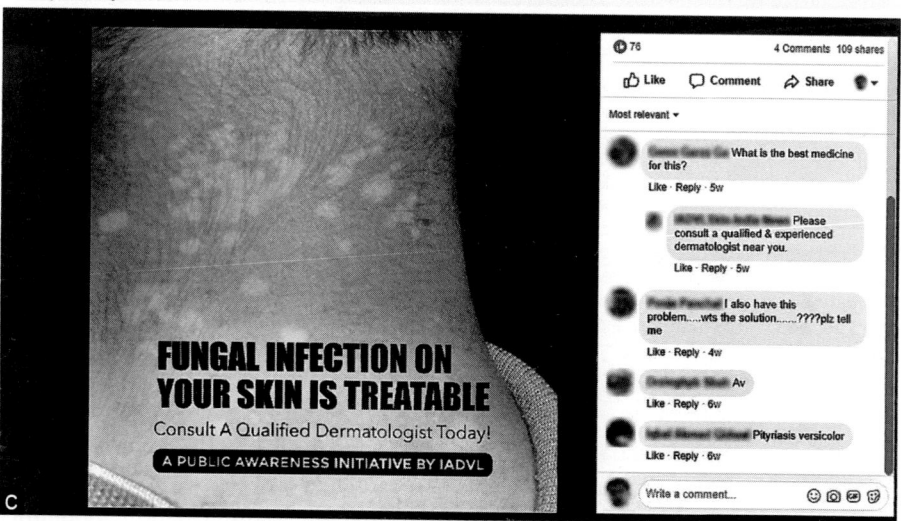

Figs. 5A to C

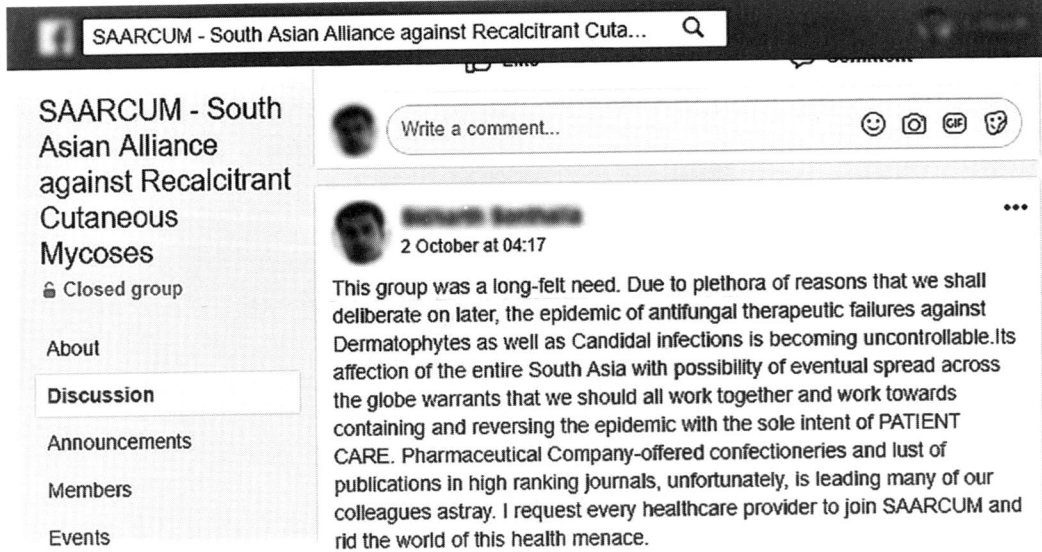

Fig. 5D

Figs. 5A to D: Facebook as a medium for (A) Sloganeering and publishing 'word of wisdom'; (B) Showcasing one's major achievements in the field; (C) Posting selfless patient awareness information; (D) Discussing contentious healthcare issues. (*For color version of Fig. 5C, see Plate 2*).

Knowledge and skill enhancement	
	Trouble shooting—Discussion forums on Facebook, e.g. the Indian Journal of Dermatology [IJD] (slow response approach), and Whatsapp/Telegram discussion groups, e.g. the DSI-IDG group (instant response approach) seeking out solution to a sticky patient situation with peer suggestions.
	Direct tutorial learning—Through procedural videos posted by peers (free/by paid-subscription), discussion forums like IADVL ACAD_IADVL (Yahoo group), IJD group (Facebook), DermaSourceIndia [DSI] - Innovative Dermatology Group (Whatsapp/Telegram) through regular featurs like Molecule of the Week, Quizzes, Posting of Updates, E-Books, sharing of Published articles, etc.
	Dedicated educational forum—The IJD FB page is primarily for trouble-shooting, in contrast, the IADVL ACAD_IADVL yahoo group is content-wise more versatile, with exchange of published material, articles, etc. and periodic selection of topics with nominated moderators and panelists. The DSI's 3 discussion groups – DSI-IDG (Innovative Dermatology Group), DSI-IDS-CDA (DSI – Cosmetic Dermatology and Aesthetic Group), and DSI-Dermoscopy group, offer, in addition to the above, other features like – Grand rounds, Daily Quiz, Dermoscopic Image Quiz, Molecule of the week, Practical Tip of the Week, Practice Management Tip and other educational paraphernalia.
	Planned learning through conferences and workshops—Dermatologist groups and Societies hold focused conferences at state/regional/national levels, with Live Demo and/or HANDS_ON training Workshops on procedures that are novel or require repeated practice. Thus Social Media offers the quickest and most wholesome dissemination about such events for interested learners.

Fig. 6: The 4 tiers of knowledge and skill enhancement on social media.

Essentially, the scope of this exchange is wide, ranging to seeking for colleagues' suggestions for an odd or difficult case management (Fig. 8A), a specific procedure, drug or molecule (Fig. 8B), or device, novel technologies, statutory and medicolegal advice, issues related to practice management, or information about upcoming CMEs or conferences or workshops (Fig. 8C)

Role of Social Media in Clinical Practice: Legal Implications

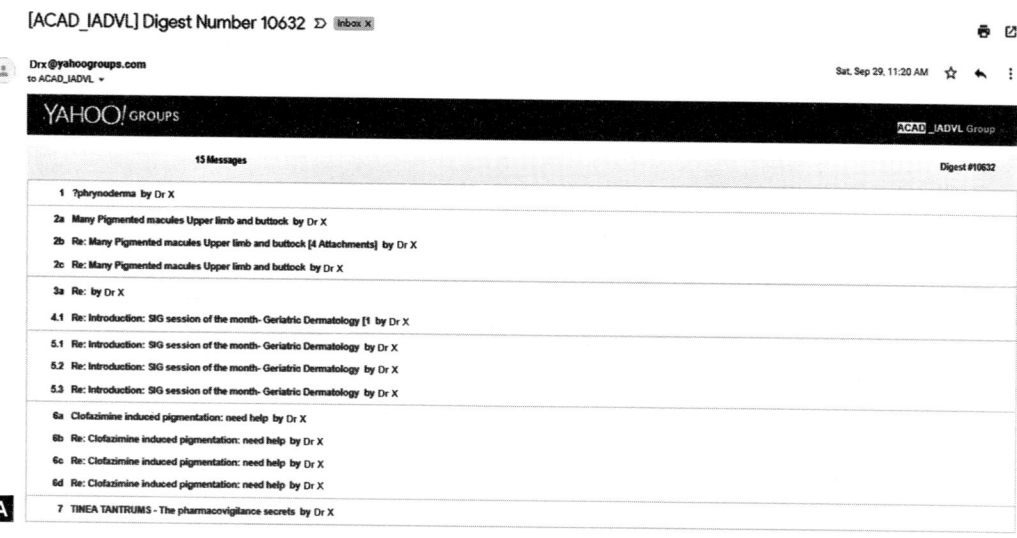

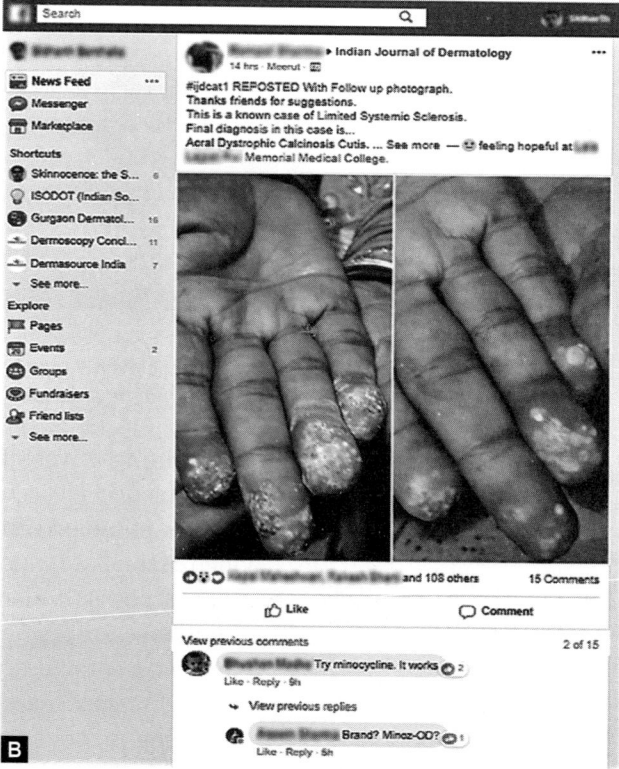

Figs. 7A and B

to name a few. The concept of dermatologists preparing and posting videos of a particular technique they are skilled in, through YouTube channels, FB video posts (Fig. 8D) and instant messenger-based portals like WhatsApp and Telegram are up trending.

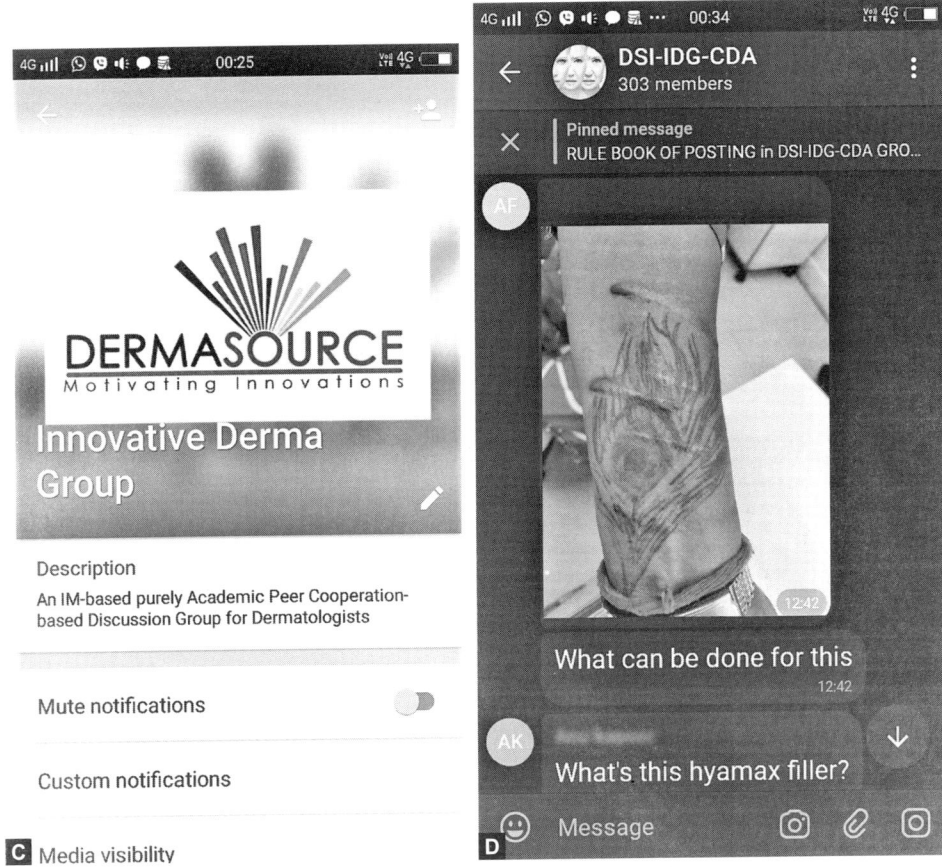

Fig. 7C and D

Figs. 7A to D: Preferential social media platforms for academic exchange: (A) Yahoo groups; (B) Facebook; (C) WhatsApp; (D) Telegram. (*For color version of Figs. 7B and D, see Plate 3*).

Essentials of Engaging in Social Media Marketing for a Dermatologist

Content creation, its presentation, and active online engagement constitute the three tenets of social media marketing. Which social platforms should a dermatologist use? Although there is no standard answer to this question, few essential guidelines may help.

- *Essential social networks worth engaging:* A bouquet of following networking portals may be the bare minimum for a dermatologist interested in maintaining prominence in social media networks – maintaining a Website and/or blog for one's practice, a Facebook Business page of one's clinic or center, a YouTube or Video channel, a Twitter account, and/or a Pinterest board. The latter assumes special importance for cosmetic dermatologists. Pinterest, a community for collecting and sharing images is an ideal platform for marketing practice, educating patients, and building brand loyalty. The site allows users to create customized "boards" on which you can "pin" pictures of your office, yourself, and your staff, as well as before-and-after images (in compliance

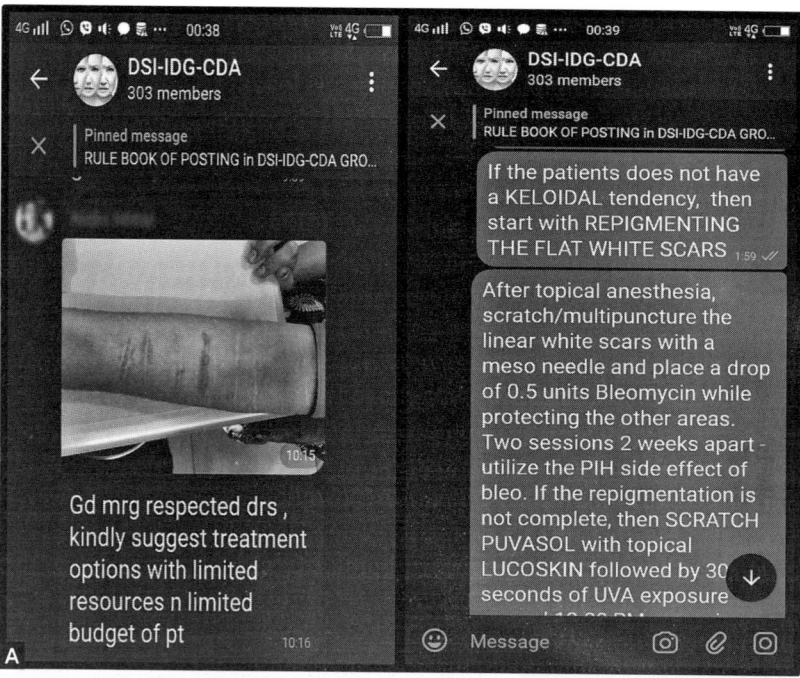
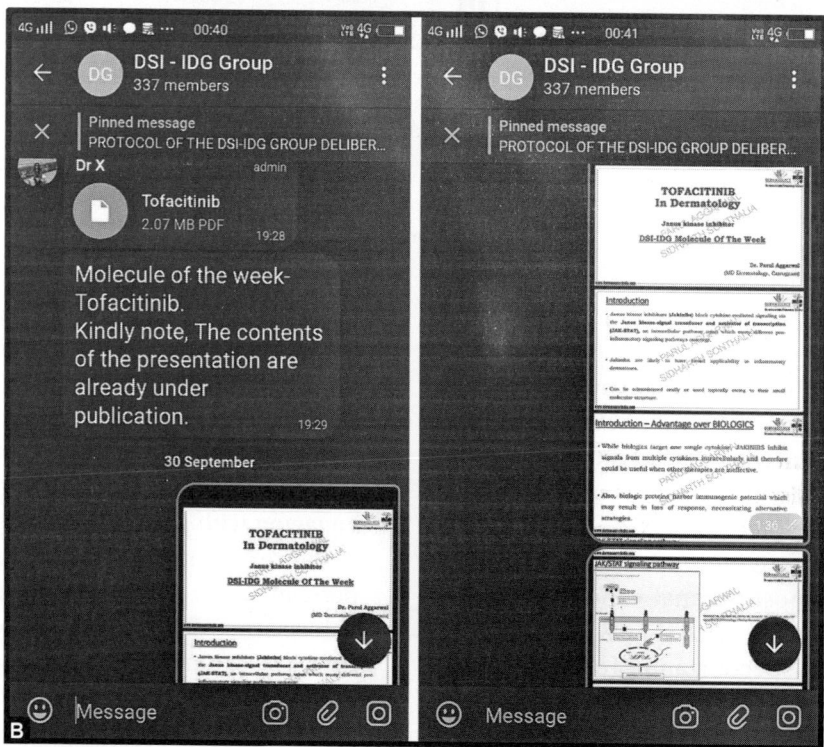

Figs. 8A and B

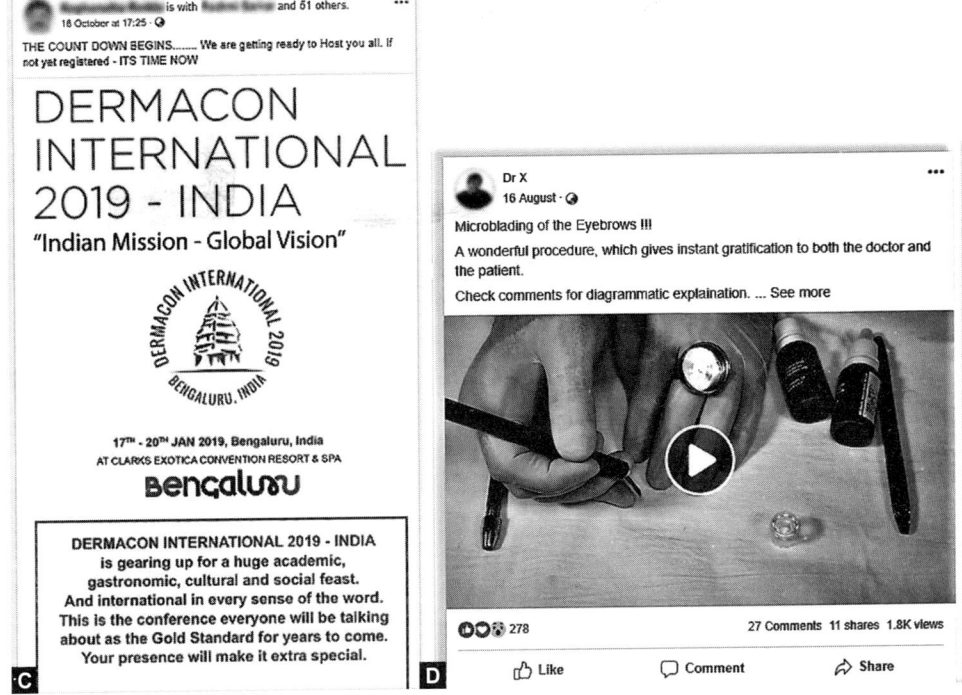

Figs. 8C and D

Figs. 8A to D: The scope of academic exchange is divided into seeking or disseminating: (A) Peers' opinion for managing a case; (B) Knowledge regarding a new drug; (C) Knowledge about an upcoming CME or conference; (D) Specific training on a procedure of academic interest. *(For color version of Fig. 8A, see Plate 3 and Fig. 8D, see Plate 4).*

with the country-specific regulation of such content), skin care protocols, product recommendations, and much more.
- *Regular updating:* The key to successful use of these portals however, is to constantly update them—whether you do it yourself (which may be difficult owing to time constraints) or delegate the task to the office assistant or manager or a professional content writer.
- *Content originality and customization:* Always post original content related to one's practice, such as areas or procedures of one's specialization (e.g. injectables for cosmetic rejuvenation, Trichology, Dermoscopy, Vitiligo surgery, etc.) features that is unique to one's practice, and useful tips and information for patients. Customized posts can drive the patient network traffic to your Website; whereas rewriting or even buying prewritten blog posts already present on the websites or webpages of your colleagues will neither improve your reputation, rather may prove counterproductive.
- *Consider seeking services from experts or professionals:* Despite the ease of engaging with social media networks, to optimize the outcome of your engagement, dermatologists can partner with professional social networking experts or companies that are experienced in social media promotions. Internet marketing firms with an exclusive focus on promoting medical practices (even specialty-specific firms) are easily available to partner with you

to create and manage a highly successful social networking campaign.

- *Social Media "Chain Reaction:"* Social media offer a dermatologist the potential to reach out to the maximum number of new patients at the lowest marketing cost per patient; additionally, it requires the least amount of time and effort compared to any other form of advertising and marketing. The power of social networks stems from the exponential transfer of any intended post through the "chain reaction" of followers and fans on each network. For example, if one follower on Twitter shares an interesting Tweet on dermatology, it will automatically reach a hundred or thousands of followers, depending on the activity of the Twitter handle of the user. And out of those 100 followers, if one other follower retweets the same tweet, the reach will grow exponentially.

Essential Notes for the Dermatologist Engaging in Social Media

Certain unforeseen issues (potential spoilers) have already started crippling the logistics of this noble academic aspect of social media in healthcare delivery. While checks and balances provided by the social media hosting companies like FB, Google, YouTube, etc. such as privacy filters for individual users, some degree of filtration of material considered universally objectionable, blocking and/or instant deletion of unlawful posts, and country-specific content vigilance are helpful to a certain extent, in essence the onus of ensuring rightful use of the content posted on these portals of a dermatologist, or any doctor or professional using social media lies on the individual.

It is imperative to discuss certain grey areas in this regard:

Online Reputation Management

The Internet is a free medium with minimum control rendering it extremely difficult to manage a dermatologist's or doctor's online image or reputation. Websites such as Yelp and Dr Score now enable patients to expand the reach of their recommendations. Doctor-rating Web sites like Dr Score are essentially social media forums that allow patients to connect and share information about a dermatologist and his or her practice.[3] While dedicated attention paid to the social media accounts can significantly enhance the dermatologist online reputation, even fake negative testimonials posted by third-party reviewers can actually counter it hugely. Ironically, there is nothing much that the dermatologist or the concerned professional can actually do about the issue. In contrast, social media networks such Facebook, Twitter, YouTube, Google Plus, Flickr, and LinkedIn provide the user with a far greater degree of personalized control through various hierarchical empowering the dermatologist or the professional to manage his or her online reputation in a much better way.

Online Consultation

Although teledermatology may be considered to be a totally separate subject, there is a definite overlap between social media networking and teledermatology. Websites and apps that facilitate "online consultation" like Icliniq have cropped up, with many of them suffering from lacunae with respect to patient confidentiality, regulations on exchange of patient pictures, and inadequate control of spammers. The "visual diagnosis" specific to Dermatology makes this issue more pertinent for skin specialists. Many online-consultation websites entice dermatologists with the proposition of making "extra money" by engaging in online consultations with patients. Many patients who use these portals also request for specific dermatologists based on their social media reputation. The doctor, on the other hand, must exercise caution in responding to such requests. Online consultations should never be solicited.[9] Matters relating to doctor or patient relationship are legally binding. Needless to say, that a proper consultation is based first on social interaction, history taking, and then employment of diagnostic tools like Dermoscopy, skin smears, biopsies, etc. prior to coming to a proper diagnosis. A doctor may be doing harm if this interaction is compromised.

Instant Messenger Consultations

For a plethora of reasons, some of which may be genuine (patient developing a reaction to prescribed topicals while he or she is out of town or country, emergency-like situation developing at an odd time, inability to physically bring an invalid patient for face-to-face consultation) patients have started using IM based portals like WhatsApp to seek a diagnosis and guidelines on management from a dermatologist by freely sharing their pictures with the dermatologist. In absence of a clear law in India and many other countries, even if the dermatologist responds with some advice other than asking for a face-to-face consultation, any untowardly consequence arising out of lack of personalized consultation, poor quality of images sent by the patient, patient's misjudgment of the symptoms, or misfit between the actual medical condition and the prescription suggested by the dermatologist on WhatsApp—the entire onus is likely to be on the doctor, rather than the patient. It is common place that many patients who sustain any postprocedure issue, (e.g. persistent redness or excessive flaking after a chemical peel, or mild burn after a laser

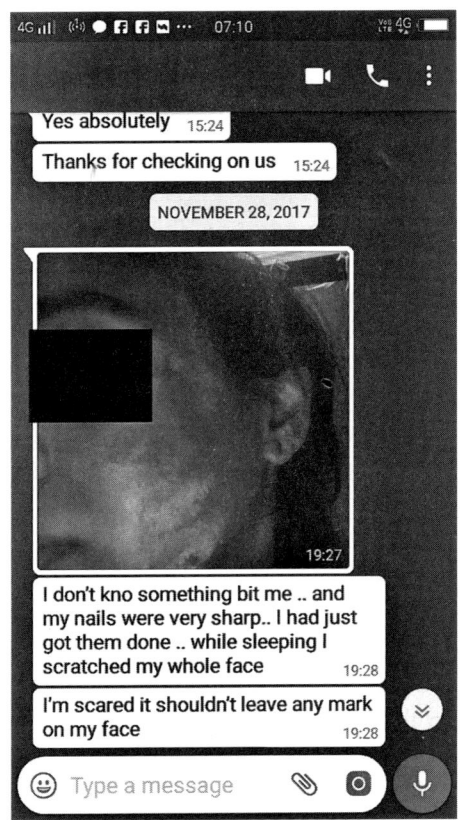

Fig. 9: A WhatsApp excerpt showing a patient attempting to gain online consultation to avoid a physical visit to the clinic. (*For color version of Fig. 9, see Plate 4*).

treatment) or an intermittent issue prefer to seek a follow-up advice on WhatsApp to avoid another physical visit to the dermatologist's clinic (Fig. 9). Some of the unjustified reasons of patients for exploiting WhatsApp and Telegram seeking dermatologist's consultation include avoidance of making the effort to physically meet the doctor as the clinic and unwillingness to pay the doctor's fees.

The "Dark Side" of Social Media Use in Dermatology

Although the proponents of social media engagement in healthcare often compare a dermatology set-up with a small or medium-sized business and base their arguments on the advantages to the dermatologists and patients, and the increasing necessity of networking with changing times, there are many potential risks of using social media in medical practice. These stem from the sense of disinhibition and anonymity in online environments that may lead to inappropriate postings, amplified immediately by the wide reach of the media.[10] Notions of privacy itself are being reconfigured through online norms, which are guiding the patient-doctor engagement. The major concerns include the risk with patient confidentiality, erosion of general faith in the medical profession through doctors posting content that contains blasphemous or discriminatory language, and/or depictions of intoxication or sexually explicit behavior.[11] Patients hold a stereotypical image of a doctor, and any depiction on social media like Facebook or Instagram which is in gross contradiction with that can tarnish the reputation of that doctor and by extension of the fraternity. Mixing up personal and professional pages by displaying to the patients, vacation photographs of doctors in a carefree attitude and unprofessional attire can be disastrous.

The above concerns make a strong point favoring the concept of *"e-professionalism"* as a distinct new paradigm requiring particular training and practice and formulation of new policies that prescribe guidelines for normative behavior to regulate and reduce social media use.[12,13] For example, The General Medical Council of the United Kingdom released a national social media policy in April 2013 that emphasizes the prohibitive on: *"If you identify yourself as a doctor, do not share identifiable information about patients anywhere, do not mix social and professional relations, and do not post anonymous material on any site."*[14]

The recent incidents from India, of patient information and contact details being leaked out by some online clinic management software (CMS) to third party vendors like online pharmacies and other doctors is an unfortunate addendum to this issue. Many developed countries have enforced strict laws to provide protection for the privacy of patients' medical records, like The Health Insurance Portability and Accountability Act (HIPAA) enacted by the United States Congress in 1996 with civil or criminal penalties on breach of privacy.[15] Similar laws are urgently required in a country like India where the influence of social media on healthcare is expanding exponentially.

Social media can also be a large distraction in the workplace. With all the perks of accessing medical records easily through different websites or applications, it is also highly tempting to use that resource for recreational purposes during work. In fact, one study showed that institutions that allowed their participants to use Facebook every day for 15 min demonstrated a decrease in work efficiency by 1.5%.[16]

Social media participants can simultaneously be viewed as empowered agents and targets for exploitation.[10] Further the "digital divide" continues to complicate genuine online outreach to aging, low-income, or rural populations, which is huge issue in developing nations like India.

SOCIAL MEDIA USE BY PATIENTS AND PROSPECTIVE PATIENTS— CONCERNS AND CONTROVERSIES

The Flip-flop of "Words of Mouth"

A detailed account with statistics about the reasons for which patients, potential patients and their family members or peers use social media for healthcare, in particular dermatology-related issues has been discussed (*vide supra*). Gone are the days when the only determinants of sick people visiting a particular doctor were—community reputation, good experience in the past, proximity to their homes and/or the "word of mouth." The "word of mouth" literally refers to the concept of one or many satisfied patient(s) recommending a particular dermatologist, e.g. *"Dr XYZ finished off my acne within 2 months,"* or *"Dr ABC did chemical peels for me before my wedding and gave me a fabulous skin," "So you must visit him or her only before your wedding preparations."* Notwithstanding the contemporary contribution of the above determinant being significant even today, a larger chunk of patients seeks out a healthcare professional based on internet search via search engines like Google, checking out their websites, reading from blogs and microblogs like Twitter, and the impression generated by the extent and style of social media marketing by the doctor. The *"word of mouth"* is rapidly transforming into *"online reviews"*. The inherent problem with this approach is the absolute untrustworthiness of the source of review checked by the patient for the doctor. It is well-known that the specific nugget of information one is searching for, on searching using the closest "keywords" also ends up generating loads of information clutter, sifting which is impractical for a nonmedical person. According to Thomas Friedman, *"Never before in the history of the planet have so many people—on their own—had the ability to find so much information about so many things and about so many other people."*

Information has too many realms. Too much of information, especially unsorted, without any weightage and credibility itself serves as the biggest barrier to communication. The misuse or rather abuse of medical information from the net and social media is the outcome of the dichotomy between "information load" and lack of "information literacy."[17]

In the following discussion, we are extrapolating the concepts of "internet savviness" basically defined for general public to that of the e-patients in order to highlight certain core issues of their understanding of medical posts on social media portals.

Visual Literacy

Digital photography, along with audio and video "casts," allow anyone, including doctors to self-publish on the Web, potentially reaching a global audience. Dermatology being primarily visual medicine is most susceptible to good use or abuse of visual imageries put up by specialists for marketing their skills. Sophisticated and relatively inexpensive image-editing software puts the power of professional image manipulation into the hands of many—if not dermatologists themselves, then their less erudite clinic or business managers. Apart from the danger of luring internet-savvy, but visually illiterate innocent patients or clients by morphed images being propagandized as a product of the dermatologist's unique skills, copyright infringement (with images downloaded and freely used from the internet) and sometimes leakage and misuse of some other colleague's real patient's pictures leading to potential medicolegal hassles constitute the dark side of the use of visual cues by dermatologists to demonstrate pre- and post-treatment outcomes.

Information Fluency

Information fluency is perhaps the most commonly used term (after *information literacy*) to describe our ability—or lack thereof—to understand today's information environment. Information fluency is similar to information literacy, though it adds stronger technology or computer literacy and critical thinking skills into the mix of desired capabilities.[17] Akin to an information-fluent student, an e-patient ideally should possess the following skills to optimize the use of Social Media (SoMe) for healthcare purposes and offset any misguidance: determining the nature and extent of the information that is needed, processing the needed information effectively and efficiently, evaluating information and its sources critically and incorporating selected information into the knowledge base, using information to accomplish a specific purpose; and understanding many of the economic, legal, ethical, and social issues surrounding the use of that information.[17]

The best example that epitomizes the web-generated malformed opinion about a drug due to patient's lack of information fluency is that of a highly educated, net-savvy and SoMe networking corporate employee who staunchly refuses to take finasteride for advanced androgenetic alopecia due to his firm belief that this drug will definitely cause sexual adverse effects. It is important to mention here that the nocebo effect (psychological perception of adverse effects of a therapy, owing to the patient being self-cognizant about it or having been told by the treating dermatologist) plays a huge role in this scheme of things.[18]

Information Credibility

While information about a health issue, e.g. psoriasis or atopic dermatitis, or a procedure, e.g. chemical peel or laser hair reduction can be accrued from multitude of sources on the net, with exchange of information with peers through blogs, Twitter and other Some portals, the accuracy and credibility of that information for an "information illiterate or nonfluent" e-patient can be high or very low. Thankfully, Google, the most popular global inter search engine has started optimizing the webpages linked to credible information sources (webmd.com, healthonline.com, mayoclinic.org, nhs.uk, aad.org/public/conditions) when one searches for a particular health/skin-related query (Fig. 10). Thus, information credibility on health-related issues from the internet and some networks is being improved.[19]

From no specific opinion to broad-based opinion (via search engines alone) to tubular opinion (via social media engagement) about the dermatologist: The transformation of dermatologist-seeking behavior from visiting someone based on "word of mouth" to a broad opinion gathered from Google to questionable opinion held steadfast due to sheer statistics or imagery presented on Instagram is unfortunate. The tool has become powerful enough that patients may quote accounts on Instagram without looking into the educational background or experience of individuals they are quoting. Facts may be taken out of context from textbooks. For some reason, when a patient sees that an account has more than 50,000 followers, they may mistakenly believe that anything written is factual.

Although "word of mouth" holds fairly good when it comes to hardcore clinical dermatology, the internet and social media generated hype is becoming increasingly more influential over the dermatologist-seeking behavior of patients looking for cosmetic, esthetic and trichology-related solutions. The proliferation of Online Clinic management Softwares like Practo, and

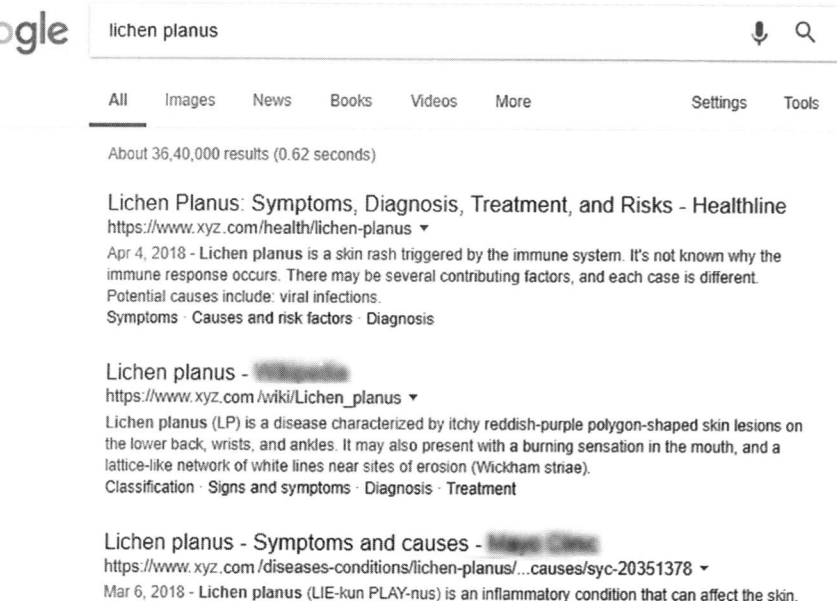

Fig. 10: Google's Search Engine Optimization to relevant websites.

Curofy, and teledermatology facilitating portals like icliniq have for better or for worse, resulted in skewed empowerment of patients complicating the whole issue. Patients post-testimonials about not just the specialist, but for the "overall quality of service" they received at the skin clinic or center; this phenomenon holds good for positive as well as negative testimonials. This trend in authors' opinion is worrisome for at least two reasons:
- Healthcare, even if pure esthetics, cannot and should not be compared to general hospitality industrial units like hotels and restaurants.
- More often than not, the dichotomy between the dermatologist's skills, experience and specific advice given to the patient and the negative testimonial posted by the patient stems from various reasons (discussion about all of them beyond the scope of this chapter) including the patient's unrealistic expectations, unwillingness to comply owing to a relatively higher cost of the suggested treatment protocol, and sometimes a psychological dislike for the specialist in nonmedical spheres of interpersonal communication.

Box 3 summarizes important precautions for medical professionals who are actively engaging or plan to engage in SoMe networking.[20]

REGULATORY STATUS OF SOCIAL MEDIA IN HEALTHCARE AND MEDICOLEGAL ASPECTS

Medical Advertising

Historical Perspective

The year 1977 was a landmark year for healthcare providers, as prior to that, State Bars (legal) in the US imposed a prohibition on attorney

> **BOX 3:** Important precautions for medical professionals who are actively engaging or plan to engage in SoMe networking.[20]
> - *Patient confidentiality:* Before putting any patient information online, the patient's express consent should be obtained, and such consent acknowledged within the post. Care must be taken to ensure that the patient is properly deidentified; the use of a pseudonym is not always enough.
> - *Fraternal ties:* Professional codes of conduct specify that doctors must not engage in behaviors that can harm the reputation of colleagues or the profession. 8°Care should be taken when commenting on any colleague or health organization in the online environment, even when using the thin layer of anonymity provided by a pseudonym.
> - *Doctor-patient boundaries:* Doctors should avoid online relationships with current or former patients. If a patient does make contact with a medical practitioner in an online context, it is appropriate to send a polite message to the patient explaining that further online interaction would be unprofessional. Another way is to create separate profiles for professional and personal use.
> - *Colleagues' online conduct:* Looking after colleagues is an integral element of professional conduct. If a medical practitioner notices the posting of inappropriate content by a colleague, he or she should let the colleague know in a discreet and appropriate manner.
> - *Maintaining online professional conduct of medical profession:* While medical students and doctors are entitled to a private personal life, online social media have challenged the concepts of "public" and "private." Once information is online it is nearly impossible to remove and can quickly spread beyond one's control. A moment of rashness could have unintended and irreversible consequences in the future—inappropriate online activities can be detrimental to patients, colleagues, your training and employment prospects, and your personal integrity.

advertising, which was extrapolated across the board to all professionals, including doctors. This ban was lifted in 1977, when a gentleman named Bates moved the ruling by the State Bar of Arizona and appealed to the United States (US) Supreme Court against the ban. Subsequent to this, attorney advertising was allowed, albeit with a few statutory conditions.[21]

Indian Scenario—the Codified Regulations and the Conundrum and Controversies on their Contemporary Interpretation

For physicians back home in India, the story unfurled in 2002, when the Medical Council of India (MCI), vide its Code of Ethics Regulations, 2002, permitted doctors to advertise only in the following capacities and situations—starting or changing a practice, changing the address, temporary absence from duty, or a public declaration of charges. The MCI maintained the embargo on solicitation, directly or indirectly, or inviting attention to a professional standing, achievements, appointments, honors, or anything resulting in "self-aggrandizement." With regards to training establishments, the name, type of training offered, type of patients admitted, and the fee structure were allowed to be advertised.

Sections 6.1.1 and 6.1.2 of Chapter 6.1 of the *Indian Medical Council (Professional Conduct, Etiquette and Ethics) Regulations, 2002 (amended up to 8th October 2016)* have spelt out the recommendations on the aspect of advertising by Medical professionals (Box 4).

Practical Points Worth Consideration

Having been framed way back in 2002, the following issues merit deliberation:
- There is no distinction mentioned in these guidelines regarding conventional advertisements on hoardings or in print media versus online advertisements (internet and/or on SoMe portals).

> **BOX 4:** Sections 6.1.1 and 6.1.2 of the amended IMC Regulations, 2002.
>
> 6.1.1 Soliciting of patients directly or indirectly, by a physician, by a group of physicians or by institutions or organizations is unethical. A physician shall not make use of him or her (or his/her name) as subject of any form or manner of advertising or publicity *through any mode* either alone or in conjunction with others which is of such a character as to invite attention to him or to his professional position, skill, qualification, achievements, attainments, specialties, appointments, associations, affiliations or honors and/or of such character as would ordinarily result in his self-aggrandizement. A physician shall not give to any person, whether for compensation or otherwise, any approval, recommendation, endorsement, certificate, report or statement with respect of any drug, medicine, nostrum remedy, surgical, or therapeutic article, apparatus or appliance or any commercial product or article with respect of any property, quality or use thereof or any test, demonstration or trial thereof, for use in connection with his name, signature, or photograph in any form or manner of advertising through any mode nor shall he boast of cases, operations, cures or remedies or permit the publication of report thereof *through any mode*. A medical practitioner is however permitted to make a formal announcement in press regarding the following:
> - On starting practice
> - On change of type of practice
> - On changing address
> - On temporary absence from duty
> - On resumption of another practice
> - On succeeding to another practice
> - Public declaration of charges.
>
> 6.1.2 Printing of self-photograph or any such material of publicity in the letter head or on sign board of the consulting room or any such clinical establishment shall be regarded as acts of self-advertisement and unethical conduct on the part of the physician. However, printing of sketches, diagrams, picture of human system shall not be treated as unethical.

- However, the 6.1.1 code also categorically uses the phrase *"through any mode,"* which, pending legal clarification may be assumed to be an all-inclusive expression, the only defense in favor of practitioners *possibly* being the dichotomy between the time of framing of the code and contemporary interpretation of "modes of advertising" including the internet and SoMe.
- One can witness the flooding of Facebook, Instagram and other SoMe portals with plethora of "self-aggrandizement" posts by clinicians including their photographs, their therapy results in the form of data and pre- and postphotographs, and glorification of an innovative approach developed by them. Such information has been posted both with the name and identification of the physician or group of physicians as well as in abstract terms, but from a validated, verified and traceable user handle of the physician and/or the involved marketing team. Excepting anecdotal law-suits that were triggered off primarily by a serious discord between the patient and the doctor, these posts (that appear in disagreement with the concepts laid down in 6.1.1) have apparently continued to benefit from innocent or ignorant or deliberate or confusion-oriented incognizance of the medicolegal system personnel.
- With respect to medicolegal cases, especially regarding grey areas like this, it is commonly said that "remain calm till your violation is challenged by someone in the court of law." But authors strongly suggest that clinicians should rather subscribe to the code (as per the closest legal interpretation) than risk a lawsuit

while continuing to violate the code under the pretentious comfort of the above paraphrase.

Social media is a new entity as for code of ethics for doctors by Medical council is concerned. Whether of ethics is applicable only to doctors or it applicable to companies which run hospitals is being debated. While medical council can act against doctors by way of suspension or removal from registry, what action it can take against hospitals is not clear. This issue of ethics of advertisement is dealt with in detail in the chapter on advertisement and code of ethics.

Another Act, called the *Drugs and Magic Remedies (Objectionable Advertisements) Act, 1954*,[22] prohibits advertisement regarding the use of drugs and "magical remedies" unless they conform to the huge list of permissible conditions detailed in the act.[23] This act has defined as advertisement as: "*any notice, circular, label, wrapper or other document, and any announcement made orally or by any means of producing or transmitting light, sound or smoke.*" While the conundrum of this act having been laid down in 1954, and not subject to revision ever since, and the transformation of the landscape of communication in the same period are confusing, one may extrapolate that it *may* include prohibition of advertisements by doctors through SoMe.

THE NOT-SO-CURIOUS CASE OF SOME CLAIMS OF "GUARANTEED CURES OR RESULTS"

Case Studies

Another thing looked down upon, and very much in vogue, is the "No Cure, No Payment" or "Guaranteed Cure" clause. As per a press release by the Indian Medical Association (IMA), this challenge or clause is in direct violation of both the aforesaid Acts. A few cases have been registered against offenders in this regard:

- In the Dr Anjali Malpani vs. The State of Maharashtra Case (Bombay High Court; 29 April, 2016), Maharashtra Medical Council (MMC) suspended licenses of a doctor couple running an "in vitro fertilization (IVF)" clinic in Mumbai. They had advertised aggressively, and promised "a guaranteed pregnancy, or money back." MMC also issued a show cause notice to 40 doctors, even suspending a few, for unethical advertising in print media and on television.
- In a similar case, the Madhya Pradesh Medical Council (MPMC) issued warning notices to nearly 50 erring doctors in the vicinity for "unethical claims to cure infertility, diabetes, obesity, and other conditions."
- The Tamil Nadu Medical Council (TNMC) took a resolution warning doctors against "online advertisements, and imposed fines on advertisements with photos, names, contact details given by doctors, even to the extent of removing a few names from their registry."

Practical Points worth Consideration

These guidelines were last amended in 2016, to include the role of media—radio, television and internet chats, wherein, lectures or information pertaining to public health can be disseminated, again, with the exception of solicitation, personal publicity, and attempts hereof. And just the mere inclusion of "Internet chats" does not clarify the use of social media, replete with its multiple platforms—Twitter, Facebook, LinkedIn, Practo, Curofy and WhatsApp. *Advertisements on personally-owned domains do not attain coverage under* any of the laws mentioned, or any, for that matter. Would that be considered unethical, even without the intent to solicit, or not! Well, the jury is out.

Online Consultation

Another controversial topic is online consultation, falling under the purview of teledermatology, wherein medical consultations are growing a dime a dozen, with "practice management" apps, viz., DocsApp, ICliniq, Lybrate, Practo, JustDoc and GroAyu ruling the roost, and becoming household names. As with advertising on social media, this area has unclear regulations and guidelines, in terms of acceptability. Vide Section 27 of the MCI Act[24] and the Malay Ganguly vs MCI case (the Supreme Court of India),[25] decided in favor of the plaintiff–"a person who is borne in the Indian Medical Register *can practice anywhere in India.*" Literally, and even figuratively, this *may* be transcribed in favor of online consultation. The last decade has seen a geometric progression in the number of agencies offering not only medical products, but services online. And needless to say, this facilitation of "transfer" of trust from a face-to-face consultation to a technology-mediated information-dissemination has been met with a mixed emotion. Without a shadow of doubt, these services have provisioned convenience, by providing doctor-to-home consultations, medical services and medicines, all at the drop of a hat, and more often than not, at a cheaper price. Its cons comprise psychosocial, ethical and legal implications.[26]

A lot of liability issues have cropped up with the advent of these modalities. By definition, a professional becomes liable in the event that he or she fails to perform a duty. In the medical profession, this translates to professional negligence, malpractice and a confidentiality breach, in a traditional patient-doctor relationship, which can invite criminal or civil liabilities. With respect to online consultations, incumbent liabilities are only civil in nature, as there is no direct physical or verbal connect between the physician and the patient, and hence, the traditional "duty-of-care" does not apply. An offshoot of this situation pertains to the fact that a doctor cannot be held liable, if he does not answer a call or reply to a requisition for an online consultation. Answering this call or text however, constitutes liability on the part of the doctor. Moreover, an omission, however, resulting in loss of life or limb, can and will amount to professional misconduct, rendering the doctor liable for prosecution. Herein, the contract breached will be a financial one, wherein a patient has paid the doctor to utilize his professional services.[26] Teledermatology applications and service providers, thus have to have rigorous guidelines and standard operating procedures in place, to safeguard the interest of the service and service provider.[27] Furthermore, to make matters more confusing for doctors in this regard—online service providers, most, if not all, do not maintain the standard employer-employee relationship, and construe medical professionals as individual entities with a no-liability-clause in the event of misconduct, misdemeanor or negligence.

A raging issue these days involves consultations through the immensely popular communication application, WhatsApp, as described previously (*vide supra*). The IMA, vide an advisory, forewarns and dissuades doctors to refrain from prescribing medication without examining patients thoroughly, and hence, never based purely on symptomatology relayed over telecommunication. As of 4th August 2018, the Bombay High Court had booked a non-bailable charge against a

Maharashtra based specialist couple for telephonic prescription that resulted in the loss of a puerperal lady. The Court observed– *"Prescription without diagnosis would amount to culpable negligence. This amounts to gross negligence from the point of standard of care and recklessness and negligence, which is a tricky road to travel."* The IMA further states that penalization under Section 304 of the Indian Penal Code may be invoked, if such a situation was to arise.[27]

Reputation Management

Sources of Defamation for a Clinician: Comments and Posts by Viewers or Visitors or Patients or Competitors

With the advent of medical informatics, there has been a recent upsurge in aggressive reputation management by most doctors, with a high degree of focus on website management and review management and other outreach programs, for which professional help is often sought. Needless to say, a negative review is taken extremely seriously and may be construed as an attempt of defamation. Unfair or unjust comments regarding a person in public domain, amount to defamation. This defamation has serious implications for the person mentioned, especially when they are public figures like a Doctor in Private Practice. Such offensive or unacceptable remarks or comments can be seen in the following forms:
- News report in Newspapers or other Print media
- Paid Advertisement or Notice in newspaper
- Social media
- Online News websites.

In the attempt to harm the Doctor, the culprit often includes the photograph obtained from SoMe online source. Every Doctor by virtue of being a public figure and will have their photograph at some location or the other online, by some third party. This amounts to theft of identity, since the picture is a unique part of the person's identity and has naturally been used without the Doctor's permission.

Defining "Defamation" and the Legal Remedial Measures—Indian Penal Code (IPC) Sections 499 and 500

- While IPC Section 499 defines Defamation, Section 500 deals with legal remedies for it.[28]
- According to *Section 499 of IPC*, whoever, by words either spoken or intended to be read, or by signs or by visible representations, makes or publishes any imputation concerning any person intending to harm, or knowing or having reason to believe that such imputation will harm, the reputation of such person, is said, except in the cases (*vide infra*) hereinafter expected, to *defame that person.*
- *Exceptions in Section 499:* These include "imputation of truth" which is required for the "public good" and thus has to be published, on the public conduct of government officials, the conduct of any person touching any public question and merits of the public performance.
- *Section 500*, which is on punishment for defamation, reads: "Whoever defames another shall be punished with simple imprisonment for a term which may extend to two years, or with fine, or with both."
- *In India, defamation is both civil and criminal offence.* The remedy for a civil defamation is covered under the Law of Torts. In a civil defamation case, a person who is defamed can move either High Court or subordinate courts and seek damages in the form of monetary

compensation from the accused. Also, under sections 499 and 500 of the IPC, a person guilty of criminal defamation can be sent to jail for 2 years.

Defamation Suit vs Right to Speech: Invoking Section 19 of the Indian Constitution

- Intense legal deliberations have happened over years with some lobbying against Section 499/500 based on their being violative of the right to freedom of speech and expression provided under Article 19 of the Indian Constitution. The provisions of section 499 challenging its constitutionality include—easy misuse by the plaintiffs, inclusion of criminal realm despite a huge lobby justifying the adequacy of civil punishment for defamation, the consideration given to even an ironical statement as amounting to defamation. Most importantly, based on the argument that *"even truth is not a defense,"* even if a patient has expressed the truth about a physician's misconduct, he can be prosecuted for defamation. And while the first exception to section 499, "the truth will only be a defense if the statement was made for the *public good"* seemingly offers a solution to this imbroglio, essentially the arbitrary understanding and court's reading of "public good" renders it more complicated. The example in Box 5 is an attempt to simplify the understanding of this legal conflict in possible real life scenario.

Direct and Indirect Redressal Measures Available to a Victimized Innocent Plaintiff Doctor

- It is important to note that *Section 199(1) the CrPC* plays a balancing act in the IPC Section 499/500 vs Article 19 conflict. By placing the burden on the complainant to pursue the criminal complaint (excluding the state machinery), many frivolous complainants get filtered out, most of whom are not willing to bear the associated monetary, logistical and physical burdens of pursuing the complaint.
- Another act, the *Prevention of Violence and Damage of Property Act, 2010* has a bye-law on "Prevention of Violence against Medicare Persons and Medicare Institutions Acts," which has a clause on verbal abuse.[29]
- Clinicians engaging in SoMe promotions (who are automatically vulnerable to its abuse against them) must also be aware of *Section 66C in The Information Technology Act, 2000* that safeguards against SoMe abuse against doctors or any individual stemming from the complainant employing fraudulent impersonation using a false identity. This Section deals with punishment for identity theft. The Section states *"Whoever, fraudulently or dishonestly make use of the electronic signature, password or any other unique identification feature of any other person, shall be punished with imprisonment of either description for a term which may extend to three years and shall also be liable to fine with may extend to rupees one lakh."*[30]

MEDIA TRIALS AND VIOLENCE AGAINST DOCTORS: THE LATEST CHALLENGE FOR HEALTHCARE FACILITIES

It is no "breaking news" anymore, any issue ranging from pest-infestation of a building to top political scandals are dug out, processed, and presented with completely premeditated and opinionated approach to the general public by news channels, the mainstream conventional mode of "media." Much before the issue reaches the courts of law, it is subject

BOX 5: Practical example to explain the inherent conflict between the clauses of IPC Sections 499/500 and Article 19 of the Indian Constitution.

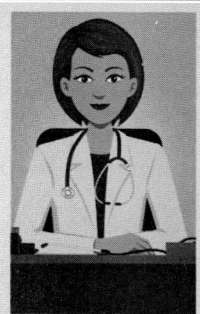

Dr ABC—Dermatologist
Plaintiff

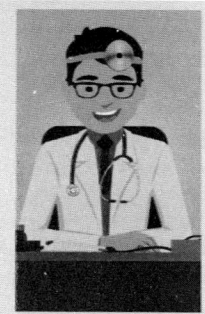

Dr XYZ—ENT Specialist
Defendant

- Consider that some patient or qualified Dermatologist (Dr ABC) notices that another medical professional, an ENT specialist (Dr XYZ) has been posting on SoMe about availability of hair transplantation at his center (backed with enticing pre- and postpictures).

- In firm view of the plaintiff (Dr ABC), Dr XYZ is "unqualified" to conduct it, (e.g., many dermatologists believe that GPs, dentists, general surgeons, ENT specialists are "unqualified" as hair transplant surgeons) and posts on the Facebook page of "*This doctor is a fake and unqualified to conduct hair transplantation.*"

- In response, the defendant confident of his qualification and skills invokes IPC Section 499/500 and files a defamation suit against.

- Now, even if it becomes established that the plaintiff is technically correct and has posted the 'truth' (although it is also a highly debated grey area of Dermatosurgery), how will the court decide whether the plaintiff should be adjugated and sentenced for defaming under Section 499/500 for his derogatory post on SoMe despite the primary assertion being "true" but not good enough to qualify for "public good" or spare him by extending the benefit of *Right to free Speech* enshrined in Article 19 of the Indian Constitution!

to multiple "Media Trials" that end with declaration of outcome and in many cases, "recommendation of punishment" as well.[31] This phenomenon in the current context assumes importance owing to a potentially sinister partnership with series of defamatory messages on social media posted by the SoMe-active members of a protesting mob that reaches a healthcare facility to "avenge" the unfortunate death or procedural complication of a relative. Emboldened by the lack of Action to the online defamation, the mob is often abusive in their protests, verbally as well as physically. There are regions in India, where mobs are even available to protest against a hospital, for a price. There is a perception that the Doctors or Hospital will agree to either pay some compensation to buy silence or at least waive of a substantial part of the Hospital bill, fearing negative publicity that comes with any mob empowered with their inflammatory posts on Facebook, Twitter, etc. and direct audiovisual media involvement who are often interested in a saleable news scoop. Such a situation may become catastrophic for otherwise innocent healthcare providers. Clinicians should be aware of the options available and what relevant action should be taken in such situations.

Onus of the Healthcare Workers to Reduce the Risk

It is the responsibility of the healthcare workers to immediately inform police in the following situations:[32]
- Death of patient where cause of death cannot be made out, deaths linked to abortions, anesthetic deaths, deaths related to violence or accidents.
- Any case of mortality where law mandates postmortem.
- Whenever there are chances that the healthcare workers may be accused of mismanagement.
- As soon as there is any hint or possibility of violence against the healthcare professionals.

Essential Information about Protective Acts

- Invoking the *Hospital Protection Act* and *Doctor Protection Act* that identify even verbal abuse as a noncognizable offense.[33]
- Unauthorized entry of people into any private property or restricted area of a government hospital amounts to trespass.
- Protesting outside the hospital gates on the road which is inevitably without police permission to protest, amounts to a punishable offense.

All such matters need help of a Lawyer well versed with the criminal Laws. Further discussion on this subject is beyond the scope of this chapter.

CONCLUSION

We are practicing dermatology during an era of great scientific advancements and technological innovations, which ultimately will benefit our patients; however, we are undergoing a significant paradigm shift and restructuring on how healthcare is delivered. Social media has transformed communication and is on its way to transforming healthcare including dermatology. When used wisely and prudently, it offers the potential to promote individual and public health, as well as professional development and advancement. Professionals must abide by the ethical codes that govern their professions as practitioners in face-to-face relationships and should be aware of the implications this has on our ethics, professionalism, relationships, and profession. At the same time, there is a pressing need for e-professionalism to be included in the contemporary curriculum on ethics and professionalism at our nation's health education institutions.

The legal territory of the use of SoMe in the practice of medicine remains undefined, and currently only vague recommendations and anecdotal case outcomes exist that unfortunately may serve as precedence (both right and wrong) in such matters. For the practicing dermatologist and other clinicians, it may be best to adhere to the basic prescribed norms by the MCI and keep a close watch on developments in this area to safeguard themselves as well as their patients.

REFERENCES

1. Hamm MP, Chisholm A, Shulhan J, et al. Social media use by health care professionals and trainees: a scoping review. Acad Med. 2013;88(9):1376-83.
2. Social Media. [online] Available from https://www.merriam-webster.com/dictionary/social%20media/. [Accessed December 2018].
3. Benabio J. The value of social media for dermatologists. Cutis. 2013;91(6):269-70.
4. Fox S, Duggan M. Health Online 2013. Washington: Pew Research Center; 2013.
5. Fox S, Duggan M. Tracking for Health. Washington: Pew Research Center; 2013.
6. Max Health Insurance. Indians are becoming more aware about their health and health care needs and are increasingly using Internet to seek answers. [online] Available from https://www.maxbupa.com/media-center/health-news/indians-are-becoming-more-aware-about-their-health-and-health-care-needs-and-are-increasingly-using-internet-to-seek-answer.aspx/. [Accessed December, 2018].
7. The Statistical Portal. (2017). Penetration of Leading Social Networks in India as of 3rd quarter 2017. [online] Available from https://www.statista.com/statistics/284436/India-social-network-penetration/. [Accessed December 2018].
8. Hamm MP, Chisholm A, Shulhan J, et al. Social media use by health care professionals and trainees: a scoping review. Acad Med. 2013;88(9):1376-83.
9. Galadari HI. Social media and modern dermatology. Int J Dermatol. 2018;57(1):110-11.
10. Fenwick T. Social media and medical professionalism: rethinking the debate and the way forward. Acad Med. 2014;89(10):1331-4.
11. Chretien KC, Greysen SR, Chretien JP, et al. Online posting of unprofessional content by medical students. JAMA. 2009;302(12):1309-15.
12. Spector ND, Matz PS, Levine LJ, et al. e-Professionalism: Challenges in the age of information. J Pediatr. 2010;156(3):345-6.
13. Cain J, Romanelli F. E-professionalism: a new paradigm for a digital age. Curr Pharm Teach Learn. 2009;2:66-70.
14. General Medical Council. (2012). Doctors' Use of Social Media. [online] Available from http://www.gmc-uk.org/guidance/10900.asp/. [Accessed December, 2018].
15. Centers for Disease Control and Prevention. (2003). HIPPA privacy rule and public health guidance from CDC and the US department of Health and Human Services. [online] Available from http://www.cdc.gov/privacyrule/Guidance/Content.htm/. [Accessed December. 2018].
16. Moqbel M. (2012). The effect of the use of social networking sites in the workplace on job performance. Texas A and M University. [online] Available from http://www.citeseerx.ist.psu.edu/viewdoc/download?doi=10.1.1.306.5775&rep=1&type=pdf/. [Accessed December, 2018].
17. Lorenzo G, Dziuban C. (2006). Ensuring the Net Generation Is Net Savvy. [online] Available from www.educause.edu/ELI/EnsuringtheNetGenerationIsNetS/156766/. [Accessed December, 2018].
18. Sonthalia S, Sahaya K, Arora R, et al. Nocebo effect in Dermatology. Indian J Dermatol Venereol Leprol. 2015;81(3):242-50.
19. Mashable. (2012). Mak Health Survey. https://admin.mashable.com/wp-content/uploads/2012/09/Mak-Health-Survey-Infographic.jpg/. [Accessed December, 2018].
20. Mansfield SJ, Morrison SG, Stephens HO, et al. Social media and the medical profession. Med J Aust. 2011;194(12):642-4.
21. Medical Council of India. (2002). Indian Medical Council (Professional Conduct, Etiquette and Ethics) Regulations, 2002. [online] Available from https://www.mciindia.org/documents/rulesAndRegulations/Ethics%20Regulations-2002.pdf/. [Accessed December, 2018].
22. The Drugs and Magic Remedies (Objectionable Advertisements) Act, 1954. [online] Available from https://indiacode.nic.in/bitstream/123456789/1412/1/A1954-21.pdf/. [Accessed December, 2018].
23. Bates v. (1977). State Bar of Arizona. U.S. Supreme Court 433 U.S. 350 (1977). [online] Available from https://supreme.justia.com/cases/federal/us/433/350/. [Accessed December, 2018].
24. The Medical Council of India Act 1965. [online] Available from http://fdaharyana.gov.in/

actpdf/Indian_medical_council_act_1954. pdf/. [Accessed December 2018].
25. Casemine. (2001). Malay Ganguly vs Medical Council of India and Others. Supreme Court of India Writ Petition No 317 of 2000; Argued February 18, 2000; Decided October 10, 2001. [online] Available from https://www.casemine.com/judgement/in/56ea8bf7607dba382a078e61/. [Accessed December, 2018].
26. George C, Duquenoy. Online Medical Consultations: Legal, Ethical and Social Perspectives. In: Duquenoy P, George C, Kimppa K (Eds). Ethical, legal and social issues in medical informatics, 1st edition. Pennsylvania: Hershey Publishing House; 2008. pp. 1-29.
27. Position Statement on Teledermatology (Approved by the Board of Directors: February 22, 2002; Amended by the Board of Directors: May 22, 2004; November 9, 2013; August 9, 2014; May 16, 2015; March 7, 2016). [online] Available from https://www.aad.org/Forms/Policies/Uploads/PS/PS-Teledermatology.pdf. [Accessed December, 2018].
28. The Indian Penal Code (IPC), 1860. [online] Available from https://indiankanoon.org/doc/1133131/. [Accessed December, 2018].
29. PRS Legislative Research. Prevention of Violence and Damage of Property Act, 2010. [online] Available from https://www.latestlaws.com/bare-acts/state-acts-rules/maharashtra-state-laws/maharashtra-medicare-service-persons-medicare-service-institutions-prevention-violence-damage-loss-property-act-2010/. [Accessed December, 2018].
30. Central Government Act. (2000). [online] Available from https://indiankanoon.org/doc/118912881/. [Accessed December, 2018].
31. Chowdhury S. Media Trials: Contradiction to Media Ethics? Conference Paper presented at: Media Ethics: Reality or Myth, Shantiniketan, West Bengal, Volume: 1. March 2013.
32. Sharma ML, Harsh R, Sharma S. Violence against doctors: a review. Ann Int Med Den Res. 2018;4(5):PE11-4.
33. Gupta MC. What should Doctors and Nursing Homes do to Prevent and Manage Violence by Patients/Relatives? Indian J Clin Pract. 2012;22:470-2.

CHAPTER 21

Avenues to Study and Apply Medicolegal Law

Satish Bhat

KEY OBJECTIVES
- Need for doctors study and be familiar with medical law
- Avenues for doctors to study and learn law
- Common avenues to apply knowledge of medicolegal laws, including simple precautions in daily work
- Current limitations in the practice of law, for a medical professional trained in law
- Right to protest by doctors: how to use this?

WHY DO DOCTORS NEED TO STUDY AND LEARN LAW?

Medical law is not yet a formal part of the medical curriculum. Problems faced by doctors as part of their regular work often need legal remedy. Medical organizations need legal help for issues they face while addressing the concern of doctor members.

When any medical dispute reaches the Court of Law, it is the Lawyers who present the matter and Judges who adjudicate. Unlike other common matters, Lawyers do not have much idea of the intricacies of health care—especially the technical aspects, and neither do Courts. In the absence of Special courts (example: Labor Tribunals) for health care/medicolegal matters, where the adjudicating authority has some exposure/training to the medicine filed, in the current scenario the Judges rely significantly on how the Lawyers present the medical matter during the Court arguments. Medical facts are fit into legal principles when presented to the Court, which needs a close understanding of the fundamentals of both medicine and law.

Many cases have been won or lost simply because of the manner in which the facts of the case were presented and argued in Court. While law can be done as an evening course after a Degree in Medicine, MBBS cannot be done as a part time course after an initial degree in law. This explains why there are a few hundred qualified doctors (medical practitioners) with an additional Law degree—in the Country; however, there is perhaps not a single person who has done an MBBS course after qualifying initially in law.

Thus, whenever there is a dispute in a medical matter, whether medical education or health care services—the person with an exposure to both medicine and law faculty is best placed to analyze and show the way ahead. This applies both to situations needing remedial measures (medicolegal cases against doctors, hospital violence), or preventive measures to improve the current scenario (health care and medical education policy decisions). Unless there is a balanced focus on the rights and duties of all the stakeholders: authorities, health care professionals and common man, the overall health care scenario of the country will not improve.

The existing Indian Education system does not have a provision to create a professional trained in both health care and law, through a single course.

WHAT ARE THE AVENUES TO STUDY AND LEARN MORE ON MEDICOLEGAL ISSUES?

Following avenues are available to acquire training in medicolegal matters:
- *One:* Do a formal Law degree: available across the country, which has ample capacity to take up new students. Graduate of any stream can register for a 3-year course in the Bachelor of Law (LLB), run by any institute attached to the various Universities across the country.
- *Two:* Do a medicolegal Diploma course, available with a couple of institutions in the country. Few institutions offering such courses include:
  – National Law School of India University (NLSUI), Bengaluru
  – Symbiosis Institute, Pune
  – Krishna Institute, Karad, Maharashtra
  – Tamil Nadu Dr Ambedkar Law University
  – Annamalai University, Tamil Nadu
  – Institute of Health and Management Studies, Delhi
  – West Bengal National University of Juridical Sciences (NUJS), Kolkata.

  These are typically 12-month distance learning program, with contact points in between. A thesis and evaluation at the end is usually done, before the Diploma is awarded.

  This is a simpler alternative for someone who does not want to consider the formal 3-year Degree course in law—LLB.
- *Three:* Be part of a medicolegal cell in any medical organization/institution: having like-minded peers, along with the support of a panel of lawyers, this is a simple way to improve awareness though regular discussions and application of law in medicolegal matters.

Few Larger Aspects
- Any graduate, including a medical graduate, can join a law college and pursue a 3-year LLB course. The Bar Council of India had announced age restrictions about 3 years ago. These have been struck down by the Supreme Court. However, this 3-year course is now only possible as a full time course, unlike earlier when it was possible even as a part time evening course. Admissions can be taken without any entrance examination to many of the courses in many states, though some like Maharashtra have a common state entrance conducted by the state Government.

- Many doctors in service face problems which end with them feeling harassed and wronged and the doctor feels like quitting service. The practical problems in finding an alternate career do not allow them to do so. If he has an LLB degree, he can immediately join the bar and start law practice.
- Practicing law is also not difficult. A doctor's capacity to understand English, analyze facts, work hard and dedicatedly are attributes that would see him through successfully in law, all provided he/she has basic interest in law.
- Getting a law degree does not mean that the doctor has to give up medical practice. That stage would come only when he would want to join the bar. There are many doctors in India today who have an LLB degree but continue to indulge in medical practice as medicolegal consultants without joining the bar. They draft replies for court cases filed against doctors and these replies are submitted and argued in the court by a lawyer associated with them.
- Even when a doctor completes LLB, he may practice law in consumer courts as an accredited nonadvocate volunteer and can even charge fees as per the provisions of the Consumer Protection Regulations, 2014.
- Assuming that a doctor ultimately joins the bar, it is unlikely that he/she will regret this decision. Going by the current trend, there are going to be more and more restrictions and burdens on doctors and small nursing homes. On the other hand, lawyers are their own Lords and have almost no restrictions on their profession. A doctor practicing law is likely to have a good name and prestige as well as good earning.

COMMON AVENUES TO APPLY KNOWLEDGE OF MEDICOLEGAL LAWS

Common aspects of health care system include:
- Healthcare services
- Medical education/training.

These have the following stakeholders:
- Healthcare professionals: Doctors, nurses, technicians, therapists, etc.
- Healthcare drug and device industry
- Medical establishments providing healthcare services:
  - Public healthcare system
  - *Private healthcare system:* Include all from the small establishments (usually <20 beds) owned by couple doctors (both husband and wife are doctors) to corporate hospitals
  - *Medical institutions:* Training and education services—both government and private
  - Patients and common man
  - Authorities; including elected leaders, Government officials and judiciary: the three pillars of democracy
  - *Media:* the fourth pillar.

Each of these has some rights and responsibilities. Only when there is a healthy balance between Rights and Responsibilities of each of these stakeholders, can the health care system serve its objective to improve the health of the Nation.

While each of the groups has their concerns, the list ahead has the concerns from perspective of Readers of this book: Individual Doctors in independent practice or as a full time job, with few having their own small to medium-sized medical establishments. Most of these have been dealt in detail, in individual Chapters of this book. This list is merely representative:

- There are multiple Government notifications allowing Hakims/Vaids to practice modern medicine, despite Court judgments to the contrary. This amounts to official sanction to quackery. How do we doctors stop this?
- When there is a complaint against a doctor following patient death—how to ensure that relevant sections of the Indian Penal Code (IPC) 80, 81, 88, 92 and IPC 93 are invoked, rather than the harsh IPC 304-A (rash and negligent act) or worse still IPC 304 (culpable homicide not amounting to murder)? How to address the concern—will the doctor be arrested—which is commonly used to pressurize and harass the doctor for compensation?
- Violence against doctors—how to respond when authorities fail to implement existing regulations? Culprit is not arrested despite the complaint being registered under cognizable and non-bailable sections of the Medicare Act?
- When it is matter of civil rights of doctors in private practice—right to professional charges—authorities have passed orders to provide services free of cost, on multiple occasions, without provisions to reimburse the same. How do we go about correcting this situation?
- Doctors (especially the trainee doctors) have been repeatedly going on strike to press for their genuine needs—what other means can doctors use, to ensure authorities fulfill these genuine demands?
- How to improve better access to the reliable health care services to the common man?
- How to improve quality and pricing of drugs and devices in the health care industry? How can unfair profiteering be addressed?
- How to improve the seats available for MBBS and PG courses across the country—better training opportunity?
- Is there any legal intervention which can result in increase in health budget allocated by the Government?

For any group of doctors concerned about the deteriorating scenario in health care, and would like to take constructive steps, this is what can be done:

- For any problem faced by the doctors, compile the existing rules and laws
- Go through them in detail to check if there are any aspect of the rules that look unrealistic
- If the rules are reasonable, next to check if there are any issues in implementing, whether by the authorities or the fraternity
- For outstanding issues, a combination of meeting the concerned people/authorities along with writing a formal letter on behalf of the association is to be done
- Letters can be followed up with queries under Right to Information (RTI) Act.
- In case matter does not proceed, even a Legal notice can be sent to the concerned
- Write ups (Articles) in Media (Print media, Online Portals and Social Media) can be done at the relevant time
- If all this fail, the option to file a case in High Court as a Writ Petition is always there, as advised by the Lawyer
- At an appropriate point of time, if there is a crisis with a possible high-handed attitude of the authorities, option to have a protest, in a legally approved manner, is always available.

To be kept in mind, is the option of taking inputs and guidance from others with more information regarding the problem, whether a Lawyer or Medicolegal Expert or another Association who has handled the problem earlier.

Common Scenarios in Day-to-Day Work

There are many precautions/safeguards that can be taken which if missed, will add to medicolegal troubles:

- *Drug prescription (generic or brand):* This is mentioned in the Professional Conduct, Etiquette and Ethics Regulations, 2002,[1] after modification on 08.10.2016 as under. "Every physician should prescribe drugs with generic names legibly and preferably in capital letters and he/she shall ensure that there is a rational prescription and use of drugs."

    Practical problems:
    - "My handwriting is not so legible": When in doubt, use Computer print-outs.
    - "With combination drugs, do we write the entire list of generic names in the combination?" When this is available as part of a Clinic management software, this can be entered in advance, selected and will be printed out.
    - "I am not sure of the quality of some of the brands": Name of any one or two brands can be mentioned in brackets after the Generic name. The Regulations do not mention anywhere that Brand names are *not* to be mentioned.
    - "I am not sure of the quality of the drug, of any random brand provided by Pharmacist": Follow the above guidelines, but mention verbally that drug quality is a critical aspect in the therapeutic response. Example: warfarin, antiepileptics, etc.

- Precaution while referring patient to another doctor, of same/different specialty for same or different problem.
    - It the referral is on record (as usually happens during treatment of a hospitalized patient), and there is some complaint about negligence with the services provided by the referred doctor, the original referring doctor is also held liable on account of vicarious responsibility.
    - One way to avoid this potential problem is by suggesting the name only verbally, but have the records show that the referred doctor was brought in only as requested by the patient.
    - This is possible with some smart documentation for hospitalized patients, and is much easier with outpatients.

- *What qualifications/expertise to display:* Outside clinic/on letterhead, as per the Professional Conduct, Etiquette and Ethics Regulations, 2002,[1] only those qualifications that are approved by the Medical Council of India (MCI) can be mentioned next to the name of the Doctor, and the Doctor can call him/herself a specialist only in only those aspect where he/she has an MCI approved specialized training, not others.

    The question often arises, "How do I convey my expertise to society in such a scenario?" One way to do this without violating current guidelines is to call oneself, for example "MD Medicine (Internist) with special interest in Cardiology/Nephrology/Rheumatology".
    - It is important to note that many overseas qualifications are not recognized by the MCI, and displaying them as qualifications is a violation of the Law. They can be only described as additional training/experience.

- *Precautions regarding resuscitation in case with local anesthesia:* Another common scenario that weakens the Doctor's position in the event of a scrutiny, and makes

situation untenable, is lack of resuscitation equipment in the event of an anaphylaxis to local anesthetic drug. A common lapse noticed in case of a scrutiny is lack of availability of the following:
- Crash cart and trolley with resuscitation equipment
- Defibrillator machine
- Pulse oximeter with electrocardiography (ECG) monitor.

There is simply no way to justify the lack of any of the above, as these are indispensable parts of the resuscitation protocol. Not having them available, but knowing the possibility of an anaphylaxis amounts to:
- Deficiency of service even if there is unrelated problem, with possible compensation for the same being awarded by a Consumer Forum.
- Willful ignorance of guidelines, if this leads to a breach, and is the cause of complications, it will be seen as gross Negligence that may be liable for criminal proceedings.

- Record that patient was discharged from Hospital (or after any treatment) in satisfactory condition, with relief from symptoms and in a positive frame of mind. A common scenario that the Doctor is forced to defend following any scrutiny, is that the patient was unhappy and in pain, despite the treatment being provided as planned. This allegation is used to substantiate other allegations/complaints that the patient has.

A simple precaution to follow regarding such matters it to collect a patient feedback on a printed form, with few lines in their own handwriting, having their opinion collected at the time of leaving the hospital/clinic after the treatment/procedure. This is invariably the time when patient is in the most receptive frame of mind, and gives a realistic opinion/feedback, which is invariably quite positive. It should have points that include:
- My presenting problems were relieved and taken care of
- I do not have any new/pending problems
- I am satisfied with the treatment provided, it was as promised to me
- I am satisfied with the other services provided
- I am happy to recommend this facility to others with the same problem.

This document with above points when produced later, in the face of complaints by the patient, makes it very clear that the patient has turned volte-face, and the onus rests completely on the patient to prove their allegations, which now will become doubly difficult.

In the absence of any such record, the sympathies of the Court invariably lie with the patient, and with the onus on the Doctor to disprove the same, the situation becomes difficult to salvage.

Value of these Safeguards

In case of any complication, complainant Lawyer will try to identify these weak points, whether or not they have contributed to the outcome. Proof that there has been a deviation from standard, is sufficient to create a bias in the mind of the adjudicating authority that some compensation is warranted even if there is no negligence by the Doctor. It is seen as deficiency of service.

CURRENT LIMITATIONS IN THE PRACTICE OF LAW, FOR A MEDICAL MAN TRAINED IN LAW

It is quite evident there are a host of issues in health care that needs to be addressed legally, and a professional trained in both Medicine and Law can play a key role. Despite this, there are certain hurdles in utilizing the services of medicolegal experts to their full potential, as per the current Indian laws.

It is quite clear there is a paucity of professionals with this unique distinction. Currently there is no single course in India that creates a professional with training in both Medicine and Law. It is also clear that this dual training is likely only for those who initially finish their training in Medicine, and not vice versa. To add to the problem, is the unfortunate ban in India on practicing doctors from registering with the Bar Council and *simultaneously* practicing law. Few details of this ban are as follows:

The ban was imposed vide a judgment dated 08.04.1996 by AM Ahmadi, CJI, SB Majmudar and Mrs Sujata V Manohar, JJ in (Dr) Haniraj L Chulani versus Bar Council of Maharashtra and Goa.[2]

- *This is despite a situation to the contrary in the United States:* They have many universities with a 7- to 8-year course in both Medicine and Law, with the initial few years of training in Medicine and last few in Law. Once they are qualified, they can register with both the Medical and Bar Councils, and simultaneously practice both Medicine and Law.
- In Indian, even if a practicing doctor does an LLB course, while practicing medicine, they are not allowed to register with the Bar Council to practice as an advocate unless they give up their Medical Council registration. Given our shortage of doctors, it is a loss to the country if a trained doctor has to give up their right to practice medicine, just to meet the technical requirement of practicing law, and represents a medicolegal/legal matter when the situation demands, despite their unique position in handling Medicolegal Matters.
- A review petition will need to be filed in the Supreme Court to have this anomaly rectified by amending the earlier judgment of 1996.

However, there are avenues for a doctor trained in law to formally handle legal matters even without registering with the Bar Council. Once such avenue is to represent either of the parties in the proceedings of a Consumer Forum, as an "Accredited Agent" in the Forum.

Rules for "Authorized Agents" were framed after the Supreme Court upheld in 2011 through its order, the legal validity of such agents within the ambit of law.[3]

In its order, the Hon'ble Supreme Court gave directions to the National Consumer Forum to frame rules for the same, to while were subsequently notified in 2014, Chapter 1 (3)—Consumer Protection Regulations 2014, mentions Rules for Accredited Agent in Consumer Forum.[4]

RIGHT TO PROTEST: DO DOCTORS HAVE THIS RIGHT? WHAT IS THE LAWFUL WAY TO PLAN A PROTEST?

Despite all provisions to address problems, authorities often fail to address issues in a logical manner or as per provisions of law. Taking the matter to Court, even as an emergency in case of a strike by Hospital staff, may end up with Courts listing the matter low in the case listing priority.

This is when a protest is useful, provided it is done with sound legal planning. Write letters to authorities initially, follow-up with RTI queries, put evasive answers by Authorities on record, give a Legal Notice on grounds of failure to reply to correspondence in a fixed time failing which the aggrieved persons will be forced to use their fundamental right to protest. This is the recommended sequence of events. All this has to be done after giving due coverage in media after a press release/conference, while ensuring emergency services are not affected.

The bane of the Medical Community with all members being intellectuals, is that they often fail to shed their internal differences even for a common cause. It is often said that it is easier to get a group of rickshaw-wallas together, but not doctors, even for a matter of injustice to the entire fraternity. A strategically sound way is for someone to approach the High Court with an appeal asking Government to fulfill the lawful demands of the protesting doctors, failure of which has precipitated a public health crisis. Failing this, within 2–3 days of the strike by doctors in a Public Hospital, it is inevitable that some individual or non-governmental organization (NGO) will file a petition [public interest litigation (PIL)] against the doctors for endangering public health. Courts being more sympathetic to patients than doctors have come down heavily on doctors in such instances. Thus, strategy decides whether the aggrieved doctors get justice or are seen as culprits. If strikes are planned without due planning, Government threatens to invoke the Essential Services Maintenance Act (ESMA) and arrest the protesting doctors.

Rajasthan: High Court asks state government to arrest doctors if they do not return to work.[5]

Resign and stay at home if you are so scared: High Court to doctors—Times of India.[6]

Most unfortunate is a recent development following a 2-day strike by Resident Doctors in King George's Medical College (KGMC), Lucknow, in May 2016. Shortly after that the Lucknow Bench of the Allahabad High Court on 02.06.2016 passed orders without hearing all the parties in question, following a petition regarding death of patients during a strike. It used rather strong language against doctors and issued directions that those who died because of the strike would be paid ₹ 2,500,000 per death and that this amount would be recovered from the salary of doctors. The hearing was in connection with a PIL filed by an advocate against the strike by doctors in Uttar Pradesh which lasted just 2 days. As per the judgment, the court ordered a special committee to be set up to find those who died as a result of the strike. The bereaved family would be given ₹ 2,500,000, to be deducted from the salary of the striking doctors. The judgment also stated that doctors have no right to go on strike in any circumstances.

Medicos Legal Action Group (MLAG), a Doctor's Association from Chandigarh, had filed a Special Leave Petition (SLP) challenging this Order of the Allahabad High Court, which was admitted by the Hon'ble Supreme Court in September 2016, and final order is still pending.

CONCLUSION

The scope of Medicolegal specialty is rapidly rising. The professional with dual training in medicine and law has a unique role in the same. A single course that gives training in both medicine and law will significantly help in increasing the numbers of such professionals. Despite the current restrictions on the practice of law, for doctors practicing medicine, the field is undoubtedly an attractive one, whose relevance will only increase in coming days.

ACKNOWLEDGMENTS

The Author is Convenor, Medicolegal Cell of the Association of Medical Consultants (AMC) Mangalore since the inception of the organization 6 years ago. It is a registered body of about 500 specialist doctors practicing in the city of Mangalore (Dakshina Kannada district) and the surrounding districts in Karnataka, as well as the adjacent Kasargod district in the state of Kerala. Though all doctors in AMC are members of the Indian Medical Association (IMA)—the parent body of Practitioners of Modern Medicine, having an independent registered body gives the local doctors a legally valid platform, to take up issues right from the Local, State or National level, without any external limitations or approvals.

AMC Mangalore is affiliated to the parent body AMC Mumbai based in Mumbai, currently having 11,000 registered specialist doctors and working since last 40 years for the welfare of doctors and the health care sector.

AMC Mangalore has been able to bring about a visible change on the ground for daily issues faced by doctors such as abuse, violence, jousting, legal notice and other issues faced by small and medium hospitals.

AMC has now set up in a dozen more cities across the country, in multiple states. All the various units work together under the common platform of FAMCI: Federation of Associations of Medical Consultants of India. Dr Lalit Kapoor is the Director and Dr Kishore Adyanthaya is the Honorary Secretary of this Federation.

REFERENCES

1. Professional Conduct, Etiquette and Ethics Regulations, 2002. [online] Available from https://www.mciindia.org/documents/rulesAndRegulations/Ethics%20Regulations-2002.pdf [Accessed December, 2018].
2. SB Majmudar and Mrs Sujata V Manohar, JJ in (Dr) Haniraj L Chulani versus Bar Council of Maharashtra and Goa. [online] Available from http://indiankanoon.org/doc/77295/ [Accessed December, 2018].
3. Supreme Court judgment regarding validity of Authorized agents in Consumer Forum. [online] Available from https://indiankanoon.org/doc/1399474/ [Accessed December, 2018].
4. Chapter 1 (3)—consumer Protection Regulations 2014, regarding rules for accredited agent in Consumer Forum. [online] Available from https://consumeraffairs.nic.in/consumer/writereaddata/CPU%20Notification.pdf [Accessed December, 2018].
5. Rajasthan: High Court asks state government to arrest doctors if they do not return to work. [online] Available from https://scroll.in/latest/862735/rajasthan-high-court-asks-state-government-to-arrest-doctors-if-they-do-not-return-to-work [Accessed December, 2018].
6. Resign and stay at home if you are so scared: High court to doctors—Times of India. [online] Available from https://timesofindia.indiatimes.com/city/mumbai/resign-and-stay-at-home-if-you-are-so-scared-hc-to-docs/articleshow/57761819.cms [Accessed December, 2018].

CHAPTER 22

A Guide for Expert Opinion: Is every Adverse Outcome a Medical Negligence?

Satish Bhat

KEY OBJECTIVES

- Missing guidelines, rising allegations and prevailing confusion
- Legal principles involved in medical negligence
- Safeguards from allegations of criminal negligence, for the Indian doctor
- Value of an expert:
  - Process of including an expert opinion in a complaint of negligence received by the police
  - Process of including expert opinion after complaint of negligence received by consumer forum
  - What is expected in the expert opinion?
  - Guidelines for analyzing severity of guilt
- Recommendations by the author and grading the spectrum of medical injury
- Significance of grading severity of guilt

MISSING GUIDELINES, RISING ALLEGATIONS AND PREVAILING CONFUSION

A recent report mentioned a 110% rise in number of medical negligence cases in India every year.[1] This is apart from the allegations made as defamatory news and reports of violence seen in Media: whether print, online, or social media. Another report in 2014 quotes a legal resource Manupatra "Medicolegal cases have gone up by 400% in the Supreme Court in the last 10 years".[2]

Given this scenario, any reputed doctor is very likely to face a major allegation of negligence sometime in their career, and a colleague will be called in to give an expert opinion on the same. Such a task brings forth many doubts in the minds of the doctors involved: the expert, the respondent-doctor, and other colleagues.

However, guidelines to judge Professional incompetence are not yet framed by the Medical Council of India (MCI) so far. Errors in adjudicating on any adverse outcome have far reaching consequences on the health of many individuals, beyond those connected with the case. Often, the allegations itself are very painful and shocking for the doctor, being untrained in the principles of law, he is at a loss at how to defend himself from the accusations made, even when he has tried the maximum for adverse situation the patient was in. This fear may in fact become a deterrent for doctors to take up any slender chance available to save a patient, when faced again with a critical illness or accident. The doctor is the only person who can stand between such a patient and death, and he needs to be empowered, and not made to feel threatened.

The process of adjudicating is also slow and painful, for the Doctor concerned and the patients involved, and the long-drawn process is itself a punishment even for those who have a favorable outcome at the end. Guidelines to make the process of scrutiny simpler and objective, with a standardized process, will ensure this concern is unfounded, delays in outcome are reduced, errors and the agony they bring are minimized. Scrutiny Guidelines also help the professional to do a good job in their regular work, without concerns of their own safety from baseless allegations and their reactions like violence. Removing this ambiguity is the need of the hour.

LEGAL PRINCIPLES INVOLVED IN MEDICAL NEGLIGENCE[3]

The essential components of negligence, as recognized, are three: (1) "duty", (2) "breach", and (3) "resulting damage" that are:
- Existence of a *duty of care*, which is owed by the defendant to the complainant;
- Failure to attain that standard of care, resulting in a *breach of such duty*; and
- Damage/injury (adverse outcome), which is both causally connected with such breach and recognized by the law, has been suffered by the complainant.

Other aspects have been detailed in the Jacob Mathew versus State of Punjab Judgment of 2005, and a complete read, understanding, and application is highly recommended for anyone in the role of an expert.

Key points in deciding on negligence:[3]
- What constitutes a reasonable level of knowledge, skill, and overall care by the service provider to the patient? This point has been settled in Para 49 (3) of the order.
  - "The standard to be applied for judging, whether the person charged has been negligent or not, would be that of an ordinary competent person exercising ordinary skill in that profession. It is not possible for every professional to possess the highest level of expertise or skills in that branch which he practices".
- What makes the negligence grievous enough to be called as criminal negligence? Para 49 (5) of the order says:
  - "Concept of negligence differs in civil and criminal law. What may be negligence in civil law may not necessarily be negligence in criminal law. For negligence to amount to an offence, the element of "mens rea" must be shown to exist. For an act to amount to criminal negligence, the degree of negligence should be much higher, i.e. gross or of a very high degree. Negligence, which is neither gross nor of a higher degree may provide a ground for action in civil law but cannot form the basis for criminal prosecution".

- What is the reference point in time for deciding average level of knowledge, skill, and care? Para 49 (2) of the order says:
  - "The standard of care, while assessing the practice as adopted, is judged in the light of knowledge available at the time of the incident, and not at the date of trial".

SAFEGUARDS FOR THE DOCTOR AGAINST CRIMINAL PROSECUTION IN INDIAN PENAL CODE

Recognizing the unique role played by doctors, there are few Sections of the Indian Penal Code (IPC) that seem to have been drafted specially to safeguard the interest of doctors.

Section 80 of the Indian Penal Code[4]

Accident in doing a lawful Act: "Nothing is an offence, which is done by accident or misfortune and without any criminal intention or knowledge in the doing of a lawful Act in a lawful manner by lawful means and with proper care and caution. *Illustration:* A is at work with a hatchet; the head flies off and kills a man who is standing by. Here, if there was no want of proper caution on the part of A, his act is excusable and not an offence".

Section 88 of the Indian Penal Code[5]

Act not intended to cause death, done by consent in good faith for person's benefit: Nothing which is not intended to cause death, is an offence by reason of any harm which it may cause, or be intended by the doer to cause, or be known by the doer to be likely to cause, to any person for whose benefit it is done in good faith, and who has given a consent, whether express or implied, to suffer that harm, or to take the risk of that harm. *Illustration:* A, a surgeon, knowing that a particular operation is likely to cause the death of Z, who suffers under a painful complaint, but not intending to cause Z's death and intending in good faith, Z's benefit performs that operation on Z, with Z's consent. A has committed no offence.

KEY POINT ONE—CRIMINAL NEGLIGENCE

- A reading of these Sections only re-emphasizes the concept of "mens rea" mentioned in the Supreme Court Judgment of 2005 (2) that will invariably be missing in the usual course of events when any doctor provides medical treatment to a patient who approaches him with an illness.
- In other words, since the intention to cause harm is invariably missing when a Doctor provides treatment to a patient, charges of Criminal Negligence will not hold.
- Even if there are grounds for Civil Negligence, police have no role in the matter, as this dealt separately by the Consumer Forum or Civil Court.

VALUE OF AN EXPERT

An expert opinion has immense value, whether by an individual Doctor or a designated Medical Board, and guides the court in professional/ technical matters, which they may find difficult to follow by themselves. Assessment of negligence involves both legal and medical aspects, and the Doctors in the role of an expert need to be familiar with the legal principles, which is not part of their usual training.

While legal principles involved are fairly constant in most cases, the principles of medicine involved will vary from case-to-case even within the same specialty. Hence, it is far more important for the medical experts to be familiar with the legal principles of negligence as vice versa is not possible. The judiciary will accept the expert opinion assuming that the legal perspective has been considered as well. Using terms in the Medical Expert Report without realizing their legal meaning or principles involved, can cause miscommunication and immense travesty of justice.

Process of Including an Expert Opinion in a Complaint of Negligence Received by the Police

This has already been prescribed in Jacob Mathew versus State of Punjab Judgment.[3] This was further discussed in a meeting of the Ethics Committee (EC), Medical Council of India (MCI) held in 2007[6] and is as follows:

- It shall be mandatory to patient/his relative that before lodging a complaint against treating doctor/hospital regarding rashness or negligence, he must obtain a credible opinion from a competent doctor qualified in that branch of medical practice on the facts mentioned in the documents supplied by the concerned doctor/hospital.
- No complaint shall be entertained by the police or investigating agency unless the allegation is specified and supported by a credible opinion of competent doctor qualified in that branch of medical practice.
- After receiving a complaint supported with a credible opinion of a competent doctor along with supporting treatment and investigation papers against the treating doctor/hospital, police, or investigating agency before registering the Crime under Section 304A IPC or under any other relevant section of law should seek an independent, impartial, and unbiased opinion from a Committee or Body constituted by Government of India or State Government comprising of uneven number of members and such committee must include an eminent senior faculty member of that branch of medical practice.
- The committee formed shall examine the complaint, opinion of the doctor in support of complaint submitted by the complainant in the light of documents related to investigation, diagnosis, and treatment considering the qualification of doctor and the circumstances of case including time and place and shall give clear opinion about whether or not the treating doctor(s) has/have been rash and negligent in their duty in treating the patient. This shall be communicated to police/investigating agency in minimum possible/reasonable duration.
- The committee, if it thinks so, shall also visit the place/hospital where patient was treated, and examine if the facilities available for such treatment/operation given to the patient or not, and if the treating doctor is duly qualified, registered with competent body/organization and whether the place is recognized or not for such treatment.
- The police/investigating agency after receiving the opinion of Government Doctor/Committee shall register a case only when, in the opinion of committee the treating doctor(s) has/have been found rash and negligent in Act of Commission or Omission.
- If the doctor accused is found not guilty by the committee then no case should be registered by the Police and in such case the patient/ relative may lodge a complaint in the appropriate court, if they feel so, and court should take appropriate action in the light of opinion given by the Government Doctor/Committee constituted for this purpose. Appointment and duties of doctor(s) or committee constituted for the purpose of giving opinion for Prosecution of Doctors for Medical Negligence under Criminal Law.

Few guidelines related to arrest of a doctor, specific to those in Government Service, have been mentioned in 2017 Judgment of High Court of Madhya Pradesh Dr BC Jain versus Maulana Saleem on 28-2-2017.[7]

> **KEY POINT TWO—IMPLICATIONS OF DIFFERENCE: CRIMINAL VS CIVIL NEGLIGENCE**
> - Understanding the Key difference between Criminal Negligence OR not, following an adverse outcome, helps the police decide whether an FIR may be registered and further criminal investigation initiated.
> - Any error of Judgment by the Expert in this aspect, whether on Legal Principles OR Medical Knowledge, can make the difference relief and agony for the accused Doctor.
> - Relief comes when complaint is dismissed as frivolous. When possible grounds for Criminal Negligence are made out, and FIR is registered to initiative investigation into the criminal motive, it is the beginning of a long distressing period for the Doctor, if the matter is eventually proved wrong later on.

Process of Including Expert Opinion after Complaint of Negligence Received by Consumer Forum

The SC in Martin D'Souza versus Mohd. Ishfaq of 2009[8] extended this Role of Expert Opinion to complaints before even the Consumer Forum. It decided that:
- "Whenever a complaint is received against a Doctor or Hospital by the Consumer Fora (whether District, State or National) or by the Criminal Court then before issuing notice to the doctor or hospital against whom the complaint was made the Consumer Forum or the Criminal Court should first refer the matter to a competent doctor or committee of doctors, specialized in the field relating to which the medical negligence is attributed, and only after that doctor or committee reports that there is a prima facie case of medical negligence should notice be then issued to the doctor/hospital concerned. This is necessary to avoid harassment to doctors who may not be ultimately found to be negligent".

This was further modified by the SC order of 2010, in V Kishan Rao versus Nikhil Super Speciality Hospital[9]. It said:
- "If any of the parties wants to adduce expert evidence before the Consumer Fora, the members of the Fora by applying their mind to the facts and circumstances of the case and the materials on record can allow the parties to adduce such evidence if it is appropriate to do so in the facts of the case. The discretion in this matter is left to the members of Fora especially when retired judges of Supreme Court and High Court are appointed to Head National Commission and the State Commission, respectively. Therefore, these questions are to be judged on the facts of each case and there cannot be a mechanical or strait jacket approach that each and every case must be referred to experts for evidence".

It also said "The question whether a medical practitioner or the hospital is negligent or not is a mixed question of fact and law and the Fora is not bound in every case to accept the opinion of the expert witness. Although, in many cases the opinion of the expert witness may assist the Fora to decide the controversy one way or the other."

> **KEY POINT THREE—EXPERT OPINION IN CONSUMER FORUM**
> Consumer Forum can decide whether:
> - Technical Matters in a given case warrant an Expert Opinion or not.
> - Opinion by Expert is to be accepted or not.

What is Expected in the Expert Opinion?

Expert help is needed primarily to decide the severity of the guilt or absence thereof. This helps the process of adjudication (by Judicial/

Quasi-judicial Authority), to help arrive at Legally valid conclusions.

Conclusions may be explicitly mentioned within the expert opinion as per the questions asked to them, OR the facts that directly reflect this opinion may be mentioned by the expert.

Usual questions that an expert may need to answer include:
- Is there any negligence?
- If so, what is the severity? Is it severe enough to be called as criminal negligence?
- What is the recommendation, if any to the authorities?
- What is the penalty that a peer body may impose for the same?

The expert body handling a case may be faced with a situation, wherein despite the key components of negligence apparently present in a particular case, is it possible there is NO negligence. Hence, the first step is to take a back seat and separate any impression of negligence from the matter presented, by looking at it as a "Medical Injury or Adverse/Unfavorable outcome". Also, there are many overlapping terms that come into the picture at this point of time, needing clarity. Failing this, there is the risk that every unfavorable outcome may be labeled/implied as negligence/incompetence/misconduct.

Guidelines for Analyzing Severity of Guilt

Are there any guidelines for such an expert body? Sadly, these are still missing. Though an effort seems to have been made by the authorities in the last two decades and some guidelines may have been proposed, the matter has not reached a logical conclusion.

Most of these overlapping terms in the context of an Adverse Outcome, were reported[10] in September, 2017, as being considered by a study group constituted by President MCI in 2017, in view of the pending action: "To prescribe guidelines regarding Professional Incompetence that are judged by a Peer Group" when there is a need to adjudication, as per the 2002 MCI Code of medical Ethics, Section 8.6.[11] Also mentioned was the need to address ambiguity regarding these similar terms that are used colloquially and in a practical sense.

Terms included in the draft prepared include:
- Adverse event
- Medical accident
- Medical error
- Medical malpractice
- Medical mishap
- Professional incapacity
- Professional incompetence
- Professional misconduct
- Professional negligence
- Untoward event.

Since the time it was reported that this report was submitted by the expert committee to the EC of the MCI, there is no update on the same. This is probably what led Delhi High Court to issue fresh directives to the MCI,[12] not only for guidelines on deciding the severity of guilt in a negligence but also on the severity of punishment to be awarded, as part of the judgment in *Ravi Rai versus Medical Council of India and Others, 2018*.[13]

Importance of the inputs of peers, on deciding matters relating to Medical Negligence came up first in the *Jacob Mathew versus State of Punjab 2005 Judgment*[3] by Supreme Court. The Honorable Court laid down the guideline regarding charging doctors or arresting them following any complaint of negligence. Details already discussed above. This was given with the rider that:
- "Statutory Rules or Executive Instructions incorporating certain guidelines need to

be framed and issued by the Government of India and/or the State Governments in consultation with the MCI. So long as it is not done, we propose to lay down certain guidelines for the future which should govern the prosecution of doctors for offences of which criminal rashness or criminal negligence is an ingredient."

Following this Judgment, it seems the matter was taken up by the MCI in 2007.[6]

- The MCI Ethics Committee considered the matter with regard to framing of guidelines for prosecution of Medical Professional under Criminal Law for possible Medical Negligence, in compliance of the Supreme Court Judgment and noted that the *draft guidelines is prepared for consideration of the Executive Committee.*

However, this matter has not progressed to reach a logical conclusion, where it could be approved by the Government and notified in the Union Gazette.

The draft that could be accessed included details of the process of handling a complaint with allegation of negligence, especially Criminal Negligence, including:

- Duties of patient/complainant
- Responsibility of the accused doctor
- Responsibility of the police while handling the matter
- Formation and duties of the committee that handles the matter.

In all the above, what was perhaps missed was to:

- Form the guidelines that can be used by the committee to actually decide the actual guilt in a given complaint (including its severity),
- Prescribe the suggested punishment for the same, in a graded manner in proportion to the severity of the guilt.

This is exactly what the Delhi High Court Judgment in *Ravi Rai versus Medical Council of India and Others*[13] aims to achieve, by reminding the MCI to respond to this matter. MCI report is awaited.

RECOMMENDATIONS BY THE AUTHOR AND GRADING THE SPECTRUM OF ADVERSE OUTCOME

In view of the above ambiguity of the situation, the author proposes to suggest the below recommendations. The focus is on the possible outcomes in the situation, that the expert body needs to consider. This is presented as a practical guide. While this may not be comprehensive, it does provide an overview.

Categories of Medical Injury OR Adverse/Unfavorable Outcome

Grading the spectrum of medical injury in an (adverse/untoward) event following medical treatment, is done in increasing severity of guilt.

All these are applicable in cases where there is a valid duty to provide care.

- *Medical Accident—no Negligence:*
  - An injury to patient in the absence of any breach in the care/skill/knowledge related to the duty
  - Incidents that have a similar implication include those which are described as Mishap, inevitable, error of judgment, or absence of causation.
- *Civil Negligence—cannot be prosecuted under Criminal Law:*
  - An injury to patient with a recognized breach in the care/skill/knowledge.
  - Incidents that have a similar implication include those which are described as malpractice, incompetence, and medical error.

- *Gross Negligence*—amounts to recklessness that can be prosecuted under Criminal Law
  - Applicable when a qualified person commits a conscious breach of guidelines despite knowing them, or
  - Any injury that results following treatment by an unqualified person

Medical Accident is a diagnosis/definition by exclusion. This is a concept poorly recognized in the Indian context. Mentioned ahead is a definition proposed by IMA, Pune and expanded by inputs on the online medicolegal forum by Professor MC Gupta up to 14-9-18.

"Any Patient, who was reasonably evaluated to be fit for the planned surgical/medical procedure with or without anesthesia or under medical treatment for an illness, dies as per HOTA (Human Organ Transplantation Act) or suffers significant trauma/injury/damage to brain or other body parts.

In an unforeseen manner, suddenly, unexpectedly, and unintentionally due to:
- Reason(s), which are unexplained, or
- Reason(s), which can be attributed to abnormal host response, or
- Reason(s), which can be attributed to equipment failure, or
- Reason(s), which cannot be attributed to normal course of the disease, or
- Reason(s) which cannot be attributed to negligence of healthcare provider/ hospital or its staff, or
- Reason(s), which cannot be conclusively determined, even after postmortem examination:
  - Which may occur again pending advances in medical science.
  - Will be termed as medical accident". Also aptly described as "An Act of God", once again to imply no human is responsible, and which can potentially happen again. Thus, this is a diagnosis/definition by exclusion.

KEY POINT FOUR—NO NEGLIGENCE: IMPLICATIONS
- Every Adverse Outcome is not a Medical Negligence.
- Medical Accident is a diagnosis of exclusion. It is due to unknown reason, and may not be preventable.
- When there is no Negligence, Doctors/ Healthcare Providers are not guilty and hence not liable for compensation in any Court.

SIGNIFICANCE OF GRADING SEVERITY OF GUILT

There is currently a trend to label any complication/adverse outcome as a negligence, not just by the patient and attenders but also the authorities and even colleagues at time. Part of this is due to inadequate focus on the possibility of a medical accident. That most allegations do not amount to negligence is perhaps reflected from the fact that more than 80–90% of the cases filed in consumer forum do not stand legal scrutiny.

Given the complexity of the medical field, and the pace at which advancements are coming, conveying a clear message to society that every adverse outcome is not a negligence by the Doctor, has many benefits to all at large. Few of these are mentioned below, not necessarily in sequence of importance:
- *Jousting*—will reduce, as ambiguity in labeling the guilt is minimized, and clarity improves. Colleagues will find it simpler to respond when asked to comment on a medical complication. Patients and Authorities will realize that a casual opinion does not mean much and a formal opinion can immensely help, given the complexity of decisions in medical treatment.

- *Patient education and responsibility*: Patients become aware that reasons other than negligence exist for an adverse or unfavorable outcome. Educated patient will cooperate, support and compliment the treatment, all for a better outcome.
- *Avoids frivolous complaints (of negligence) and violence*: Being a consequence of the first two, its chances also minimizes. Rather than simply deny the possibility of a negligence, it is now simpler for the hospital authorities/doctors to explain the alternative scenarios that lead to a complication/adverse outcome. A healthy discussion dissipates the anger, an informed patient is less likely to be unhappy, and reduces the chances that they go hunting for a Lawyer, and ultimately a complaint to the authorities.
- Decrease in Patient hostility will mitigate the chances that the doctor is harassed by authorities or patient attenders; whether based on genuine/biased opinion. Pressure on doctor to settle the matter by monetary compensation will reduce.
- Once the concept of medical accident is well-established and accepted by the system, there are other major improvements possible—"No-fault Compensation".

In the conventional system though the Consumer Forum, once established that there is no negligence, there is no further possibility of any benefits for the patient, despite the injury they may be left with. On the other hand, other aspects in life where accidents are common (deaths outside a hospital), say following road accidents and natural disasters, there is a predecided amount as compensation—simply because they have been recognized as an accident since ages. When these victims of accident can get a compensation from the System/Government, then why should victims of a medical accident be deprived of similar benefits? All that is needed is to create a separate corpus for the same, on the lines of no-fault compensation for road accidents. When this is possible for one scenario, why is it not possible for another? If it were possible to set up a system to provide compensation for medical accidents, there are many further benefits possible. One example is seen with the system of compensation followed in New Zealand for Medical Injury at large[14], called "No fault compensation". Currently in India, Principle of Torts is applied for adjudicating medical compensation, which has many shortcomings; where negligence has to be proven, and extent of loss has to be argued. This deprives the most needy from the benefit of a compensation, for example:
- Those without strong legal aid
- Elderly and invalid who cannot wait till the final outcome of the proceedings.

On the other hand, if the aggrieved person so choses, they should have the option to get compensation whether or not someone was negligent and responsible for the adverse outcome/medical injury or not. The same Medical Accident Corpus can then provide them with the compensation. It may be a fanciful dream, for the Indian system to completely move away from the prevailing system of tort to system of no-fault compensation, for unless the Government initially arranges funding of healthcare, how will it arrange for the funding for accidents arising out of the same? However, having "No-fault" as an option, in addition to the option of compensation through the Consumer Forum, may be worth for addressing the prevailing shortcomings in the Consumer

Forum system, where over 90% claims are rejected, and the aggrieved person gets no compensation at all.

- *Improvement in patient safety*: By getting the focus to the concept of "Medical Accident", it will be possible to put to scrutiny issues in the process, products, and anything else involved in providing a healthcare service. Take just quality of drugs or medical devices as an example of issues that lead to an unfavorable outcome.
  - *Complications involving drugs:*
    "With cases of medical negligence on the rise, more and more families are getting angry. Not only because of hospital's negligence but also their complete ignorance on the kind of medicines that should be prescribed.[15] In the past, such cases have led to the death of a patient or severe side effects." This is how media usually reports adverse outcomes after medical treatment.
    The need to be countered with the scientific facts—"Expert Speak: All drugs have side effects, so are all doctors legally guilty?"[16]
    Corrective comment by news portal: "As Dr Satish Bhat has rightly pointed out, we here at the better Indian did not fully explore all possible fallouts of a new judgment."
  - *Surgical devices*:[17] The Indian arm of Johnson and Johnson, one of the leading global Medical Industry majors, "suppressed" key facts on the harmful aftermath of surgeries conducted on hundreds of patients in the country using "faulty" hip replacement systems it imported and sold.
    In a "clear abdication of responsibility", it did not inform the national regulator about the exact number of patients who used these devices, the adverse reports following such surgeries and the corrective operations subsequently conducted. It also "did not provide any compensation" to those affected. That Johnson and Johnson could get away without paying compensation after implanting faulty hip replacement devices points to a regulatory deficit, and lack of medical ethics.
  - *Drugs contamination*: "Eleven women die after sterilization surgeries in Chhattisgarh. Chief Minister Raman Singh visited the victims at Bilaspur hospitals and suspended four health officials, including Health Director Kamalpreet Singh and Bilaspur Chief Medical Officer Dr SC Bhange".[18] This is how the events initially unfolded. The doctor was held responsible and even arrested.[19] Ultimately, it turns out the Government administrators are responsible for this gory negligence—the true cause of negligence was rodenticide contamination in the antibiotic tablets.[20] But were the real culprits ever hauled up? The victimized doctors were quietly released, no mention of any compensation for the needless harassment as the fall guy, unlike the victim families who got compensation for their misery. No discussion of the real culprits or pinning responsibility subsequently, not any mention of preventive strategy.
  - *Drug quality testing*: August, 2018—Irregularities in the Health Department of the previous Karnataka Government has cost the state exchequer a loss of Rupees 5352.2 million revealed a Comptroller and Auditor General (CAG) report. According to the CAG

Section 1: General Medical Law

report on social and general sector, the health department during 2014–2017 procured drugs chemicals and miscellaneous items which failed basic quality checks.[21]

The items were procured by the Karnataka State Drugs Logistics and Warehousing Society, which come under the Health and Family Welfare Ministry. The CAG reports shows that 14,209 batches of drugs were to be tested, however, only 6,776 batches of drugs were tested, leaving 7,433 batches untested. These drugs were then supplied to patients without testing/quality assurances. These drugs were also distributed to various Government Hospitals and primary healthcare centers across the state, risking the lives of many patients.

As per the Drugs and Cosmetics Act, 1940 the purchased items have to be tested in an approved laboratory. However, the department failed to conduct any such test. The CAG report also notes that the fact that the drugs were not of standard quality (NSQ), and was not communicated to the respective medical institutes in time and hence, many were never replaced as prescribed as per standard procedure. Worse still, the contractors supplying these items got full payments and were never blacklisted.

It is not known, if there was any complication following use of these untested drugs, though it was confirmed that they were distributed and consumed by unsuspecting patients.

Only once the focus of an adverse/unfavorable outcome or complication is widened, away from the current focus on "Negligence by Doctors" as a cause, will the real problem get the due attention. Unless this happens, tendency to make the treating doctor as the fall guy for any lapse, will continue unabated. If this is not achieved, the current tendency to hold the doctor responsible for every shortcoming in the healthcare system will continue.

KEY POINT FIVE—GRADED SEVERITY OF GUILT OR ABSENCE THEREOF: BENEFITS

Benefits from deciding graded severity of guilt or absence thereof:
- Professional jousting can reduce
- Better patient education
- Avoids frivolous complaints
- Focus on patient safety
- Focus on causes for adverse outcome not due to negligence—Products and processes in healthcare like:
  - Drugs
  - Surgical devices

SUMMARY

While the above suggested guidelines may not be perfect, it hopes to create a sense of order in a matter that is very pressing, and pending since the time of:
- Professional Conduct, Etiquette and Ethics Regulations, 2002
- Supreme Court Judgment of Jacob Mathew versus State of Punjab, 2005.

Whatever may the best guideline, it is of no use unless it is simple to use and accepted by the fraternity. Inability to speak in one voice has been our bane, since a long time, even for matters that are in the best interest of our patients. It is this failure of self-regulation and formulating guidelines by the Fraternity, that forces the authorities to step in and frame guidelines from their perspective. This often ends up with disappointment for the Medical Fraternity, and eventually the patients we are meant to serve. Whether it is healthcare policy, healthcare corruption, hospital violence, treating healthcare as a consumer service, the list is endless.

This Guidelines on Severity of Guilt may be even more relevant for those who occupy positions of authority, in the Medical Boards that are called to give expert opinions. Unless the concept of medical accident is well-appreciated, it may be difficult to keep away the tag of negligence from any medical injury or adverse outcome, when the matter comes up for opinion. This is besides appreciating the nuances of the process and composition of the board itself.

Imagine the disservice that would result, if an innocent doctor is held responsible for an unfavorable outcome that is completely beyond his/her control. On the other hand, having the focus on medical accidents should not imply that this can become an option to escape responsibility by those genuinely guilty.

Grading the severity of the guilt, when one does exist, is will help to suggest a graded punishment for the guilty Doctor. Ultimately, punishment is meant to reform an individual who has committed an offense, and must be in proportion to the violation, neither more nor less. Unless there is an objective mechanism to identify breach in safety and responsibility for the breach, punishment prescribed for the breach cannot be an effective means at restitution or to prevent safety breach once again.

However, unless the breach is adjudicated in a fair and logical manner, and penal measures imposed only on genuine lapses, punishing the wrong ones may act as a deterrent for future generation doctors from taking up risks in the interests of patients in an emergency. If the patient succumbs despite all heroic efforts, who will take up such a case again, if the risk of being unfairly penalized are high?

Unless this issue is appreciated and these guidelines acknowledged, considered, and tried out by the fraternity, the prevailing chaos will continue. Only when the fraternity speaks more and more on "medical accidents", can a change be possible. Perhaps then, it may be possible to turn the tide that currently seems to be against us.

CASE EXAMPLE

The author has been a victim of the prevailing scenario himself in 2011. Following the unexpected death of a burns patient, a 37-year-old lady with about 20% burns, there was a huge hue and cry alleging negligence and demands of compensation. While this did not help, defamatory and malicious reporting was seen in the Media. When this also did not help, a complaint was lodged with the local police station. The Author first got to know of all this when he was summoned to the police station, and threatened with "arrest" following FIR (Number 03/2012, dated 5-1-2012, Mangalore East PS, Dakshina Kannada District, Karnataka) under IPC 304A,[22] after the complaint—that too for a bail-able section! What saved the day was the basic knowledge of law, and the presence of mind to ask "Which are the sections applied?" It turns out IPC 304A for a "Rash and Negligent Act" is the same section applied for the common road accident, where a motor vehicle hits any pedestrian leading to death. Compare this to the language used by the police "I may have to arrest you"!

It took more than a year for the Author to follow-up with each stage of the investigation—collecting an expert opinion, ensure progress of the investigation, and the final submission of the report with "No Negligence" to the Magistrate. All this was done without any expenses beyond that prescribed by law.

If the concept of a medical accident been accepted by all, and not just the medical fraternity, the author, patient family, police, and the Magistrate would have been spared the trouble of the process of litigation!

As told by the Supreme Court in *Ravi Rai versus Medical Council of India and Others*,[13] "Before punishing someone, can we please decide who really is guilty?"

CONCLUSION

The medical fraternity needs to quickly form guidelines for evaluation of technical aspects of medical profession, in the face of rising allegations and ramifications. Failure to do so, with end up with some nonrepresentative authority framing these guidelines and then it will be too late to rectify any aberrations.

REFERENCES

1. http://www.indiamedicaltimes.com/2016/11/20/110-rise-in-number-of-medical-negligence-cases-in-india-every-year-study/.
2. http://indiatoday.intoday.in/story/litigation-doctors-medicine-law-national-accreditation-board-for-hospitals/1/394983.html.
3. Jacob Mathew vs State of Punjab 2005. [online] Available from: https://indiankanoon.org/doc/871062/.
4. Section IPC 80: Accident in Doing a Lawful Act. [online] Available from: https://indiankanoon.org/doc/602933/.
5. Section IPC 88: Act not intended to cause death, done by consent in good faith for person's benefit. [online] Available from: https://indiankanoon.org/doc/862963/.
6. The MCI Ethics Committee recommendations, minutes of its meeting held on 19-3-2007. [online] Available from: http://www.mciindia.org/meetings/Ethics_/2007/Minutes%20Ethics%20Committee%2019.03.2007.pdf.
7. Dr BC Jain vs Maulana Saleem on 28-2-2017. [online] Available from: https://indiankanoon.org/doc/93902571/.
8. Martin D'Souza versus Mohd. Ishfaq of 2009. [online] Available from: https://indiankanoon.org/doc/1092676/.
9. V Kishan Rao vs Nikhil Super Speciality Hospital. [online] Available from: https://indiankanoon.org/doc/1920027/.
10. MCI defines Professional Incompetence, issues Guidelines. [online] Available from: https://medicaldialogues.in/mci-defines-professional-incompetence-issues-guidelines/.
11. Professional Conduct, Etiquette and Ethics Regulations, 2002. [online] Available from: https://www.mciindia.org/documents/rulesAndRegulations/Ethics%20Regulations-2002.pdf.
12. https://www.vakilno1.com/legal-news/medical-negligence-delhi-high-court-directs-mci-to-formulate-guidelines.html.
13. Ravi Rai versus Medical Council of India and Ors. [online] Available from: https://indiankanoon.org/doc/142469582/.
14. No Fault Compensation in New Zealand. [online] Available from: http://content.healthaffairs.org/content/25/1/278.long.
15. https://www.indiatimes.com/news/india/bengaluru-doctor-has-to-pay-rs-90-000-fine-for-prescribing-wrong-medicine-to-neurological-patient-337764.html.
16. https://www.thebetterindia.com/128643/expert-speak-all-drugs-have-side-effects-so-are-all-doctors-legally-guilty/.
17. https://indianexpress.com/article/india/johnson-johnson-buried-key-facts-on-faulty-hip-implant-surgeries-kept-regulator-in-dark-5322149/.
18. https://www.thehindu.com/news/national/other-states/8-women-dead-in-botched-surgeries-at-chhattisgarh-govt-camp/article6586425.ece.
19. https://www.thehindu.com/news/national/other-states/bilaspur-sterilisation-deaths-doctor-arrested/article6594051.ece.
20. https://www.indiatoday.in/india/story/chhattisgarh-sterilization-deaths-due-to-medicines-contaminated-with-rat-poison-227268-2014-11-15.
21. https://www.news18.com/news/india/cag-report-exposes-irregularities-in-karnataka-health-dept-says-patients-given-sub-standard-drugs-1874449.html.
22. Section IPC 304A: Cognizable and Bailable. [online] Available from: https://indiankanoon.org/doc/1371604/.

CHAPTER 23

Who Can Do What?

Putta Srinivas

"Beauty is the gift of God"

—Aristotle

KEY OBJECTIVES

- Introduction
- Dermatologist
  - Dermatologic Surgery
  Plastic Surgeon
  - Plastic Surgery
- Cosmetology/Cosmetologist
  - General Cosmetology
  - Cosmetic Dermatology (Medical/Clinical Cosmetology)
- Aesthetician/Aesthetic Medicine
- Trichiatrist/Dermatotrichologist, Trichologist
- Abolition of Quackery in Cosmetology, Aesthetics, Trichiatry
  - Public Education
  - Statutory Regulations
  - Setting of statutory panels for standards for all the procedures of cosmetic dermatology, aesthetics, and trichiatry

INTRODUCTION

Advances in medical science have led to development of many specialties and Dermatology is the branch of medicine concerned with the diagnosis and treatment of skin disorders.

However, many subspecialties have evolved mainly as lifespan has increased, control or reduction/elimination of many common infectious and nutritional diseases, people started showing more concern particularly regarding "beauty, appearance, to look younger, to reduce the weight", etc. Consequently, subspecialties such as dermatosurgery, aesthetic medicine, cosmetology have developed. Unfortunately, there is lot of commercialization, and to make the matter worse, many self-styled institutions have sprung and started training even nonmedical persons and making money, just to exploit the situation taking advantage of lack of regulations and monitoring statutory authorities.

Common people including highly educated and professionals like software engineers are psyched by bombardment of advertisements in print and electronic media, sometimes creating panic and made to believe in quackery by aggressive use of social media, dubious websites, YouTube, Facebook, etc. Hence, there is a definite need to educate the people about the "who are the actual eligible experts?" That is what this chapter is meant for.

The following are the specialists who deal with skin, appendages, dermatosurgery, cosmetology, aesthetics, and reconstructive surgery.

DERMATOLOGIST

What a dermatologist can do? Advances and application of science and technology has completely changed the field of dermatology ranging from treatment of skin diseases to surgical and cosmetic procedures, making dermatology to reach new frontiers.

The syllabus of postgraduate (PG) degree in dermatology includes surgery in dermatology including, chemical peels, dermabrasion, lasers, skin punch grafting, substances for soft tissue augmentation (Fillers, etc.), cryosurgery, nail surgery, hair transplantation, and alopecia reduction, Mohs micrographic surgery.[1]

Dermatologic Surgery

- Chemical peels
- Dermabrasion
- Laser
- Skin punch grafting
- Wound dressings
- Cryosurgery
- Nail Surgery.

Although these dermatosurgical procedures were part of curriculum, unfortunately in many medical colleges, they were not implemented, in Government colleges due insufficient budget allocation and in private colleges as the managements were not concerned as they were not part of mandatory requirements during Medical Council of India (MCI) inspections for grant or recognition of PG courses in Dermatology. The matter was brought to the notice of MCI in 2014, by this author when he was a member of MCI, PG Committee, and then and now these dermatosurgical procedures were made mandatory as a part of Standard Assessment Forms (SAF) during inspections and throughout India. Consequently, now the equipment required is procured by all the departments and PG students are now having direct hands on experience in:

- Acne surgery[2]
- Cryosurgical procedures
- Chemical peels
- Skin grafting procedures
- Keloid treatment
- Nail surgeries
- Laser procedures
- Laser hair reduction
- Laser scar revision
- Laser pigment removal
- Cosmetic surgical procedures.

Plastic Surgeon—Plastic Surgery

Plastic surgery is the specialty of reconstructive surgery, performing operations to repair or replace skin, which has been damaged, or to improve people's appearance. The field of plastic surgery is very vast:
- Breast augmentation, reconstruction with breast implant, with flap surgery
- Rhinoplasty
- Lip surgery
- Cheek surgery
- Ear surgery
- Liposuction
- Fat filling
- Scar revision surgeries
- Replantation surgeries (microsurgery)
- Endoscopic plastic surgery
- Facelift
- Flap transfer
- Skin grafting
- Acute burn care
- Trauma
- Tendon transfer
- Nerve repair (brachial plexus nerve repair)
- Hair transplant.

COSMETOLOGY/COSMETOLOGIST

Cosmetology is the science of beautifying skin and its appendages[3] and can be broadly classified into two main types. They are:
1. *General/nonclinical cosmetology*
2. *Cosmetic dermatology (medical/clinical cosmetology).*

General Cosmetology

General cosmetology is all about using skin and hair care practices, which are usually followed at salons, beauty parlors, spas, and hair care centers. In India, many private beauty centers are conducting training courses/programs for individuals with minimum educational qualification of 10+2.

Cosmetic Dermatology (Medical/Clinical Cosmetology)

Cosmetic dermatology is a broad subspecialty encompassing a range of topics, including colored cosmetics, camouflaging techniques, basic skin care, cosmetic fashion trends, nail manicuring practices, surgical techniques, hair care, cosmeceuticals, allergic and irritant contact dermatitis.[4]

Cosmetic dermatology is all about advanced medical practices related to hair and skin. Since hair and skin care is part of dermatology PG course, the minimum qualification should be diploma or degree in Dermatology.

Unfortunately, many individuals and institutions, with the sole intention of making quick money are training, MBBS, BDS, BHMS, BAMS, BUMS graduates and giving certificates, which are neither approved and recognized by MCI nor registered with State Medical Councils, but are accredited by certain foreign associations such as International Society of Aesthetic Physicians and World Society of Interdisciplinary of Aesthetic and Anti-Aging Medicine.

AESTHETICIAN/AESTHETIC MEDICINE

Aesthetic medicine comprises all medical procedures that are aimed at improving the physical appearance and satisfaction of the patient, using noninvasive to minimally invasive cosmetic procedures. Some aesthetic medicine procedures are performed under local anesthesia while some procedures do not require anesthetics at all.

The exciting field of aesthetic medicine is a new trend in modern medicine. Patients not only want to be in good health, they also want to enjoy life to the fullest, be fit, and minimize the effects of normal aging. Indeed, patients are now requesting quick and noninvasive procedures with minor downtime and very little risk. As a general rule, the needle is increasingly replacing the scalpel.[5]

This recent trend explains the current success of aesthetic medicine around the globe. These aesthetic procedures consist of:
- Injections of neurotoxins and dermal fillers
- Chemical peels
- Cosmetic dermatology treatments
- Microdermabrasion
- Body contouring and treatment of cellulite
- Nutrition
- Hair transplant
- Hair reduction
- Fat grafting/platelet-rich plasma
- Lasers
- Scar management
- Venous treatment
- Cosmetic gynecology.

Dermatologists are the eligible specialists to perform all aesthetic procedures.

TRICHIATRIST/ DERMATOTRICHOLOGIST, TRICHOLOGIST

Trichiatrist/Dermatotrichologist is a medical physician dealing with hair and scalp in health and disease.[6]

Trichologist is a nonmedical person, is associated with laity and cosmetics,[6] and advise the application of a particular cream or lotion to the scalp or the use of nutritional therapy and appropriate counseling.[7] However, trichologists are not medically qualified, and they can neither prescribe medicines nor perform any surgical procedures. All the trichologists are nonmedical persons.

Dermatologists are the eligible specialists to treat Hair disorders since it is a part of their curriculum.

ABOLITION OF QUACKERY IN COSMETOLOGY, AESTHETICS, TRICHIATRY

The professional association bodies of dermatology and plastic surgery have social responsibility to focus on abolition of quackery and take necessary steps.

Public Education

We have to reach to people, by conducting seminars and discussions, involving different sections of people, intellectual groups, administrators, policy makers, medical associations, like Indian Medical Association (IMA) and other different specialty associations.

Statutory Regulations

Many people are becoming victims of cosmetic quackery, and are getting cheated. On the other hand, genuine specialists are facing litigations, sometimes, cases filed just to exploit.[8,9]

Trichology

The current need of the hour is enactment of acts/regulations for uniform scientific standards, regarding, eligibility criteria of the experts, setting of scientific standards of procedures, and infrastructure requirements and selling of highly technical instruments like lasers, etc. which in the hands of unqualified can lead to disasters.

There shall be regulatory boards to supervise, control the effective implementation of acts/regulations and, if necessary, to have powers to act on those who violate the regulations.

KEY MESSAGES

- People are brainwashed by advertisements in print and electronic media, sometimes

creating panic and made to believe in quackery by aggressive use of social media, dubious web sites, You Tube, Facebook, etc.
- There is a definite and urgent need to educate the people about the who are the actual eligible experts.
- Dermatologists are the eligible specialists not only to treat skin diseases but also eligible to perform many dermato-surgical and cosmetic-surgical procedures.
- Plastic surgeons are the eligible specialists to perform reconstructive surgery, performing operations to repair or replace skin which has been damaged, or to improve people's appearance.
- There is a urgent need for setting of Statutory panels for enactment of acts/regulations for uniform scientific standards, regarding, eligibility criteria of the experts, scientific standards of procedures, and infrastructure requirements and selling of highly technical instruments, like, Lasers, etc.

REFERENCES

1. National Board of Examinations (2006). Syllabus of Postgraduate Degree/Diploma Training Programs, MCI, 2006. [online] Available from: http://www.natboard.edu.in/notice_for_dnb_candidates/dermatology.pdf. [Accessed December, 2018].
2. mciindia.org/helpdesk/download/SAF_PG/Dermatology.doc
3. Savant SS. Textbook of Dermatosurgery and Cosmetology, 2nd edition. Indian J Dermatol Venereol Leprol. 2005;71(4):493.
4. Draelos ZD. Cosmetic Dermatology. USA: Wiley; 2005.
5. American Academy of Aesthetic Medicine (2014). What is aesthetic medicine? [online] Available from: https://www.aaamed.org/aesthetic_med.php. [Accessed December, 2018].
6. Treb et al. Skin Appendage Disorders DOJ May 07.2018. Pages 1-6.
7. Mysore V, Khopkar U. Check if your trichologist is a doctor: Need for educating the public. Indian J Dermatol Venereol Leprol. 2007;73(3):147-8.
8. Jitender Kumar Joshi vs. General Hospital on 13 September, 2011, SCDRC, UT, Chandigarh.
9. State Consumer Disputes Redressal Commission (2005). Dr. Bhramaramba S.A.V. vs Tln Anusha on 24 August, 2017, Telangana. [online] Available from: https://indiankanoon.org/doc/193268809/. [Accessed December, 2018].

SECTION 2

Dermatology

- The Changing Face of Dermatology Practice

   Part A: General Dermatology
- Is Dermatology a Safe Subject? Pitfalls and Safeguards during the Practice of General Dermatology
- Consent for Drug Administration: It is Necessary?
- Investigations and Law
- Medicolegal Issues in Cutaneous Adverse Drug Reactions
- Legal Issues in HIV and STD Patients
- Legal Aspects of Leprosy
- Photography and the Law
- Setting up a Pharmacy in a Clinic

   Part B: Aesthetic Dermatology
- Special Features of an Aesthetic Patient
- Medicolegal Aspects of Hair Practice
- Special Aspects of Dermatosurgery Practice
- Handling Difficult Patients in Dermatology
- Consent for Injectables in Cosmetic Dermatology
- Medicolegal Aspects of Lasers
- Consent in Procedures with Less Evidence and Off-label Indications

CHAPTER 24

The Changing Face of Dermatology Practice

Venkataram Mysore, Madhulika Mhatre

INTRODUCTION

Medicine and specifically dermatology are undergoing enormous changes in the way in which it is practiced. Many advances have made treatment options possible in a way that could not have been imagined two decades back. Dermatology and dermatosurgery are more interventional now. Patients, attitudes have also changed and expectations are higher. With the advent of more advanced telecommunication, imaging capabilities and information transfer, the very ways in which we examine patients, develop diagnoses and plan treatments as dermatologists, have changed dramatically. Changes in patient attitudes and social norms too have contributed to this epochal shift.

At the core, medicine and specifically dermatology are being practiced in much the same manner today as in centuries past: a patient presents to the concerned physician, a detailed history is elicited, a thorough physical examination is performed, an assessment is made, and appropriate treatment is recommended. However, the level of complexity of each of these steps has changed dramatically over the course of years, as have both the spectrum of recognized diseases/disorders, as well as treatment options. Much of this change can be attributed to the way technology has evolved in this field of dermatology, and also the patients' own sense of self and prerogative to seek out procedures and treatments on their own. The role of social media and other mass media in promoting and highlighting this field, has also contributed to this massive rise that dermatology practice has so lately observed.

Introduction of technology while enhancing efficiency have also meant for raising costs, with increased efforts to recover the costs. Increasing technology has also lead to simplification of procedures leading to safer, less invasive procedures with far less complications and downtime than earlier.

This has in turn led to jumping into this foray, of individuals seeking to capitalize

> **BOX 1:** Scope of this chapter.
> - Cosmetic versus clinical dermatology
> - Rise of untrained individuals/quacks
> - Role of technology in dermatology
> - Client versus patient
> - Desire dermatology
> - Violence against doctors
> - Role of media
> - Role of pharmaceutical companies
> - Rising incidence of medicolegal cases
> - Response of dermatologists

on this huge potential, qualified or not. Dermatology has, more than any other specialty, attracted a huge number of "quacks" or untrained professionals claiming to have the said qualifications required to manage and treat skin and hair problems.

We examine these factors in detail, as listed in Box 1.

COSMETIC DERMATOLOGY VERSUS CLINICAL DERMATOLOGY

The last few decades have seen a sharp shift of physicians having degrees in dermatology shift their focus toward the glamorous field of cosmetology over the traditional art of practicing clinical dermatology. The paradigm seems to have shifted from clinical dermatology to cosmesis, and from temperament and diathesis, patient history taking and treating for the individual, to new-age, over-the-top therapies and short-stop, quick acting shortcuts, all in the name of a fatter paycheck. This has had an alarming consequence on, not only the doctor's perspective of a patient (or rather, a client), but also on the perceived image of a practitioner, in the eyes of the patient. This can be vastly attributed to the monetary profits that can be made in a short span of time compared to establishing a clinical practice that can take years. A complete shift of perspective has also lead to the rise of unqualified physicians completely focused on finding an aesthetic solution (procedure-driven) for all skin/hair problems! Moreover, this has paved a way for a hoard of salons and unqualified therapists putting up centers and clinics offering skin-related services, thus promoting quackery and duping ignorant patients in the bargain.

Clinical dermatology is an art, the training of which is hard-achieved through rigorous training and patient interaction. Whereas, cosmetology, albeit skillful, is fast becoming an art form acquired with premature knowhow and near-absent training. Needless to say, the golden adages—"patient first", "primum non nocere", and "a doctor, a God" hold far less meaning in this day and age, and may only spiral down further, in times to come.

RISE OF UNTRAINED INDIVIDUAL PRACTICING COSMETOLOGY (QUACKS)

Over 25% of patients who first visit their primary care doctor annually do so for a problem related to skin and over a period of 2 years the number climbs to 50%.[1,2] Overall, 6–7% of outpatient visits to all physicians are for a complaint regarding the skin and although many of these are simple, straightforward, self-limited problems, skin disease is a leading cause of disability.[3] Even common maladies, such as acne or psoriasis, may affect the quality of life of a patient dramatically.[4]

Of late, there has been a significant rise in the number of non-dermatologists practicing as skin specialists or cosmetologists. These physicians surely lack sufficient training during medical school and postgraduate training to qualify them as expert in matters that pertain to skin diseases.[5] They possess limited dermatologic diagnostic and therapeutic skills and have little confidence in their own ability to diagnose and treat skin disorders, including skin cancer. Despite their deficiencies, perceived or not, they continue to treat patients with skin disorders of all kinds, charging hefty amounts not because they believe they possess expertise, but because it generates revenue and being the primary point of contact, they have already established the necessary rapport with the patient. More alarmingly, they do not understand enough about skin disease and its physical and psychological implications to really know the difference.[6]

In an effort to supplement their limited diagnostic skills, non-dermatologists tend to order inappropriate tests. Unfortunately, however, these physicians lack insight into the importance of interpretation of many of these tests and their implications in skin disease pathology. The number of non-dermatologists or untrained professionals carrying out laser procedures has also increased, and with half-knowledge of the required parameters to be used, these procedures cause more harm than help. These quacks are a larger threat to the society due to their inadequate skills and thus more often putting the patient in harm's way in the process.

In India, multiple systems of medicine exist such as Homeopathy, Allopathy, Ayurveda, etc. and though strict laws are in place to limit illegal practice of medicine, the implementation of these laws is inadequate. However, the scenario is somewhat different in case of "skilled quackery" in which a physician or a dentist practices dermatology or cosmetology including invasive procedures without having sufficient training for the same. Sometimes, for it to look more authentic, they advertise having certain qualifications, which are not recognized by any governing bodies. Also, there is lack of clear-cut guidelines regarding who can perform certain procedures and with what qualification. Doctors with just a basic MBBS degree or non-medical diploma in cosmetology or dentists, homeopaths, general surgeons are rampantly conducting hair transplants, liposuction, injectables, etc. Even an educated patient at times finds it extremely difficult in identifying a qualified competent doctor and gets duped in the process.[7] In light of these upsurges, the Indian Association of Dermatologists, Venereologists and Leprologists (IADVL) set up a task force against quackery (ITAQ) in the year 2017, which has, relentlessly and tirelessly, been targeting both in-house dermatologists who are training other realms of medicine, as well as quacks who are foraying into this field.

There is a significant role played by general physicians, who have been prescribing unregulated topical preparations, and thereby promoting pharmaceutical companies to dish out, by the dozen, unethical preparations, mostly steroid based. This has resulted in the last two decades seeing a rise in the abuse of topical steroids, and its ensuing sequelae. Another initiative by IADVL, the task force against steroid abuse (ITATSA), has been addressing this issue for over half a decade now.

An offshoot of all these is the fact that patients are at difficulty in distinguishing genuine from the fake, and an expert from the charlatan. This has fuelled a sense of suspicion about medical profession among patients and the tendency to repeated second consultations.

TECHNOLOGY IN DERMATOLOGY

The advances in technology have revolutionized modern medicine on many levels. Telemedicine has made it possible to deliver healthcare to even the remotest locations. As tools for diagnosis become more advanced, our reliance on technology becomes more and more addictive. With the advancement of knowledge and expanding facilities everyday, no medical practitioner can keep up without help. By adopting high-tech medical communication, high-performance computers, high-resolution cameras, diagnostic tools like dermatoscopes, advanced methods for histopathology, the field of dermatology has seen a drastic revolution; wherein, the entire world of medical science remains placed at the fingertips of even the most isolated rurally situated doctor.

The strides in technology have not only made diagnosis and treatment more accurate and prompt, but it also has a definitive role in prognosis and therapeutic monitoring.

Today, most medical practitioners are accustomed to having patients who are well-informed or perhaps even overinformed, having done research on the Internet regarding their own medical symptoms and/or diagnoses. These individuals represent a dramatic shift from traditional physician–patient encounters, with patients now asking detailed and probing questions regarding diagnosis, treatment, and alternative options. Many patients have been empowered by the ease and availability of medical information via the Internet and have assumed a much more active role in their medical care.

For although the Internet does allow access to information of all kinds, it is often unfiltered and can include information that is biased or erroneous. Some patients may find it difficult to sort fact from fiction.

Teledermatology and the Dermatologist

Virtual conferences and webinars have paved the way for continued medical education without having to be physically present. Thus, this advancement in dermatology has gone a long way in benefiting dermatologists who can improve their knowledge and skills without having to miss their clinic days.

Teledermatology and Privacy

As with any new advancement, comes the question of safety and protection of rights. A number of medical forums and social networking sites or groups on various social apps have come up as a forum for discussing cases and treatment and sharing patient-related information. We indeed benefit from discussing difficult cases and learn from each other's experiences; however, the right to patient's privacy and confidentiality is a much-debated issue. These issues are dealt in greater detail in the first section of the book.

CLIENT VERSUS PATIENT

With the rapid boom in cosmetology over the last couple of decades, the authors have seen an upward rise in the number of "retail clinics" and "medical spas" cropping up all over the country. Cosmetology has been more of a "need"-based intervention, wherein due to media propagation, highly disposable income in the middle-class population, increased awareness of cosmetic procedures or peer pressure, women and men alike are pushed toward various cosmetic procedures thus contributing to the upward trend of these medical spas and clinic. This is where the distinction between a patient and client comes into play, a patient being someone with a skin/hair disorder that has a medical implication, whereas a "client" being someone seeking treatment just to enhance their cosmetic appearance. This attitude, more so, festers the ideology that doctors are mere service providers and the age-old respect for the noble profession is somewhere lost in translation.

This has led to an increased number of "clients" being dissatisfied with the "service provided", even if there is no negligence, and an increase in the number of litigations. There is a tendency to treat lack of results as a deficiency in service. Deficiency in service is then being treated as negligence. The result of this attitude is that a lot of young doctors are overcautious in their diagnosis, management, and therapeutic approach, given the fear of this dissatisfaction. As a result, patient expectations are seldom met. Both sides of this attitude are detrimental, and the need of the hour is to strike a balance and establish a fulcrum between explicit, uncontrolled therapy, and the "one-step-back-approach".

DESIRE DERMATOLOGY[8]

Cosmetic surgery is concerned with the "maintenance, restoration, or enhancement of one's physical appearance through surgical and medical techniques". Common phrases such as "beauty is in the eye of the beholder" and "beauty is only skin deep" are testaments to our belief that attractiveness is ephemeral. For example, the philosopher David Hume is often quoted for making the argument that "beauty is no quality in things themselves: it exists merely in the mind which contemplates them; and each mind contemplates a different beauty". Social pressures to look good and desirable are other huge motivating factors. In this case, even though the motivation is external, the required cosmetic procedure may be undertaken to uplift the patient's confidence and self-image. This self-awareness, and a heightened perception of self, has further aggravated the paradigm shift, discussed previously. And for obvious reasons, this "desire dermatology" or practicing according to the patients' whims and fancies, causes further dissatisfaction, and culminates in a vicious circle.

VIOLENCE AGAINST DOCTORS

Violence is increasingly being used against doctors and other medical personnel, and a general estimate of three-fourths of practitioners has faced some form of aggression at some point in time. China was the forerunner, till a few years back, but India has been catching up, stealthily. As discussed earlier, the nobility of the medical profession is largely at stake owing to both endogenous and exogenous factors.

Countries in the European Union, the National Health Service (NHS) of the United Kingdom, and other developed nations have deployed a "Zero-Tolerance" policy for this issue, under the aegis of WHO. Back home, we have guidelines in place as well, even though it will be a long time gone before they take shape. With the sad portrayal by all forms of media, patients and their relatives and informants are becoming more and more daring, with reports surfacing every other week, of destruction to hospital property, in addition to the gruesome violence against doctors.

The news-hungry media seek out sensational stories of organ theft, medical negligence, prescription of expensive branded drugs, and malpractice, sometimes even supported by our politicians and bureaucracy. And this lack of support, coupled with the perils of daily practice, add to the burden of lengthy periods of studying, and existing reservations. And this multifactorial net has seen a sharp decline in people willing to opt for medicine after secondary school. According to the authors, this is the number one priority that needs to be addressed at the earliest to avoid brain-drain and a reduction in the general and specialist medical pool.

ROLE OF PHARMACEUTICAL COMPANIES

Due to this ever-expanding sector, pharmaceutical companies have assumed a bigger role than before. First and foremost, with the trend of patients considering themselves as "consumers", rather than needy patients, has spewed hatred against our community. There, undoubtedly, are a few black sheep on the inside, who accept monetary gratitude, sponsorships, workshops, gifts and so on, oft at the expense of patients, by prescribing unnecessary medications, advising needless procedures. As a result, pharmaceutical companies are at the helm of the stock market, and are considered to be in a constant boom in the 21st century. The ill-effects of the other side of this seesaw have been discussed at length, throughout this chapter. This image of doctors as money makers is rampant and needs to be checked right at the grassroot level, till the higher echelons.

ROLE OF THE MEDIA

Media, in all its forms: print, mass, video, and even social, have since the turn of this millennium shown doctors in extremely poor light. This blasphemy has left medical professionals, worldwide, at the beck and call of outrage from patients and relatives. Doctors seem to, also, have become bashing-posterboys (and girls) for politicians and ministerial staff, who instead of downregulating this blasphemy, join in on the action and make rules more stringent for us. The pen is mightier than the sword, and very soon, than the stethoscope too! Doctors and even paramedical staff are being vilified—often without concrete proof or even a basis. Negative reviews, based out of thin air, are left on professional websites. In certain countries, *fatwas* are issued left, right and center against our profession. As long as these insinuations continue, we will bear the brunt of media, its negative propaganda, and its gullible audience.

RISING INCIDENCE OF MEDICOLEGAL ISSUES IN DERMATOLOGY

It is ironic that dermatology, once regarded as a safe specialty, should turn into an unsafe specialty. While this is largely due to the advent of cosmetic dermatology, even traditional dermatology has not been immune to medicolegal challenges. A case in point is the fact is that the highest ever compensation was given to a skin patient of Steven-Johnson syndrome (SJS) (in 2011). Drug-induced side effects, use of drugs for off-label indications, and drugs with potentially serious side effects for nonserious indications all have the potential for medicolegal challenges. In fact, SJS has been one of the main reasons for medicolegal claims—either because the patient blames the doctor for the adverse reaction or the poor outcome, which can happen in severe cases of SJS.

RESPONSE OF DERMATOLOGISTS (PHYSICIANS)

The medical profession, generally lagged behind in adjusting to these changes, has shown a tendency to withdraw into a shell and play victim. The doctors have, in general, lacked the communication skills, ability to engage, or spend the time and effort needed for educating the community and take on the offenders. It is only of late that the profession has shown a desire to respond to the challenges. It is important for the doctors and the associations to adapt to these changes and come up with strategies.

CONCLUSION

To conclude, the face of dermatology has changed manifold over the past two decades, with an increasing shift toward procedural treatment, quick results, and lesser and lesser clinical practice and old-school consultation. The upsurge of blasphemy by the media, the aggressive intervention by pharmaceutical companies, and other factors has led to a stark increase in violence against doctors and a reduction in patient tolerance.

REFERENCES

1. Branch WT Jr, Collins M, Wintroub BU. Dermatologic practice: Implications for a primary care residency curriculum. J Med Educ. 1983;58(2):136-42.
2. Lowell BA, Froelich CW, Federman DG, et al. Dermatology in primary care: prevalence and patient disposition. J Am Acad Dermatol. 2001;45:250-5.
3. Allen AM. Skin disease in Vietnam, 1965-72. In: Ognibene AJ (Ed). Internal Medicine in Vietnam, Volume 1. Washington, DC: Medical Department US Army, Office of the Surgeon General and Center of Military History; 1977. pp. 2, 29-30, 34-35, 42.
4. Finlay AY, Coles EC. The effect of severe psoriasis on the quality of life of 369 patients. Br J Dermatol. 1995;132(2):236-44.
5. Ramsey DL, Mayer F. National survey of undergraduate medical education. Arch Dermatol. 1985;121(12):1529-30.
6. Whited JD, Hall RP, Simel DL, et al. Primary care clinicians' performance for detecting actinic keratosis and skin cancer. Arch Int Med. 1997;157(9):985-90.
7. Amrendra K, Chouhan K. Challenges in aesthetic dermatology: Quackery and spa dermatology. In: Mysore V (Ed). ACS(I) Textbook of Cutaneous and Aesthetic Surgery, volume 2. New Delhi: Jaypee Brothers Medical Publishers (Pvt) Ltd.; 2017.
8. Kapoor MC. Violence against the medical profession. J Anaesthesiol Clin Pharmacol. 2017;33(2):145-7.

Part A
General Dermatology

CHAPTER 25

Is Dermatology a Safe Subject? Pitfalls and Safeguards during the Practice of General Dermatology

Rakesh Bharti, Ameesha Mahajan, Vipan Bhasin

KEY OBJECTIVES
- To understand how everyday doctor-patient relations can turn into a medicolegal issue.
- Tips to save your own skin from legal bites.

BACKGROUND

Today, the field of dermatology is the most sought-after specialty among medical practitioners due to its extensive scope of treatment, earnings, and self-possessed approach. It has now matured into various specialists and further its subspecialist. In today's world, the mindset of most people is that "than a profession medicine is more of a business than a profession"; whereas, patients mindset is that "they are buyers and we are sellers". These different ways of perception or understanding sometimes lead to law-court, therefore, few practitioner specialists take extra guard and look for safer options of practice. Dermatology in their perception is one such branch. Even those who are dermatologists consider that practice of general dermatology is a safer option compared to other subspecialists of our field. How much of it is the truth and how much is a myth, in this conviction of our brethren, is a matter of introspection and we will try to demystify the same in the following few pages.

Clinical dermatologists treat diseases of young and old, men and women, which may be serious. The ammunition we use is like a double-edged sword. On one edge, our drugs—steroids, antimetabolites, and biologicals all require constant monitoring for their safety, while on the other edge this makes us prone to lawsuits, which were almost unheard of till a few years back. The loud and clear proof in one of the landmark court judgements in which Indian rupee (INR) 110 Million as compensation was offered against a hospital and the reputation of a senior dermatologist was maligned during the treatment of toxic epidermal necrolysis (TEN).

This has become the most "talked about" judgment during medicolegal talks in our country, at least. In the present context, we must equip ourselves with the knowledge of possible pitfalls, as this can prove as a measure against fury of "Jurisprudence" against the clinical dermatologists.

The following few case studies can exemplify the pits in which we can fall and sustain serious injuries. We should try to avoid falling into such pits.

CASE STUDY 1

Mr Sudhir Gupta (name changed) a middle-aged man with a maculopapular rash all over the body went to a senior dermatologist (one of the authors of this chapter) with complaints of severe itching and fever. He also gave history of taking some antibiotics (cephalosporins) prior to coming to him. Initially the dermatologist's first thought was the possibility of a drug rash, however he kept viral exanthem as a second differential. A routine total leukocyte count (TLC), differential leukocyte count (DLC), liver function test (LFT), and urine examination was requested urgently. After the reports, he zeroed down (on the basis of clinical examination and tests) to the diagnosis of viral exanthem. He prescribed antihistamines and a soothing lotion and also advised to see an internal medicine specialist. Next day, he got a frantic call from the attendants of the patients. They informed him that ever since his medication, the condition of patient had deteriorated and he was having difficulty walking and talking and presently in a serious condition. The dermatologist requested them to visit the clinic immediately. Subsequently during physical examination of the patient and discussions, he found that the patient was having hemiplegia.

He reiterated his earlier written command of consulting an internal medicine specialist—an internist.

He told the attendants that he had already warned and advised the patient to consult a medicine physician and the medicine (levocetirizine), he prescribed had nothing to do with his present deterioration.

The attendants took the patient to a medicine specialist who later on informed him that the patient had hemiplegia which may have been due to the viral infection and has already been admitted. The viral infection after admission turned out to be HIV.

The written prescription of consulting an internal medicine specialist became a savior for the dermatologist, or else the attendants were threatening him to law-court.

CASE STUDY 2

Ms Shilpa (name changed), a young girl went to a dermatologist with nodulocystic acne on her face and back. During the discussions, this 2nd year college girl had informed that she had no plans to marry soon and gave her consent to use contraception (even if she gets married) up to minimum of 3 months after stopping isotretinoin, being prescribed for her acne. It was at the ripe moment of writing the prescription that the dermatologist observed some hesitation marks on her wrist. A further probe would unearth a history of an attempt of suicide and it was further revealed that she was on antidepressant medicine for the last 1 year. This is an example, which advises that each dermatologist should always be alert before prescribing drugs, which has an effect on the psyche of the patient, for example, isotretinoin.

CASE STUDY 3

In another case of acne, a young girl was prescribed Minocycline by a dermatologist for her acne. The girl, after a few days, reported yellow-colored urine and itching. She was taken to a physician who told the father of the girl that she has jaundice, which has been caused by the medicine she was taking. On knowing his daughter's condition, the father went to the dermatologist at an odd hour and threatened him to bear the expenses of the treatment as the physician had told him that the cause of jaundice was the medicine prescribed by him for acne. With great difficulty, the dermatologist was able to convince the father and the physician that autoimmune hepatitis can occur with this medicine and it was not his fault.

CASE STUDY 4

Mrs Shanti (name changed), a doctor by profession came as a patient of Dr Bharti with eczema of palms and soles. She was asked to undergo a skin biopsy so as to rule out psoriasis. The histopathology (H/P) examination proved it to be a case of eczema. Dr Bharti prescribed her oral corticosteroids but before she could take the treatment, her husband (an Indian Army Captain) got transferred to another city. She consulted a skin specialist at the place of her husband's posting. The skin specialist made a diagnosis of psoriasis (despite H/P examination proving otherwise) and prescribed Acitretin to her by which she was completely cleared of the disease.

A recurrence after 3 months or so, however, brought her back to Dr Bharti. Once again Dr Bharti prescribed her steroids, but she and her husband were reluctant, as they were planning a pregnancy and scared of steroids. Since she had come after a long gap, on enquiry, she explained about her earlier treatment. Immediately Dr Bharti informed the couple about the wash-out period of Acitretin and suggested them not to conceive till at least 3 years from stopping the medicine. The couple was very upset and approached the doctor who failed to advise them of the complete side effects of the medicine. The whole experience of Dr Shanti, a patient, as expressed to Dr. Bharti in a Whatsapp message, can be an eye-opener for all of us. It went like this:

"Sir, we hear a lot about negligence but being a doctor I faced it as well. I did not have any clue that this medicine was teratogenic for this much period. Usually, Sir I read about the drug before consumption but that time I did not read about it because my problem was flared up and I was not in a state to search about it. Moreover Sir I got that drug from skin department only because in cantonment mostly drugs are being provided by them and there is no need to purchase. I was just told that there was a form which should be filled before starting Acitretin but overall the skin specialist didn't bother to ask the status of my kids and completion of my family or take my consent."

It was a long session of counseling, which restrained her from filing a law-case. She is now waiting for 3-year wash out period to conceive.

CASE STUDY 5

The antifungal medication- Terbinafine, was prescribed by a faculty of a tertiary care hospital in double dose (not USFD approved dose) to another dermatologist suffering from a fungal infection without first enquiring what other medications he was already on. The dermatologist, a patient, was on beta-blockers and it led to severe bradycardia. Timely caution by the patient, a doctor himself prevented a cardiac catastrophe.

CASE STUDY 6

A patient of psoriasis was advised 15 mg Methotrexate, weekly, after baseline complete blood count (CBC) and LFTs. After 1 week, the patient was admitted in emergency with severe oral ulcers, falling blood count, and deteriorating health. During the detail discussions, the patient admitted to taking Methotrexate daily. She was transfused with 28 units of blood and luckily survived.

The case illustrates the importance of explaining the intake of medicines prescribed. The dosage schedule should be well-explained to the patient and written in vernacular language to avoid such situations.

CASE STUDY 7

A reputed dermatologist from Uttar Pradesh was in trouble after one of his old patients on dapsone suddenly succumbed to severe anemia. His arrest warrant was issued. He could wriggle out from the bad scenario, just because he was prescribing regular investigations and that too he was keeping a complete record of the same. Thanks to his alertness and knowledge that he had advised her glucose-6-phosphate dehydrogenase (G6PD) done and was regularly doing CBC. The clear-cut lesson is to keep investigating even chronic long-term patient on drugs like dapsone and keeping a record as well.

CASE STUDY 8

Biologicals: Wonder Drugs?

A patient diagnosed with severe pemphigus vulgaris was prescribed rituximab therapy with the consent of family. The patient's family was extremely hopeful even with the higher cost of therapy. They thought that by providing their son with the best and most expensive treatment option available, he will not only survive but also will have a better quality life ahead. Despite the dermatologist counseling them about the severity of the disease and poor prognosis, they believed that such an expensive drug was sure to do wonders. As fate would have it, the patient developed severe septicemia following the first dose of rituximab and succumbed to it. The patient died, but the dermatologist survived without having a court case, thanks to the transparency by the concerned dermatologist, who kept the family informed throughout the period of his admission after the infection and taking the family into confidence during the course of his deterioration while being in the hospital. No hospital panes were ever broken, no court case filed—just because of good communication skills of the dermatologist. Lesson is that errors can occur but do not run away from the situation. Be transparent and keep the family informed of the true situation.

CASE STUDY 9

A worried couple consulted a number of dermatologists available in their town for white patches that had developed on their 7-year-old girls skin. One of the dermatologists consulted used dermatoscopy and showed them the images on her laptop to rule out vitiligo—the couple's main cause of concern. Treatment on the lines of *pityriasis alba* was initiated. When there was no therapeutic relief in a couple of months, the parents and patient visited another dermatologist. Based on biopsy report, vitiligo was confirmed and treatment initiated. The parents were not very happy due to loss of time before the initiation of correct treatment and filed a case in the district consumer court against the doctor who ruled out vitiligo by dermatoscopy and wasted precious time. Later on, the case was withdrawn after a lot of persuasion and counseling by the second dermatologist consulted (who diagnosed vitiligo).

CASE STUDY 10

A dermatologist was about to remove a small mole of a patient but got quite a scare when the patient developed an adverse reaction to xylocaine given as local anesthesia. After 15–20 minutes, when situation was brought under control, the patient confessed that she had a similar reaction earlier in a dentist's chamber. The doctor could have simply avoided the reaction by asking a simple question "Have you ever been given anesthesia?" This case also demonstrates the need for basic resuscitation facilities in the clinic even if performing minor procedures.

All the above case studies are based on actual facts and situations faced by the authors or their colleagues. This can happen to any practicing dermatologist. To avoid law-court cases in similar circumstances, everyone should know the following facts:

"In the court of law, to accuse a person of negligence, one must establish a connection between the doer and the negligent act. Further to hold that person liable, the damage caused must be the direct result of this negligent act."

- The element of negligence in a doctor-patient relationship can be attributed at various stages such as:
  - History taking
  - Clinical assessment
  - Prescribing investigations which in the opinion of doctor are essential
  - Suggesting names of labs and diagnostic centers
  - Making a diagnosis
  - Guidance in use of ancillary aids, if any, necessary for better and quicker prognosis
  - Instructing the patient on dos and don'ts including postoperative instructions.
- The conspicuous areas, which could fasten liability on a doctor are:
  - Negligence by way of not recording proper history and complaints of the patient
  - Failure to carry out essential investigations
  - Wrong diagnosis
  - Incorrect advice
  - Negligence by way of not cautioning the patient with clarity on what activities the patient could undertake and what should be avoided
  - Negligence in the management of the preoperative procedure
  - Negligence during the surgery, how so ever minor, e.g. biopsy or wart removal
  - Negligence in the management of the postoperative follow-up
  - Introducing untrained, inexperienced, and unreliable staff in the team of the doctor's aides.
- The slight difference between a wrong diagnosis, which may be termed negligence and simple error of judgment, has been recognized by the courts. An honest error of judgment does not make a doctor liable and similarly a well-established known complication of the procedure does not make the doctor liable.

Against the above background, some of the defenses available to the doctor are that the patient:

- Has not revealed his history in entirety and accurately
- Did not give an opportunity to examine the case properly
- Did not cooperate with the doctor in getting investigations done as advised

- Did not take his medication as prescribed
- Had not inadvertently or otherwise disclosed related information necessary for proper diagnosis and treatment of the case
- Did not carry out all the instructions as regards rest, diet, weight bearing, etc.
- Failed to follow-up as advised.

Based on the experiences of the authors from time-to-time during dealing with the patients, we recommend the following steps which will prevent the dermatologists from falling into pits and getting seriously injured in the process!

- It is very important to choose the right dose of the drugs, being careful about comorbidities and coprescribed drugs by others. The list of drugs and situations, which can put the dermatologists in trouble, is long. To quote a few, drugs like cyclophosphamide, azathioprine, cyclosporine, methotrexate need constant monitoring. Before starting any immunosuppressive drug, do consider any pre-existing medical condition like diabetes, hypertension, tuberculosis, etc.
- Always prescribe routine tests at regular intervals when patients are on such drugs, which need monitoring. Instruct and counsel the patient, make a note and write in patient's language regarding this.
- Write about contraception in patient's language, while prescribing teratogenic drugs.
- Prior testing of few investigations such as G6PD, lipid profile, liver, renal, and cardiac functions, Mantoux, etc. is a must while prescribing medicines requiring them as per guidelines. Thiopurine methyltransferase (TPMT) for azathioprine can be considered variably, especially in economic constraint situations but one can get CBC regularly and monitor.
- Always think about drug interactions and always cross-check on apps like drug checker or Medscape or Epocrates.
- Always recommend ophthalmologist check-ups before prescribing drugs like hydroxychloroquine for lupus erythematosus (LE) and other ailments. This can cause permanent damage to retina.
- Avoid giving pulse therapy in OPD, if facilities for monitoring and emergency drugs are not available. Always consider this in IPD.
- First dose of biologics like omalizumab, adalimumab, etc. should also preferably be given in IPD.
- One must confirm from the patient about earlier exposure to xylocaine, even for a wart removal or biopsy procedure. Make sure resuscitation facilities are available in the clinic.
- Dermatoscopy can be used an adjuvant only and cannot stand legally as a confirmatory diagnostic test as it is still developing and not yet standardized. Clinicohistopathological correlation is a must is a must to support dermoscopy.
- Before starting phototherapy or any therapy, consent from the patient should preferably be taken on record.
- If an issue has surfaced due to your prescription then accept it. We all know that complications are inevitable. When things go wrong, do not avoid the patient or distance yourself from potential negative feelings. It is better to acknowledge any patient complaint and express sympathy. One should embrace the situation, express genuine concern, and help the patient through an unfavorable outcome. Do not let the patient feel abandoned. This will make it much easier to overcome the hurdles of the complication and create an environment of trust. Remember that

patients are more likely to initiate litigation over bad feelings than bad outcomes.
- Try to follow the consensus guidelines or the accepted professional practices, when dealing with high-risk cases or high-risk medicines. In case you deviate from them then there should be sufficient justification. Consensus guidelines act as evidence in your favor in the court of law.
- Do not criticize your colleagues or their treatment verbally as well as non-verbally (your gestures sometimes speak louder than your words). This is true every single time and irrespective of the fact that you are in agreement to another doctor's diagnosis/treatment, or not. A lot of times, medicolegal hassles occur because we doctors speak against each other. If your diagnosis or treatment line is different, you should treat to the best of your abilities and not criticize the other doctor.
- It is advisable to have a professional life insurance (PLI), also known as professional indemnity insurance (PII) or as Errors and Omission (E and O). This liability insurance cover protects individuals from professional risks and related legal expenses. It provides indemnity in case a third party sustains injury, harm, death, or damage to property due to the professional service or advice provided by the insured. Some of the leading insurance providers of such policies in our country, are Tata AIG, New India Assurance, HDFC Ergo, Bajaj Allianz, United India Insurance, ICICI Lombard, and National Insurance Company. The scope of each can be compared at www.bankbazaar.com.

Fortunately, our own association, The Indian Association of Dermatologists, Venereologists and Leprologists (IADVL), the largest representing society of Indian Dermatologists also provides one such scheme under the name of DVL welfare trust—details of which are available at www.dvlwelfaretrust.org. Authors strongly recommend readers to opt for this.

We recommend to remember CCD (counseling, communication, and documentation) rules so as to avoid medicolegal hassles:
- *Counseling*: Role of counseling can never be overemphasized. One should ensure involvement of patient in planning his or her treatment. Patient should be informed about pros and cons of treatment offered, in a language, which patient can understand and it should always be recorded.
- *Communication*: It is a key which can open any locked mind. One should never lose one's cool and get irritated about answering patient's queries (howsoever silly and repetitive they may sound). A good communicator can always be successful in all walks of life. We are no exceptions. Addressing patient by name or suitable adjectives is a bridge, which helps in crossing any difficult terrain.
- *Documentation*: Documentation is the single most important step to avoid medicolegal hassles. It can be in form of consent as well as writing important instructions on the prescription itself. Verbal instructions must be written down on the head of the prescription, preferably in patient's language, bold/different ink, or highlighted with a marker.

Further, we are quoting few medicolegal cases where lack of documentation led to compensations granted against doctors and medical negligence was established based on the principle of *res ipsa loquitur* which termed as:

In medical negligence cases, res ipsa loquitur can be invoked only when: (1) the patient suffers an injury that is not an expected complication of medical care; (2) the injury does not normally occur unless someone has been negligent; and (3) the defendant was responsible for the patient's well-being at the time of the injury. For example, assume that a portable X-ray is ordered in an intensive care unit on a young, otherwise healthy patient recovering from peritonitis. After the technician leaves, it is found that the patient has a dislocated shoulder. This is not an expected complication of an X-ray; there are no explanations for the injury other than mishandling or failing to restrain the patient properly, and the defendant was responsible for the patient's well-being at the time the injury occurred.

- In the case of Dr Shyam Kumar versus Rameshbhai Harmanbhai Kachhiya, I (2006) CPJ 16 (NC) the National Commission held that an operation was conducted for glaucoma and cataract but the retina was weakened and eye sight was lost, it was held that conducting the operation without obtaining informed consent was improper. A patient cannot be deprived of this information. Not even medical records were produced; hence, the patient was entitled to claim compensation.
- In the case of Meenakshi Mission Hospital and Research Centre versus Samuraj and Anr., I (2005) CPJ 33 (NC), the National Commission held the hospital guilty of negligence on the grounds that the name of the anesthetist was not mentioned in the operation notes though anesthesia was administered by two anesthetists' at 10 am and 10.30 am. The child was pulseless and the doctor who administered anesthesia was not produced before the Commission. Two progress cards about the same patient on two separate papers were produced. What the two anesthetists were doing inside the OT was not explained. The hospital is accountable for whatever happens in the hospital and was held liable to pay the compensation and cost. It is relevant to note that in this case the District Forum found the hospital negligent and awarded a compensation of ₹ 300,000 and cost of ₹ 2000. Thereafter, the State Commission had dismissed the appeal with a cost of ₹ 500.

CONCLUSION

Clinical dermatology is neither immune nor safer than any other branch of medicine as far as law-courts are concerned. To avoid this, we must be balanced in our approach to our patients. It is not a good idea to be a good doctor and not to be a good human being. Better to be a good human being and a doctor, only then you are safe and true to your patient during practicing general dermatology.

CHAPTER 26

Consent for Drug Administration: It is Necessary?

Kiran Godse, Anant Patil

INTRODUCTION

According to the Indian constitution, every person has different rights including right to autonomy, self-determination, and right to live with dignity.[1] Under this context, a patient can refuse treatment, even if it is important for his health, hence obtaining consent is one of the important and critical issues in routine clinical practice as well as clinical research from the point of view of medical ethics and human rights.

Consent to treatment indicates permission given by the patient before he/she receives any type of treatment or undergoes any investigation or examination.[2]

Obtaining consent before providing treatment to the patient is a legal and professional obligation for the healthcare provider. Consent helps to respect patient's autonomy for the treatment decision.[3] Obtaining consent before treatment also helps to provide protection to the medical practitioner in terms of legal implications.

Therefore, doctor should obtain consent for all types of treatments including:[3]
- Therapeutic care
- Preventive care
- Palliative care
- Diagnostic procedures
- Cosmetic treatment, or
- Other health-related procedure.

VALID CONSENT

Consent is considered valid, if it is:[2]
- Voluntary,
- Informed, and
- The person giving consent has a capacity to make the decision.

The components of the informed consent are shown in Figure 1.[4]

Types of Informed Consents

An important question doctors often have is that should the consent always be documented in writing on a mandatory basis. In order to understand this, one needs to know different types of consents.

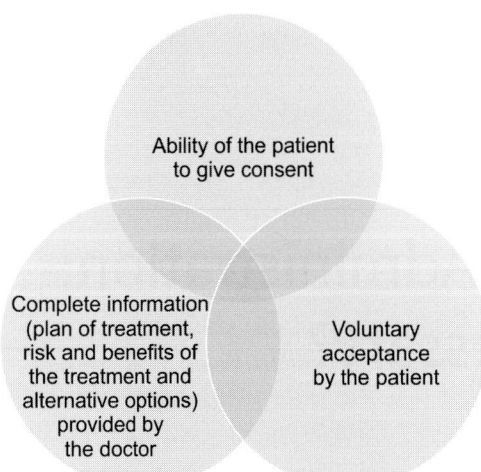

Fig. 1: Components of the informed consent.

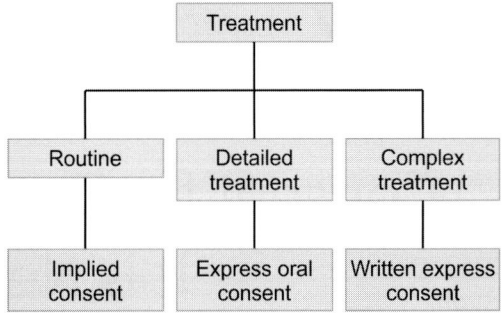

The consent for treatment can be expressed or implied.[1] In an express consent, the terms are stated or described in distinct and explicit language;[5] hence, it is also known as explicit consent. Implied consents is also known as implicit consent.[3]

Implied Consent

The consent is called as "implied" based on the conduct of the patient. Following are the examples of implied consent:
- Taking an appointment of doctor[5]
- Patient coming to a doctor for consultation on his/her own[1]
- Subject himself to the physical examination[5]
- Patient holding arm for blood test implies that he/she is agreeable for the treatment.[2]

If physician is relying on implied consent, it is important to note that other person should be able to interpret the actions of patients as implied for the action taken by the physician.[6]

Types of Express/Explicit Consent

Expressed consent can be either oral or written.

- *Oral consent*: For specific intimate examination (e.g. vaginal examination), in addition to implied consent, doctor should ideally take another consent (e.g. oral consent).[1]
- *Written consent*: For invasive examination, such as an incision or collection of samples of body fluids, a written consent is ideally needed.[1]

In day-to-day clinical practice for routine treatment, implied consent may be sufficient. For detailed treatment, one has to ideally take express oral consent. For complex treatment, written express consent is needed (Flowchart 1).[1] Written consent from the patient is required before performing an operative procedure.

If the patient can give consent, he/she should give it. In case of children, consent from parent is required. It is not necessary that during routine clinical practice, doctor should always obtain written consent from the patient. However, if obtained, it greatly helps in case of litigation.

Where consent is not necessary?
In some instances, consent is not necessary.
- Treatment in an emergency (e.g. treatment to save life of an unconscious patient).
- While performing a surgery, if an additional emergency procedure is required.

In both the cases, doctor should explain the reason for treatment/procedure to the patient after he/she is recovered and surgery is performed respectively.

- Severe mental disorder resulting in inability to give consent for the treatment
- Patient posing risk to the public health because of transmission of infections such as rabies, cholera, or tuberculosis.[2]

SUMMARY

- Physicians must ensure that they obtain consent from the patient before any treatment or examination.
- The risk to the patient and potential for pain and discomfort to the patient should be considered for deciding the type of consent needed.
- The consent should be voluntary, informed, and given by the patient who has capacity to give it.
- For routine treatment, implied consent may be sufficient.

REFERENCES

1. Nandimath OV. Consent and medical treatment: The legal paradigm in India. Indian J Urol. 2009;25(3):343-7.
2. NHS (2016). Consent to treatment. [online] Available from: https://www.nhs.uk/conditions/consent-to-treatment/. [Accessed December, 2018].
3. College of Physicians and Surgeons of Ontario (2015). Consent to treatment. Policy Statement #3-15. Issue 2, 2015. [online] Available from: http://www.cpso.on.ca/CPSO/media/documents/Policies/Policy-Items/Consent-To-Treatment.pdf?ext=.pdf. [Accessed December, 2018].
4. Bhute A. Informed consent in obstetrics and gynecology: Indian Scenario. Int J Recent Surg Med Sci. 2017;3(1):67-71.
5. Aggarwal KK. Real consent and not informed consent applicable in India. Indian J Clin Pract. 2014;25:392-3.
6. College of Physicians and Surgeons of Nova Soctia (2016). Professional standard and guidelines regarding informed patient consent to treatment. Available from: https://cpsns.ns.ca/wp-content/uploads/2017/10/Informed-Patient-Consent-to-Treatment.pdf. [Accessed December, 2018].

CHAPTER 27

Investigations and Law

Satyanarayana Rao KH

INTRODUCTION

Doctors are often blamed for advising unnecessary investigations. On the other hand, doctors are worried that in case of litigation, they may face the charge of being negligent in not advising all necessary tests. So, they may resort to what is referred to as "defensive medicine" to varying degrees.[1,2] Among other things such a practice involves ordering unnecessary tests, which increase the cost to the patient and puts a strain on the scarce resources in case of public hospitals. Therefore, it is important to understand the balance between what is essential investigation and what may be perceived later as over or under investigation.

LEGAL LIABILITIES

- In cases of alleged medical negligence, legal forums may adjudicate, with or without expert opinion, whether standard care has been provided or whether there has been negligence in not investigating properly or not repeating investigations when indicated:
    - To arrive at a diagnosis
    - To plan and administer treatment
    - To look for side-effects of drugs during treatment
    - To pick up post-procedure complications, if any, as and when they appear.
- A doctor can be held guilty of professional misconduct, if he/she:
    - Refers patients to a particular laboratory/imaging center and gets referral commission[3]
    - Fails to provide reports of investigations to facilitate follow-up by a different doctor.

When to investigate?
The decision to order a test must be solely based on its utility for diagnosis, management, early identification of postoperative complications or better outcome.[4] Some tests may have to be repeated during the course of treatment to

rule out side-effects of drugs, to assess progress or revise diagnosis in case there is less than expected or no improvement.

Cosmetic/plastic surgeons should refrain from ordering a battery of tests to all patients as a part of preoperative assessment. If it is being practiced as an institutional policy, anesthesiologist's requirement, medicolegal concerns, general trend, or lack of guidelines, it needs to be changed. Several studies, especially in case of clinically healthy individuals undergoing ambulatory surgery, have shown that such a strategy is of little or no benefit in deciding to go ahead with the procedure or in predicting postoperative complications.[5-8] Avoiding unnecessary investigations will reduce the cost to the patient without compromising patient's welfare.

How much to investigate?
In deciding the tests to be done, several factors need to be considered—age, sex, past medical history, condition to be treated, comorbidity, treatment/procedure planned, etc. For example, electrocardiography (ECG) and chest X-ray may be needed in case of comorbid cardiopulmonary disease. Coagulation profile may be indicated in case of invasive procedures and in patients with bleeding diathesis. Liver function tests and renal function tests are in order while hepatotoxic or renotoxic drugs are to be administered. Pregnancy test is mandatory in case of treatment with drugs like isotretinoin, thalidomide, etc.

What tests to do will have to be decided on a case-to-case basis and nothing can be labeled as "routine" preoperative investigations.

CONSENT FOR INVESTIGATION

For routine blood tests, patient's willingness to give blood sample may be taken as implied consent. But for HIV test, pretest counseling and expressed written consent are mandatory. There may be situations when patients refuse to undergo tests, which are medically indicated. For example, biopsy to rule out leprosy, lupus vulgaris, basal cell carcinoma, malignant melanoma, repeat biopsy to rule out malignant transformation in a premalignant condition, etc. Such patients have to be counseled with care, so that they understand the risks involved in not undergoing the tests and document it in the form of "Informed Refusal" to undergo investigations.

DISCLOSURE OF REPORTS OF INVESTIGATION

Patients have the right to get the reports of all investigations that they undergo. The reports form a part of the patient's medical record and hence confidentiality has to be maintained.[9] Disclosure of test reports to other healthcare providers must be on "need to know" basis. Unauthorized disclosure of sensitive test reports like HIV positivity can lead to legal liability for breach of confidentiality.[10]

Reports of investigations done in the past cannot be denied to the patient, if he/she decides to go to another doctor for second opinion/follow-up/further treatment.

DERMATOLOGIST AS A DERMATOPATHOLOGIST

Dermatologists study dermatopathology during their Post-Graduation and spend considerable but variable number of hours in learning dermatopathology. It is part of theory examination and slide interpretation is part of Postgraduate practical examination. Several dermatologists take active interest in learning and also interpreting biopsy slides. Most dermatopathology books have been written by clinical dermatologists with knowledge of dermatopathology. Several dermatologists have undergone certificate programs, fellowships, and have even acquired qualification, and regularly report on biopsy specimens.

A question has often been asked whether dermatologists can report and interpret slides. The following can be stated:
- Reporting on biopsy specimens sent by other dermatologists would need significant training/qualification in the field. However, there are no prescribed guidelines to define such qualification or experience.
- However, if a dermatologist chooses to interpret his own biopsy slide in view of the clinical picture and the dermatopathology report, that would be acceptable.

CONCLUSION

Legal liability risk of under investigation can be taken care by ordering investigations, which are essential for diagnosis and management after careful history taking and clinical examination. But patient's benefit should be kept in mind at all times. Cosmetic/plastic surgeons in collaboration with anesthesiologists should tailor the preoperative investigations on case-to-case basis rather than ordering a battery of so-called "routine" tests. Confidentiality of reports of investigations should be ensured.

REFERENCES

1. O'Dowd A. Doctors increasingly practise "defensive" medicine for fear of litigation, says regulator. BMJ. 2015;350:h87.
2. Silberstein E, Shir-Az O, Reuveni H, et al. Defensive medicine among plastic and aesthetic surgeons in Israel. Aesthet Surg J. 2016;36(10):NP299-304.
3. Indian Medical Council. (2002). Indian Medical Council (Professional Conduct, Etiquette and Ethics) Regulations, 2002, published in Gazette of India, No.14, Part III, Section 4 dated 6.4.2002. [online] Available from https://www.mciindia.org/documents/rulesAndRegulations/Ethics%20Regulations-2002.pdf. [Accessed December, 2018].
4. Fischer JP, Shang EK, Nelson JA, et al. Patterns of preoperative laboratory testing in patients undergoing outpatient plastic surgery procedures. Aesthet Surg J. 2014;34(1):133-41.
5. Brown SR, Brown J. Why do physicians order unnecessary preoperative tests? A qualitative study. Fam Med. 2011;43(5):338-43.
6. National Institute for Health and Care Excellence Guideline. (2016). Routine preoperative tests for elective surgery. [online] Available from https://www.nice.org.uk/guidance/ng45. [Accessed December, 2018].
7. Benarroch-Gampel J, Sheffield KM, Duncan CB, et al. Preoperative laboratory testing in patients undergoing elective, low-risk ambulatory surgery. Ann Surg. 2012;256(3):518-28.
8. Nicholas N. Confidentiality, disclosure and access to medical records. Obstet Gynaecol. 2007;9(4):257-63.
9. Rao K. (2008). Safer practice of dermatosurgery. [online] Available from http://www.ijdvl.com/text.asp?2008/74/7/75/42298. [Accessed December, 2018].
10. Trehan SP, Sankhari D. Medical Professional, Patient and the Law: the Institute of Law and Ethics in Medicine, 2nd edition. Bangalore: National Law School of India University; 2002. pp. 57-68.

CHAPTER 28

Medicolegal Issues in Cutaneous Adverse Drug Reactions

Lalit Kumar Gupta, Vaishali Masatkar

KEY OBJECTIVES

- Ensuring drug safety is of paramount importance to every clinician. Owing to the perceived benign nature of skin diseases, the distress resulting from side effects of medication is relatively less expected and accepted by the patients with dermatologic diseases.
- It is important to keep in mind that all drugs, even those taken safely in the past, may have serious side effects that can prove dangerous in certain patients.
- Cutaneous adverse drug reactions (CADR) or drug allergies are common in clinical practice. Most of them are benign and seldom require aggressive treatment. Drug withdrawal and supportive treatment are usually sufficient to alleviate the symptoms and patients do not resort to legal action in most cases.
- Medication error is the most common preventable cause of CADR. The ordering or administration of the wrong drug, at the wrong dosage, via the wrong route, or to the wrong patient are errors and hence constitute negligence for which there is no justification and defense.
- Proper counseling, disclosure, and documentation are the pillars in reducing the risk of lawsuit as well as in dealing with them.
- Awareness of high-risk situations, high-risk drugs, banned drugs, off-label drugs, drug interactions, and a detailed enquiry about past history of drug allergy cannot be understated.
- A healthy, respectful, and honest relationship with patient goes a long way in reducing the likelihood of being sued if something goes wrong.

INTRODUCTION

The safety of patient is of prime importance and every clinician has an obligation to fulfill the Hippocratic admonition—"first of all be sure that you do no harm" (*primum non nocere*). Fact, however, remains that despite executing extreme caution, a physician may encounter adverse drug reactions (ADRs) and "to err is human" is rarely an excuse when it comes to treating patients. ADRs may be considered as an inevitable price we pay for the benefits of modern drug therapy. The World Health Organization has defined an ADR as "an appreciably harmful or unpleasant reaction, resulting from an intervention related to the use of a medicinal product, which predicts hazard from future administration and warrants prevention or specific treatment, or alteration of the dosage regimen, or withdrawal of the product".[1] CADRs are common, milder, and self-limiting ones are more common in comparison to severe and the mere occurrence of an ADR does not implicate a doctor for medical negligence. However, failure to diagnose the drug reaction and manage them appropriately in time can lead to a liability for medical negligence. Counseling of the patient forms an important step in dealing with a case of drug reaction.

CURRENT SCENARIO

Dermatologists globally enjoy lower malpractice rates in comparison to many other specialties.[2] However, there is a rising trend in medical litigations over recent years with the advent of cosmetic procedures, biologics, and targeted therapies. The most important sources of legal liability risks for dermatologists include:[3]
- Failure to obtain the patient's valid consent before engaging in a medical intervention
- Misdiagnosis or delayed diagnosis
- Improper performance of operative procedures on the skin
- Errors in pathology specimen processing
- Failure to obtain consultation or refer the patient to another physician even when it is indicated, and
- Failure to timely communicate to patients the results of biopsies and other tests.

The premiums paid by dermatologists have also trended upwards in past years. According to the Physicians' Insurers Association of America (PIAA) data from 1985 to 2001, the most prevalent "medical misadventure" was operative procedure on the skin (289 claims), followed by malignant neoplasms (93 claims) and malignant melanoma (77 claims).[4] Interestingly, ADR to oral medication contributed to only two claims (<1%). Likewise, a record analysis of 5–30 years in 10 Canadian provinces reported that seven dermatologists and five other specialists faced lawsuits relating to dermatology, of which two were due to drug rash.[5] A reputed Indian newspaper reported that three out of 10 doctors are facing a medicolegal issue each year and this is on the rise. The maximum number of cases occurs against gynecologists and surgeons followed by orthopedics and dermatologists.

Saha's case (discussed later) is a frequent and a potent reminder to dermatologists of the cautious use of steroids, following proper guidelines, the compensation, and reputation at stake.

One of the undesirable consequences of medical malpractice claims is *defensive medicine*, which can be defined as the modification of clinical practice solely to reduce exposure to legal challenges by patients rather than for direct clinical reasons.[6] There is also a risk of focus shifting from what is customary to do to what ought to be done and resulting in a slaving adherence to clinical guidelines.[7]

Nonetheless, the factor that predominantly decides whether a patient will resort to litigation is a prior poor relationship with the clinician and the feeling that the patient is not being kept informed. Thus developing a good rapport with the patients and involving them in decision-making is very helpful in preventing such mishaps.

What constitutes negligence in relation to ADRs?

Does the mere occurrence of a CADR implicate the doctor for professional negligence?[8] The answer to this question is certainly "No". There are certain drugs that are relatively safer and others that involve a greater amount of risk of adverse reactions, but the fact is that any drug can cause any rash and it is not always possible to predict the adverse reaction in a given patient. Therefore, simply because a CADR has occurred by itself will not indicate negligence on the part of the treating doctor. The factors, which play a role in constituting medical negligence, are described below:

- *Medication error*: Medication error is the most common and preventable cause of medical injury.[9] It is defined as an error in ordering, transcribing, dispensing, or administering a drug or medicine.[10] A medication error may or may not cause injury. *The components of medication error are*:[11]
  - Wrong drug or dose
  - Wrong route of administration
  - Administered to the wrong patient or at the wrong time
  - Decline in hepatic or renal function requiring dosage modification
  - Ignorance of previous history of drug allergy to same medication class or with drugs having cross-reaction potential
  - Using the wrong drug name, dosage form, inappropriate abbreviation, and incorrect dosage calculations
  - Ignorance of potential drug interactions.

  It is estimated that there are 5.3 medication errors/100 prescriptions. These include missing dose (53%), dose errors (15%), frequency errors (8%), and route errors (5%), but only 1% of them were associated with adverse drug events (ADEs).[12]

- *Failure to diagnose CADR timely and appropriately*: The clinical spectrum of drug reactions is very wide and ADRs can practically mimic any inflammatory dermatosis. The most common presentation of CADR is in the form of urticaria and maculopapular rash, which are benign in nature and seldom requires aggressive therapy, but the possibility that these benign-appearing rash may be the forerunner of a more serious reaction and hence get converted into a serious reaction should always be kept in mind. For instance, toxic epidermal necrolysis (TEN), erythroderma, and drug hypersensitivity syndrome (DHS) may initially begin as maculopapular rash before turning in to a more ominous rash. The failure to diagnose these reactions and delay in management can constitute negligence on doctor's part.

  Ochronosis due to hydroquinone, hyperpigmentation due to minocycline, steroid facies due to long term use of topical steroids, and lichenoid rash due to antihypertensive drugs are some of the examples of ADRs due to chronic use of drugs. Inability to diagnose these conditions, failure to stop the causative agent, and institute appropriate treatment can amount to medical negligence.

- *Failure to recognize and treat accurately and promptly*: It is the responsibility of a clinician to make the correct diagnosis, administer the right treatment, and to relieve the patient of his illness. Reaching a definitive diagnosis is sometimes not possible on clinical examination alone and a series of investigations are required. It is important to keep in mind that drugs like steroids, other immunosuppressive agents and biologics should not be used lightly and recklessly till it is certain that the drug will do more benefit than harm. A written consent may be obtained for the drugs in the "orphan drug" category when there is no sufficient evidence to use the drug in that particular indication.

For the drugs that are approved or fall under the "off-label" category for which enough literature is available in the standard journals and textbooks, a written consent may not be necessary. The risk and benefits of the potentially toxic drugs should be discussed with the patients/attendants and documented in writing in their medical records. This becomes even more important when prescribing costly drugs like biological agents, off-label, or orphan drugs. Not following the recommended dose, the tapering schedule and management guidelines can account to medical negligence. For example, corticosteroid is a double-edged sword; if used promptly in appropriate doses and tapered fast in Stevens-Johnson syndrome (SJS)-TEN, it is life-saving; failure to do so, however, can have fatal consequences. Saha's case is the prototype example of such negligence. Similarly, female patients in reproductive age should be asked to avoid pregnancy by using double contraceptive methods and this should be instructed in writing in their records. Likewise in patients on immunosuppressive agents, a clear instruction about baseline and repeat blood counts, liver or renal function tests and other relevant tests should be provided in writing and properly documented.

- *Unauthorized practice*: The Supreme Court of India has held that a person qualified in one system of medicine cannot practice another system of medicine. This amounts to medical negligence per se (without any further proof of negligence), i.e. "*res ipsa loquitur*" which in Latin means "the thing speaks for itself". In India, the encroachment in the field of dermatology and cosmetology is rampant with nonallopathic practitioners and other specialty allopathic practitioners prescribing for skin diseases, performing aesthetic procedures and hair transplantation. There are many such cases where specialists of other fields (ophthalmologist, pediatrician, etc.) have been held responsible for medical negligence because of improper treatment and insufficient care to patients of SJS-TEN. One such case is discussed below. IADVL (Indian Association of Dermatology, Venereology and Leprosy) Task Force against Quackery (ITAQ) is dedicated to curb the menace of quackery in dermatology.

PREVENTIVE MEASURES

Prevention is better than cure and dermatologists must save their as well as patients skin. The measures which are useful in avoiding medicolegal issues can be alphabetically classified into anticipatory approach, baseline evaluation, counseling, documentation, evidence-based approach, futuristic approach, guidelines, high-risk management, interactions, insurance, judgment, knowledge, learner's approach, and management[13] (Table 1).

MANAGING A LAWSUIT

Facing a malpractice lawsuit can be a daunting and traumatic experience for healthcare practitioners, with most clinicians naive to the legal landscape. The general Dos and Don'ts after receipt of a legal claim, during the deposition, and during the trial phases are listed in Table 4.[24]

In context with medicolegal issues related to CADR, the following specific points should be kept in mind:
- To be thorough with the drug class, its pharmacodynamics and pharmacokinetics,

TABLE 1: Ways to prevent the risk of lawsuit associated with cutaneous adverse drug reaction (CADR).	
Anticipatory approach	A proactive approach and all-time preparedness toward development of CADR to any drug.
Baseline evaluation	• Detailed interrogation about the intake of drug, both prescriptional as well as nonprescriptional, previous episode(s) of reaction to drug(s) in patient as well as family members, and presence of comorbid conditions. • Relevant baseline investigations should be undertaken before commencing therapy (e.g. G6PD for dapsone, chest X-ray, and Mantoux for TNF-α inhibitors). • Testing for drug sensitivity should be carried out "every time" before drug administration such as penicillin and local anesthetic agents).
Counseling	• Establish a "therapeutic relationship" with patient • Patient should be provided very clear and unambiguous written instructions regarding dose, frequency, and duration of medications by the treating clinician or his support staff/pharmacist. In India, by convention, the doctor has to do the job of counseling, unlike in West where pharmacist is responsible for explaining the side effects of medications. • Ensure adherence and compliance • Instruct clearly regarding strict avoidance of pregnancy during use of teratogenic, mutagenic, or high-risk drugs (e.g. retinoids or cytotoxic drugs) • Inform the patient about the warning signs of drug reaction and common adverse effect of drugs (e.g. drowsiness with antihistamines and avoidance of driving or operating dangerous machines) • Instruct the patient in writing to report immediately in case of any unexpected event • Discourage telephonic consultations.
Documentation	• Episode of drug reaction should be documented clearly and legibly in the medical records • Electronic prescribing and use of information technology systems[14-16] • Baseline and serial photographic documentation • Reporting to the related drug regulatory authorities.
Evidence-based approach	• Integrating one's clinical expertise with the best external evidence from systemic research[17] • Use of unconventional and "off-label" medications should be avoided and the references be kept ready. • Simple and topical treatment should be tried first before resorting to potentially risky and systemic therapy in recalcitrant cases.
Futuristic approach	• Remain updated with the recently introduced medications and their potential toxicities • Details of banned drugs must be known and their use should be avoided • Patient should be provided with ADR card for future use.

Guidelines	• Remain updated with the latest guidelines on treatment of disease as well as drug reactions. Some of the useful guidelines on the subject include:
	  – British Society for Allergy and Clinical Immunology (BSACI) guidelines (2008) for the management of drug allergy[18]
	  – The UK guidelines (2016) for the management of SJS/TEN[19]
	  – The Indian guidelines (2016) for the management of SJS/TEN,[20] and
	  – The top 100 drug interactions 2016 guideline.[21]

Contd...

Contd...

High-risk assessment	• Probability of developing reaction to drug(s) differs in an individual depending on several factors such as age, gender, nature of the drug, concomitant medications, genetic susceptibility of a person, and comorbid conditions. • It is important to be aware of black-box warning and list of banned drugs • High-risk drugs and high-risk situations are listed in Table 2.
Interaction	• Thorough knowledge about interactive potential of drug-drug, drug-food, and drug-herbs can help to prevent the complications resulting from coadministration of drugs. • Drug interactions usually follow 80/20 rule, i.e. 80% interactions result from 20% drugs.[22] It is very helpful to be aware of this fact. • Common drug interactions, which are relevant in dermatology, are mentioned in Table 3.
Insurance/professional indemnity	• Obtain suitable malpractice insurance and get acquainted with the terms of your insurance policy, which ideally contains a "consent to settle" clause. • If there is impending/possible legal "trouble", promptly contact the insurer, who will connect you with legal counsel.
Judgment	• Whether the rash is due to the administered drug or exacerbation of primary disease or appearance of a new dermatosis is very important, though difficult. • Recognize the warning signs (Box 1). • Whether the ongoing treatment needs to be "carried through" or "abruptly stopped" is very relevant. • In situations that require disruption of therapy, a decision on which drug to stop and which alternative substitute to use is very important.
Knowledge	• Maintain your medical license. • Keep up with the latest advances in disease management, newer drugs, their interactions and side effect profile. • Subscribe to medical journals or related publications.
Learner's approach	• Consult the current literature, database, and other resources in the field of ADRs and remain constantly updated.
Management	• *Avoidance*: Use of precipitating drugs (e.g. NSAIDs and ACE inhibitors in urticaria/angioedema), drugs having cross-reaction potential, strong drug interactions. • *Supplementation*: For example, folic acid with methotrexate and calcium, vitamin D3 and bisphosphonates with prolonged use of corticosteroids. • Avoiding rapid infusion of drugs may help to reduce chances of complications of therapy, e.g. "red man syndrome" due to vancomycin. • *Temporary cessation*: Stopping aspirin or anticoagulant therapy before dermatosurgical procedure may reduce the risk of bleeding during and after the procedure. • Observation and carry through approach for benign CADR. • Hospitalization, supportive, and specific treatment for serious cutaneous adverse reactions (SCAR). • Drug challenge to be carried out as per protocol where indicated. • A clear written instruction in the form of card mentioning the details of suspected drug(s) should be issued to the patient. The patients are instructed to always carry this card and show it to the treating physicians every time.

(ACE: angiotensin-converting enzyme; ADR: adverse drug reaction; G6PD: glucose-6-phosphate dehydrogenase; NSAID: nonsteroidal anti-inflammatory drug; SJS: Stevens-Johnson syndrome; TEN: toxic epidermal necrolysis; TNF: tumor necrosis factor)

TABLE 2: High-risk drugs and high-risk situations for adverse drug reaction (ADRs).[23]

High-risk drugs	High-risk situations
• Nonsteroidal anti-inflammatory drugs (NSAIDs) • Sulfonamides • Antibiotics • Antiretroviral drugs • Antitubercular drugs • Antiepileptics • Allopurinol • Antihypertensives • Antimalarial drugs	• Previous reaction(s) • Elderly • Polypharmacy • Immunosuppression (100 times risk with sulfa drugs in AIDS patients) • Collagen vascular diseases (Sjögren's syndrome, rheumatoid arthritis, SLE, etc.) • Genetic predisposition (certain HLA associations) • Renal impairment • Hepatic impairment

(AIDS: acquired immunodeficiency syndrome; HLA: human leukocyte antigen; SLE: systemic lupus erythematosus)

TABLE 3: Common drug interactions relevant in dermatology.

Drugs	Interaction	Important remarks
Methotrexate with NSAIDs	Increased risk of renal toxicity	—
Methotrexate with sulfa drugs	Increased risk of hematological toxicity	—
Methotrexate with oral retinoids	Increased risk of hepatotoxicity	—
Azathioprine with allopurinol	Increased hematological toxicity of azathioprine	Febuxostat can be used safely with azathioprine
Itraconazole with lovastatin or simvastatin	Rhabdomyolysis	Rosuvastatin and fluvastatin may be used safely
Cyclosporine and ketoconazole	Enhanced CsA toxicity	—
Oral contraceptive pills (OCPs) with rifampicin or broad-spectrum antibiotics	Failure of OCPs	—

(CsA: cyclosporine A; NSAIDs: nonsteroidal anti-inflammatory drugs)

BOX 1: Warning signs of serious adverse drug reactions (ADRs).

- *Mucocutaneous*: Skin tenderness, centrofacial erythema and edema, atypical target lesions, purpura, bullae, and widespread erosions
- *Systemic*: Anxiety, malaise, fever, lymphadenopathy, arthralgia/arthritis, jaundice
- *Laboratory*: Cytopenias, eosinophilia, impaired liver, and renal function.

uses, adverse effects, contraindications, and interactions of the implicated drug.

- To have in-depth knowledge of the type of CADR, drugs commonly implicated, incidence, and management.
- Literature documenting the association of drug and CADR should be kept ready.
- Patient's medical records with details of previous drug reactions/allergies, comorbidities, specific indications, clinical details of the primary disease and the reaction, treatment given (name of drug, dosage, route, etc.), warnings and protection

TABLE 4: The general Do's and Don'ts when dealing with a lawsuit.	
What to Do's	*What not to Don'ts*
• Contact your lawyer immediately after receiving a summon or any legal document • Locate the patient's file and documents and keep them in a secure place • Spend time with the attorney teaching them about medical facts and also preparing for anticipated cross-examination question • Consider settlement if responsible for an unfortunate medical outcome and if the legal process will cause significant emotional and psychological burden • Give clear, concise, direct answers without medical jargon, if possible	• Do not alter the documents, it is illegal and will be held against treating clinician • Do not confront the patient or attendants directly, do not give explanation or admit fault • Avoid playing blame game • When in court, avoid giving details, which are not directly related to the question • Do not answer "compounded" questions that have two or more questions in one or queries with double negatives

advised, investigations advised with reports should be maintained and securely kept ready for evidence.

- Relevant guidelines on the management of disease and reaction in support of the protocol followed.

Recently several new drugs have become available such as biological which are expensive and which may also have serious side effects such as biological. Likewise, some drugs may have serious side effects such as immunosuppressives in pemphigus, isotretinoin in a young lady, finasteride for young men. Some drugs are used for off-label indications, e.g. azathioprine for lichen planus/vitiligo. In these instances, while there is no law to state that written consent is necessary, it will be helpful to record that side effects have been discussed either on patient's prescription or a separate paper.

CASE EXAMPLES AND LEARNING ESSENTIALS

Case 1: Medication Error—The 11 Crore Compensation Saga: Anuradha Saha's Case[25]

A wife of a doctor settled in the United States came to India on a holiday. She developed some skin rashes for which she presented to a doctor who diagnosed her ailment as "vasculitis". As the condition of the patient continued to worsen, she was hospitalized to a tertiary care center. She was diagnosed to be having TEN. However, the cause of TEN could not be ascertained. When the condition further deteriorated, the patient was flown to Mumbai. The patient later died of septicemia. The husband filed a complaint before the National Consumer Disputes Redressal Commission claiming compensation for the negligence on the part of the doctors in the medical management. The National Commission dismissed the complaint. The husband challenged its decision before the Supreme Court.

The Supreme Court verdict revealed that the deceased patient was prescribed tablet prednisolone in the dose of 120 mg/day for 7 days and injection Depo-Medrol intramuscular twice a day for 3 days prior to commencement of prednisolone. Depo-Medrol is a depot preparation and is not administered twice daily as per the opinion of the experts. The Supreme Court held the doctor negligent for prescribing a long-acting steroid and an excessive dose of corticosteroid without foreseeing its implication. The medical literature was filed before the Supreme Court, which noted two schools of thoughts pertaining to the use of corticosteroids in TEN. It also noted that the pro-steroid group recommended the use of corticosteroids in the *initial stage of the disease only* as there is a higher risk of side effects of corticosteroids with continued use. As per the medical records, appropriate lifesaving supportive care was not administered and the nursing care was abysmal. The medical records were also not maintained properly.[26]

Learning Essential

This case highlights the importance of drug prescription by duly qualified doctor as per accepted professional norms and that the doctor would be held responsible, if there is failure of duty of care toward a patient. Steroids and other immunosuppressive agents should be used cautiously, after performing necessary baseline investigations, under careful monitoring and as per standard protocols.

Case 2: Unauthorized Practice, Failure to Diagnose Accurately and Promptly[25]

In a case decided by the National Consumer Disputes Redressal Commission (referred to as National Commission in short), a boy of about 8 years with fever, cough, and cold presented to a general physician who prescribed him a sulfonamide along with antihistaminic and antipyretic. The child developed swelling of the lips and blisters in the mouth and over different parts of the skin. A diagnosis of measles was made. Later, a referral was made to a pediatrician who concurred with the opinion of the general physician that the child was suffering from measles. As there was no improvement in the condition of the child, he was advised to be hospitalized. Nearly 36 hours following the hospitalization and further deterioration, a referral was made to an ear, nose, and throat (ENT) surgeon who made the diagnosis of SJS. A dermatologist was then called in for the management of SJS. There was permanent damage to the eyes leading to severe impairment of vision and inability to even keep eyes open.

A complaint was filed before the State Consumer Disputes Redressal Commission claiming a compensation of ₹ 9.95 Lacs. The State Commission held the pediatrician liable for medical negligence and awarded compensation in favor of the complainant. An appeal was filed before the National Commission. The National Commission after perusal of the medical records and the medical literature arrived to a conclusion of negligence on the part of the general physician, the ophthalmologist, and the hospital and awarded a compensation of ₹ 5 lacs along with interest. In this case, the dermatologist and the ENT surgeon were not made party to the complaint. In fact, they had made the diagnosis in time and appropriate therapy had been commenced.

Learning Essential

The above case law highlights the importance of making a referral to a specialist in time. Failure to diagnose a CADR may not be a negligent act but failure to refer to a specialist in time may result in a finding of negligence. TEN and SJS require a multidisciplinary management strategy and therefore referral to ophthalmologist and dermatologist would be essential. Management in an intensive care setting would be also required.

Case 3: Liability of Pharmaceutical Manufacturer

A patient suffering from rheumatoid arthritis was prescribed indomethacin and he developed SJS and died. The state commission observed that the drug manufacturer had failed to warn the users of the drug in a prominent manner about the contraindications on the container/receptacle of the capsules taken by deceased and was liable to pay compensation. It was fought in the court that as per material published on systemic NSAIDs, SJS is rarely caused by indomethacin. No evidence on record was found to substantiate that the said drug caused SJS to deceased on account of which she died. State commission erred in fastening liability on the pharmaceutical company and the order was set aside.

Learning Essential

Manufacturers must ensure that the indications, dosage, interactions, common side effects, contraindications, and date of expiry are prominently displayed on all medications supplied by them. And it is prudent for the prescribing doctor to warn the patient of the side effects mentioned on the package insert. Failure to do so can make ground for medicolegal action.

Case 4: Dapsone-induced Liver Failure in Lichen Planus[27]

Complaint: Patient was suffering from lichen planus and was prescribed dapsone, a drug for treating leprosy. No pathological test was done prior to initiating dapsone. On follow-up, the patient was not given any instructions except to continue dapsone. Patient eventually succumbed to the side effects of the drug causing liver failure.

Verdict: Doctor was acquitted.

The doctor conducted baseline blood and urine test prior to initiating dapsone. Viral markers for hepatitis virus were positive and hence cause of death was "viral hepatitis with hepatic encephalopathy". Evidence for validity of clinical diagnosis of lichen planus and dapsone as one of its treatment was also presented in the court.

Case 5: Lamotrigine-induced SJS/TEN[28]

Complaint: Dr Nirmal (neurologist) prescribed lamotrigine for bipolar disorder, following which the patient developed SJS/TEN. Despite prompt admission to intensive care unit (ICU) and Medrol 4 mg, patient succumbed to the disease. No opinion of dermatologist was asked.

Verdict: Doctor was acquitted.

Minimal care was delivered, patient was diagnosed with SJS and admitted to ICU and given supportive care.

KEY MESSAGES

- Adverse drug reactions (ADRs) to medications are common and at times inevitable. Attempts to prevent them from occurring are the best management strategy.
- A proper evaluation including detailed history of reactions in the past, high-risk assessment, comorbidities, relevant laboratory investigations, and drug sensitivity testing wherever relevant should be carried out.
- As far as possible, "evidence-based practice" should be adopted. In children and elderly, topical and less aggressive treatment approach is helpful.
- Prompt diagnosis by recognizing the warning signs of serious drug reactions and abrupt stoppage of all suspected drugs in cases of serious reactions is an important aspect of management.
- A proper documentation of reactions including photodocumentation of serious drug reactions should be done in medical records. Patients must be warned not to consume the suspected drug(s) again and

issued a drug alert card with clear written instructions to carry this card all the times and to show it to the treating physician.
- Obtain suitable malpractice insurance and get acquainted with the terms of your insurance policy. If there is impending/possible legal "trouble", promptly contact the insurer, who will connect you with legal counsel. During trial give clear, concise, direct answers without medical jargon, if possible. Answer just the question asked and avoid giving details that are not directly related to the question.

ACKNOWLEDGMENT

We are highly thankful to:
- Dr Jagdish Singh (Ex Senior Professor and Head, Department of Pediatrics, SMS Hospital, Jaipur and legal advisor to medical institutions and trainer for Government medical officers and visiting faculty at IIHMR, Jaipur) in providing useful inputs in the preparation of this manuscript.
- Dr Manasa in contributing Case 4 and 5.

REFERENCES

1. Edwards IR, Aronson JK. Adverse drug reactions: definitions, diagnosis, and management. Lancet. 2000;356(9237):1255-9.
2. Resneck JS. Trends in malpractice premiums of dermatologists: results of a national survey. Arch Dermatol. 2006;142(3):337-40.
3. Elston DM, Taylor JS, Coldiron B, et al. Patient safety: Part I. Patient safety and the dermatologist. J Am Acad Dermatol. 2009;61(2):179-90.
4. Read S, Hill HF. Dermatology's malpractice experience: clinical settings for risk management. J Am Acad Dermatol. 2005;53(1):134-7.
5. Nasseri E. Disciplinary and legal actions against dermatologists in Canada. J Cutan Med Surg. 2016;20(1):29-34.
6. Miller RA, Sampson NR, Flynn JM. The prevalence of defensive orthopaedic imaging: a prospective practice audit in Pennsylvania. J Bone Joint Surg Am. 2012;94(3):e18.
7. Hurwitz B. How does evidence-based guidance influence determinations of medical negligence? BMJ. 2004;329:1024-8.
8. Sirur SP. Drug eruptions and drug reactions. Indian J Dermatol Venereol Leprol. 2003;69:248-9.
9. Oyebode F. Clinical errors and medical negligence. Med Princ Pract. 2013;22(4):323-33.
10. Aggrawal A. Drug induced injury, accidental and iatrogenic. In: Payne-James JJ, Byard RW, Corey TS, Henderson C (Eds). Encyclopedia of Forensic and Legal Medicine, Volume 2. London: Elsevier Academic Press; 2005. pp. 230-8.
11. Lesar TS, Briceland L, Stein DS. Factors related to errors in medication prescribing. JAMA. 1997;277(4):312-7.
12. Bates DW, Boyle DL, Van der Vliet MB, et al. Relationship between medication errors and adverse drug events. J Gen Intern Med. 1995;10(4):199-205.
13. Gupta LK, Khare AK. Ensuring drug safety in dermatology practice: an overview. In: Gupta LK, Martin AM, D'souza P, Pande S (Eds). IADVL's textbook on Cutaneous Adverse Drug Reaction—A comprehensive guide, 1st edition. New Delhi: Bhalani Publishing House; 2017. pp. 64-71.
14. Gandhi TK, Weingart SN, Seger AC, et al. Outpatient prescribing errors and the impact of computerized prescribing. J Gen Intern Med. 2005;20(9):837-41.
15. Bates DW, Cohen M, Leape LL, et al. Reducing the frequency of errors in medicine using information technology. J Am Med Inform Assoc. 2001;8(4):299-308.
16. Devine EB, Wilson-Norton JL, Lawless NM, et al. Characterization of prescribing errors in an internal medicine clinic. Am J Health Syst Pharm. 2007;64(10):1062-70.
17. Sackett DL, Richardson WS, Rosenberg Q, et al. Evidence-based Medicine. How to Practice and Teach EBM. London: Churchill Livingstone; 1997.
18. Mirakian R, Ewan PW, Durham SR, et al. BSACI guidelines for the management of drug allergy. Clin Exp Allergy. 2008;39(1):43-61.

19. Creamer D, Walsh SA, Dziewulski P, et al. UK guidelines for the management of Stevens-Johnson syndrome/toxic epidermal necrolysis. Br J Dermatol. 2016;174(6): 1194-227.
20. Gupta LK, Martin AM, Agarwal N, et al. Guidelines for the management of Stevens-Johnson syndrome/toxic epidermal necrolysis: An Indian perspective. Indian J Dermatol Venereol Leprol. 2016;82(1):1-23.
21. Hansten PD, Horn JR. The Top 100 Drug Interactions 2016: A Guide to Patient Management, 17th edition. Freeland: H&H Publications, LLP; 2016.
22. Shapiro LE, Shear NH. Drug interactions. In: Wolverton SE (Ed). Comprehensive Dermatologic Drug Therapy, 3rd edition. Philadelphia: Saunders; 2013. pp. 730-46.
23. Breathnach SM. Drug reactions. In: Burns DA, Breathnach SM, Cox NH, Griffiths CEM (Eds). Rook's Textbook of Dermatology, 8th edition. Oxford: Blackwell Publishing; 2010. pp. 75.1-177.
24. Shah VV, Kapp MB, Wolverton SE. Medical malpractice in dermatology part II: what to do once you have been served with a lawsuit. Am J Clin Deratol. 2016;17(6):601-7.
25. Sirur S. Legal issues and counseling in cutaneous adverse drug reaction. In: Gupta LK, Martin AM, D'souza P, Pande S (Eds). IADVL's textbook on Cutaneous Adverse Drug Reaction—A comprehensive guide, 1st edition. New Delhi: Bhalani Publishing House; 2017. pp. 507-10.
26. Jain RC, Naik SK. National Consumer Disputes Redressal Commission, New Delhi: Original Petition no. 240 of 1999-2011. [online] Available from http://ncdrc.nic.in/. [Accessed December, 2018].
27. Santosh Gupta and others vs Dr GG Dhir and others (May 21st, 2007). National consumer dispute redressal. III (2007) CPJ 322 NC.
28. Dr Nirmal Kumar Bera vs Sh Dibyatam Subba (Feb 21st, 2011) SC case No. FA/115/2010 (Bench—Justice Mr PK Samanta, Mrs S Majumdar, Mrs Corai).

CHAPTER 29

Legal Issues in HIV and STD Patients

Yogesh S Marfatia, Reema Baxi, Kajal Mehta

INTRODUCTION

Responsible sexual behavior includes making informed decisions and safer sex choices, having open communication with partner about all forms of sexual activity and taking precautions against transmission of sexually transmitted infections (STIs) and human immunodeficiency virus (HIV). Such behavior is desirable to prevent transmission of HIV or other STIs and undesirable conception.

In reality, irresponsible sexual behavior is more frequent in vulnerable population. Females bear the brunt of unsafe sexual behavior because of conducive biologic and socioeconomic factors. Power in equation makes inmates of refuge homes or shelters susceptible to sexual abuse. All this results in a large quantum of nonconsensual sex, coercive sex, and rape. Such sexual activities are usually unprotected and high risk with potential for STI and HIV transmission. Consequences of such behavior include morbidity, mortality and potential for certain malignancies, effect on long-term health of the individual and vertical transmission.

Undesirable sexual activities have a lot of legal, moral and ethical connotations.

What is the Recent Legislative Act Related to HIV or AIDS in India?

The Human Immunodeficiency Virus and Acquired Immune Deficiency Syndrome (Prevention and Control) Act, 2017[1] (Government of India)

Prevention and control of the spread of HIV-AIDS and for the protection of human rights of persons affected by the said virus and syndrome and for matters connected therewith or incidental thereto.

What are the Provisions under HIV and AIDS Prevention and Control Act, 2017 Relevant to Medical Professionals?

Prohibition of Discrimination
- No person shall discriminate against the protected person on the basis of

denial from employment or occupation, procurement of healthcare services or right to reside.
- No person can publish, propagate, advocate or communicate the feelings of hatred against any protected persons.
- In case of *termination from employment*, the protected person is terminated when he or she poses a significant risk of transmission of HIV to other people in the workplace, or is unfit to perform the duties of the job.

Informed Consent

- Informed consent is defined as voluntary authorization, by a patient or research subject with full comprehension of the risks involved, for diagnostic or investigative procedures, and for medical and surgical treatment.

Under this provision:
- No HIV test can be performed or no person can be subjected to medical treatment, interventions or research, without the informed consent of such person or his representative.
- HIV test includes pre-test and post-test counseling.

When is informed consent for conducting an HIV test not required?
- Where a court orders HIV testing.
- For procuring, processing, distribution or use of a human body, tissues, blood, semen or other body fluids for use in medical research or therapy.
- For epidemiological or surveillance purposes where the HIV test is anonymous and is not for the purpose of determining the HIV status of a person.
- For screening purposes in any licensed blood bank.

Disclosure of HIV Status

- No person can be compelled to disclose his HIV status except by an order of the court stating that the disclosure of such information is necessary in the interest of justice.
- Disclosure of HIV status can be done only with the informed consent of that individual.

When is informed consent for disclosure of HIV-related information not required?
- By a healthcare provider to another healthcare provider who is involved in the care, treatment or counseling of such person, when such disclosure is necessary to provide care or treatment to that person.
- By an order of a court.
- In suits or legal proceedings between persons, where it is necessary in filing suits or legal proceedings or for instructing their counsel.
- For statistical purposes.
- To the officers of the Central or State Government or State AIDS Control Society for the purposes of monitoring, evaluation or supervision.

When and to whom can healthcare providers disclose HIV Status?
- Only a *physician or a counselor* shall disclose the HIV-positive status of a person to his or her partner.
- A healthcare provider, who is a physician or counselor can disclose the HIV positive status of a person to his or her partner, if:
  – Partner is at significant risk of transmission of HIV from such person
  – Such HIV-positive person has been counseled to inform partner
  – Has informed consent from HIV-positive person.

- The healthcare provider shall not be liable for any criminal or civil action for any disclosure or non-disclosure of confidential HIV-related information made to a partner.

Case 1: Subhash Mohanrao Pachlore versus Apex Hospital

- *Complaint:* Patient, a lawyer by profession, was diagnosed with cerebral venous thrombosis with HIV infection. A single HIV test by enzyme-linked immunosorbent assay (ELISA) was done by the doctor, after informing the patient's wife. He tested reactive, but the test was not repeated. The HIV positive status was then disclosed to the patient, his wife and immediate relatives at the hospital. This caused severe mental agony; also, as the news reached the bar association, it affected his reputation and thus his legal practice. The patient repeated the tests at another pathology center and was tested non-reactive repeatedly. He requested for a compensation of 10 lakh rupees for the same.
- *Verdict:* The doctor was held negligent and directed to compensate 5 lakhs.
- *Comments:* **Why was the doctor wrong?**
    - It is mandatory to offer pre-test counseling and take informed consent from patient which was missed in this case.
    - Result can be declared through post-test counseling to the patient.
    - Except wife, the HIV positive status cannot be disclosed to other relatives.
    - The result was declared on the basis of only one positive test. As per World Health organization (WHO) guidelines for HIV testing (2015), HIV test is considered positive only after 3 consecutive tests.
    - In this case, repeat ELISA was non-reactive. Therefore, the loss of income and reputation was transient, and hence the compensation money was lowered.[2]

Message: Every treating doctor should follow the protocol of pre-test and post-test counseling and disclose HIV status to spouse only. It is essential to ensure that the testing laboratory is following standard guidelines of testing and reporting.

Case 2: Mr "X" versus Hospital "Z"

- *Complaint:* The complainant was tested HIV positive during blood donation, following which the doctor informed the fiancée of the complainant. The marriage was then called off by the fiancée. The right of the hospital to disclose to the fiancée was questioned. Also, detail on the "suspension of right to marry" was also questioned upon.
- *Verdict:* It was open to the hospital or the doctor concerned to reveal such information to persons related to the girl whom he intended to marry and she had a right to know about the HIV positive status of the appellant. If a person suffering from HIV(+) contracting marriage with a willing partner after disclosing the factum of disease to that partner will not be considered as committing an offence.[3]
- *Message:* It is the duty of the HIV positive patient to disclose his status to wife or prospective spouse or sexual partners. The doctor should motivate sero-positive client through counseling to disclose his status and if not done, doctor can do so strictly in limited scenarios like this.

Obligation of Establishments

- *Ensuring confidentiality of information by* adopting data protection measures and procedures to ensure accountability and liability of persons in the establishment.
- *To provide a safe working environment by* training, education and information about use of *Universal Precautions and Post Exposure Prophylaxis (PEP)* to all persons who may be occupationally exposed to HIV.
- *Strategies for reducing risk of HIV transmission by providing* information, education and counseling services relating to prevention of HIV and safe practices and by provision of safer sex tools including condoms; drug substitution and drug maintenance; and provision of comprehensive injection safety requirements.

What is the legal provision for child sexual assault in India?

Protection of Children from Sexual Offences (POCSO) Act, 2012

An act to protect children from offences of sexual assault, sexual harassment and pornography and establishment of special courts for trials.[4]

What is the role of medical professionals for providing emergency medical care in cases of child sexual assault?
Protection of Children from Sexual Offences Act 2012 states that emergency medical care is to be provided by any medical facility—private or public and no legal or magisterial requisition shall be demanded as a prerequisite to rendering such care.[4]

Is there any law under Indian constitution applicable for doctors treating STI?
Transmission of STI occurs not only from symptomatic cases but also from asymptomatic cases or carriers. In fact, the latter is more frequent. Infections like HPV and HBV can cause malignancy, whereas HIV can cause morbidity as well as mortality. Many infections can be vertically transmitted from pregnant female to the fetus. These factors make STDs a special group of disorders necessitating more involvement of treating physician beyond drug therapy. Though not legally bound, anybody treating STI is morally and ethically bound to offer counseling to the sufferer regarding inherent health risk and potential of transmission to the novice.

The doctor must counsel and educate the patient and his or her partner regarding risk of asymptomatic transmission, undesirable sequelae and consequences of untreated STD and safe sex measures. The patient must be motivated to disclose his or her infection status to the partner.

Is it the treating doctor's duty to disclose about STD status to the spouse or partner?
There is no law per se, but as an analogy to disclosure clause of HIV and AIDS act, it can be stated that it is the duty of the doctor to disclose STI status and possible risks of transmission to the partner or spouse if sought for.

Is STD a ground for divorce?
Under Hindu Marriage Act 1955, if one of the spouses is suffering from a serious disease that is easily communicable (STD/HIV), a divorce can be filed by the other spouse.[5]

What is Section 377 of Indian Penal Code (IPC)?
Section 377 of the Indian Penal Code (1861) introduced during the British rule of India, criminalized sexual activities "against the order of nature" including homosexual activities.[6]

377. Unnatural offences: Whoever voluntarily has carnal intercourse against the order of nature with any man, woman or animal shall be punished with imprisonment for life, or with imprisonment of either description for a term which may extend to 10 years, and shall also be liable to fine.[4]

What is the current verdict of Section 377?[7]
- Delhi High Court decriminalized Section 377 in July 2009.
- Supreme Court of India (SC) overturned the judgment on 11 December 2013 with the Court repealing that section 377 should be a matter left to Parliament, not the judiciary.
- On 24 August 2017 in a landmark judgment known as the Puttaswamy judgment, the SC had upheld the Right to Privacy as a fundamental right under the Constitution.
- On 10 July 2018, a five-member constitutional bench of the SC commenced hearing of the pleas challenging the constitutionality of section 377.
- Consensual sex between adults in a private space which is not harmful to women or children cannot be denied as it is a matter of individual choice. Section 377 results in discrimination and is violative of constitutional principles.[5]
- *On 6th September 2018, the Supreme Court decriminalized section 377 IPC and gay sex is no longer a punishable offence.*

CONCLUSION

Taking into account the nature of STI transmission and undesirable health consequences, the treating doctor, though not legally but morally and ethically, is bound to assume a greater role beyond being a drug prescriber.

He or she is supposed to counsel the patient to follow a self-protective sexual behavior and advise to protect the partner. Motivating patients to disclose infection status to their partners and bring them for management is a part and parcel of counseling.

Rather than stigmatizing and discriminating HIV or AIDS cases, promotion of universal precautions in healthcare settings will go a long way in preventing such infections.

Though little is defined in books of law regarding STD's, it is the social responsibility of STI physicians to do the utmost to curtail the menace of sexually transmitted diseases.

REFERENCES

1. The Human Immunodeficiency Virus and Acquired Immune deficiency Syndrome (Prevention and Control) Act 2017. (Ministry of Law and Justice). Part 2; Section 1. Available from: http://naco.gov.in/sites/default/files/HIV%20AIDS%20Act.pdf.
2. Apex Hospital vs Subhash Mohanrao Pachlore. FA/65/2011.2014. p 65 of 2011. Available from: https://indiankanoon.org/doc/110666943/
3. Indiankanoon.org. (2018). Mr. 'X' vs Hospital 'Z' on 21 September, 1998. [online] Available at: https://indiankanoon.org/doc/382721/ [Accessed 3 Jan. 2019].
4. The Protection of Children from Sexual Offences Act 2012. Ministry of Law and Justice. Part 2; Section 1. Available from: http://wcd.nic.in/sites/default/files/childprotection31072012.pdf
5. The Hindu Marriage Act 1955 (High Court of Punjab and Haryana). Available from: https://highcourtchd.gov.in/hclscc/subpages/pdf_files/4.pdf
6. Indiankanoon.org. (n.d.). Section 377 in The Indian Penal Code. [online] Available at: https://indiankanoon.org/doc/1836974/ [Accessed 3 Jan. 2019.
7. The Times of India. News I. Supreme Court reserves verdict on Section 377.[Internet]. 2019 [cited 2 January 2019]. Available from: https://timesofindia.indiatimes.com/india/supreme-court-reserves-verdict-on-section-377/articleshow/65020367.cms

CHAPTER 30

Legal Aspects of Leprosy

Nanda B Kishore

INTRODUCTION

Leprosy is a disease of antiquity and has been known to have been prevalent in India, China and Africa. More than 2,000 years ago, *Sushruta Samhita*, which is one of the ancient books on medicine probably compiled in 600 BC gives a detailed account of the various manifestations of leprosy. "*Manusmriti*" is another ancient Indian literature believed to be of antiquity, but dated around 500–1,300 BC by the European scholars, also describes a disease "*Kushtha*". Manu lists some diseases which if some one suffers from, as a ground for refusal to accept alliance in marriage of which "*Kushtha*" is one. Therefore this particular law of Manu may be considered as the most ancient legal aspect of leprosy.[1]

In India, the laws pertaining to leprosy were framed by the British Government which appeared relevant during that period as leprosy had no specific treatment and the sequelae of the disease was severe and deforming. With the advances in the treatment of leprosy and the various surgical procedures available to correct the deformities, all these laws framed before independence became obsolete requiring drastic modifications.

Let us see some of these old and outdated laws:[2]

- The Hindu Marriage Act of 1955, Christian Marriage Act of 1872, and the Muslim Marriage Act of 1939 permitted divorce on the grounds of leprosy if one among the spouse is suffering from this disease. However, the Parsi Marriage Act of 1936 does not allow divorce.
- The Hindu Succession Act of 1956, however, permits inheritance of ancestral property which is not allowed till then based on the ancient codes.[3]
- Motor Vehicle Act of 1939 does not permit driving license to leprosy patients.
- The Indian Railway Act of 1890, although prohibits leprosy patients to travel in train with other passengers, gives concession in the travel fare to go to other places for the purpose of treatment.

- The Tenancy Act does not allow renting out of houses to these patients.
- Prevention of Begging Act 1959 permits arrest of leprosy patient who are found soliciting alms in public places. Such patients are to be kept in the leprosy asylums.

In the darkness of all these draconian laws, the light at the end of the tunnel appeared in the form of United Nations Convention on the Rights of Persons with Disabilities 2007 (UNCRPD), which was unanimously adopted in the United Nations General Assembly 2010.

Accordingly the Law Commission prepared a model draft legislation titled "Eliminating Discrimination Against Persons Affected by Leprosy (EDPAL) bill 2015. This bill contains principles of nondiscrimination and equal protection before law that must be guaranteed to all persons affected by leprosy. The Leprosy Mission Trust India (TLMTI) identified 14 laws that are discriminating in nature and when the present Central Government decided to repeal these obsolete laws in September 2014, took the initiative in convincing the Government of this urgent need. Accordingly, the Law Commission submitted its "Report No 256 on EDPAL" dated 7th April 2015.[4]

KEY ASPECTS OF THE DRAFT LAW

- *Repeal and amendment of certain laws*: Besides the repeal of the Lepers Act, 1898, the Law Commission recommends the repeal of discriminatory provisions in various personal laws. It also recommends including persons affected by leprosy among the list of persons eligible for legal aid under the Legal Services Act, 1987.
- *Measures against discrimination*: The Law Commission recommends that persons affected by leprosy and their family members must not be discriminated against in any institution. It also guarantees to such persons the right to access healthcare, adequate housing, education, employment, and other such basic amenities.
- *Land rights*: Persons affected by leprosy are usually made to relocate to "leprosy colonies" in India, but they do not have land rights, and are constantly under fear of eviction. The Law Commission recommends that title and ownership of property in leprosy colonies should be legalized, and if land rights cannot be given, alternative settlement options must be explored.
- *Right to employment*: Many employers misuse existing employment laws to terminate services of persons who are diagnosed with leprosy. The draft law prohibits the termination of employment of such persons solely due to their association with leprosy.
- *Educational and training opportunities*: The Law Commission recommends that the draft law should ensure the admission of persons affected by leprosy and their family members in schools, colleges, and other institutes, as educational qualifications are necessary to allow them access to employment opportunities.
- *Appropriate use of language*: The use of the term "leper" and similar terms carries negative connotation, hampers efforts for the inclusion of persons affected by leprosy into society, and affects their sense of dignity as human beings. The Law Commission recommends that the term "leper" and other such terms in all government and private documents should be replaced with "persons affected by leprosy" or a similar term.
- *Right to freedom of movement*: The draft law ensures that persons affected by leprosy

are guaranteed the right of travel in public transport and the right to obtain a driving license.

- *Concessions during treatment*: The draft law seeks to provide relevant concessions and monetary benefits to persons affected by leprosy who are undergoing treatment, for their travel, lodging during treatment, and medicines.
- *Social awareness*: Creating awareness regarding the cure and transmission of leprosy is the best way to address the discrimination and stigma against persons affected by leprosy and their family. The Law Commission recommends that awareness about the disease, its treatment, and curability should be conducted through campaigns and programs in schools, hospitals, government institutions, and private establishments.
- *Welfare measures*: The draft law imposes specific duties upon establishments to execute certain welfare measures to foster an environment for financial and social growth of persons affected by leprosy and their families. It also creates Central and State Commissions to strictly enforce such measures, and provides for accountability measures in case of nonenforcement.

The "EDPAL" is only a bill at present and its journey towards being an "Act" may be long. A bill becomes an Act only when it is passed in both the houses of the parliament. But the nature of the bill is such that no party can oppose this despite any kind of political affiliations or obligations.

Let us look at the implications. When the bill is approved and the "Act" gets notified in the Central Government Gazette:[5]

- *Equality and nondiscrimination*: No person establishment or government shall discriminate against a person affected by leprosy or members of his family (spouse, parents, children, and siblings) on the grounds of the disease or its disabilities.
- *Duty to uphold rights*: Nondenial of any rights guaranteed in the constitution.
- *Right to health and treatment*: Entitlement for multidrug therapy and other health care facilities.
- *Disclosure of medical records*: Maintaining confidentiality of the medical records.
- *Right to ownership of property*: Every right to own, reside, purchase or rent any property.
- *Right to access public goods and services*: Any privileges of the general public or customarily available to the public should be made available to a person with leprosy.
- *Right to movement*: Travel in public transport and obtain driving license.
- *Right to education*: No denial of the right to education, training, and resume education after duly furnishing a certificate by an authorized person that attests that the person has been started on multidrug therapy or completed the course of therapy.
- *Right to employment*: Person affected by leprosy or his family members can continue their appointment in a public or private organization after furnishing a medical certificate issued by a registered medical practitioner.
- *Right to form family*: No person shall be denied the right to marry and form a family including through access to adoption or assisted procreation.

The bill has also made provisions for leprosy patients to file case against any one who are found to violate the above mentioned laws and provides legal aid wherever necessary. This provision comes under section 25 of the Act, and if the court comes to a conclusion that any person or establishment has breached or not complied with the provision of this Act, it shall award to the person affected by leprosy, compensation and damages of not less than ₹ 25,000 along with all cost incurred in litigation.

CONCLUSION

The EDPAL bill 2015 is a much awaited, revolutionary bill which is going to bring a silver lining in the lives of the person affected by leprosy transforming their lives from frustration and despair to satisfaction, fulfillment, and hope. As per the newspaper reports (TOI 11-08-2018 and NIE 23-08-2018) the central government has finally initiated steps to remove from statutes leprosy as a ground for divorce, separation, and annulment of marriage. Additional solicitor general informed Supreme Court that the process for drafting a comprehensive legislation to repeal various discriminatory laws against people afflicted with leprosy was underway and government may need 4 months to complete the process. Let this bill become an "Act" in the near future.

REFERENCES

1. Dharmendra. Leprosy in ancient India medicine. Int J Lepr. 1947;15(4):424-30.
2. The Society for the Eradication of Leprosy seminar on the legal aspects of Leprosy. Indian J Lepr. 1989;61(3):351-4.
3. Muthuswamy S. Legal aspects of Leprosy. Indian J Lepr. 1990;62(3):402.
4. https://blog.ipleaders.in/leprosy-is-curable
5. Law Commission of India. Report No. 256: Eliminating Discrimination against Persons affected by Leprosy; 2015. pp. 52-9.

CHAPTER 31

Photography and the Law

Feroze Kaliyadan, Karalikkattil T Ashique

> **KEY OBJECTIVE**
> - To appraise the reader regarding medicolegal issues related to clinical photography and tips on how to deal with them.

INTRODUCTION AND BACKGROUND

With the advent of digital photography, it has become routine and very easy to capture clinical images of patients. Dermatologists use clinical photography for various purposes including pre- and post-treatment evaluations, patient counseling and scientific publications/presentations.[1] The popularity of internet, social media and smartphones in the last few years have made it very easy to share clinical images of patients.[2] This opens a way to inadvertent dispersal of patient data and possible breaches in patient confidentiality. It is therefore very important for the dermatologists to be aware of pertinent ethical and legal issues related to clinical photography and it use of such images.

PRACTICE: RELEVANCE AND SIGNIFICANCE

Recent years have seen many instances when medical practitioners both in India and abroad have had to face legal issues related to sharing of patient images, especially in the ever-burgeoning social media.

LEGAL PRINCIPLES

The most serious issue the dermatologist might face is patient complaints regarding breach of confidentiality and as a corollary the most sensitive images are the ones where identifiable facial features are present.

The code of conduct of the Medical Council of India (MCI) explicitly states that patient consent is essential for publication of clinical photographs. The MCI Code of Ethics Regulations, 2002 Chapter 7, Section 7.17 states that a registered medical practitioner shall not publish photographs or case reports of his/her patients without their permission, in any medical or other journal in a manner by which their identity could be made out. If the identity is not disclosed, the consent is not needed.[3] Although MCI gives leeway to the medical practitioner for publication of photographs without consent, as far as identity is not discernible, it should be noted that most scientific journals now insist on patient consent even in cases where the patient identity is not discernible.[4] Also, while not explicitly mentioned, "publication" can be extrapolated to any means of sharing of patient data, including presentations and social media, although this is one area which needs more clearly defined rules and regulations to be set down by the MCI. It should be understood that the ethics of clinical practice are also governed by principles of trust in the healthcare team and this implies certain unsaid ethical practices need to be followed including taking permission for photographs even in cases where identity is not an issue.

Another related issue, which comes under the realm of publication ethics, is image tampering and image plagiarism.[5]

As of now neither the MCI nor the government of India have clear guidelines specifically on the sharing of clinical images on social media, although a general framework for government organizations was published by the Department of Information Technology which can be extrapolated to some extent to health care too.[6-8]

CASE REPORT

A surgeon posted the surgical photographs of a 45-year-old male patient on his Facebook® page without patient's consent. Besides being a gross violation of privacy, the incident was traumatic to the patient because of the comments posted, which poked fun at the image. The surgeon had apparently assumed that since the photograph was of internal organs, patient identity would not be compromised. The concerned surgeon later apologized to the patient and removed the images from social media platforms. In this particular case, the surgeon was lucky that the patient did not seek further legal recourse.[9]

The key message is that while legally informed consent is only essential for images where identity is discernible, in other cases too, the medical practitioner is ethically bound to obtain consent before publishing patient images in any forum.

REMEDY AND PREVENTION

The key to prevent legal issues related to publication of patient images is a clear informed consent, even in cases where patient identity is not compromised. Some institutions have blanket consent forms, which cover procedures, investigations and medical photography. We would however recommend a separate exclusive form for photography consent. It is also important to ensure that the patient is verbally explained the content of the consent form, especially the point that "publication" can include both scientific publication and social media.[10]

Each practitioner can customize their photography consent forms as per their requirements. An example of an ideal, comprehensive yet simple, consent form for clinical photography, used by the NHS, UK is available at: https://www.rlbuht.nhs.uk/media/2188/consent-to-clinica-photography-form-v202.pdf.
Another example is available on the website of the Indian Dermatology Online Journal (http://www.idoj.in/contributors.asp).

In all cases, the practitioner must try to conceal identity as much as possible [for example, by cropping out or blackening identifiable features and ensuring that patient tags are removed from items like radiographs and electrocardiography (ECG) readings]. Tattoos and named rings are often neglected marks of identity, which should not be missed.

The practitioner in charge must be careful regarding storage of patient images, as for any other sensitive patient data, ensuring that the images can be accessed and shared only with authorized, responsible persons.[11]

Acceptable image editing includes—cropping, background correction, changing image resolution, some amount of color, brightness-contrast and sharpness correction (except in pre-post images where uniform parameters must be applied to both set of images). Major tampering with pixels to partially or completely enhance or obscure specific features to deceive the viewer is a form of scientific misconduct. The same applies true for image plagiarism of any kind.[5] Using images from the internet or received from social media from other doctors, without permission and due acknowledgment, will also come under the purview of plagiarism. Although the MCI does not specifically cover this in its code of ethics, this kind of plagiarism would amount to major ethical misconduct. To some extent, this form or plagiarism can be prevented by using watermarks on the clinical images to show the original source.

Other general aspects and etiquettes, as for any medical procedure, are to be kept in mind for clinical photography too—ensuring patient confidentiality and comfort during the process, using appropriate chaperones in case of female patients (in case the photographer is male) and ensuring a sterile environment in the context of surgical procedures.[11] It is always a good practice to show the photographs to the patients whenever possible.

It is within the patient's right to refuse being photographed and all patients should be assured that their medical care will not be affected in any manner due to this refusal (this excludes imaging which are part of the patient record file—like X-rays for example). However, other than in emergency situations, it should also be the right of the doctor to refuse further treatment to such patients, especially in cases where photographic documentation is crucial (for example, pre and post images in elective aesthetic procedures like hair transplantation). Consent for serial documentation should ideally be covered in the initial consent form itself. Proper consent and serial documentation also helps in cases where patients might falsely claim lack of improvement after treatment, either based on their subjective feeling or on the basis of photographs taken (or edited) by themselves. It is important that doctors maintain a properly arranged database and adequate back up of the raw images to deal with any medicolegal issues in the future.

Broadly, clinical photographs are used in two contexts—one as part of the clinical records of the patient and the second for academic purposes (which includes teaching, scientific presentations/discussions and research). Another use, which is increasingly seen, is in the context of advertising—especially pre and post images of aesthetic procedures. The same general guidelines apply for commercial photography too—informed consent and ethical photography to ensure that the viewers are not deceived by the images. There are arguments against the use of patient photographs for commercial purposes like the fact that patients might be coerced to participate due to the inherent vulnerability of their position.[12] When used ethically, pre and post images have good value in educating patients regarding various procedures.

PEARLS

- Use dedicated forms for photography consent.
- Show the images to the patient/guardian whenever possible.
- Try to remove identifying features as much as possible, even if consent is taken.
- Understand scientific ethics related to image editing and image plagiarism.
- In general, share images on social media only if really necessary and if you sincerely feel that it will benefit the patient(s).

SUMMARY AND KEY POINTS

Clinical imaging and sharing of images by dermatologist is on the rise and is likely to increase in future. The most important aspect in avoiding medicolegal issues related to clinical photography is taking an explicit informed consent, even when the images do not compromise patient identity. Clear guidelines and regulations on the sharing of clinical images in social media is also an urgent need of the times.

REFERENCES

1. Kaliyadan F. Digital photography for patient counseling in dermatology—a study. J Eur Acad Dermatol Venereol. 2008;22:1356-8.
2. Kaliyadan F, Ashique KT, Jagadeesan S, et al. What's up dermatology? A pilot survey of the use of WhatsApp in dermatology practice and case discussion among members of WhatsApp dermatology groups. Indian J Dermatol Venereol Leprol. 2016;82:67-9.
3. Medical Council of India. Indian Medical Council (Professional Conduct, Etiquette and Ethics) Regulations, 2002. Published in Part III, Section 4 of the Gazette of India. New Delhi, India; 2002.
4. Smith R. Informed consent: edging forwards (and backwards). BMJ. 1998;316:949-51.
5. Kaliyadan F. Image manipulation and image plagiarism—what's fine and what's not? Indian J Dermatol Venereol Leprol. 2017;83:519-21.
6. Ministry of Electronics and Information Technology. (2018). Framework and guidelines for use of social media for government organizations. [online] Available from: http://www.meity.gov.in/writereaddata/files/Approved%20Social%20Media%20Framework%20and%20Guidelines%20_2_pdf. [Accessed December, 2018].
7. Srivastava SK. Adoption of electronic health records: a roadmap for India. Healthc Inform Res. 2016;22:261-9.
8. Padmanabhan S. What's Up(App) Doc? J Indian Orthod Soc. 2018;52:87-8.
9. Where are the ethics? Surgeon posts pictures of patient's internal organs on Facebook. [online] Available from: https://www.firstpost.com/india/ethics-surgeon-posts-pictures-patients-internal-organs-facebook-2179891.html. [Accessed December, 2018].
10. Palacios-González C. The ethics of clinical photography and social media. Med Health Care Philos. 2015;18:63-70.
11. Supe A. Ethical considerations in medical photography. Issues Med Ethics. 2003;11:83-4.
12. Bhattacharya S. Clinical photography and our responsibilities. Indian J Plast Surg. 2014;47:277-80.

CHAPTER 32

Setting up a Pharmacy in a Clinic

DA Satish

OBJECTIVES

The article discusses rules and regulations of setting up a pharmacy in a clinic setting, medicolegal issues involved in dispensing medicines without a license and current status of online or e-pharmacies in India.

Setting up a pharmacy in a clinic setting is a good value-added service we can provide to our patients. The rules and regulations are governed by the Drugs and Cosmetics Act, 1940 and rules 1945. The broad guidelines and regulations for opening a pharmacy are applicable in all states of India except Jammu and Kashmir.

PROPRIETORSHIP OR PARTNERSHIP

Any individual including a doctor can open a pharmacy either as an individual proprietor or in partnership with another person. If you have a partner in the pharmacy, you should set-up partnership firm. This partnership firm is to be registered for example in Karnataka, in the office of the Registrar of firms, Government of Karnataka, under the Indian Partnership Act 1932 (Section 58). A current account has to be opened in a bank under the name of the pharmacy.

RETAIL LICENSE FROM THE DRUG CONTROLLER

Retail license has to be obtained from the Drug Controller and Licensing Authority, in Form 20 and Form 21. The License is granted for a period of 5 years, which is renewable.

Some of the other licenses granted by the Drugs Control Department by respective Jurisdictional delegated licensing authorities are:
- Wholesale drug license in Form 20B and Form 21B
- Licenses to sell drugs under Schedule X (in Form 20F for retail and Form 21G for wholesale).
- Restricted licenses in Form 20A and Form 21A.

Details on forms, fees and checklist of documents required can generally be obtained from website of the Drugs Control Department.

Minimal Prerequisites for Retail License

- Adequate premises—10 m² (107.63 sq ft)
- If you want to be a dispensing chemist (compounding and dispensing) you need 15 m² (161.44 sq ft). This point has to be particularly noted by dermatologists who want to compound and dispense formulations.
- Adequate storage facilities—racks, refrigerator, etc. The refrigerator should be on 24 hours.
- Should be in charge of a competent person, who should be a registered pharmacist.

The drug license and registered pharmacist certificate should be prominently displayed in the pharmacy.

There is no separate license required for sale of cosmetics by the retail chemist.

It is an offense to stock physician samples inside the pharmacy premises and should never be done.

Fresh license has to be obtained if there is any change in premises or change in constitution of the firm. Also if there is change in the registered pharmacist, relevant documents of the new person have to be submitted to the concerned licensing authority and necessary endorsement on the license has to be obtained immediately.

In case application is made for both wholesale and retail licenses, minimum floor area required is 15 m². If you want to run a 24-hour pharmacy, minimum 3 registered pharmacists have to be employed.

Unlike in a retail pharmacy where drugs must be sold in the presence of a registered pharmacist, the sale of drug by wholesale can be made either in the presence of registered pharmacist or in the presence of a competent person who can be a graduate with 1-year experience in dealing in drugs or a person who has passed SSLC with 4 years' experience in dealing in drugs, especially approved by the department for this purpose.

GST (Goods and Services Tax) Registration Certificate

Vat certificate has now been replaced by GST certificate. This can be obtained from the Commissioner of Commercial Taxes, of the respective state. Monthly, quarterly and annual GST returns have to be compulsorily filed in commercial taxes department as per existing rules which keep changing often. If pharmacy is proprietorship, then same GST number used in cosmetology practice can be used for pharmacy. If it is a partnership deed than a separate GST number will be required.

Now if the turnover of the sale of goods of pharmacy is within state and is less than 20 lakhs, it is not required to register under GST and neither to levy GST on sale of goods. But if sale of goods is outside state then irrespective of turnover of goods, it is required to register under GST and required to levy GST on sale. Though the rules are like this, it is always better to take GST number for pharmacy as it is near impossible to purchase goods from wholesaler or stock lists without the same.

A person can opt for composition tax of 1% for turnover of up to 1.5 crore business per year.

Professional Tax

A yearly professional tax has to be paid separately by the owners of the pharmacy, per person, which varies from state to state. In Karnataka, the rule comes under Karnataka Tax on Professions, Traders, Callings and Employment Rules, 1976. There is no professional tax for persons above 60 years of age. In Karnataka, the current Professional tax rates are 1,000 rupees per person if turnover per year is less than 10 lacs, 1,500 rupees if turnover is between 10 lacs and 25 lacs and 2,500 if turnover is above 25 lacs per year.

Other Requirements in the Pharmacy

A good desktop computer and pharmacy software is a must. You will need adequate staff, telephone, credit card machine, closed circuit television (CCTV) cameras (to monitor), printer, stationary, backup power and a store room to keep your inventory.

Recurrent Expenditure Involved in Running Pharmacy

The recurrent expenditure involved includes salaries to the employees, software maintenance and upgradation charges, fees to sales tax consultant and auditor.

Dispensing of Medicines by Doctors without License

There is controversy and confusion regarding whether registered medical practitioners can dispense medicines to their patients without a license. This happened because a doctor in Kollam, Kerala in August 2014 was found guilty of running a pharmacy without license by the State Drugs Control Department. Kollam Additional Session's Judge issued a sentence of one-day imprisonment and slapped a fine of 1.20 lakhs rupees on a doctor running a single-doctor clinic in Sasthamkotta in Kollam District. The doctor served the sentence by remaining in there till the rising of the court.

Qualified Private Medical Practitioners Association (OPMPA) and the Indian Medical Association, Kerala Chapter have defended the doctor and said the State Drugs Control Department was misinterpreting the Act.

This is what the Drugs and Cosmetics Act 1940 (Schedule k, item 5) says about prescribing and dispensing medicines by doctors:

"Drugs supplied by a registered medical practitioner to his own patient or any drug specified in Schedule C supplied by a registered medical practitioner at the request of another such practitioner if it is specially prepared with reference to the condition and for the use of an individual patient, provided the registered medical practitioner is not (a) keeping an open shop or (b) selling across the counter or (c) engaged in the importation, manufacture, distribution or sale of drugs in the provision of Chapter IV of the Act and the Rules there under:

- The medicine shall be labeled with the name and address of the registered medical practitioner by whom it is supplied.
- If the medicine is for external application, it shall be labeled with the words "for external use only" or if it is for internal use with the dose.
- The name of the medicine or ingredients of the preparation and the quantities thereof, the dose prescribed the name of the patient and the date of supply, maintenance of a register.
- The entry in the register shall be given a number and that number shall be entered on the label of the container.
- The register and the prescription if any on which the medicines are issued shall be preserved for not less than 2 years from the date of the last entry in the register or the date of the prescription as the case may be."

The drug will be stored under proper storage conditions as directed on the label.

All the provisions of Chapter IV of the Act and the Rules made thereunder, subject to the following conditions:

- The drugs shall be purchased only from a dealer or a manufacturer licensed under these rules and records of such purchases showing the names and quantities of such drugs together with their batch numbers and the names and addresses of the manufacturers shall be maintained. Such records shall be open to inspection by an Inspector appointed under the Act, who may, if necessary, make enquiries about purchases of the drugs and may also take samples for test.

So, basically a doctor can dispense a drug to a patient and has to be personally given by him to patient without any intermediaries. He has to maintain proper records as above.

But to avoid unnecessary hassles, it is always better to take a drug license and follow the rules accordingly.

Patient Counseling by Pharmacist

The Pharmacy Council of India allows patient counseling by registered pharmacist with regard to the prescription. While dispensing the patient should be explained:
- How to take the medications and for how long?
- When to take medicines–before food or after food, etc.
- Possible side effects and how to manage them
- What to do if doses are missed
- Any other precautions to be taken.

Prescription Writing by Doctors

The Medical Council of India before it got dissolved recently issued a notification for all allopathic doctors on the format of writing a uniform standard prescription for patient safety.

The comprehensive format includes the doctor's full name, his or her qualification, patient's details and name of the generic medicine or its equivalent along with the dosage, strength dosage form and instructions. The names of the medicines should be in capital letters. Name of medical store, pharmacist's name and date of dispensing should be mentioned. The doctor's signature and stamp is a must. The new format was till recently available on the website of Medical Council of India (MCI). The website has now been taken off online with the dissolution of MCI by Government of India.

The Uttarakhand High Court on 15th September 2018 issued a direction to all government and private doctors in Uttarakhand to give computer-generated prescriptions to enable patients and their attendants to understand the same. It has also directed the government to provide adequate infrastructure for same to the government doctors. It has to be seen whether in future the same rule will be applied to all over the country.

Online or E-Pharmacies: Current Status

Of late, there has been a tremendous surge in online pharmacies where the patients can order medicines online with valid prescriptions and they are supplied to the consumer at their doorstep. But till now there are no government rules and regulations governing these e-pharmacies and they are rapidly mushrooming offering up to 25% discount on medicines with widespread advertisement in the media.

This has led to outcry from offline or brick and mortar pharmacy associations as there business is gradually getting eroded. There have been raids on a few online medicine offices and duplicate and spurious medicines have been recovered. The All India Association of Chemists and Druggists (AICOD) observed a day long All-India strike on 28th September 2018 to protest against the center's move to regulate online pharmacies. There concerns include sale of fake and spurious drugs, sale of habit forming drugs leading to drug abuse, threat to their business and loss of employment at offline pharmacies.

The Ministry of Health and Family Welfare has published new draft rules in June 2018 for information of all persons likely to be affected and notice was given that the said draft rules will be taken into consideration on or after 45 days after expiry of the date of publication. Some highlights of the draft rules are given below:

- These rules will be called the Drugs and Cosmetics (Amendment) Rules, 2018 and will come into force after their final publication in the official gazette.
- There will be only one central agency providing e-pharmacy license and regulating the same. They need not apply to state authorities.
- License will be issued for 3 years with a fee of 50,000 rupees.
- The retailer has to keep a record of the e-prescriptions of patients. They should run the pharmacy for at least 12 hours in a day 7 days in a week. They should have customer support and grievance redressal of all stakeholders with a registered pharmacist in place.
- The e-pharmacies should comply with provisions of Information Technology Act, 2000. They should maintain strict secrecy with regard to patient prescriptions with disclosure only to central and state governments as the case may be when required for public health purposes. Data shall not be sent to any third party or outside the country.
- They should comply with the provisions of Narcotic Drugs and Psychotropic Substances Act, 1955. The drugs covered under these acts should not be sold in e-pharmacies.
- To maintain quality of the drugs, updated information on all medicines, vendor lists and supply chain should be available on websites.
- They are not allowed to advertise any drugs over media such as radio or television.

According to a report published by The Federation of Indian Chambers of Commerce and Industry (FICCI), e-pharmacies are expected to account for 5–15% of pharma sales in our country. The new regulations definitely addresses quality issues, privacy issues, narcotic drug abuse issues and may actually herald a new beginning in sale of medicines in the healthcare industry.

Meanwhile a writ petition has been filed in Delhi High Court by South Chemists and Distributors association in October 2018 to close down so called 'illegal online pharmacies' and the court has issued notices to the center for responses. The matter has been posted for hearing on February 2019. So, the wait for regulation of e-pharmacies continues.

SUGGESTED READING

1. Drugs Control Department, Karnataka. (2012). [online] Available from: https://drugs.kar.nic.in/. [Accessed December, 2018].
2. Ficci.in-last mile access to medicines–a report.
3. Financial express online October, 2018,
4. Hindustan times online September, 2018.
5. Ministry of Health and Family Welfare. [online] Available from: https://mohfw.gov.in. [Accessed December, 2018].
6. Times of India online August, 2014.
7. Times of India online September, 2018.

Part B
Aesthetic Dermatology

CHAPTER 33

Special Features of an Aesthetic Patient

Namitha Chathra, Venkataram Mysore

INTRODUCTION

We live in an era of increasing focus on physical appearance and the pursuit of perfection, an idea that has been reinforced by the media and the marketing agencies peddling innumerable services and products catering to health and beauty.[1]

It comes as no surprise that there is an exponential upswing in the demand for cosmetic procedures.

According to the statistics released by the American Society of Plastic Surgeons in 2009, more than 12 million people underwent aesthetic surgery in 2008, which shows an increase of 63% since 2000 and a whopping increase of 234% since 1992. These numbers have raced to 14.6 million in 2012.[2]

India is ranked 4th in the world cosmetic procedures' market, according to a survey by The International Society of Aesthetic Plastic Surgery (ISAPS). The statistics reflect a rising demand of cosmetic procedures in the country owing to better affordability and growing aspirations of the middle class population to achieve a perfect body image.

Individuals seeking a cosmetic procedure are referred to as "clients" or "customers" as they are otherwise healthy. However, in this chapter, we prefer to use the term "patient" for those who seek advice.[3]

DEMOGRAPHY OF AN AESTHETIC PATIENT

Typically, patients desiring aesthetic treatment in an urban dermatology practice are middle-aged women, highly educated, and mostly employed with a high monthly income.[4]

According to the 2009 Consensus of American Academy of Cosmetic Surgery, the percentage of women patients seeking cosmetic surgery is around 85.7%.[5]

Although at present, women outnumber men in an aesthetician's clinic, an increase in the number of men seeking treatment is being observed. Furthermore, a recent study has shown that patients wanting aesthetic treatment showed higher quality of life, especially health-related quality of life, when compared with controls.[6]

Marital status or motherhood status has been proven to be an insignificant motivating factor for treatment.

Interestingly, a prospective demographic study opines that, majority of the patients interested in aesthetic treatment are either older or younger than their partners. Those who are the same age as their partners seldom seek cosmetic surgery and represent only 16.7% of all cosmetic surgery patients.[7]

In the patient population, both employment and education are significantly higher than the normal population, and this may reflect a greater ability to access the procedures, as also to take legal action when the demands are unmet.

CLASSIFICATION OF AESTHETIC PATIENTS

Sachidanand et al. have classified patients encountered by the aesthetic physician under following categories:
- *Professional need-based clients:* Professions involving the service sector, visual media, marketing, etc. make it necessary that individuals look their best all the time. However unrealistic, this pressure nudges the individuals toward the doorstep of an aesthetician's clinic.
  Most of the professional need-based clients are often specific in their approach and have a realistic expectation of the outcome. However, as they are constantly in the lime light, a procedure gone wrong can have deleterious effect on everyone involved.
- *Look good-feel good clients:* These are individuals who are self-assured about their appearance and visit an aesthetic physician only for specific indications that they want rectified, e.g. removal of Dermatosis Papulosa Nigra (DPNs) or acrochordons, Botox and fillers for wrinkles.
- *Emotional need-based clients:* Very often, aesthetic physicians do come across patients with poor self-esteem which may be due to a rough patch in life, e.g. midlife crises, neglected housewives, broken marriage. These patients tend to fixate on certain physical aberrations and seek treatment for the same hoping to rectify the low self-esteem. Such patients are heavily dependent on the doctor for emotional support and require constant hand holding.
- *Clients of special occasion:* The societal pressure to look impeccable on special occasions such as marriage, graduation, job interviews makes patients seek the help of an aesthetic physician. A cautious approach and avoidance of aggressive treatment is necessary here, as in the event of an adverse effect, most patients do not have adequate time to recuperate.
- *Clients with underlying psychiatric problems:* This is the population that requires utmost caution as they feel easily victimized and are perennially dissatisfied as the real problem is in their minds! It is necessary for the aesthetic physician to know the spectrum of presentation of patients with psychopathological conditions.[3]

UNDERSTANDING THE PSYCHOLOGY OF THE AESTHETIC PATIENT

Approximately 47.7% of the patients consulting for cosmetic procedures meet criteria for a mental disorder; commonest being body dysmorphic disorder, narcissistic personality disorder, and histrionic personality disorder.[8,9] Given this magnitude, it is essential for the aesthetic physician to be aware of the red flags suggestive of these disorders or traits. If psychopathology is suspected, it is necessary to refer to a mental health specialist prior to initiation of treatment, as these patients, when met with dissatisfaction, may seek legal action or even show violent behavior towards the treating physician.[10] A basic understanding of the characteristic features of these conditions and preoperative interview questions are valuable to dermatologic surgeons.

Body Dysmorphic Disorder or Body Image

Body dysmorphic disorder (BDD) is defined in the DSM-IVTR™ as "the preoccupation with an imagined or exaggerated defect in physical appearance."[11]

Body dysmorphic disorder is observed in 5–15% of aesthetic surgery patients.[12,13] More often, patients with body dysmorphic disorder (BDD) approach dermatologists or plastic surgeons for treatment rather than psychiatrists.[14]

Patients with BDD often have poor outcome following aesthetic procedures, which can result in a dangerous situation for the surgeon.[15]

In a survey of American Society for Aethetic Plastic Surgery Members, 40% of respondents indicated that a patient with BDD had threatened them. One-third of the respondents reported being threatened legally, 2% were threatened physically and 10% were threatened both legally and physically.[16]

Thus, it is imperative that an aesthetic physician be able to identify the red flags using simple screening tools. One such tool is the Body Dysmorphic Disorder Questionnaire-Dermatology Version, first put in use by Dufresne et al.[17] As a screening tool for body dysmorphic disorder in an aesthetic dermatology setting, was shown to have 100% sensitivity and 92.3% specificity.

Narcissistic Personality Disorder

As defined in the Diagnostic and Statistical Manual of *Mental Disorders-IV* (DSM-IV)-TR™, narcissistic personality disorder is "a pattern of grandiosity, need for admiration, and lack of empathy."[18]

Narcissistic personality disorder is observed in 25% of cosmetic surgery patients.[19] These patients may strive to perfect their bodies through aesthetic surgery in an attempt to garner attention, establish superiority, or to amplify a grandiose but unstable sense of self.[20,21]

To the aesthetic physician, narcissistic perfectionists are particularly challenging. It is nearly impossible to satisfy a vain, entitled, and grandiose patient demanding a perfect (and therefore unrealistic) outcome—even if the outcome obtained is objectively successful and aesthetically pleasing.

However, it should not be assumed that all cosmetic surgery patients intensely pursuing bodily perfection are afflicted with narcissistic personality disorder. A realistic and healthy view of themselves and others around them differentiates individuals with healthy personality from narcissists, who can be diagnosed with the help of criteria in the DSM-IV-TR™ for the diagnosis of narcissistic personality disorder.[18]

Histrionic Personality Disorder

As defined in the DSM-IV-TR™, histrionic personality disorder is "a pattern of excessive emotionality and attention seeking."[18] Histrionic personality disorder is observed in 9.7% of cosmetic surgery patients.[19] These patients tend to have unrealistic expectations when it comes to themselves and results of cosmetic procedures.[22]

Personality Trait: Neuroticism

Unlike temporary reactions, personality traits are relatively stable over time and a good indicator of patient's acceptance of results and coping mechanisms.[23] Individuals characterized by high neuroticism are generally more anxious, self-conscious, and susceptible to stress compared with individuals with low levels of neuroticism.[24] Furthermore, neuroticism has previously been found highly correlated to ineffective coping strategies such as hostile reactions and indecisiveness.[25]

Screening for Psychological Issues

A thorough medical and social history including psychiatric history is an absolute must. History of numerous procedures performed by many clinicians, particularly in those patients who were unsatisfied with the results, along with a history of lawsuits or violence towards previous physicians should be obtained in a delicate manner.[22,26]

Ritvo et al. has suggested to assess for the following features:
- History of noncompliance with previous treatment plans
- Use or misuse of emergency contact mechanisms with their physician
- Unreasonable or unreachable expectations of the proposed procedure
- Response to education or the informed consent process
- Spending money that is beyond their means.[22]

Malick et al. have described easy to implement interviewing techniques, to explore the possibility of the above-mentioned psychological disorders.[27] When there is suspicion of an underlying psychological illness, the patient should be referred to psychosocial counseling at an early stage. Without this step, initiating aesthetic treatment in such patients can result in legal and rarely violent complications for the doctor.

WHAT MAKES A PATIENT PURSUE LEGAL ACTION?

It is not always the surgical outcome of a procedure that propels a patient to seek legal action against a doctor. Most often, the patient's perception of his or her relationship with the doctor is the pivotal factor that determines whether or not legal action will be pursued. In aesthetic medicine, appearance of pigmentation or scarring and lack of results are the commonest causes for dissatisfaction among patients. Perceived lack of empathy, poor communication skills, hasty or absent counseling and improper handling during the procedure contributes further to patient's dissatisfaction.

Heightened expectations in a patient always leads to disappointment and therefore should be tuned to realistic level before the procedure. A cliché, but always to be remembered is the dictum "promise less, deliver more." The presence of a downtime, the risk of adverse effects such as pigmentation and instructions to avoid its occurrence have to be reinforced at every possible occasion.

Case Example 1

Complainant No.2 (Patient), who had some unwanted hair on her face and neck, approached OP-1 (X hospital) for permanent removal of the same through laser technology, which was to be done in four sittings, i.e. on 13.09.07, 24.10.07, 21.11.07 and 02.01.08 by Dr Y. Complainant No.1 (Patient's spouse) paid 1,000 rupees per sitting to Dr Y, who was later on transferred from the X Hospital, where after OP-2 (Dr Z), a private medical practitioner, was engaged on contractual basis by OP-1. It was alleged by the complainants that after treatment by OP-2, the condition of complainant No.2 started deteriorating within a few days after treatment on 17.09.08 when OP-2 used the laser machine at a frequency of 50, as recorded in the outpatient card. Her skin was burnt and scars appeared on her neck. It was alleged that complainant No.1 was planning to arrange the marriage of her daughter (complainant No.2) but under mental tension and due to disfigurement of her face, he chose to take her to the private clinic of OP-2 for her treatment. She attended the sitting of OP-2 on 03.12.08, 20.02.09 and 16.03.09 after paying huge fee, but there was no improvement. It was alleged that the scars on the face and neck of complainant No.2 were caused due to medical negligence and deficiency in service on the part of OPs, which ruined her personality and caused mental pain and agony besides financial loss, which prompted her to pursue legal action.

OP-1, in its reply, admitted that Dr Y was transferred from OP-1 Hospital and Dr Z (OP-2) was engaged on contract basis. It was denied that OP-2 had given treatment to complainant No.2 in four sittings on 14.03.2008, 21.05.2009, 16.07.2008 and 17.09.2008 as he joined the hospital on 13.06.2008 only. It was pleaded that the last sitting through laser technique was given to complainant No.2 by OP-2, a qualified Dermatologist and Specialist in Hair Removal Laser Treatment, having more than 6 years experience, and she was advised to follow some instructions and to visit OP-hospital for follow-up treatment on alternate days but she visited the hospital on 27.09.08 after 10 days of the last sitting. It was averred that complainant No.2 failed to follow the instructions like use of sun screen, to avoid the sun exposure, regular use of medicines, etc. and, thus, complainant No.2 was herself negligent. It was pleaded that the treatment was given by OP-2 to the complainant No.2 by adopting laser technology and using the laser machine on 50 J/cm^2 which was recommended in Savant's textbook of Dermatosurgery and Cosmetology on page 457. It was stated that the complainants never made any complaint regarding the treatment given by OP-2 and rather started taking treatment from the private clinic of OP-2. Remaining averments were denied being wrong. Pleading that there was no negligence on its part, prayer for dismissal of the complaint was made.

The complaint was dismissed by the district forum.[28]

In the above example, documentation and adherence to standard operating procedure turned the tide in favor of the doctor and the hospital.

WHAT TO DO WHEN SOMETHING GOES WRONG?

Mistakes can happen even with experienced hands and even the most skilled aesthetic physician can have a bad day!! In such a case, it is wiser to acknowledge the issue and politely listen to the patient's complaints. It is necessary to counsel the patient and instil confidence and trust, without resorting to panic. The patient should be offered treatment, free of cost, until resolution of the issue. Acknowledging may result in a temporary hassle, but will avoid the problem snowballing into a lawsuit. When a physician shows compassion, gentle authority and determination to solve the patient's problem, chances of the patient resorting to lawsuits are lesser. If the defense is weak, it is more sensible to attempt an out of the court settlement, to save the reputation as well as the economic loss due to the time spent in attending the courthouse.[29]

In India, as the medical profession has been brought under the provisions of the Consumer Protection Act, 1986, patients have an easy method of litigation. In the year 1995, the Supreme Court ruled that for any service charged by the doctor, he or she can be sued in consumer courts, only exemptions being the hospitals providing free service. A complaint can be filed in (I) the District Forum, when the value of services and compensation claimed is less than 20 lakh rupees; (II) before the State Commission, when the value of the goods or services and the compensation claimed is not more than 1 crore rupees; or (III) before the National Commission, when the value of the goods or services and the compensation exceeds more than 1 crore rupees.

An aggrieved patient can approach the consumer forum with a complaint of medical negligence within a period of 2 years from the date of cause of action. Once the complaint is filed, the forum decides whether the complaint is maintainable before it. If it is, it issues a notice to the doctor ("the opposite party"), who is required to reply within 30 days. This is called as a written statement or version of the opposite party. The complainant is then allowed to file a rejoinder. Cross-examination is permitted in appropriate cases and affidavits can be filed. Whenever necessary, the forum may summon an expert to give evidence. It is always advisable to seek the advice of a legal advisor.[30] A proper legal reply from the doctor's side can alleviate the need to visit the courthouse, in case the patient has the intension of mere monitory gain.[3]

STEPS TO PREVENT LEGAL ACTION

- *Selection of the patient:* The most crucial step of smooth aesthetic practice is choosing the right patient for a cosmetic procedure. First and foremost, it is necessary to assess whether the expectation of the patient from the desired procedure matches the expected outcome of the procedure. Patient's age, indication for the procedure, possible complications and ability to cope with it, psychological assessment are some other basic considerations before any procedure.

  Teenagers may bow down to peer pressure and seek cosmetic surgeries, sometimes with parental support. It is better to defer cosmetic procedures until the patient attains 18 years of age as teenagers are prone to changing ideas and may also possess difficult coping mechanisms. However, an exception can be made in medical issues such as gynecomastia or hirsutism secondary to PCOS, because the symptoms and signs of these conditions, if not treated, can be devastating to the teenager's self-esteem.[31]

  It is useful to review past history of cosmetic interventions, and avoid patients who have had numerous procedures performed by several practitioners, particularly those who are unsatisfied with the outcome. Any history of legal proceedings or threats or overt violence towards treating consultants should serve as a warning.

- *Counseling:* This stage is the cornerstone for building a healthy patient doctor relationship. Hence, adequate time should be assigned for counseling the patient, preferably in the presence of a trusted relative or friend.

  Counseling should involve detailed discussion about the advantages, disadvantages and adverse effects and the generally expected outcomes of the procedure chosen for the patient. Patient responsibilities such as postprocedure care, regular follow-up, fees payable, etc. should also be discussed. It is necessary to disclose important information, e.g. if a better or cheaper or safer procedure is available elsewhere.

- *Informed consent:* Informed consent, obtained in the presence of a witness, is vital for ethical and legal reasons, as well as to improve patient satisfaction and quality of care.[32,33] The consent form should include the indication, need for treatment, description of the procedure, other modalities of treatment, duration of treatment, number of sittings, expected outcome, pre and postprocedure instructions and possible side effects. The consent should be comprehensible and in the language, which the patient understands, and should always be taken prior to the procedure, by the treating doctor only. For patients in the teenage group (13–18 years), it is better to take the consent of both the minor and the parent. It should be borne in mind that a patient has the liberty to revoke his/her consent at any time. Failure to obtain informed consent is one of the commonest allegations in medical malpractice suits.[34]
- *Preprocedure work up:* Detailed medical history, relevant drug history, occupational and recreational history, and appropriate investigations have to be asked for and documented. Photographs in several angles and in good lighting have to be taken during preprocedural work up, and subsequently during every follow-up session.
- *Procedure:* Standard of care provided by the dermatologist should always be based on the best evidence available at the time.[35] He or she should obtain adequate training to perform a procedure, by attending specific workshops or conferences and hands on training. It is important to communicate with the patient during the procedure as she will be conscious throughout. Unnecessary, irrelevant communication with other doctors or support staff should be avoided in the patient's presence. Adequately trained assistants or nurse, referred to as "Physician extenders (PE)," are eligible to assist the dermatologist.[36] However, it should be remembered that, in the event of a complication, the vicarious responsibility lies with the dermatologist.
- *Postprocedure care:* Patient responsibilities following the procedure should be communicated clearly to the patient, with stress on the "downtime" of each procedure and need for follow-up. Patient should be advised to review without delay, in the event of an adverse event, and should be treated with empathy.
- *Documentation:* Complete and accurate documentation of the proceedings is as important as the verbal communication.[37] Medical records should contain documentation of counseling provided, operation notes, informed consent, advice given, follow-up visits and serial photographs. The operation notes should list all the steps, the materials used and also the date, time of the procedure and should contain the signatures of the treating dermatologist. It is considered as an important evidence in the court of law.

CURRENT SCENARIO IN AESTHETIC PRACTICE

The boom in demand for aesthetic procedures has led to the mushrooming of several beauty clinics or aesthetic centers across the nation, more so in urban areas. Some of these clinics hire qualified dermatologists on paper. However most often procedures are performed by untrained assistants in the absence of the dermatologist. These clinics do not adhere to even the basic standard of care and compromise on the safety of the patients as well as their staff. Unfortunately, the price paid is quite heavy, and is evident in the recently reported cases of HIV following "Vampire facials" in clients of a Spa in New Mexico.

According to the Drugs and Magic Remedies Act, 1954, doctors are prohibited from advertising in any media. Claims of guaranteed treatment by doctors amounts to violation of medical ethics under the Indian Medical Council (Professional conduct, Etiquette and Ethics) Regulations, 2002. However, these laws are restricted to medical professionals only and are not applicable to the beauty clinic or spas. The lack of regulations on such establishments has resulted in blatantly exaggerated advertisements that have roped in celebrities to lure gullible patients. Claims of guaranteed results, refunds on failed results are commonplace; some of them have gone to the extremes of unethical practice by offering freebies such as car, bumper prizes with every procedure. Patients, who are serenaded constantly with this brand of marketing, approach a dermatologist with expectations of similar outcome, ultimately turn disgruntled when faced with reality.

Case Example 2

Vimal (name changed), who was seeking treatment for baldness, spotted an advertisement by X beauty clinic promising complete hair regrowth after 24 months of treatment and approached them for treatment. When he did not notice any regrowth after 20 months of treatment and payment of 198,628 rupees as nonrefundable fee, he demanded a refund from the facility. On being denied of the refund, Vimal lodged a complaint with Bangalore 4th Additional District Consumer Disputes Redressal Forum, seeking compensation. After a 2 year litigation process, the court was of the opinion that the facility should have given an expert opinion on whether he would respond to treatment or not before accepting the money. The forum ordered X clinic to refund the amount with interest to the complainant.

KEY MESSAGES

- Weighing in the personality traits and psychological evaluation of the patients seeking aesthetic procedure is important.
- It is better to avoid patients who have had numerous procedures performed by many practitioners.
- Documentation of communication and communication of documentation is an absolute necessity.
- It is wiser to promise less and deliver more.
- In case of adverse effects, empathizing and treatment of the complication until resolution goes a long way in avoiding a lawsuit.

REFERENCES

1. Gangestad SW, Scheyd GJ. The evolution of human physical attractiveness. Ann Rev Anthropology. 2005;34:523-48.
2. Honigman R, Castle DJ. Aging and cosmetic enhancement. Clin Interv Aging. 2006;1(2):115-9.
3. Sacchidanand SA, Bhat S. Safe practice of cosmetic dermatology: avoiding legal tangles. J Cutan Aesthet Surg. 2012;5(3):170-5.
4. Alharethy SE. Trends and demographic characteristics of Saudi cosmetic surgery patients. Saudi Med J. 2017;38(7):738-41.
5. American Academy of Cosmetic Surgery. American Academy of Cosmetic Surgery 2009 Procedural Census. [online] Available from: http://www.cosmeticsurgery.org/media/2009_full_report.pdf/. [Accessed December, 2018].
6. Scharschmidt D, Mirastschijski U, Preiss S, et al. Body image, personality traits, and quality of life in botulinum toxin A and dermal filler patients. Aesthetic Plast Surg. 2018;42(4):1119-25.
7. Schlessinger J, Schlessinger D, Schlessinger B. Prospective demographic study of cosmetic surgery patients. J Clin Aesthet Dermatol. 2010;3(11):30-5.

8. Ishigooka J, Iwao M, Suzuki M. Demographic features of patients seeking cosmetic surgery. Psychiatry Clin Neurosci. 1998:52(3):283-7.
9. Ritvo EC, Melnick I, Marcus GR, et al. Psychiatric conditions in cosmetic surgery patients. Facial Plastic Surg. 2006:22(3):194-7.
10. Phillips KA, McElroy SL, Lion JR. Body dysmorphic disorder in cosmetic surgery patients [letter]. Plast Reconstr Surg. 1992:90:333-4.
11. França K, Roccia MG, Castillo D, et al. Body dysmorphic disorder: history and curiosities. Wien Med Wochenschr. 2017;167(Suppl 1):5-7.
12. Wilson JB, Arpey CJ. Body dysmorphic disorder: suggestions for detection and treatment in a surgical dermatology practice. Dermatol Surg. 2004:30(11):1391-9.
13. Veale D. Body dysmorphic disorder. Postgrad Med J. 2004:80(940):67-71.
14. Koblenzer CS. The broken mirror: dysmorphic syndrome in the dermatologist's practice. Fitz J Clin Dermatol. 1994;14-9.
15. Sweis IE, Spitz J, Barry DR Jr, et al. A review of body dysmorphic disorder in aesthetic surgery patients and the legal implications. Aesthetic Plast Surg. 2017;41(4):949-54.
16. Sarwer DB. Awareness and identification of body dysmorphic disorder by aesthetic surgeons: results of a survey of american society for aesthetic plastic surgery members. Aesthetic Surg J. 2002;22(6):531-5.
17. Dufresne RG, Phillips KA, Vittorio CC, et al. A screening questionnaire for body dysmorphic disorder in a cosmetic surgery practice. Dermatol Surg. 2001:27(5):457-62.
18. American Psychiatric Association. Diagnostic and Statistical Manual of Mental Disorders, 4th edition. Text Revision. Washington: American Psychiatric Association; 2000.
19. Napoleon A. The presentation of personalities in plastic surgery. Ann Plast Surg. 1993:31(3):193-208.
20. Raskin R, Terry H. A principle-components analysis of the Narcissistic Personality Inventory and further evidence of its construct validity. J Pers Soc Psychol. 1988;54(5):890-902.
21. Hewitt P, Flett GL. Perfectionism in the self and social contexts: conceptualization, assessment, and association with psychopathology. J Pers Soc Psychol. 1991;60(3):456-70.
22. Ritvo EC, Melnick I, Marcus GR, et al. Psychiatric conditions in cosmetic surgery patients. Facial Plastic Surg. 2006:22(3):194-7.
23. Bazana P, Stelmack R, Stelmack R, et al. Stability of personality across the life span: a meta-analysis. In: On the Psychobiology of Personality: Essays in Honor of Marvin Zuckerman. New York: Elsevier Science; 2004. pp. 113-44.
24. Costa PT Jr, McCrae RR. Neuroticism, somatic complaints, and disease: is the bark worse than the bite? J Pers. 1987;55(2):299-316.
25. McCrae RR, Costa PT. Personality, coping, and coping effectiveness in an adult sample. J Pers. 1986;54(2):385-404.
26. Castle DJ, Honigman RJ, Phillips KA. Does cosmetic surgery improve psychosocial wellbeing? Med J Aust. 2002:176(12):601-4.
27. Malick F, Howard J, KOO J. Understanding the psychology of the cosmetic patients. Dermatol Ther. 2008;21(1):47-53.
28. Jitender Kumar Joshi. vs General Hospital on 13 September, 2011 Indiankanoon.
29. Hagihara A, Hamasaki T, Abe T. Association between physician explanatory behaviors and substandard care in adjudicated cases in Japan. Int J Gen Med. 2011;4:289-97.
30. Sirur SP. Consumer courts. Indian J Dermatol Venereol Leprol. 2004;70(1):52-3.
31. Singh K. Cosmetic surgery in teenagers: to do or not to do. J Cutan Aesthet Surg. 2015;8(1):57-9.
32. Goldberg DJ. Legal issues in dermatology: Informed consent, complications and medical malpractice. Semin Cutan Med Surg. 2007;26(1):2-5.
33. Brezis M, Israel S, Weinstein-Birenshtock A, et al. Quality of informed consent for invasive procedures. Int J Qual Health Care. 2008;20(5):352-7.
34. Rathor MY, Rani MF, Shah AM, et al. Informed consent: A socio-legal study. Med J Malaysia. 2011;66(5):423-8.
35. Gittler G, Goldstein EJ. The standard of care is not so standard. Clin Infect Dis. 1997;24(2):254-7.
36. Leshin B, Hauser D. The role of a physician assistant in dermatologic surgery. Dermatol Surg. 1999;25(2):148-50.
37. Arndt M. Physician's errors-legal advice for physicians accused of malpractice. MMW Fortschr Med. 2004;146(5):25-9.

CHAPTER 34

Medicolegal Aspects of Hair Practice

Manjot Marwah, Venkataram Mysore

KEY POINTS

- Hair transplant has become popular as it has become safer and widely available with the advent of follicular unit extraction (FUE).
- Misleading aggressive advertisements in this field are the root cause of litigation cases.
- Issues like duties of a hair transplant surgeon, preoperative counseling, informed consent, standard of care, confidentiality of medical data, medical negligence, and civil, criminal and professional liabilities need proper attention.
- The importance of good doctor-patient relationship and communication skills need to be emphasized.
- Indemnity insurance is a must for any hair transplant surgeon.

INTRODUCTION

Medicolegal situations arise in every medical practice, but are more likely in esthetic practice. It is also true of hair practice, wherein expectations are high, fees are also high, and there are high-voltage advertisements on all forms of media.

Hair transplantation (HT) is a cosmetic surgery. Hence there is no need or urgency to do the procedure and the patient is in complete well-being before surgery. In such cases, if there is even a minor complication or unsatisfactory results, the patient regards this as a point to complain, since he was better off without the surgery. Despite knowing that hair transplant is a surgery and results are not guaranteed, there is a lot of pressure on the surgeon to deliver his best results in every patient to avoid such complaints. Patients nowadays are increasingly aware about their consumers' rights too. Unrealistic expectations often result in dissatisfaction among them which may end up in litigation. The enactment of the Consumer Protection Act (CPA)[1] in 1986 and its subsequent interpretation by the Supreme Court that it applies to medical practice[2] as well has changed the attitude of patients towards doctors. Consumer forums provide a quick, simple and cheap pathway for the aggrieved clients to claim compensation for deficient service in place of prolonged, cumbersome and expensive civil or criminal court procedures.[1]

Below is a list of a few of the reasons why hair transplant practice has a higher potential for medico legal situations:

- It is a cosmetic surgery hence there are always high expectations.
- Zero tolerance for complications since it is a cosmetic surgery.
- Exaggerated and often misleading advertising highlight only the best results. Terms such as permanent results or scarless surgery or unlimited grafts or guaranteed results are partly the root cause of most litigation cases in HT.
- Surgeons often take consultation via email or phone and this may lead to a wrong diagnosis or estimation of grafts.
- Few clinics employ counselors from non-medical field to counsel the patients, suggest the type of surgery they should go for and give an estimate on number of graphs.
- Entire surgery is not done by the doctor himself and it is a team work between the doctor and his technicians. If the patient is not explained this during the counseling, then he is bound to accuse the doctor of negligence for not doing the entire surgery himself. While there is some work that can be safely delegated to assistants, in many clinics most of the work is delegated to the assistants, which is unacceptable.
- Medical tourism is common in HT; many times the patient is travelling the next day and not available to follow-up. There are also some patients who come by online consultation and hence patient-doctor relationship may be lacking. Hence avoidable complications become bigger issues due to lack of follow-ups and check-ups.
- Results are not instant, they are seen over a period of 1 year and an impatient patient may feel cheated to see inadequate growth before 1 year.
- Cost of hair transplant is not covered by any insurance agencies.
- These patients are also internet savvy and active on social media—there are forums for such patients where in every case may be discussed. Dissaftisfied patients may also give bad reviews on online sites.
- Hair transplantation is an evolving field. New techniques and technologies get introduced, and some time is needed before evidence becomes available for such treatments. Surgeons often try these procedures, without any evidence.
- Hair transplantation like all surgeries is both a science and an art. Techniques vary and often there is no one single technique. Such wide variations make it difficult for assessment. Several controversies exist regarding utility of several areas such as platelet-rich plasma (PRP), laser, FUE versus follicular unit transplants (FUT), stem cells, etc. Guidelines are therefore lacking. Indian Association of Dermatologists, Venerologists and Leprologists (IADVL) formulated standard guidelines of care in HT (Box 1).[3]
- This area is perceived to be simple and yielding financially. Hence doctors of all specialties, dentists have ventured in to these. MCI has not taken any stand on this issue. In a Right to Information (RTI), asking who can do hair transplant? Medical Council of India (MCI) has mentioned that hair transplant is included in the syllabus

> **BOX 1:** Guidelines for hair transplantation by Indian Association of Dermatologists, Venerologists and Leprologists (IADVL).
>
> - *Patient selection:* Patterned hair loss, with good donor area and reasonable expectations is the ideal patient for hair transplantation. Patients with early alopecia or extreme cases with Norwood grade VI or VII with poor density and patients with unrealistic expectations should be dealt with caution.
> - *Anesthesia:* 2% lignocaine with adrenaline is generally used for anesthesia; tumescent technique is preferred. Bupivacaine may be used.
> - *Donor dissection:* Strip dissection in follicular unit transplantation (FUT) should be done by a single blade for donor area. Stereomicroscopic dissection is recommended for dissection of hair units in FUT.
> - *Recipient insertion:* Graft placement can be done by stick and place, premade slits or via implanters depending on the operating surgeon's choice.
> - *Density:* Minimum density of 35–45 grafts/cm² is recommended. Results depend on donor characteristics, technique used and individual skills of the surgeon.

> **BOX 2:** Guidelines for prescribing finasteride.
>
> - Patient information brochures with proper counseling regarding the efficacy and side effects needs to be provided before starting finasteride.
> - The patients should contact the doctor for any advice, should he or she experience a side effect.
> - The intake of the drug is voluntary and cannot be forced by the doctor. If they choose to avoid the drug, they should be prepared for further progression of baldness.
> - The treating physician should provide full information about the drug in order to enable the patient to make an informed decision.
> - It is better to avoid the drug in patients who have had history of oligospermia or infertility or in an anxious patient worrying about its sexual adverse effects.
> - In apprehensive patients, it is worthwhile to consider administration of lower or staggered doses of the drug to enhance patient compliance.

of plastic surgeons and it did not take any clear stand on who can and who cannot do transplants. The International Society of Hair Restoration Surgery (ISHRS) Guidelines mention that, HT can be performed by any licensed physician in the field of medicine and with adequate training in hair restoration. Association of Hair Restoration Surgeons (AHRS) India has taken a much stronger stand and specified the specialties that can perform HT. In October 2015 AHRS India resolved that the only specialties eligible to become members of AHRS India would be MCh. Plastic Surgery, MD or postgraduate in Dermatology, MS or postgraduate in ENT surgery and MS General Surgery.[4]

- Androgenetic alopecia (AGA) is an evolving condition with progressive hair loss; so while grafted hairs may be permanent, existing hairs are lost, and this may disturb the patient unless patient is informed well and documented properly about need for medical treatment.
- The options in medical therapy for AGA are limited and need to be taken for a long time. Finasteride has special issues of perceived side effects and patients are reluctant to take it, leading to future hair loss. IADVL has released specific guidelines for finasteride consumption (Box 2).[5] United States Food and Drug Administration (US-FDA) has stated separate guidelines for healthcare professionals and patients. The FDA states that there is no clear cause and effect relationship between finasteride and the sexual adverse events may continue in some patients after stopping the drug. Healthcare professionals should consider this information when deciding best treatment options. It has also urged patients not to discontinue the medication without first consulting the healthcare provider and

- discuss its pros and cons with the healthcare provider before starting treatment.
- Patients before and after photos are often displayed on websites without specific permission from patients.
- Several issues can come up during counseling such as age of patient, patient with keloids, patient with medical problems and patient on blood thinners, HT for medical conditions such as pseudopelade, vitiligo, and psoriasis. These depend on individual judgments.
- Use of the word "stem cells" for hair regeneration has been used widely in recent years to entice patients into getting treatments without any evidence or scientific bases. The National Guidelines for Stem Cell Research prohibit stem cell therapy and consider its use for any other purpose outside the domain of clinical trial unethical in India. As per the National Guidelines for Stem Cell Research (2013), at present, there are no approved indications for stem cell therapy other than the hematopoietic stem cell transplantation (HSCT) for hematological disorders. AHRS India also condemns the use of the word "stem cells" for any marketing or promotional activity.[6]
- Artificial hair fibers: USFDA has banned the use of artificial hair fibers since 1983, while ISHRS has refused to endorse them and left the approval on the regulatory authorities of the respective countries. Despite the recent advances in artificial fibers, they have been known to cause several side effects and it is therefore controversial to use them.[7]

Given these liability risks in hair restoration practice, few suggested points for safe practice include:

- Stick to procedures or methods or options that have evidence.
- With newer procedures, make sure patient is aware that this is a new treatment yet to garner full evidence, and document the same. Read the chapter on off-label treatments for more details.
- Avoid assurances that are not possible to deliver.
- Highlight what the treatment cannot achieve, e.g. permanent restoration, original density, total coverage to entire area.
- Be realistic in promoting through advertisements.
- Maintain a good doctor patient relationship.
- Consult the patient personally before surgery explaining the entire procedure, sequence, progress and complications of the surgery.
- Take detailed history and preoperative tests before the surgery.
- Have a detailed and thorough consent form (Box 3).[3]
- Follow evidence-based medicine and stick to the guidelines provided by IADVL, AHRS India or ISHRS to avoid legalities.

> **BOX 3:** Salient points to be mentioned in a hair transplant consent.
>
> - Discussion on the process of pattern hair loss, and different management options available.
> - Detailed explanation about the surgical procedure, possible postoperative complications.
> - Specific instructions that results would be seen only after 8–9 months.
> - In young specific instruction that the existing hair may be lost in future and that continued drug therapy is necessary to preserve existing hair.
> - Patients should not expect to get the same amount of hair that they had before balding.
> - Patients should understand that hair transplantation is a cosmetic procedure and will not affect the underlying process of baldness, which may continue in future.
> - Any allergies or medical condition that the patient may have should be recorded.

- Maintain regular follow-ups.
- If there is any area without adequate growth, provide a touch up session.

One of the highly debated aspects is the role of technicians in HT. It is generally agreed that technicians and assistants should not do any procedure which involves injury to patient. Technicians cannot therefore perform; scoring in FUE. Strip excision in FUT, and recipient site creation. These should be done only by the physician.

However, a technician or assistant can do the following:
1. Extraction after scoring in FUE.
2. Arranging grafts.
3. Grafts insertion.

Below are examples and discussion of few cases which had legal issues.

CASE 1: LACK OF IMPROVEMENT

In 2007, a student from was being treated by the city-based treatment center for falling hair. He alleged that he met Dr ABC at their Chandigarh center of XYZ clinics, who along with other staff of the clinic and assured him that after availing the treatment for 1 year, his problem would be solved. Under the "Gold plan" (1 year), the clinic asked for 5,900 rupees which he paid. However, after 1 year of treatment he noticed no change as his problem persisted compelling him to knock at the consumer forum's doors. In his complaint, he maintained that he went to the clinic after reading advertisements in newspapers claiming that the doctors of the Opposite Party were specifically trained in Trichology by international experts and had successfully treated over 100,000 hair patients by using cutting edge technology like video Microscopy. Patient continued treatment for 2 years and paid additional amount of 6,500 rupees and 6,700 rupees at two separate occasions. Throughout the treatment, patient kept complaining that there was no improvement and he kept losing hair on his eyebrows also and he suffered from depression for the same. He was also given "laser comb," but no improvement was seen. He asked for a refund from the clinic, which he was declined. Hence a case was filed with the consumer court in view of misleading advertisements, mental agony, medical negligence and unfair trade practices. The patient filed a complaint under the Consumer Protection Act, 1986 directing the Opposite Party to refund 18,700 rupees spent on treatment; pay 50,000 rupees spent on special diet; 4,00,000 rupees as compensation for harassment and mental agony, 11,000 rupees towards Counsel fee and 3,300 rupees as cost of litigation, was filed.

After both the parties submitted their evidence, the district forum concluded that the opposition party (clinic) was responsible for the misleading advertisements. The doctors available at the clinic were homeopaths and had no training in trichology. It is against the law for a homeopathy doctor to give advertisements itself. Secondly, it was ruled after an expert opinion that the use of a laser comb is out of the scope of homeopathy. The court accepted the complaint of the complainant (patient) partly and directed the opposition party (clinic) to refund the amount of 18,700 rupees given by the complainant to it. It shall also make payment of a compensation of 100,000 rupees to the complainant for mental agony and harassment on account of unfair trade practice and deficiency in service. It shall also make payment of litigation expenses of 11,000 rupees to the complainant.

The case was instantly appealed by the opposition party (clinic) with an affidavit from the owner of the chain of clinics claiming that the doctor was trained in trichology, however this was regarded insufficient evidence and the appeal was dismissed.[8]

Discussion

- Adequate training and education in trichology is a must before starting practice. Differentiate between alopecia totalis and androgenic alopecia is a part of syllabus in dermatology, hence ideally cases of alopecia should only be treated by a dermatologist.
- In the above case, the compliant escalated because of false advertising. Making false claims to lure patients should be avoided. Using words like "permanent" and "cure" in terms of hair fall are medically incorrect. There is no permanent cure for a process that may be physiological or pathological.
- During counseling, the terms and conditions need to be explained in detail to the patient. Ideally, the patient should be given time of a day or two and then follow-up for starting treatment. All treatments which are given as a package should have a consent, informing in detail about each type of medicine and procedure to avoid conflict.
- Counseling should be done by a doctor, not a counselor.
- It is important to preserve medical records for at least 3 years post-treatment and in case of settlement cases, till the case it settled. These records are helpful in evidence to show that adequate care was taken and there was no negligence.[9] However, the Consumer Court has the power to allow the consumer to file a case even after several years in special cases. Ministry of Health and Family Welfare, Government of India has published standards for Electronic Medical Records.[10]

CASE 2: ALLERGIC REACTION AND FOLLICULITIS AS A COMPLICATION

A television script writer approached a clinic for this receding hairline after seeing their advertisements, and underwent a hair transplant surgery there. The complaint stated that the doctor had assured him that the procedure would be carried out by highly skilled and learned medical practitioners and surgeon. But the entire procedure was carried out by an assistant and a nurse and there were no certified doctors present in the operation theatre during the surgery. The script writer filed a case with the civil court claiming that his hair transplant went "horribly wrong" as he started suffering from frequent allergic reactions and folliculitis on his face and beard postsurgery. This folliculitis was not controlled by antibiotics and he was forced to depend on steroids. He alleged offences of fraud, cheating, criminal breach of trust under the Indian Penal Code, and offences under the Drugs and Magic Remedies (Objectionable Advertisements) Act and the Maharashtra Medical Practitioners Act.

In defense, the accused doctor defended that the allergies were not caused by the surgery and that the patient has allergic tendencies, which he should get checked, but he refused to do so. Also, he stated that they always perform such surgeries in the presence of a plastic surgeon and a dermatologist. In this case the metropolitan magistrate observed that serious allegations of cognizable offences were made, hence they directed the police to carry out a preliminary inquiry into the incident.

The proceedings of this case are unknown as there is no record of the police report or outcome available by any source. It is not known if there was an out of court settlement or the case was withdrawn.[11]

Discussion

- Folliculitis can occur after any hair transplant but excessive folliculitis may occur due to the surgeon's errors such as

excessive transection rate, burrowing of grafts, deep implantation, and incorrect slits made in implantation, etc. Always have a detailed consent form, mentioning the side effects in detail and giving the patient adequate explanation for them. Special care has to be taken during beard extraction, to use smaller punch sizes and to extract with proper training so that the transection rate is low.
- It is important to have a CCTV in the operation theatre (OT) to avoid false claims that the surgery was done by technicians. Anesthesia, extraction, designing hairline and making slits are the job of the surgeon. The technicians are only supposed to implant. As per Indian legislation, absence of the doctor from the operation theatre in defined as medical negligence. This is a very important issue that needs to be addressed by every hair restoration association or it could increase the number of litigation cases considerably. So ideally a doctor has to be present even during implantation in the OT.
- Consent form should mention what is the role of doctor and what is that of technician. Guidelines by IADVL and AHRS India clearly mention all the steps that can be performed by the doctor and those that can be done by the assistants. The surgeon is responsible for marking the hairline, giving anesthesia, making the slits, implanting if it is with an implanter, and extraction of grafts. Assistants can only dissect, pick up, arrange and implant the grafts and help keep them hydrated.[4]
- If negligence occurs on behalf of his staff or technicians, the doctor is held responsible. Hence trusted trained staff is a must for HT.

CASE 3: DEATH AFTER HAIR TRANSPLANTATION

Case 3A

A medical student underwent a hair transplant surgery at a clinic in Chennai and died 2 days later. The family did not file any police compliant and no case was registered but the case came to light 1 week after the incident when his batch-mates urged the Directorate of Medical Education to look into the matter. Case was forwarded to the Director of Medical Services and the center was sealed. The body was exhumed and after a postmortem analysis, doctors concluded he could have died of toxic shock syndrome or septic shock or anaphylactic syndrome. The operating clinic was registered as a saloon and did not have license to perform the surgery. They had license for hair styling and hair cutting only. There were two operating doctors performing the surgery, one of them was an MBBS graduated from China and the other an anesthetist and he was present for only part of the surgery, not the entire surgery. There was no infrastructure to deal with any emergency complications in the clinic. The patient had started developing discomfort during the evening of the surgery and he was taken to the operating anesthetist in a private clinic set up elsewhere, the anesthetist examined him and reported it as a routine case and gave symptomatic care. After this the patient returned to his village and brought to a tertiary care medical intensive care unit (ICU) on the 2nd day with multisystem failure, where he died.

Two days post the death, suspecting foul play by the hair transplant center, a police complaint was lodged. The police, however, refused to file the complaint due to lack of evidence since the body was buried without a postmortem. Hence the body was exhumed 2 days later and a postmortem was conducted. The postmortem report has not been released to the public. The case was then highlighted to the Director of Medical Sciences, who took strict action and sealed the center immediately. The drug controller has recovered a huge stock of medicines kept without license.

The state medical council has sent a notice to the owners while the health department is recommending using a tough law to regulate such centers dealing with surgical procedures masquerading as beauty parlors, spas and hair treatment centers.

Two years after the incident, the State Medical Council suspended the licenses of the anesthetist and operating doctor involved for 6 months and 1 year respectively.[12]

Discussion

- Multiple factors went wrong in this case, starting with the licensing of the premises. Surgeries cannot be performed in saloons. Adequate sterilization and crash cart set-up is a must. Licensing of the doctors is equally important. A licensed registered doctor has to be present throughout the surgery.
- No test dose for anesthesia was given. This step is a must in cases that have never had any prior injections of local anesthesia. A trained doctor in HT will be aware of the maximum dose of lignocaine and shall not administer above it. Untrained doctors can do this mistake in Mega/Giga session cases.
- Anaphylaxis to lignocaine may arise in any patient however, it is important to identify it. If a patient complaints of discomfort postsurgery, it is better to record all the findings and tests, to address why the discomfort happened. Continuous monitoring is a must during surgery too. It was an anesthetist doctor who examined the patient during his discomfort, this was the best case scenario and an escalating anaphylactic shock could have been picked up. This amounts to medical negligence if not identified by the doctors.
- Patients residing far away from the operating center, should be informed priorly the importance of visiting the next day. Well-being of the patient can be documented the next day too.

Case 3B

A similar case was reported in Pakistan, where an Army captain died within a few hours after hair transplant done at a private clinic in Lahore. He failed to follow-up when he developed uneasiness and died at his residence at night. The case was not highlighted enough in media and most of the scientific facts are unknown. The entire staff of the center was reported as absconding and unavailable for comment.

CASE 4: "BAD JOB" OF HAIR TRANSPLANTATION

A diabetic patient entered into an agreement with a clinic to transplant 6,000 strands of hair for 140,000 rupees. Following the first transplant of 500 strands on day 1, the patient suffered from headaches, giddiness, and diarrhea and wanted to discontinue the treatment. However, as he had already paid for the transplant, he underwent a second session on day 2, which lead to boils on his head and left him unsteady on his legs. He later approached the Consumer Disputes Redressal Forum seeking compensation and refund of total amount paid for surgery.

The forum observed that the consumer suffered and was put through unnecessary medical expenditure entirely on account of complete negligence and gross deficiency in service. They stated that the clinic's "entire conduct in the matter so far has been totally unethical, unprofessional, highly casual and unconcerned and regardless towards complainant and his health." The forum has directed the clinic to pay a compensation of 1 lakh rupees for harming a consumer with "illegal activities of hair transplant." The clinic has also been directed to refund the consumer 95,000 rupees for the pending 5,000 hairs that were not transplanted and pay 20,000 rupees towards cost of litigation. The Directorate of Health Services informed that the clinic has not taken any license to operate under the State Medical Practitioner's Act, 2004 and Rules 2011, as a health clinic.[13]

Discussion

The case filed in this case was for unethical and unprofessional practice leading to unnecessary medical expenses. In this case the doctor or center failed to give standard care to the patient. There is no defined "standard of care" which is universally applicable or acceptable. In this regard is the standards established by a professional body of similarly qualified esthetic surgeons in a country or region is regarding as the standard of care. Other resources are also helpful are textbooks, peer-reviewed journals, evidence-based guidelines, etc. Generally, when the medical care is alleged to be substandard by a client, courts take the opinion of expert esthetic surgeons. But, the stand taken by such an expert is not binding on the court. Court will see whether the deposition of the expert is logical, reasonable and responsible before taking a decision as to its acceptability.[10,14,15]

CASE 5: COMPLICATIONS IN A DIABETIC PATIENT

A diabetic patient lost his eye after hair transplant surgery. According to the patient no preoperative tests were done before the surgery to determine his blood sugar levels. The State Medical Council claimed that the doctor is an MBBS and does not have the qualification to perform hair transplant surgery, however Medical Council of India does not give clear definitions that who is certified to do hair transplants. The doctor claimed he is a member of ISHRS and Asian Association of Hair Restoration Surgeons. The State Medical Council has suspended the registration of the doctor for 2 years and debarred him from practicing hair transplant surgery. The doctor filed an appeal in the Medical Council of India stating that he was not at fault and obtained a stay against the order.[16]

Discussion

Infections in a diabetic patient can always occur. The doctor could have protected himself by getting the preoperative tests done beforehand. Who can perform hair transplant needs to be defined by the Medical council. There are many dentists who are performing hair transplant now. Without clarity, such instances will keep growing. The Associations of Hair Restoration Surgeons India does not recognize dentists as hair transplant surgeons.[4]

CASE 6: SURGERY DONE BY DENTIST AND CLINIC NOT REGISTERED

An ex-Army man underwent an FUE procedure for 136,800 rupees at a hair transplant clinic. The clinic had included the service tax amount in the above said fee. The patient during the surgery realized that the surgery was being done by untrained staff and not a doctor. Postsurgery the patient was forced to buy medication worth 20,000 rupees from the center itself which would felicitate his hair growth. Postsurgery, the patient filed a RTI to the Assistant Commissioner of Tax Commissionerate Division, seeking information on service tax payment by the clinic and was told that no service tax was paid on any invoice raised. Also a second RTI was filled to the District Health and Family Welfare Officer and was sent a reply that the clinic was not registered under the State Medical Establishment Act.

The patient then filed a complaint with the consumer forum against the clinic. It includes:
- For unfair trade practice as it was not registered with the State Medical Establishment Act and collecting service tax without filing it.
- Untrained professionals were doing the surgery.
- Furthermore there was failure to transplant 6,000 follicles as claimed, which amounts to deficiency in service as defined by Consumer Protection Act.
- The medicines that were forced to purchase inside the clinic were available outside at a cheaper price, hence this amounted to monopolistic trade practice.

The clinic (opposition party) replied to the notice with each of the complaints as false. They stated that:
- They agree that the clinic was liable to be registered under the State Medical Act and that had applied for the same and everything about the process was completed from their side. They also had been filing service tax under the health clubs, spa and saloon category.
- They submitted the degree of the doctor operating. She was a Bachelor of Dental Surgery (BDS).
- They stated that they had never claimed 6,000 grafts will be implanted and it was mentioned that the number of grafts depends on the donor area and accordingly 1,500–2,000 grafts were implanted.
- They claimed that the medicines advised were supplements specially made by Zode pharmaceuticals and should not be mistaken with par with the medicines available in the market as they are far superior.

The court finally ruled that, the opposition party (clinic) had misled the complainant by advertisements by unskilled ordinary person, treated by a dentist and was treated by unscientific use of medicine. Complainant suffered from financial loss and mental agony and bodily pain due to unprofessional treatment given by untrained staff. The court stated that the complainant deserves the relief as sought in the complaint due to unfair trade practices and deficient service. The court directed the opposition party to refund the entire amount of 136,800 rupees and also 20,000 rupees paid for medicines. Furthermore, opposition was asked to pay 200,000 rupees towards unfair trade practice, 150,000 rupees towards deficiency in service and 100,000 towards mental agony and 5,000 rupees towards cost of proceedings. A total said amount of 455,000 Rupees to be paid with 18% interest from the date of filling till the date of payment. Failure to comply with the judgment, the opposition shall face imprisonment.[17]

Discussion

There are many aspects of the case that went wrong. The clinic did everything possible to avoid the harsh judgment but failed because the type of practice was wrong. Firstly a dentist cannot do HT, secondly there was no registration with the State Clinical Establishment Act, this would amount to unfair trade practice and is an unavoidable situation to get out of. It is always better to be transparent about the number of grafts being transplanted to maintain a fair practice. There should be a justified scientific reason behind prescribing medicines postsurgery. It is best to stick to FDA approved medications to avoid legal issues.

CASE 7: FALSE CLAIMS IN ADVERTISING

The Consumer Complaints Council (CCC) of the Advertising Standards Council of India (ASCI) has banned as many as 100 advertisements out of 152 complaints it received across segments during November 2016. Out of 100 advertisements against which complaints were upheld, 43 belonged to the healthcare category.

One of India's well-renowned multicenter hair clinics came under this scanner. Points objected in the advertisements were: "Grow your own hair for just Re.1", "Fight 5 signs of hair thinning for just Re.1," "Worlds first hair thinning treatment with plant stem cells" and "Anagrow is a treatment for hair volume and density. It does not grow new hair."[18]

Discussion

- The advertisement's claim was prominently displayed in the headline as "Grow your own hair for just Re.1," with a visual of 1 rupee coin. It was concluded that the claim offering the service at 1 rupee is misleading by ambiguity.
- "Fight 5 signs of hair thinning for just Re. 1," after review it was concluded that it is misleading to say that five signs of hair thinning are scanty hair, decreased volume, lack of hair growth, decreased density and hair loss.
- "World's first hair thinning treatment with plant stem cells," was not substantiated with supporting evidence and with comparative data versus other hair thinning treatments available worldwide, and is misleading by exaggeration.
- Further, it was also concluded that the claim, "Anagrow is a treatment for hair volume and density. It does not grow new hair," was inadequately substantiated, and is misleading by ambiguity.

CASE 8: MULTISESSION HAIR TRANSPLANTATION

In or around February 1989, Boggs contacted Bosley Clinic regarding treatment for his hair loss problem. Boggs claims that, during his initial consultation, it was represented that only two surgical treatments would be required to correct his problem. However, after the two surgical procedures on February 21, 1989, and July 17, 1989, Boggs claims that his scalp was badly scarred and his hair density was not as promised. Boggs returned to Bosley and claims he was told that one more surgical "touch-up" procedure was required. Following surgery on April 25, 1990, however, he still had not achieved the promised results. Between June 18, 1990, and November 11, 1993, five more surgical procedures were performed by Bosley physicians. Boggs claims that, prior to each such surgery he was informed that only one more treatment was required to correct the problem.

On February 23, 1996, Boggs sued Bosley for fraud, claiming that it had intentionally misrepresented the number of procedures required to correct his hair loss problem. He also asserted a malpractice and fraud claim against Bosley and Phillips, the physician who performed one of his surgical procedures, alleging that such procedure was negligently performed.

Bosley stated that it was entitled to summary judgment on the fraud claim because, prior to each surgical procedure, Boggs signed a form acknowledging that "no guarantee or promise regarding the eventual appearance or permanence of results has been made" and that "no guarantee or assurance of results has been made by anyone regarding the operation which I have herein requested and authorized." Bosley contends that Boggs thus could not have reasonably relied on Bosley's representations. Hence the fraud claim could not stand in court and malpractice claim has a time frame of 2 years to be filed. Boggs' injuries from such procedure manifested themselves no later than November 11, 1993, when he underwent a subsequent procedure to correct the hematoma caused by the previous surgery. Boggs did not file suit until February 23, 1996, well outside the statute of limitation. Accordingly, the trial court did not err in granting defendants' motion for summary judgment on this claim.[19]

Discussion

This case was in favor of the hair transplant clinic only because of a good thorough consent form. It is not just sufficient to have a detailed consent form, it is important to explain it to the patient in detail, in his preferred language too. Details on how a consent form for hair transplant should be prepared are mentioned in a different chapter.

CASE 9: WIDE FOLLICULAR UNIT TRANSPLANT SCAR AND NECROSIS IN FOLLICULAR UNIT TRANSPLANT—COMPLICATION

The 25-year-old patient underwent an FUT hair transplant in 2012 at a plastic surgery clinic in Seoul. Postsurgery, the patient developed an infected wound that was not given adequate postoperative care by the operating surgeons. After the surgery, the patient developed a skin infection that left a 22/3 cm scar on his scalp. As the hair did not grow due to the scar, the patient became almost bald.

According to the court, the hospital had excessively cut the scalp during the operation, and did not give proper treatment until the skin had already died. Scalp incisions are regarded as requiring extra care, since they can spark skin infections and damage skin cells. The court said in its ruling that the hospital was responsible for paying for a new cosmetic surgery, so that the patient can recover. The Seoul Central District Court ordered the two doctors who performed the surgery to pay 54 million Won ($65,000) in compensation to the patient.[20]

Discussion

- This is a case of a large FUT scar with improper closure and necrosis. This can happen in any case of FUT if the surgery is done by untrained staff or doctor. Who can do a hair transplant is a very debatable topic and not clearly defined by any law. However, adequate training is of utmost importance. If a staff member is being trained on a patient, it is important to mention in the consent and inform the patient.
- Such cases can be easily avoided by sticking to the literature and not trying overzealous extraction. FUE is the most commonly performed surgery and overextraction has become a regular practice in most clinics. Overextraction and dense packing of grafts is always hand in hand. Necrosis is an easily avoidable complication if there is proper technique and aftercare followed.

- Many patients tend to travel postsurgery and do not follow-up and these are the cases which usually lead to litigation, as there is failure to follow-up. The documentation of the patient should also have provision to note the postprocedure consultations, neglect of precautions and noncompliance of instructions, if any.

CASE 10: A PATIENT WHO WANTED ₹ 2,00,000 COMPENSATION

A patient accused a doctor of:
- Not performing the procedure properly
- Lack of results
- Prescribing laser comb leading to additional expense.

History: Patient, aged 25 years underwent surgery in 2007, with 1,200 grafts. He was satisfied with results and recorded the same in feedback. However, he stopped drugs, as he was afraid of side effects and this lead to loss of existing hairs.

He came back for a second session. He was told not to hurry and take drugs. He refused. Repeated counseling was done not to hurry for surgery, and this was recorded in documents. He still insisted and a second session was performed with express documentation that:
- He is unwilling to take drugs and will be responsible for consequences.
- Surgery will not give full results if he does not take drugs.

Six months later, he continued to have hair loss and wanted a third session, Doctor refused surgery. Patient then went to court with above complaints.

The consumer court squashed the case with following observations:
- There is no negligence as surgery has been performed and documented properly.
- Lack of results is because patient did not take drugs, and this has been documented. So patient is negligent not doctor.

- There was no prescription produced for laser comb.

Lessons

Documentation has to be full and proper. In this case, doctor had separate consents for each procedure, drugs, and also a feedback form. The case also demonstrated the need to be diligent, in work, ethics and documentation.

CASE 11: REJECTION OF ARTIFICIAL HAIR FIBERS

A female patient suffering from alopecia totalis, consulted a doctor for artificial hair fiber treatment. She agreed to pay 5 lakh rupees for 10,000 Italian "Biofiber." Two patch tests were done initially and one of them gave an adverse reaction and rejected the implanted grafts. Despite the rejection, on the patient's persuasion the artificial hair fiber implantation was done. Two months after the procedure the patient developed multiple pus filled lesions. The fibers had to be removed within a few months to stop the reaction. The patient filed a complaint of medical negligence with the consumer court after their removal.

The consumer commission however dismissed the appeal stating that the doctor cannot be held responsible for an unsuccessful transplant. There was no sufficient or cogent evidence to hold the surgeon negligent. The skin of the patient was unable to accept the hair fibers, was considered as the reason for the unsuccessful procedure by the court.[21]

Discussion

Artificial hair fibers is not US-FDA approved[7] and using them requires good documentation and thorough consent. Doing a patch test in such cases can help to avoid a big disaster like in this case. There should be sufficient documentation as evidence to show that the patch test failed. If despite this the patient wants the procedure, an agreement stating that the patient will not hold the doctor responsible for any complications or rejection of fibers should be signed.

SUMMARY

Multiple measures can be taken or are being taken by doctors to counteract these issues. Despite this there are some situations which become unavoidable. The above-mentioned cases only give a gist of the things that can go wrong during a hair transplant surgery. The most important points that should be included in training of trichology are how to maintain doctor patient relationship, drafting a consent form, documentation and maintaining ethics while advertising. Guidelines provided by the national and international associations should be followed strictly to be protected. And once a patient does complain in the clinic about any procedure, it is wise to be compassionate and sympathetic towards the patient's complaints. Showing empathy initially can actually avoid a law suit completely. Lastly, in case one does land up with such a case professional indemnity insurance is a must to have for all hair transplant surgeons (Box 4).

CONCLUSION

Under the best of ethical situations, one may still have to face legal issues. What a patient thinks or how he reacts cannot be predicted but it can be controlled with empathy from the time the counseling starts. Avoiding patients, who undergo complications, will actually worsen the situation for the doctor by increasing the patient's discomfort. Raising patient's expectations by giving unrealistic advertisements is the root cause of most of these legal suits.

BOX 4: Tips to avoid medicolegal cases for hair transplant surgeons.
- Practice evidence-based medicine.
- Do not give false claims or hide facts while advertisements or counseling.
- Maintain a good doctor patient relationship.
- Consult the patient personally before and after surgery explaining the entire procedure, sequence, progress, complications and post-operative care of the surgery. Explain the consent form in detail personally (Box 3).
- Take detailed history and preoperative tests before the surgery.
- Take photographic documentation and patient's signature on all follow-up records and make notes about patient's views on every follow-up.
- Give free touch up session if any patient feels that a particular area has lesser density.

REFERENCES

1. State Legal Services Authority Chandigarh. The Consumer Protection Act, 1986, published in Gazette of India, Extra-ordinary, Part II Section I dated 26.12.1986 amended by Act No. 34 of 1991 and 50 of 1993. [online] Available from http://chdslsa.gov.in/. [Accessed December, 2018].
2. Legal Services India.com. (1996). Indian Medical Association v V.P. Shanta, AIR 1996 SC 550. [online] Available from http://www.legalservicesindia.com/article/1097/Indian-Medical-Association-V-V.P.-Shantha.html/. [Accessed December, 2018].
3. Patwardhan N, Mysore V; IADVL Dermatosurgery Task Force. Hair transplantation: Standard guidelines of care. Indian J Dermatol Venereol Leprol. 2008;74 Suppl:S46-53.
4. Haircon 2019 Beyond Scalp. Association of Hair Restoration Surgeons of India (updated October 2015; cited 2018 Aug 02). [online] Available from http://www.ahrsindia.org/. [Accessed December, 2018].
5. Mysore V, Shashikumar BM. Guidelines on the use of finasteride in androgenetic alopecia. Indian J Dermatol Venereol Leprol. 2016;82(2):128-34.
6. Ministry of Health and Family Welfare. (2013). National Guidelines for Stem Cell

Research and Therapy. [online] Available from http://pib.nic.in/newsite/PrintRelease.aspx?relid=116030/. [Accessed December, 2018].
7. Mysore V. Synthetic hairs: Should they be used? Indian J Dermatol Venereol Leprol 2006;72(1):5-7.
8. State Consumer Disputes Redressal Commission. Dr. Batra vs Harjot Singh on Sept 13, 2013. [online] Available from https://indiankanoon.org/doc/157599954/. [Accessed December, 2018].
9. Nanda L. The need for a computerized patient-record system for the public hospitals in Andhra Pradesh. Journal of the Academy of Hospital Administration. [online] Available from http://www.indmedica.com/journals.php?journalid=6&issueid=17&articleid=122&action=article/. [Accessed December, 2018].
10. Satish M, Menon R, Rao KV. Professional Accountability and Patients' Rights, 2nd edition. The Institute of Law and Ethics in Medicine, National Law School of India University, Bangalore; 2002.
11. The Indian Express. Hair transplant gone wrong, court asks police to probe (April 2nd 2014). [online] Available from https://indianexpress.com/article/cities/mumbai/hair-transplant-gone-wrong-court-asks-police-to-probe/. [Accessed December, 2018].
12. Chennai Medical Student Dies after Hair Transplant Surgery. [online] Available from https://www.ndtv.com/chennai-news/chennai-medical-student-dies-after-hair-transplant-surgery-1416981/. [Accessed December, 2018].
13. The Times of India. (2017). Court orders cosmetic clinic to pay client Rs 1 L for bad job. [online] Available from https://timesofindia.indiatimes.com/city/goa/court-orders-cosmetic-clinic-to-pay-client-rs-1l-for-bad-job/articleshow/59922279.cms/. [Accessed December, 2018].
14. Dogra TD, Gupta S. Medicolegal Aspect of Health Care Delivery. [online] Available from http://www.indmedica.com/journals.php?journalid=6&issueid=72&articleid=910&action=article/. [Accessed December, 2018].
15. Goldberg DJ. Legal issues in laser operation. Clin Dermatol. 2006;24(1):56-9.
16. The Times of India. Patient loses eye after hair transplant surgery; doctor's registration suspended. 15th Feb 2018. [online] Available from http://timesofindia.indiatimes.com/articleshow/62925131.cms?utm_source=contentofinterest&utm_medium=text&utm_campaign=cppst/. [Accessed December, 2018].
17. Casemine. (2017). Kishore Kadam v. M/s Ego Wellness Pvt. Ltd. and another. [online] Available from https://www.casemine.com/judgement/in/596f27834a9326202bf93d75/. [Accessed December, 2018].
18. Moneylife News and Views. (2017). ASCI upholds complaints against 62 Advertisers including P&G, Snapdeal, TV 18 and Hyundai Motors. [online] Available from https://www.moneylife.in/article/asci-upholds-complaints-against-62-advertisers-including-pg-snapdeal-tv-18-and-hyundai-motors/40295.html/. [Accessed December, 2018].
19. FindLaw. (1997). Boggs vs Bosley, 23rd February, 1996. [online] Available from https://caselaw.findlaw.com/ga-court-of-appeals/1172087.html/. [Accessed December, 2018].
20. Asia One. (2014). Korean Hospital Responsible Faulty Hair Transplant Court. [online] Available from http://www.asiaone.com/health/korean-hospital-responsible-faulty-hair-transplant-court/. [Accessed December, 2018].
21. The Times of India. (2014). Doctor not to blame for hair transplant going awry. [online] Available from https://timesofindia.indiatimes.com/city/mumbai/Doctor-not-to-blame-for-hair-transplant-going-awry/articleshow/36177264.cms/. [Accessed December, 2018].

CHAPTER 35

Special Aspects of Dermatosurgery Practice

Savitha AS, Venkataram Mysore

INTRODUCTION

Dermatologists are no more considered as pure skin physicians. The present day dermatologists are also cutaneous surgeons. Dermatosurgery has become an integral part of current dermatology practice. Dermatosurgery has been defined as the practice of dermatology that specializes in surgical procedures and minimally invasive treatments to improve the health, function, and appearance of skin.[1] Dermatosurgical procedures have the following characteristics:

- May be diagnostic (skin biopsy), therapeutic (removal of cysts, tumors, and vitiligo surgeries), and cosmetic (hair transplantation, liposuction, skin grafting, and acne scar revision).
- Most procedures are performed under topical and local anesthesia, however, few procedures may require general anesthesia.
- Most are simple, can be done in day care theatres and patients can go back home.
- Serious side effects are rare, but may occur.

Though the surgical risks are relatively less in cutaneous surgery, possibilities of medicolegal situations and aesthetic complications always exist. High degree of standard care has to be maintained in these patients, as most of the procedures are aesthetic and done on previously healthy individuals.[2] The key steps to ensure medicolegal safety are obtaining informed consent (IC), meticulous documentation, and good communication with the patient. In the following chapter, few points, which help to ensure medicolegal safety, are enumerated.

While the procedures are considered minor, the following probable scenarios where medicolegal situations may arise in dermatosurgery should be kept in mind:

- Scarring, hypertrophic scars, keloids, or post-inflammatory pigmentation after a procedure.
- Cobblestoning, hyperpigmentation, or inadequate pigmentation after vitiligo surgery.

- Inadequate response to procedures done.
- Drug reactions and lignocaine toxicity.

COMPETENCY OF THE DOCTOR

Dermatosurgery and lasers are now a part of the Masters in dermatology syllabus in most universities.[3] However, few dermatology departments have a separate operation theatre providing primary exposure to postgraduate students for basic dermatosurgical procedures. Also, dermatosurgery is not routinely taught during postgraduation and students fresh after completing post-graduation from most colleges, may not be competent enough to perform surgeries. The level of training varies greatly from center to center. Only few centers train postgraduate students even in routine dermatosurgical procedures like subcision, acne scar surgeries, minipunch grafting, excisions (lipomas, sebaceous cysts, and mole), curettage, cryotherapy, sclerotherapy, and nail biopsies. Often these are therefore learnt in specialized centers, workshops, and conferences. It is therefore important for dermatologists to ensure proper training and also certification as proof of having learnt those procedures. In this context, below case illustrates this requirement:

Case 1: A dermatologist performed Q switched neodymium-doped yttrium aluminum garnet (Nd:YAG) laser treatment for removal of a pigmented lesion, which lead to depigmentation of the skin. The patient complained to the consumer court. In the court, the judge asked for proof of training that the dermatologist had undergone. The dermatologist replied that he was an MD in Dermatology. The question was; yes you are an MD, but

- *Was this part of your syllabus?*
- *Do you have a certificate that you were taught this?*

The doctor could not provide such proof and patient was awarded compensation.

Lesson: All doctors preferably should have a certificate of what they have learnt from their professor or head of the center.

Case 2: A dermatologist in an interior town performed a chemical peel for a patient who was from Bengaluru. Patient underwent the procedure on a weekend when he visited his hometown.

The clinic was a busy general dermatological clinic, without a proper procedure room and the assistant was not a nurse. The patient developed post-inflammatory pigmentation—patient sent notice to the doctor that:
- *Doctor was negligent*
- *Risk of pigmentation was not explained*
- *Procedure was performed by an assistant who was not trained.*

The doctor contacted the senior author for advice. It was found during the discussion that consent indeed had not been taken. It was explained to the doctor that this is a lacuna and he was told to refer the patient to the senior doctor for counseling. The senior doctor counseled the patient, explained the reason for pigmentation, it being a temporary phenomenon, and managed the patient without charging the patient. The pigmentation faded over 8 weeks and patient was happy.

Lesson: Aesthetic procedures are done to satisfy a desire, and hence the facility should be equipped properly. This may be difficult to do in a busy clinic seeing 100 patients. No procedure should be performed without consent. A dermatologist should always have a mentor whose help he should seek in such situations. Most side effects after routine dermatosurgical procedures are temporary and it is important not to panic. Counseling is vital.

Physicians who perform advanced dermatosurgical procedures should have a certification course or get trained adequately under an expert. National associations like Indian Association of Dermatologists, Venereologists and Leprologists (IADVL), and Association of Cutaneous Surgeons of India offer 1-month observership programs at multiple centers for physicians after their postgraduation. There are university recognized 1-year fellowship courses in dermatosurgery in India and abroad. As 1 year is dedicated to dermatosurgery exclusively, physicians are trained to perform advanced procedures such as flaps for reconstruction, vitiligo surgeries, ear lobe surgeries, circumcision, fat grafting, and nail procedures. Dermatologists can further update themselves by attending workshops and hands-on training courses. The procedures can be performed under the guidance of experts initially, before taking them up independently. If the physician is not confident about the procedure, it is better not to attempt it. The dermatosurgeon should be aware of the possible complications and should possess the necessary skill to deal with it.

Observational workshops where a doctor sees a procedure on television (TV) is not adequate certification to perform a procedure. Hands-on certificates are necessary. The senior author is aware of a case where a doctor tried to perform liposuction after watching the procedure on YouTube. This is strongly discouraged. Just as dermatologists invest in machines, they should invest time, effort, and money in training.

No surgical procedure is without a risk. The dermatosurgeon should have a training and regular course on advanced life support (ALS). ALS refers to a set of clinical interventions for the urgent treatment of cardiac arrest, stroke, and other life-threatening medical emergencies.

DOCTOR-PATIENT RELATIONSHIP

The relationship between a cosmetic surgeon and a patient differs from the traditional physician-patient relationship. This is essentially due to the distinction, between elective and non-elective forms of medical treatment. Cosmetic surgery, as an example of elective surgery, is a treatment, which comparatively, the patient can afford not to undergo.[4] The treatment selection is most often determined and guided by the patient's wishes. Communication between the cutaneous surgeon and the patient takes place on a different level as the patient typically expects to relate more democratically with the surgeon. In the case of therapeutic or non-elective operations, the patient is often reluctant to consent to surgery and must even be persuaded by the physician, whereas the cosmetic surgery patient requests the operation and sometimes actually talks the surgeon into performing it.[5] The cutaneous surgeon can minimize his or her exposure to medical malpractice by avoiding the certain legal pitfalls mentioned below. When patients do sustain injuries because of the surgeon's actions, many factors contribute to the patient's decision whether to take legal action. The behavior of the physician in dealing with the patient often determines whether postoperative problems are interpreted by the patient as unfortunate complications or errors by the physician. An open, truthful, and caring approach by the physician can avoid unnecessary trips to the courthouse.[6]

PATIENT SELECTION

The objectives of patient selection and counseling are ultimately to enhance successful outcomes. There is currently no consensus as to what defines therapeutic success. In its simplest form, a successful surgery may be defined as the ability to complete an operation. Success may also be defined by patient satisfaction, lack of dissatisfaction, lack of complications, lack of recurrence, or by many other definitions. A truly successful outcome is one that is patient-centered and focuses on achieving an optimal result based on the presenting condition and treatment expectations.[7] While performing diagnostic procedures or therapeutic procedures like excisions, patient selection need not be based on his or her psyche. Caution has to be maintained when choosing patients for cosmetic procedures. A cutaneous surgeon should know when to say no to a patient for a procedure. Choosing the right patient for a procedure is crucial. Patients with depression and dysmorphophobia need a psychiatric opinion and thorough counseling before subjecting them to aesthetic procedures.[8] To further help identify patients who are at high risk for dissatisfaction, a previously published mnemonic is recommended—CURSED patient (compulsive or obsessive, unrealistic, revision, surgeon shopping, entitled, denial, and psychiatric).[7]

A typical example is vitiligo surgery—here surgery is performed for an autoimmune disease, when it is stable. However, criteria to define stability are not adequately defined. IADVL adopted a definition of 1-year duration to define stability. A dermatosurgeon while performing procedure should record these facts specifically in the consent form. Otherwise, relapse of the disease can lead to litigation.

Counseling

Counseling the patient is the most crucial pre-operative procedure. Surgeons should spare adequate time for this step. It is an opportunity for the dermatologist to understand the needs of the patient and also to build up a rapport. The doctor's explanation and the patient's understanding of this explanation have been shown to improve the patient compliance. One should put forth the available options to the patient and allow them to choose. In this stage, important information should not be withheld, e.g. if a better or cheaper or more effective or safer procedure is available elsewhere. A detailed discussion about procedure goes a long way in winning their confidence as well as giving them the comfort of knowing the procedure beforehand. Doctor should discuss the advantages, disadvantages, and adverse effects and the generally expected outcomes of the procedure chosen for the patient. Patient responsibilities such as post-procedure care, fees payable, etc. should also be discussed. One should encourage the patient to clarify their doubts.[9] For cases like acne scars, multiple sessions may be required and in spite of the best care, 100% results cannot be promised. Unless these are documented, disputes can happen. During history taking prior to any procedures, relevant information regarding drug allergies, concomitant drug intake, keloidal tendencies, recurrent herpes infections, known bleeding diathesis, diabetes, previous treatments for the same condition, and pacemakers (for electrosurgery) should be elicited.

The below case illustrates this situation:

Case 3: A patient underwent a chemical peel 1 week before the marriage of her daughter for melasma thinking that the peel will remove the pigmentation in 1 week. She developed dryness, which is expected. Lack of information leads to this misunderstanding. The author recommends a checklist for documentation, in addition to history, wherein patient is asked to answer a series of questions and then signs it (Annexure 1). This puts the onus of disclosure on the patient and is thus helpful.

Consent

Informed consent (IC) is important for ethical and legal reasons as well as to improve quality of care and patient satisfaction. Presence of a witness is always preferred while taking IC. It should include the condition, need for treatment, other modalities of treatment, duration of given treatment, number of sittings, and expected results; need to follow instructions before and after the procedure and possible side effects.[9] When taking IC for a diagnostic procedure like biopsy, inform the patient regarding the need of the procedure, method, post-operative wound care, possibility of scar and complications. For ease of recall of what is considered "adequate", a mnemonic "PARCODE" has been suggested (Box 1).[10] The consent should always be taken prior to the procedure and by the doctor only. It should be written in simple and comprehensible sentences and in the language, which the patient understands better. It should be signed by the patient, parent or guardian in case of minors. In the case of teenagers (13–18 years), it is better to take the consent of both the minor and the parent. The patient should have the liberty to revoke his consent at any time.

Consent forms for common dermatosurgery procedures are available from *https://www.iadvl.org/consent-forms.php*. The same has been attached as Annexures 2 to 5.

Note: Since dermatosurgical procedures are repetitive, signatures should be obtained for each visit. A separate consent should be taken even if minor changes in procedures (which are common) are made; e.g. If in a patient undergoing chemical peel, if the peel is changed from salicylic acid peel to glycolic acid peel, a separate consent should be obtained. If during laser hair removal, laser is changed from diode to Nd:YAG the same should be informed.

Preoperative Workup

- Detailed history taking as mentioned above
- Routine hematological and biochemical investigations
- Drug history to ensure there is no interaction with the anesthesia or postprocedure medications
- Lignocaine test dose.

DERMATOSURGERY OPERATION THEATER

Dermatosurgical procedures are office based except for a few major surgeries like hair transplantation and advanced vitiligo surgeries. The operation theater (OT) should be well-equipped and in compliance with the standard guidelines published.[11] A high degree of standard of care is needed for dermatologic surgical procedures as many of them are aesthetic and are done in a previously healthy patients. Possibilities of medicolegal situations and aesthetic complications always exist and therefore dermatologic surgeons should adopt checklists and standards of care in their practice. In June 2008, the World Health Organization (WHO) announced the "Safe Surgery Saves Lives (SSSL)" initiative

---

BOX 1: Mnemonic of PARCODE.

PARCODE:
- Procedural details
- Alternate treatment options
- Risks involved
- Complications
- Outcome expected
- Duration of treatment or downtime
- Expenditure involved.

to reduce surgical error and thereby promote patient safety.[12] The aim of the WHO surgical safety checklist is to ensure that key safety elements are incorporated into the operating room. Though few points on this checklist may not be wholly applicable to dermatosurgical procedures, this can yet be used as a guide to prevent complications.

No surgery is risk free, therefore emergency resuscitation equipment should be handy and the physician should be trained in basic life support. Facilities to shift the patient in situations of emergency should be in place.

Procedure

The procedure, no matter how small (even punch biopsy) should be performed under aseptic precautions. Following aseptic precautions and safe disposal of biomedical wastes is mandatory. All precautions should be taken to avoid mishaps. Avoid using spirit swabs during electrosurgical procedures to avoid fire mishaps. When the grounding pad is loose, this may cause heat generation and sparking at the contact site, without providing an appropriate exit for the current to pass safely through the circuit. There are many reports of burns due to this.[13] The IADVL taskforce on dermatosurgery has published standard guidelines of care for procedures.[14] Communication with the patient remains vital during the procedure as the patient is conscious throughout. A qualified assistant or nurse, referred to as "physician extenders (PE)", is a valuable asset to a dermatologist. When adequately trained, they prove handy in the present day busy schedule of most practitioners. PEs are highly prevalent in dermatologic surgery practices and are playing direct roles in the delivery of dermatologic care. Not only are they trained to handle the patients and perform procedures assigned to them, they should also be encouraged to report errors, when they occur and not hide the facts for the fear of litigation. This facilitates the early appropriate intervention that could address the origin of poor quality practices. The treating dermatologist would be vicariously liable, if such events are not properly handled.[15]

It is easy for a dermatologist to take some procedures lightly, since they are minor in nature. However, side effects can be serious even in minor procedures. An anaphylactic shock in a simple biopsy can be life-threatening and consequences serious, if the clinic does not have the minimum required facilities to handle it. The authors recommend fingertip monitors in all cases. Dermatologists work in single doctor clinics and hence should have a proper referral system in place to handle these situations.

Post-procedure

Clear written instructions should be handed over to the patient along with verbal instructions after the procedure including care of the operated site, dressing, medications, and follow-up visits. The possible complications should be explained and they should be informed to report back immediately, if they notice any danger signs. In case of any unexpected development or complication, patient must have access to expert advice.[8]

DOCUMENTATION

One of the crucial steps which help in medicolegal situations, is accurate documentation. Pre-procedure work-up, counseling, instructions given to patients, the surgical steps, and materials used should be documented in detail. If any untoward incidents happen or any complications arise during the procedure, they also should be documented with date and place.

Medical records must be accurate, clear, chronological, and legible. They must be kept confidential and preserved for at least 3 years. Before and after photographs are vital in case of aesthetic procedures.[16]

WHEN SOMETHING GOES WRONG

Due to the increase in the practice of dermatosurgery and aesthetic medicine, dermatologists are now at higher risk for frequent medical malpractice insurance claims. Untoward incidences do happen occasionally. In such a case, it is better to acknowledge it. Be polite to the patient, listen to his complaints, counsel if necessary, and redo or treat the patient. Above all, do not charge the patient once again. By acknowledging, you may have a hassle on your hands, but you may not get to a lawsuit. Try to make an out of court settlement, if your defense is weak. Seek the help of a mentor and your association. This saves your reputation as well as the economic loss due to the time spent in attending the courthouse.[17]

Insurance: As every medical malpractice insurance policy is different, it is important for dermatologists to review the policy exclusions and the additional coverage that is offered before selecting an insurance company. Select a policy which covers all the procedures, which you perform. Dermatosurgical procedures are not covered by routine insurance schemes. It is important that this be clarified before taking the policy. Companies should be asked to specify the procedures, which are covered.

CONCLUSION

The cutaneous surgeon can minimize his or her exposure to medical malpractice by avoiding the legal pitfalls outlined in this chapter. When patients do sustain injuries because of the surgeon's actions, many factors contribute to the patient's decision whether to take legal action. The behavior of the physician in dealing with the patient often determines whether post-operative problems are interpreted by the patient as unfortunate complications or errors by the physician. An open, truthful, and caring approach by the physician can avoid unnecessary trips to the courthouse.

REFERENCES

1. American Society for Dermatologic Surgery. What is dermatologic surgery? [online] Available from: https://www.asds.net/ [Accessed December, 2018].
2. Mysore V, Anitha BS. Checklists for Surgical Safety in Dermatosurgery. J Cutan Aesthet Surg. 2009;2(1):1-3.
3. RGUHS. MD Dermatology Curriculum. [online] Available from: http://www.rguhs.ac.in/cdc/2015-16/OrdinanceGoverning/MDPreClinFin-ver1.2.4%20(1).pdf [Accessed December, 2018].
4. Healy "Duties of Disclosure and the Elective Patient: a Case for Informed Consent" 1998 Medicolegal J Ire 26; Nugent "Cosmetic surgery on Patients with Body Dysmorphic Disorder: the Medical, Legal and Ethical Implications" Available from: http://works.bepress.com/cgi/viewcontent.cgi?article=1004 [Accessed December, 2018].
5. Wright MR, Wright WK. A psychological study of patients undergoing cosmetic surgery. Arch Otolaryngol. 1975;101(3):145-51.
6. Coleman WP, Guice WL. Office surgery and the law. Adv Dermatol. 1987;2:207-27.
7. Ziegelmann M, Köhler TS, Bailey GC. Surgical patient selection and counseling. Transl Androl Urol. 2017;6(4):609-19.
8. Satyanarayana Rao KH. How to practice dermatosurgery safely? J Cutan Aesthet Surg. 2014;7:121-3.
9. Sacchidanand SA, Bhat S. Safe practice of cosmetic dermatology: Avoiding legal tangles. J Cutan Aesthet Surg. 2012;5:170-5.
10. Satyanarayana Rao KH. Medicolegal issues in esthetic surgery. In: Venkataram M (Ed) ACSI Textbook on Cutaneous and Aesthetic Surgery,

1st edition. New Delhi: Jaypee Brothers Medical Publishers (P) Ltd; 2012. pp. 876.
11. Rajendran SC, Omprakash HM. Standard guidelines for setting up a dermatosurgery theatre. Indian J Dermatol Venereol Leprol. 2009;75(8):76-82.
12. WHO. (2009). WHO—Safe surgery saves lives. [online] Available from: https://www.who.int/patientsafety/safesurgery/tools_resources/9789241598552/en/ [Accessed December, 2018].
13. Saaiq M, Zaib S, Ahmad S. Electrocautery burns: experience with three cases and review of literature. Ann Burns Fire Disasters. 2012;25(4):203-6.
14. Mysore V. Standard guidelines of care for dermatosurgical procedures. Indian J Dermatol Venereol Leprol. 2008;74.
15. Leshin B, Hauser D. The role of a physician assistant in dermatologic surgery. Dermatol Surg. 1999;25:148-50.
16. Rao K. Safer practice of dermatosurgery. Indian J Dermatol Venereol Leprol. 2008;74:S75-7.
17. Hagihara A, Hamasaki T, Abe T. Association between physician explanatory behaviors and substandard care in adjudicated cases in Japan. Int J Gen Med. 2011;4:289-97.

ANNEXURE 1: CHECKLIST FOR LASERS OR AESTHETIC TREATMENTS (IADVL CONSENT FORMS)

Name:　　　　　**Age:**　　　　　**Date:**　　　　　**Phone No:**

- What is the nature of your work?
- Do you have important meeting or functions in the coming week?
- Are you allergic to any medication or ointments?
- Are you sensitive to light (i.e. do you have itching, burning sensation, and redness while going out in sunlight)?
- Have you had an episode of herpes (blisters over lips)?
- Have you had anesthesia before?
- Do you suffer from an infection or inflammation that you are aware of if so, what?
- Are you pregnant?
- Are you lactating?
- Do you have tendency to scar, pigment, keloid, vitiligo, and psoriasis?
- Have you undergone facials, bleaching, or any other chemical treatment in this week?
- Are you on painkillers, vitamin E, herbal medicines, and anticoagulants?
- Do you have any systemic illnesses?
- Are you on treatment for any health issue, if so what treatment?
- Do you use sunscreen?
- What are your expectations from the procedure?

Witness:　　　　　**Dr Sign:**　　　　　**Patient Sign:**

ANNEXURE 2: CONSENT FORM FOR ACNE SCARS (IADVL CONSENT FORMS)

I have been informed that:
- The purpose of this procedure is to reduce some or most of facial acne scars and may require multiple sequential treatments.
- Prior to treatment, the area to be treated will be anesthetized with a topical numbing cream or lidocaine injection. You may be given diazepam for your comfort prior to treatment.
- Following treatment, you may experience pain, swelling, and redness and bruising.
- Risks of this procedure include but are not limited to the following:
  - *Pain:* Stinging or sharp pain may be present after the procedure and throughout the healing process.
  - *Bruising:* This treatment will cause significant bruising of the treated area. The bruising may be present for weeks.
  - *Swelling:* Swelling will be present after the procedure and should likely resolve after 1–2 weeks.
  - *Pigmentary changes:* The treated area may heal with altered pigmentation, either darker or lighter skin.
  - *Scarring:* There is a risk of scarring with this procedure any time during healing process. Nodules may form at surgery insertion sites.
  - *Bleeding:* The procedure will cause bleeding, sometimes significant which should stop within few minute without any lasting effect when pressure is applied. The bleeding may not reach upper level of the skin and may result in bruises of the skin. The red color will darken to purple and purple yellow and will disappear in 1–2 weeks.
  - *Scabbing:* A scab may be present at some of the subcision sites. The scabbing will disappear during natural healing.
  - *Infection:* Infection of the wound is always possible. Any significant infection must be brought to our attention as soon as possible. Such signs are excessive pain, swelling, redness, or drainage or pus. Any infection could last for 7–10 days and could lead to scarring.
- It is very possible that this procedure may fail to achieve your desired results. Strict adherence to preoperative and postoperative instructions is essential. You may need to repeat your treatments to achieve desired results.
- After getting the procedure done, I will follow the instructions given by doctor.
- Clinical results may vary between individuals, sessions, and scars. I am fully aware that it is to improve the healing of scars eventually.

I was also informed about:
- The other alternative methods of acne scars as well as their benefits and disadvantages.
- No guarantee, warranty, or assurance has been made to me as to the result that may be obtained.
- I am also aware that follow-up is necessary and multiple sessions are required for optimum healing of scars.

Additionally:
- I agree that any pictures taken of my treatment site may be used for publication or teaching purpose; however, my name or identity will not be disclosed and complete confidentially will be maintained.
- By signing below, I acknowledge that I have read the adverse reactions above and feel that I have been adequately informed of the possible risks of the procedure.
- I have informed the doctor about any or all drug allergies that I have.
- Before each treatment, I will inform the doctor, if I have taken any new medications since my last visit.
- I also agree to comply with the recommended aftercare instructions.
- My questions regarding the procedure have been answered satisfactorily.

Consent

I authorize Dr .... and her or his designated staff to perform procedure. Further my signature below indicates my consent to the treatment described and my agreement to comply with the requirements placed on me by this consent form.

I hereby release Dr .... and her or his designated staff from liability associated with above procedure.

Signature of patient or his authorized representative   **Signature of operating Doctor**

Date: **Time:**

ANNEXURE 3: INFORMED CONSENT FOR MOLE REMOVAL AND BIOPSY (IADVL CONSENT FORM)

Mr/Mrs/Miss:
Age:
Date:
Reg. no:
Address:
Phone no:
Mobile:
Diagnosis:
Name of procedure:

- The doctor has explained to me the potential benefits of the procedure of mole removal and biopsy. However, I understand there is no certainty that I will achieve these benefits.
- No guarantee, warranty, or assurance has been made to me regarding the outcome of the procedure.
- The reasonable alternative(s) to the procedure, as well as the risks of alternatives have been explained to me by the doctor. The alternatives include, but are not limited to leaving the mole or tissue in place, which may or may not be cancer.
- The doctor has explained to me that there are risks and possible undesirable consequences associated with this process including, but not limited to blood loss, transfusion reaction, infection, heart complications, blood clots, loss of or loss of use of body parts, other neurological injury, recurrence, scarring, and reaction to the local anesthetic if used and/or death.
- In the event any of the inherent complications mentioned above, may occur, my doctor and his team will take appropriate and reasonable steps to help manage the clinical situation and be available to me and to my family to address our concerns and questions.
- Any of the above risks or complications may require further surgical interventions during or after the procedure, which I expressly authorize. In the event any of the inherent complications mentioned above, may occur, my doctor and his team will take appropriate and reasonable steps to help manage the clinical situation and be available to me and to my family to address our concerns and questions.
- I understand that if I need blood or blood products, these carry a risk of contracting Human immunodeficiency virus infection or acquired immunodeficiency syndrome (HIV or AIDS), hepatitis, or other diseases.
- I have been explained that clinical results may vary between individuals, sessions, and scars. I am aware that it is to improve the healing of the scars eventually.

Additionally:

- I .... hereby authorize Dr .... and any associate or assistants, the doctor deems appropriate to perform mole removal with biopsy.

- I also authorize the administration of sedative and/or anesthesia as may be deemed advisable or necessary for my comfort, well-being and safety.
- In permitting my doctor to perform the procedure, I understand that unforeseen conditions may be revealed that may necessitate change or extension of the original procedure or different procedure(s) than those already explained to me. I therefore authorize the doctor and his team, perform such procedure(s) as necessary and desirable in the exercise of his or her professional judgment.
- In the event any of the inherent complications mentioned above, may occur, my doctor and his team will take appropriate and reasonable steps to help manage the clinical situation and be available to me and to my family to address our concerns and questions.
- I authorize the doctor or hospital to utilize or dispose the removed tissues, parts of organs resulting from the procedure authorized above.
- I consent to my photographing or video graphing of the procedure that may be performed, provided my identity is not revealed by the pictures or the descriptive texts accompanying them.
- I consent to the admittance of students or authorized equipment representatives to the procedure room for purpose of advancing medical education or obtaining important product information.
- I have informed the doctor about any or all drug allergies that I have. I also agree to comply with the recommended aftercare instructions.

By signing below, I certify that I have had an opportunity to ask the doctor all my questions concerning anticipated benefits, material risks, alternative therapies, and all of my questions have been answered to my satisfaction.

I hereby release Dr .... and his or her designated staff from liability associated with the above procedure. I authorize Dr .... and his or her designated staff to perform procedure.

Signature of patient or his   **Signature of the Doctor**
authorized representative

ANNEXURE 4: CONSENT FORM FOR SCAR REVISION (IADVL CONSENT FORMS)

Mr/Mrs/Miss..
Son/Daughter/Wife of ....
Age: .... Sex: ....
Date: ....
Case record No: ....
Address: ....
....

Phone No: ....   Mobile: ....

Diagnosis: ....

Site and brief description of scar: ....
....

Name of the procedure: ....

I have been informed that:
- It is impossible to completely remove the scar.
- The aim of the surgical procedure is to replace an ugly or more apparent scar to a less apparent and aesthetically better scar.
- There are many different techniques of scar revision surgery. The type of surgery may depend on the type of scar, site of scar, and surgeons expertize. In addition to surgery, there are other modalities such as laser therapy, dermabrasion, microneedling, chemical peels, etc. I have been offered the option to discuss these various therapies before opting for surgery.
- This procedure is performed under local anesthesia. A few injections will be given at the site of surgery to make the area numb. There after the procedure is expected to be painless.
- The operated site will be secured with help of sutures (stitches) in one or multiple layers and a small bandage will be put to cover the wound.
- Any surgery can have potential complications. They include pain, swelling, bleeding, infection, scarring, discoloration of skin, irregularity of contour of skin, allergic reaction to the suture material, delayed wound healing, hypertrophic scar, keloid formation, etc. These complications do not occur in all patients and can be minimized to some extent with surgical expertise. Some amount of pain, swelling, and discomfort is expected at the site of operation. For this, a course of antibiotics and painkillers will be prescribed to you. In case, pain or swelling is severe, please contact your doctor immediately.
- Very rarely serious cardiac, pulmonary, or neurological complications can occur.
- During postoperative period, avoid any activity which can produce tension at the operated site.

- Also try to keep the area dry.
- You will be called after 5–7 days after surgery for stitches removal.
- In the initial stages, the scar is red and elevated above the skin. In due course of time, the scar becomes more or less skin colored and also tends to flatten with time. This process may take up to a year.
- Clinical results may vary between individuals.
- No guarantee, warranty, or assurance has been made to me as to the results that may be obtained.
- I am also aware that follow-up treatments may be necessary for desired results.
- Smoking, tobacco products, and nicotine products (patch, gum, or nasal spray) are at a great risk for significant surgical complications of skin dying, delayed healing, and additional scarring. Individuals exposed to second-hand smoke are also at potential risk for similar complications attributable to nicotine exposure.

Please indicate your current status regarding these items below:

- .... I am a nonsmoker and do not use nicotine products. I understand the risk of second-hand smoke exposure causing surgical complications.
- .... I am a smoker or use tobacco/nicotine products. I understand the risk of surgical complications due to smoking or use of nicotine products.

Additionally:
- I agree that any pictures taken of my treatment site may be used for publication or teaching purposes; however, my name or identity will not be disclosed and complete confidentiality will be maintained.
- By signing below, I acknowledge that I have read the adverse reactions above and I feel that I have been adequately informed of the possible risks of scar revision.
- I have informed the doctor about any or all drug allergies that I have.
- Before each treatment, I will inform the doctor, if I have taken any new medications since my last treatment.
- I also agree to comply with the recommended aftercare instructions.
- I consent to the disposal of any tissue, medical devices, or body parts, which may be removed.

I hereby release Dr .... and his or her designated staff from liability associated with the above procedure.

My questions regarding the procedure have been answered satisfactorily.

I authorize Dr .... and his/her designated staff to perform scar revision surgery for my ....

The payment and fee structure have been informed to me and I agree to abide by the same.

Signature of patient or his   **Signature of the Doctor**
authorized representative

ANNEXURE 5: CONSENT FORM FOR VITILIGO SURGERY (IADVL CONSENT FORMS)

I (name) ...., aged .... years, residing at (address) ....
.... have been advised to undergo surgery for my skin condition, vitiligo.
I hereby give consent after being explained in a language that I understand about the procedure by Dr ....

I am aware that vitiligo is a disease with a chronic, recurrent course.
- I am aware that surgery is only a cosmetic procedure and other concomitant medical treatments may be essential. Surgery will not alter the course of the disease or prevent any recurrence. I am aware that the practice of medicine and surgery is not an exact science, and I acknowledge that no guarantees have been made to me as to the results of the operation or procedure.
- My disease has is not increasing in size or number for the last............months. I have no tendency for keloids.
- I am aware that the exact course of the disease cannot be predicted and, though the disease is stable at present, flare-ups and recurrences may occur at any time, in any part of the body.
- I have been explained the procedure of the operation as follows:
  - The procedure will be done under topical or local anesthesia.
  - The donor area is from back or thigh or gluteal area or inner arm.
  - The donor graft will be taken by punch or suction blister or grafting knife or dermatome.
  - Recipient area will be abraded by dermabrader and then the graft applied, covered by dressing.
- I am aware that avoiding movements and taking care of the recipient area is essential for optimal results.
- I am aware that I may experience some pain postoperatively and may need to take analgesics.
- Donor area will need dressing; the donor area may take 2–3 weeks to heal.
- I am aware that for optimal cosmetic results, it may take 6 months to 1 year. I may need to take medical treatment and phototherapy during this period.
- I am also aware that the grafted area may not match in texture and appearance with the surrounding skin. A perfect match with the surrounding normal skin may not always be possible.
- I consent to be photographed or videographed before, during, and after the treatment; that these photographs or videos shall be the property of the above doctors and may be published in Scientific Journals and/or shown for scientific reasons.
- I agree to keep the above doctors informed of any change of address so that they can notify me of any late findings, and I agree to cooperate with the above doctors in my care after surgery until completely discharged.
- I am not known to be allergic to anything except: (mention if any....)

I have read the above consent. I fully understand the contents of the consent and authorize and request the above doctors to perform this surgical procedure on me. The consent form has been signed by me when I was not under the influence of any drugs.

Signature of patient or his authorized representative   **Signature of the Doctor**

CHAPTER 36

Handling Difficult Patients in Dermatology

Govind S Mittal, Venkataram Mysore

INTRODUCTION

Receptionist: "*Sir, Mr X has come and has been creating a fuss in the waiting area.*"

Doctor: "*Oh! He is a "difficult" patient and always behaves like that, please make him sit in room number 2, I will see him shortly!*"

This is a common scenario in today's practice and it is not unusual for us to come across such a patient! It is important to handle them because they provide warning signs that may indicate a potential medicolegal situation.

Before we understand the ways to handle a difficult patient, it is important to understand as to why some patients are "difficult" or behave difficult in certain encounters. Factors leading to "a difficult encounter" with patients may be associated with the *physician, patient, a situation or a combination of these*. The patient may be "difficult" due to personality disorders, multiple and poorly defined symptoms, nonadherence to medical advice, apprehensions related to treatment costs, unmet needs, unfulfilled expectations, treatment-associated complications, perceived negligence, and unresolved medical issues. The added tensions of patients' personal lives, including but not limited to the impact of the disorder in question on their day-to-day life, adds to some patients being "really tough to deal with". Contributing to this, there could be physician factors such as poor communication skills, a very busy schedule leaving very less time for individual patients, negative bias toward certain disorders, etc. Situational or circumstantial factors would include time pressures during visits, cost of technology and admissions, patient and staff conflicts, or complex social issues. Many such "difficult encounters" and "difficult patients" play as nidus for potential lawsuits against doctors for negligence or malpractice.

The following tips can help in preventing patients becoming difficult patients:
- Be sensitive to the patients' needs. This would include things like helping an elderly patient to get up or sit, helping a patient in tears with a tissue, calling in another female staff in the room for the comfort of a female patient and so on and so forth. It may be even helpful sometimes

to have a good sense of humor, especially in breaking the ice with some patients.
- *Communication*: It must be the doctor's fundamental approach to maintain full disclosure or an open and honest communication with the patients. The doctor must communicate clearly, avoiding much of technical jargon. Illustrations can be useful tools to help a patient visualize their diagnosis or show how a medication or treatment will improve a condition. One must also avoid making tall commitments/promises to patients.
- Involve patients in their own care and decision making. It is often noted that a particular disease may not have one single solution, but multiple possible treatment options. It is always better to explain the relevant ones to the patient and discuss their opinion in going ahead with a suitable line of treatment. Use patient-centered communication to reach a mutually agreed upon plan. A patient is less likely to file a suit for a complication from a procedure that he willfully chose over another in an informed manner!
- *Consistency is the key*: Being consistent in your care is equally important. The same level of care and protocol should be administered to each patient you see.
- *Stay updated*: Lawsuits against doctors may sometimes focus or evaluate whether the latest standards of medical treatment were followed or not. It is important for doctors to update their training and knowledge in their branch of specialization and must be aware of the recently published standards of care.
- Detailed documentation, photography, and informed consent—while these are discussed in detail in a separate chapter, the importance of documentation cannot be emphasized enough. Always document all necessary facts regarding the patients' complaints, examination findings, diagnosis, management plan, pre-procedure counseling, informed consent form, and procedure details. It goes without saying that pre- and post-procedure photographs are of paramount importance. After each sitting of any procedure performed, record necessary details regarding improvement in the condition perceived by the patient, and if there was any complication noted or any deviation from the normal, during the procedure.
- *Maintain patient confidentiality*: With rising standards of privacy policies across the world, maintaining patient confidentiality is as important as maintaining medical records and photographs. Do not share any patient's photographs or information with another patient without prior consent, especially if the photo or information is identifiable. Leak of any patient information is deemed unprofessional and may form a basis for a lawsuit against the doctor.
- Another common "difficult" patient is the "Google patient". These are patients who read up the disorder and medicines prescribed, on the internet and have irrelevant concerns and excessive questions and doubts. One of the best ways to tackle such patients is to guide them with selective literature that you can provide to them that they can themselves read up on the internet without wasting too much of the consultation time. It is also important to make them understand that a lot of information on the internet may not be regulated and accurate and must always be verified by a qualified specialist.

Understanding and managing the factors above will definitely lead to a more effective and satisfactory experience for the physician and the patient in reducing difficult encounters. If difficult encounters with patients are avoided then lawsuits can be kept at bay.

How to handle difficult patients and potentially prevent patients from filing a lawsuit?

- Try and attend to a "difficult" patient on priority, or move them to a separate room! They often tend to spoil the atmosphere in the waiting area by creating a ruckus or raising their voice or refusing to pay for services that the patient has received or demanding a refund. This has an obvious negative impact on the reputation of the clinic and the doctor.
- *Listen! Be patient and genuine*: Listening to a patient sufficiently solves half of the problem for many. This is understandably tough for any practitioner with a busy OPD, but the doctor's patience indeed builds the first impression about the doctor in the patient's mind. The doctor must be empathetic and genuinely interested in understanding the patient's problem while maintaining a caring yet nonjudgmental attitude at all times. This will help the doctor to build functional, trusting relationships with the patients. However busy the OPD is—mere clearing of the crowd should not be the doctor's motive at any point in time. If the patient is going astray while narrating the history, it may be necessary to ask certain leading questions rather than jumping to the diagnosis and handing over a prescription! From the patient's point of view, the consultation is often perceived incomplete and unsatisfactory, if the patient has not got a chance to narrate his side of the story. If a doctor is not able to spare that much time, any other staff such as nurse, reception staff, or a manger can talk to the patient till the doctor is free.
- If a complication has occurred, explain the same to the patient and the possible reason behind it rather than ignoring it, or trying to cover it up. Offer honest apologies for any mistakes due an act of omission or performed.
- Waiving off your consultation fee while treating a complication may go a long way in preventing an impending lawsuit. You could also offer the patient samples of medications for treatment, which would reduce the economic burden of the treatment.
- *Timely referral*: It is important for the doctor to realize when the patient with a certain disorder is beyond his limits or specialty of management and must seek opinion of his colleagues where necessary and refer the patient to another center or a higher center without delay.
- In case of negligence or an inadvertent complication, patients tend to be more forgiving when they realize that their doctors truly had their best interests in mind and have been caring and truthful in their approach. According to the Medical Protective Company's chief medical officer, Graham Billingham, the number of malpractice lawsuits reduced considerably in the past few years since doctors had given honest explanations when faced with unexpected outcomes.[1] Also, it is important to realize that an unexpected outcome is not always synonymous with or due to poor care or malpractice. However, poor communication combined with a bad outcome usually drives patients toward litigation. Thus, the importance of effective communication with full disclosure between doctors and their patients cannot be stressed enough.

It is important to remember that although the doctor may not have direct control over inadvertent complications (that are sometimes seen as medical negligence), the manner in which the situation is handled can indeed modify the fate of an impending lawsuit. It is obvious that medical personnel who are rude and unhelpful can quickly and easily trigger the level of discontent required for a patient to file a malpractice suit, if anything untoward were to occur while that person is in a medical practitioner's care.

CLINICAL CASE SCENARIOS

Scenario 1

A young lady with psoriasis presented to the clinic of a senior dermatologist with exfoliative dermatitis. She had been treated elsewhere and was extremely anxious about treatment with immunosuppressants including methotrexate, steroids, and cyclosporin. She was counseled in great detail about the need for hospital admission and intensive care unit (ICU) care, with initial treatment with steroids and later with cyclosporin/other systemic agents after investigations. The patient was thus sent to the hospital accompanied by a junior dermatologist. The patient's sister, a senior government officer, who accompanied the patient, was explained in detail about management. Her husband who was an IAS officer landed at the hospital later where the patient was to be admitted and had several doubts that could not be adequately handled by the junior doctor. This delayed the admission. The senior dermatologist had to finally intervene and ask the patient to be admitted first and managed effectively and all the doubts could be solved later as the treatment process is initiated.

Learning Point

A doctor may be unnerved by several factors including the patients' half knowledge about the disease and treatment as well as influential and persuasive relatives of the patient, which can in-turn delay the process of treatment. Some patients in senior positions may be dominant and often young doctors find the situation difficult to handle. It is thus important for the doctor to be firm and maintain authority with polite but a "no-nonsense" attitude and addressing the patient's medical problem must be prioritized.

Scenario 2

A lady from USA came to a dermatologist Dr X with a list of about ten doctors from different towns and cities whom she was meeting enquiring about hair transplantation for her son who was in USA. She requested for the credentials of Dr X saying that she needed to do a "background check". Dr X told her that all details are available online and requested her to do the "background check" in the background, rather than in front of the doctor and asked her to tell her son to e-mail the doctor directly his doubts regarding the procedure. The lady further went on to ask if her son could ask Dr X about his credentials. Dr X politely refused and told her that he need not answer details about his credentials to the patient as everything is already available on the internet.

Learning Point

With this incident, we understand that how patients or their relatives can be very intimidating and direct to the doctor. It is best that the doctor maintains his calm and need not justify himself to each and every patient for no particular need. Also in this tech-savvy world, a doctor must take out time to put up his credentials online, so that all this need not be discussed during precious consultation time. He should recognize that while such discussions may be distasteful to the doctor, the patient has a right to get the information, which has to be available to the patient.

Scenario 3

A patient with chronic urticaria had been treated with almost all the drugs over a period of time, except Omalizumab. He was told about Omalizumab and advised to consider the same and he came back after few days saying that he wanted to use the drug. He was informed about the cost of the medication, and was asked to get it directly from the company. He found the cost to be a limiting factor and wished to know if it was covered by insurance. He was told that it is unlikely that it would be covered by insurance but was asked to verify with his insurance agent. His insurance agent said that he would try to get it covered, if the patient was given the medication with an inpatient admission. Unfortunately, the patient developed a severe episode of urticaria on the day of admission and thus Omalizumab was given only on the 3rd day. Since the patient was kept in the ICU after admission, his total bill escalated to ₹ 40,000. When the patient came back to the treating dermatologist for the second injection, he said he had no money for the second injection as all his money had been exhausted and blamed the doctor and wanted the second injection to be given to him free of charge. He was counseled but with no avail. Finally, Dr X found out that there was another company marketing the drug at a lesser cost and the second injection was administered to the patient.

Learning Point

In the field of dermatology, we see several patients with chronic diseases and many patients behave "difficult" due to the chronicity of the disease and economic factors involved and often end up blaming the doctor for the same. The only way that this problem can be tackled is that the patient is counseled from time to time in detail about the disease and its prognosis.

Scenario 4

A patient came for liposuction and, during the counseling, he asked for treatment of the chickenpox scars on his face. He was offered fat transfer as a treatment option since he was undergoing liposuction. He was counseled about the results that could be expected and that chickenpox scars are not easy to treat. Patient agreed and the fat transfer for the scars was done at a discounted price. The patient later came back saying that he was happy with the results of liposuction but not with that of the chickenpox scar treatment. He later sought repeated consultations for the chickenpox scar treatment and his unhappiness about the scars was more than the happiness of the results of liposuction for his primary problem.

Learning Point

In this case, the doctor thought he was helping the patient with an additional procedure; the patient interpreted that he had spent money unnecessarily. If a secondary procedure is being clubbed with a primary planned procedure, the patient must be counseled in detail about the secondary procedure as well so that patient knows what to expect and decide, if he really wants to go in for the secondary procedure or not.

Scenario 5

A patient with tear trough deformity came for treatment with fillers and was given all information about the procedure and treatment. After the procedure, the patient developed a bruise that lasted for almost 3 weeks. The patient was upset that the doctor had told her that the bruising if occurs may last for a few days but had lasted much longer in her case. The patient also read the Indian Association of Dermatologists, Venereologists and Leprologists (IADVL) guidelines regarding the procedure and pointed out that it mentioned that "bruising may last for a few days" and not few weeks. However, patient was managed with patience and the bruising disappeared and patient was comfortable.

Learning Point

Preprocedure counseling with the patient must be effective and complete. It is also important to understand the patient's perception about the side effects mentioned in the consent form and explained to the patient by the doctor. It is essential to drive home the point to the patient that individual variations may exist and shall be handled as necessary. Also, patients require a lot of handholding, which is especially needed at the time of any complication.

Scenario 6

A 75-year-old lady with lichen planus had been treated on multiple occasions with various medications by the doctor who was the neighbor of the patient. The patient was finally started on Azathioprine. She happened to develop bone marrow suppression after a week and was admitted to the hospital. Her daughter, who was a doctor, flew down from USA. Meanwhile, the patient was extensively investigated in the hospital and a bone marrow biopsy was also performed. The daughter searched all medical records of her mother and found the prescription for azathioprine and thus the cause for bone marrow suppression was ascertained. She went back to the dermatologist whom she had seen since childhood and questioned him if he should have actually prescribed the drug to her elderly mother who was staying alone. Since the dermatologist and the patient were neighbors and knew each other well, the case did not reach the court.

Learning Point

Dermatologists commonly have to prescribe immunosuppressants. Adequate counseling about potential side effects, baseline and monitoring investigations and follow up is very essential. It may be beneficial to ask some history about patient's family and background, so that the doctor can decide if a particular medication is especially suitable and safe for that patient.

In today's practice of dermatology, the chances of coming across "difficult patients" and "difficult encounters" are several. It is the doctor's responsibility to take measures to avoid such encounters, wherever possible, and take necessary corrective measures as discussed above, if the need arises. These would indeed pave way for healthier rapport between the doctor and the patient and help in preventing a potential medicolegal situation case did not reach the court.

KEY MESSAGES AND PEARLS

- Several factors contribute to a difficult patient-doctor encounter
- Always maintain an empathetic, compassionate, and caring attitude
- Follow the principle of full disclosure and maintain effective communication with the patient
- Do not forget the three magic words— "please", "thank you", and "sorry!"
- Educate patients about their treatment and involve them in the decision making
- Maintain patient data including informed consents and photographs and maintain confidentiality
- Stay updated with latest developments in your field and incorporate them in your practice.

REFERENCE

1. Doctors can prevent medical lawsuits. [online] Available from http://care-ins.com. [Accessed December, 2018].

CHAPTER 37

Consent for Injectables in Cosmetic Dermatology

Rasya Dixit

BACKGROUND AND INTRODUCTION

Facial injectables are set to witness a new fold growth globally with predicted Compound Annual Growth Rate (CAGR) of 10.42% during the next 5 years.[1] The factors fuelling this exponential growth include increasing demand for nonsurgical treatments as well as growing awareness and acceptability of facial injections. However, as the people electing for these treatments are well individuals, it becomes of vital importance to not reduce these medical procedures to mere beauty treatments, and hide the potential pitfalls from the patient.

As the demand for these injectable procedures increase, so do the problems arising from mismatched expectations to delivery. Most malpractice claims in cosmetic plastic surgeries are not a consequence of technical faults but because of inadequate selection criteria of the patients and lack of adequate communication between the patient and the physician.[2] The increased awareness of these options has paved the way for patients easily accepting the procedure when it is suggested to them. However, the physician needs to spend time in understanding the correct concern of the patient, and explain that the results may not correct all that they desire. A written informed consent form remains an integral part of the communication between physicians and patients and importantly can facilitate the professional protection.[3] A consent form also allows the patient to digest the information a second time and ask questions if they arise.

How is an injectable consent form different from a regular consent form?

When there is a desire for a cosmetic treatment, it is equally important to inform the patient of the likely pitfalls but not scare them away from the procedure. So the consent form should always be preceded by a detailed consultation. The consultation should encompass all the treatment options available to the patient, as well as the possible costs, advantages and pitfalls of these. In some patients, the awareness of the treatment is restricted to only the name of the treatment. They may not be aware that complete remedy to the problem may not be achieved. The consent form should document that the patient seeks treatment for the particular problem area which can be mentioned in lay people language, (e.g. frown lines, crow's feet) and the name of the product being used.[4] It is better to document the name, batch number and the units used in the treatment in the consent form itself. The need for repeat treatments, and the need for touch ups, the cost involved in the initial treatment as well as for the touch ups has to be documented in the consent form. It is important to note as a treating physician to be aware of the approved indications in the country where they practice and not to deviate from these guidelines, as the line of law can only protect them when they follow these.[5]

Most malpractice claims in cosmetic plastic surgery are not consequences of technical faults but because of inadequate patient selection criteria and lack of adequate communication between patient and surgeon. Proven efficient training, careful utilization of computer imaging techniques in association with the adoption of simple precautions and guidelines and adequate communication along with a completed patient's consent form are important essentials in case of medical litigation.[6] In cosmetic procedures, taking an informed consent is based upon the patient's autonomy. The reason for consent is information and understanding of a patient about treatment modalities and finally choosing one of the several options for treatment. Unfortunately, these days, physicians neglect precounseling and inform incomplete data for patients and taking consent that is not an informed consent.[7]

Photography and videography consent are another vital part of this form. As the rejuvenation techniques affect the animation of the face, it is important to get photos of patient in neutral and with full animation of the face or area that is to be treated. Many patients desire reassurance of a natural look when seeking facial aesthetic treatments. An example is to avoid the frozen look after botulinum toxin treatment. For some, naturalness may be defined as facial expression that is without tell tale signs of treatment, characterized by visibility of product, abnormal surface contour, or incomplete movement of the facial area. An improved appearance would be suggested by better symmetry of the facial expression, a more youthful appearance, or reduction in aging signs. Considering that facial expressions are integral psychosocial interactions, some propose that assessment of impact of treatment on facial dynamics ought to become part of evaluation of an optimal treatment.[8] A desire for natural-looking results is often described but assessment of naturalness is still subjective, and the treating physician needs a valuable tool to define the results.

In both these variations of photography, the physician should observe and point out any preexisting discrepancy or asymmetry to the patient and document the same before treatment. If possible, a video of the face in animation should also be taken as post-treatment, the change or improvement could only be visible on animation. Care should be taken to standardize these photos and videos as far as possible, so the post-treatment photos can be replicated in a similar manner.[9]

Once the patient chooses the injectable treatment, the most common as well as the rare side effects should be explained to the patient. No concern should be dismissed as very rare problem which does not occur. The physician should explain common events like bruising and what steps will be taken to minimize them. However, as this can occur even with the best injectors, do ask for social events in the near future so the treatments can be planned accordingly. The consent form has to capture that the patient is aware of the possible side effects so they can plan the time of injection.

The emergence of widespread information on the internet means that the well-informed patient has access to variety of sources of information regarding the injectable treatment. So during the consultation as well as in the consent form, it is better to be concise and clear and not avoid mentioning side effects. For example, if the patient questions about vascular event possibility or eyelid or brow ptosis, the physician can explain the high risk areas and the steps they may be taking to avoid this possibility. But the consent form should encompass this possibility.[10]

Side effects of injectable treatment may arise immediately after or present after a delay. The patient may not be able to recognize some of the side effects as related to the injectable immediately.[11] A post-treatment form which provides information about the treatment, how to recognize a potential problem and how to reach out to the treating physician should be handed over to the patient. The consent form should capture that this form has been handed over to the patient after treatment. The consent form should also encompass that the patient should not delay contacting the physician and follow the post-treatment instructions as advised by the physician.[12]

A few case reports below illustrate a few possible medicolegal scenarios arising from the use of injectables and discuss how to approach them.

Case Report 1

A patient, a Caucasian man, visited the clinic asking for botulinum toxin (BTX) for forehead wrinkles. He had undergone these treatments regularly in a clinic abroad. Examination revealed that his procerus and orbicularis muscles were hyperactive. Forehead lines also needed to be treated. After assessment, he was told that he would need about 16 units of the toxin to frontalis, and 12 units to procerus and additional treatment to his orbicularis oculi. The patient consented and pretreatment photos were taken in animation and at rest. Post-treatment, on 3rd day the patient called the clinic saying he did not see any improvement. When he was told that it can take up to 2 weeks, he got angry and said that during the previous treatments, he had got improvement in 1 day- and he accused the doctor " you have not given BTX, you just injected water."

Then 3 days later, he called again, saying that there was no improvement, and wanting a refund of the treatment cost, again accusing that water was injected. This went on for 2 weeks; at this time, an assessment was done. The photos in animation found that he had improved partially, and he needed a touch up for his procerus. He again got angry and wanted money back. He threatened that he would go to court. His photos were then sent to an expert who agreed that all protocols had been followed and he needed a touch up which is expected in any patient, particularly someone who had previously taken sessions of BTX. The patient was counseled again and explained about all these measures. He understood the situation, and accepted the touch up procedure.

Lessons

In this case, the doctor should have mentioned that the precise dose estimation may not be possible in view of past BTX injections. The post-treatment counseling should have included not only the side effects and complications, but also time taken to developing the results. Often, when patients come in for repeat treatments, it is possible that full recounseling is not done. The doctor may assume that the patient remembers all the side effects or the post-treatment care and precautions as they have had the treatment earlier. This needs to be avoided. In this patient, a full counseling would have pointed out that though results are seen as early as the third day, full results may take 2 weeks to develop, and a follow-up session is needed to assess and give any touch up dose if residual muscle action is seen.

Good photographs and ability to take the help of the expert helped in countering his claims. Proper documentation including the batch of BTX, date of dilution was also helpful. Patient should also be shown that these have been documented along with the treatment dose, which helps not only track the results so the good results can be replicated, but also refute false claims of patients like in the above case.

Following Food and Drug Administration (FDA) approved indications also allows the parent company to support the doctor, and the doctor to substantiate his claim in the case of a medicolegal issue. So, avoiding non-FDA approved indications will help the beginner doctor avoid these pitfalls.

Case Report 2

A patient who had treatment for tear trough with fillers developed mild lumpiness in the first week post-treatment. She was very upset, even though she was counseled earlier that mild lumpiness could happen immediately post-treatment and that it would soon subside. She was subsequently managed with counseling and assurance. She was also shown Indian Journal of Dermatology, Venereology and Leprology (IJDVL) guidelines to substantiate the opinion. Ultimately, it subsided after 3 weeks and she was comfortable.

Lessons

Patients need to be counseled about common side effects like bruising and lumpiness. This would allow them to plan ahead for social events. Gentle but firm counseling post-treatment and doctor initiated proactive follow-up helps patients to deal with side effects. Often patients seek these cosmetic procedures for enhancement and are very vexed when they encounter side effects, even though the side effects are temporary. Explaining the temporary nature of these side effects during counseling helps allay their fears.

Case Report 3

A patient was treated for smile lines with filler. During the procedure, patient did not experience any pain, excessive bleeding or blanching. On the first day after the procedure, the patient did not report any side effect during doctor initiated review. The third day, the patient called the clinic and reported bruising over the right nasolabial fold area and nose area. Since the nose area was not injected, the possibility of a vascular event was thought of and the patient was asked to come to the clinic for assessment and treatment. The patient was seen with erythema and bruising over the nasolabial area and over the nose. Hyaluronidase was injected into the whole area. The skin healed without event.

Lessons

Since during the procedure, the counseling included possibility of such a vascular event, and also stressed upon need to inform the doctor if something unusual arose, the patient contacted and reviewed with the doctor in time to avoid any significant sequelae. This means discussion of rare side effects during counseling in such a way to inform and empower the patient. This builds trust in the treating doctor so even if there is a problem or complication arising from the treatment the patient chooses to come back.

Case Report 4

A patient who wanted correction for the tear trough was suggested fillers. During counseling, the patient was very apprehensive as she had seen the possibility of vascular complications including blindness happening due to the treatment. The doctor explained that though this was indeed documented, it was rare. And the precautions to prevent the possibility of this event like using a large bore blunt tipped cannula and using safe points for treatment, emergency protocols were explained to the patient. The patient was also given time to make the decision for going ahead with the treatment. She went back and considered the options and during her second appointment went ahead with the filler.

Lessons

It is important to be honest and transparent with the patient. Discussing the treatment options and side effects confidently and that increases the confidence the patient has in the doctor. Allowing the patient time to make their decisions also improves the patient physician relationship.

Sample consent form for injectable filler and botulinum toxin has been attached (Annexures 1 and 2). What needs to be appreciated is the fact that while the treatments are noninvasive, expectations are high, acceptance of even minor side effect is low, and hence all aspects of the procedure, however minor, should be documented properly.

There is a special situation with fillers- cases of visual problems and even blindness has been reported. This needs to be mentioned in the consent. Of course, if blindness does happen, even if there is no negligence, it is likely that the case for compensation will be viewed seriously, and hence the doctor should be prepared with good amount of insurance. Importantly, the insurance should cover the cosmetic treatments.

It is also important to use products from well established companies as a number of fake products or products with poor background are often marketed. Otherwise use of such nonapproved products can be an issue of negligence.

SUMMARY

The esthetic industry is clearly moving from surgery to nonsurgical or minimally invasive techniques for rejuvenation. As dermatologists, we enjoy the benefits of being poised to be pioneers in this field of injectables. But we need to be also torch bearers of evidence based esthetic medicine and practice safe medicine. Empowering ourselves and our patients make us both benefit. The consent form is the basis of discussion, documentation and validation of the esthetic process to a medical procedure.

REFERENCES

1. Researches and Markets. Available on www.researchandmarkets.com, June 29, 2017.
2. Maio G. [Is aesthetic surgery still really medicine? An ethical critique]. Handchir Mikrochir Plast Chir. 2007;39(3):189-94.
3. Mavroforou A, Giannoukas A, Michalo-dimitrakis E. Medical litigation in cosmetic plastic surgery. Med Law. 2004;23(3):479-88.

4. Foucault P, Meklat H, Vial D. Botulinum toxin and medical liability: is the patient sufficiently informed? Ann Readapt Med Phys. 2005;48(2):71-6
5. Korman JB, Jalian HR, Avram MM. Analysis of botulinum toxin products and litigation in the United States. Dermatol Surg. 2013;39(11):1587-91.
6. Mavroforou A, Giannoukas A, Michalodimitrakis E. Medical litigation in cosmetic plastic surgery. Med Law. 2004;23(3):479-88.
7. Mohindra R. Medical law handbook. United Kingdom: Radcliff publishing; 2008. pp. 34-9.
8. Michaud T, Gassia V, Belhaouari L. Facial dynamics and emotional expressions in facial aging treatments. J Cosmet Dermatol. 2015;14(1):9-21.
9. Philipp-Dormston WG, Wong C, Schuster B, et al. Evaluating perceived naturalness of facial expression after fillers to the nasolabial folds and lower face with standardized video and photography. Dermatol Surg. 2018;44(6):826-32.
10. Wollina U, Konrad H. Managing adverse events associated with botulinum toxin type A: a focus on cosmetic procedures. Am J Clin Dermatol. 2005;6(3):141-50.
11. Haneke E. Managing complications of fillers: rare and not-so-rare. J Cutan Aesthet Surg. 2015;8(4):198-210.
12. Rzany B, DeLorenzi C. Understanding, avoiding, and managing severe filler complications. Plast Reconstr Surg. 2015;136(5 Suppl):196-203S.

ANNEXURE 1

CONSENT FORM FOR BOTULINUM TOXIN A INJECTION

Name of Patient:

Age: dd dd mm mm yy yy   Sex: ☐ Male ☐ Female   Phone Number:

Address:

I .... state that I have been informed about the treatment with Botulinum toxin (Botulinum Toxin Type A) for facial lines/ .... (indication).

I know that Botulinum toxin is injected into the muscle and acts by relaxing the wrinkle causing muscle. I am aware that the onset of effect is within 48–72 hours, with its peak within 7–15 days and the effect lasts up to 4 months. New applications may be done once in 4 months.

I have been informed about Botulinum toxin's proven safety, efficacy and long experience with its use. As with any drug or treatment, there are chances of side effects though very low, like mild pain, bruising, headache or temporary relaxation of the eyelid, etc. These events are transient and last for 5–7 days to 2 weeks. I confirm that I am neither pregnant nor lactating as I understand that pregnant or lactating mothers are not supposed to take Botulinum toxin.

I have been instructed about the care that has to be taken after the injection.

The doctor has fully explained the procedure to me.

I consent to co-operate fully with my doctor and to the best of my ability follow his/her instructions and recommendations about my care and treatment.

....
Signature   Date

CONSENT FORM

Photography/Video Release

I, the undersigned, voluntarily consent to the taking, copyright, publication, and use of my picture and/or video footage (my face may be identifiable) and likeness by my Doctor. I only agree to the following uses of these photographs or video footage:

I agree that these photographs or video footage will be used for training, education, publication, research & discussions with peer experts.

Patient's Signature: ....

Patient's Name: .... Date: ....

Doctor's Signature: ....

Doctor's Name: .... Date: ....

Clinic Name: ....

Clinic Address: ....

Please take the time to read this carefully and to understand any accompanying information.

ANNEXURE 2

CONSENT FORM FOR HYALURONIC ACID FILLER TREATMENT

To the patient:

It is important that you are informed about your skin condition and proposed treatment including the potential benefits and risks involved. This disclosure is not meant to scare or alarm you; it is simply an effort to inform you better so that you may give or withhold your consent to the treatment program.

I..of (address) .... have requested that Dr .... attempt to improve my facial appearance with Hyaluronic Acid (HA) filler treatment. Hyaluronic Acid filler injectable gel is made of HA in the form of a gel. Hyaluronic Acid is a natural substance (a complex sugar) that stabilizes the skin structure, attracts and binds water, and contributes to the elastic properties of the skin that allow it to remain tight. Injections of Hyaluronic Acid into the skin are thought to replenish its natural support structures damaged by aging. Dermal fillers, such as Hyaluronic Acid filler injectable gel, are commonly used for filling in facial wrinkles and hollows, restoring facial volume to areas such as the cheeks and for lip augmentation.

Over time, Hyaluronic Acid filler injectable gel is gradually and naturally degraded in the human body. The effect of Hyaluronic Acid filler generally lasts for at least six months and in many circumstances longer. Follow-up treatments are needed to maintain the effects of Hyaluronic Acid filler.

Your doctor has prescribed Hyaluronic Acid filler injectable gel which may or may not contain a local anesthetic (0.3% lidocaine). Lidocaine is added to the formulation to increase comfort during injection and treatment. Your doctor will inform you which Hyaluronic Acid filler formulation has been prescribed for your treatment.

You should not apply make-up for 12 hours after the injection and should avoid prolonged exposure to sunlight, UV light, freezing temperatures or using saunas or Turkish baths for two weeks after the injection. You should also avoid massaging and/or putting pressure on the injection site for a few days following treatment.

Injections of Hyaluronic Acid filler may cause some of the risks listed below. Although the risk of developing a serious complication is small, your doctor will monitor you closely, and, should a complication occur, they will use their best medical judgment to do whatever is necessary to treat the problem.

Risks associated with the use of Hyaluronic Acid filler treatment are redness, swelling, bruising, tenderness or itching sensation in the treated area. These common side effects typically resolve within a few days. Occasional cases of bumps and pimples, sometimes accompanied by redness, may occur a few days to a few weeks after the injection. These common side effects are temporary and generally disappear spontaneously in a few days. Very rare cases of reversible discoloration at the injection sites have also been described after Hyaluronic Acid injections. In addition, rare cases of abscess (hard and swollen sore that may contain pus), granuloma (small accumulation of tissue) and blocking of blood vessels causing damage to surrounding skin have been reported. If you experience any inflammatory or other reactions that last more than 1 week, you should notify your doctor immediately, appropriate treatment may be prescribed.

(PTO)

Please take the time to read this carefully and to understand any accompanying information.

If you have previously had a dermal filler (permanent or non-permanent) implanted, you should notify your doctor prior to receiving treatment with Hyaluronic Acid filler injectable gel. The possibility of unknown risks exist. The safety of Hyaluronic Acid filler for use during pregnancy, in breastfeeding females or in patients under 18 years has not been established and therefore Hyaluronic Acid filler should not be used under these circumstances. Please notify your doctor if you have epilepsy, porphyria (enzyme disorder), any allergies (including hypersensitivity to Hyaluronic Acid or lidocaine), an autoimmune disease, a tendency to develop keloid scarring or are taking any medications (including anti-coagulant treatment or aspirin in high doses), herbal or vitamin supplements.

The practice of medicine is not an exact science and no guarantees can be or have been made concerning the expected results. I agree that this constitutes full disclosure, and that it supersedes any previous verbal or written disclosures. I certify that I have read, and fully understand, the above paragraphs, and that I have had sufficient opportunity for discussion and to ask questions. I consent to this Hyaluronic Acid filler injection procedure today and for all subsequent treatments.

Patient's Signature: ....   Date: ....

Doctor's Signature: ....   Date: ....

Photography/Video Release

I, the undersigned, voluntarily consent to the taking, copyright, publication, and use of my picture and/or video footage (my face may be identifiable) and likeness by my Doctor. I only agree to the following uses of these photographs or video footage:

I agree that these photographs or video footage will be used for training, education, publication, research and discussions with peer experts.

Patient's Signature: ....

Patient's Name: ....   Date: ....

Doctor's Signature: ....

Doctor's Name: ....   Date: ....

Clinic Name: ....

Clinic Address: ....

Please take the time to read this carefully and to understand any accompanying information.

CHAPTER 38

Medicolegal Aspects of Lasers

Sanjeev J Aurangabadkar

INTRODUCTION

Lasers and energy-based devices have become an integral part of dermatology practice. With continuous evolution in technology, newer devices are being developed that are better than the earlier generation they replace. All this innovation and technology comes with a hefty price tag, which has to be borne by the dermatologist. Whether it is individual or group practice, buying a machine involves large initial investment along with high cost of maintenance. Along with the primary equipment, ancillary devices such as uninterrupted power supply (UPS), servo stabilizers, smoke evacuators, and air conditioning all need to be in place and in good working condition to ensure optimal performance of the laser system.

The field of lasers is an evolving one- new technology and new machines keep getting introduced, often with no or little evidence. They are introduced with approval by a regulating agency such as FDA (Food and Drug Administration) or CE (Conformite Europeenne)

Therefore evidence gets accumulated with usage of the laser. Also, early in introduction, machine may not work well or may produce side effects. Therefore usage of machines need both proper assessment and also proper information.

With ever increasing range of technologies and machines, it has become a daunting task for a dermatologist to choose the one that best suits a practice. Compounding the fact is the wide price ranges of these laser systems, often confusing the buyer further. Buying is just the initial step, maintenance and after sales service form a vital part of a successful laser practice. This involves service contracts, insurance, documentation and financial planning. A proper informed consent is an essential prerequisite for laser and aesthetic procedure that becomes an important medicolegal record.

This chapter will attempt to throw some light on critical aspects of medicolegal aspects of lasers–both patient handling as well as buying lasers.

SETTING UP A LASER THEATER

Laser surgery can be performed in either a dermatologist's minor operating room or controlled area designated procedure room. An exception to this is surgical laser procedures such as full face ablative laser resurfacing that requires an operation theatre (OT) or operating room(OR). The ideal size of the laser room is about 12 feet by 12 feet to accommodate the machine, a trolley with essentials, cooling device and smoke evacuator. Reflective surface should be avoided in the laser room. Warning signs should be in place cautioning unauthorized or accidental entry while laser procedure is on.[1] A dermatologist often uses several lasers[2-6] and hence he should be aware of requirements of these systems, their goggles, smoke evacuators, etc.

Physician and Non-physician Operator Qualification

Medical Council of India (now superseded by Indian Medical Council) has included lasers in the syllabus of postgraduate dermatology training. Lasers have now become an integral part of a dermatology-training curriculum. Any dermatologist with diploma or degree in dermatology [Diploma in Dermatology Venerology and Leprosy/Diploma of Venerology and Dermatitis (DDVL/DVD/MD)] with some basic knowledge and training in laser physics and laser tissue interaction can perform a laser procedure. Training could be obtained during postgraduation, or from dedicated workshops and conferences. Since each device is different, some basic training needs to be obtained from the device manufacturer either in designated centers or with the aid of an expert in the field in the dermatologists' office.

Many lasers (particularly nonablative ones) are easy to operate and a nurse or nonphysician assistant can perform a laser procedure provided he or she has been trained in it and preferably under a dermatologist's supervision and never independently.

It is important to understand that legally, the responsibility of the results and side effects of treatments done by a nonphysician operator lies with the physician only. Certain guidelines have been proposed by the clinical establishments act (clinicalestablishments.gov.in) and these needs to be taken into consideration and it are mandatory to register one's clinic under this Act.

Consent for Laser

Laser procedures have witnessed an exponential growth over the past decade. There are over 800 Dermatologists in the country using one or more lasers in their practice. (Data obtained from laser machine vendors from India) thousands of laser procedures are being performed every year in our country thanks to the availability and accessibility of systems, increased awareness amongst general population and affordability of patients. Correct patient selection remains of paramount importance whereby problems can be avoided. Proper communication between physician and patient, explanation of the treatment and adverse effects, other options need to be discussed. A consent form bolsters this communication further, where the patient gets a chance to go through the information again and get back with any further doubts or questions, if any. These can be clarified and then laser procedure can be taken up.

From a medicolegal standpoint, obtaining a proper informed written consent is mandatory before taking up the patient for a laser procedure. After thorough counseling, the procedure should be explained in a language that the patient understands explaining the pros, cons, average outcome expected and possible adverse effects. The consent should cover all these points; alternatives to the procedure and signature of the patient, witness and treating physician should be taken. A proper consent is hugely important as it can save a doctor in case of any litigation and even act as a deterrent as the patient knows that detailed instructions were given.

Consent for lasers has to be laser specific as multiple laser systems with different wavelengths and specifications are available. Consent will have to be indication specific too, due to unique purpose the laser is made and used for. For example, consent for laser hair removal will be different from a fractional carbon dioxide laser meant for acne scars. Even the adverse effects will vary with laser and indication.

The consent form should include patient details (including, full name, address, mobile number, email ID) laser system to be used, person performing the procedure, anesthesia if any, photography at every session (possibility of use of the photographs for scientific purposes or publishing also needs to be taken), average number of sittings and financial considerations for the said procedure. Details of the possible adverse effects should also be mentioned and follow-up schedule. Signature of patient, guardian (if patient is minor) and witnesses should be included.

Consent is not needed for each session if the original consent mentions that multiple sessions may be needed. But it is a good idea to take a signature during each successive session on the same consent for with date, as parameters change and sometimes additional wavelengths or different modes may be used. If more than one machine is used then it is advisable to take a separate consent for that procedure.

Some examples of medicolegal cases in relation to laser treatments are mentioned below:

Case 1: A female patient approached a dermatologist for laser hair removal on upper lip. The patient developed 2–3 blisters following long pulse Nd:YAG laser treatment that later turned keloidal. The patient had no keloidal tendency. The doctor showed that the fluence used was within the recommended protocol and hence was acquitted.

Lession: Always document parameters and take a good history and take a proper written informed consent.

Case 2: A patient underwent laser hair removal and developed burns and scars. Patient complained to consumer court. However the doctor was able to demonstrate that the patient did not follow-up regularly and did not follow postoperative instructions hence the doctor was not held responsible. To avoid such situations it is better to hand over written postoperative instructions to the patients so that the doctor can avoid such legal hassles.

Case 3: A patient visited the clinic, where laser hair removal was done by the assistant of the doctor, who was not a doctor by himself. It resulted in burns and hyperpigmentation. Following this 50% glycolic acid + Mesoglow was recommended, but it further caused burn at the chin. The whole procedure costed ₹ 10,000 and the receipt for consultation was not given. The patient demanded a compensation of 50 lakhs.

Verdict: Court dismissed the plea as the compensation asked for was very high, giving an option to file a new case again with request for lower compensation.

Case 4: A patient went for laser hair removal. She alleged dissatisfaction following the treatment and complained of new hair growth. She asked for the refund of money and compensation for the same.

Verdict: In spite of going for 2 years, no improvement was seen. Instructions following procedure were not clearly documented. In each visit, the joules given were incremented. But again, there was lack of documentation for the reason for this increase and no note on condition (progress notes) was made. The doctor was negligent and liable for refund and compensation.

Some consent forms of common laser procedure are enclosed in Appendices 1 to 5.

Laser training and understanding of the machine can be obtained in any of the below mentioned ways:

1a. Becoming members of societies dedicated and focused on laser and aesthetic dermatology; attending their meetings and interacting with experience users, listen to lectures, attend hands-on workshops, etc.
1b. Educational and marketing material provided by the company, and journal articles published in peer reviewed journals.
1c. Training provided by the company on their machines-either on-site or at an expert's center.
1d. The buyer should check the company's website for details such as specifications, the scientific and white papers and testimonials.
1e. Check the local companies' website, parent organization, weather it is registered firm or registered in the Indian Companies Act. Check the facility, manpower and number of installations.
2. Published articles in peer-reviewed journals on the laser technology-to access the efficacy, side effects profile of a given system. The articles can give a clue to parameters used which can serve as a starting point for new users.
3. Peer opinion and experience with the said laser system can be valuable to access stability, performance and cost-effectiveness.
4. *Demonstration:*
   - Try to obtain a demo machine to evaluate it first hand, observe the response, ergonomics, ease of use and check out the parameters.
5. *Engineer's training and expertise:*
   - Verify if the service engineers are well-trained and well-equipped for service.
6. *Power meter:*
   Ensure that the service engineer has a *power meter* for the laser which is critical to ensure correct output and the parent company always suggest this for the dealer. Other requirements that need to be ensured while buying a laser:
   - *Electrical and power back-up:*
     - A three phase electrical connection is suitable if multiple lasers or devices are being planned.[1]
     - Uninterrupted power supply (UPS) online and offline is recommended and the UPS should be of 3 kVA or more with 16 batteries of 60 amps each.[1,7-9]
   - Air conditioning is essential for laser equipment as most lasers require an ambient temperature of 18–24°C for proper functioning. This also ensures a dust free environment.[9]
   - *Cooling:* Most laser treatments for dark skin require some form of cooling to prevent epidermal injury. Cooling can be either air cooling, contact cooling or dynamic cooling. Cooling can be pre, parallel and postcooling.

- *User manual:* Each machine comes with an elaborate manual with trouble shooting guide and frequently-asked questions. Always read the manual thoroughly and familiarize with it and store it in a place where it is easily accessible.
- *Safety eye glasses and corneal eye shields for lasers:* All lasers are shipped with their specific eye protecting glasses with the recommended optical density (OD) to block out the harmful rays from entering the operator's eyes. These are to be worn during the laser procedure by the operator and any other person present in the laser room. External metal or plastic opaque eye shields are also provided with the laser to be worn by the patient during the procedure.

It is advisable not to compromise on quality of the systems.[10] It is essential to evaluate each technology and decide on the one which will add value to the practice.[11]

Check-list of the documents needed for procuring a loan for medical equipments:[12]

- Quotation from the company
- Purchase contract
- Income tax returns
- Registration documents of the clinic
- Clinic building documents
- Medical council registration
- Personal documents such as identity, address proofs, taxation documents.

Purchase Contract[12]

Having a purchase contract on paper signed by the buyer and distributor is essential. Many distributors take a brief one page *purchase order* (PO) from the customer, but this is insufficient as full details of the deal are not mentioned. The purchase contract should include:

- *Advance to be paid:* Once a price is negotiated, and a contract is signed, either an advance amount is sought by the company or they may seek full amount. Generally the advance should not be more than 25% of the total amount. A proper receipt clearly stating the cheque number and the amount needs to be obtained.
- Clause for balance payment, with date of repayment; installments, if any, need to be specified.
- *Foreign currency value:* Since most machines are imported, the price often depends on the price of dollar or other currency which are subject to market fluctuations. This should be properly discussed and proper understanding should be reached with respect to market fluctuations of currency as to who will absorb the difference in case of major change in value.
- Check the cost of the machine mentioned and note if there is any undervaluation. Avoid any undervaluation of the system.
- *Total cost:* Check if the final cost of the machine includes all taxes, customs, transportation and insurance while transportation and installment costs.
- *Warranty:* Warranty should include all parts of laser; check the fine print and see if there are any exclusion clauses. Check the frequency of service and any free services during the warranty period. Mention any extra warranty if any offered by the company in writing in the contract.
- *Repair and maintenance:* How soon can a breakdown being attended? Rough estimate of time frame required in order to repair or replaces the parts? Installation of a standby system while the machine is being repaired so that work will not be affected that should be asked for.

Transportation: Taxes can be levied while transporting the machine from the port to the place of installation. Proper documentation needs to be done for this and done accurately. Lasers are delicate systems and check if they can be transported to various centers if it is being considered. Check the robustness of the system with other colleges.

Installation: This should be done from the company representative or engineer himself. A satisfactory detailed installation report should be sought and kept for records.

Import Export Code

- The contract of purchase always should be under the IEC (*Import Export Code*) of the doctor.

Serial Number

- Prior to purchase, one should communicate with the parent organization via phone or email regarding the *serial number of the device* and the date of manufacture.
- The serial number on the machine at the time of purchase should be noted and mentioned on purchase bill. At the time of taking insurance this number should be mentioned on insurance form. Note the dates of manufacture of the machine and handpieces separately.
- The serial number of hand piece should also be noted and mentioned separately on purchase bill. In case hand piece needs replacement, it has to be proved that it was bought with laser.

Service Report and Spares

- Ensure that the service engineer gives a *service report* after each visit signed by him with comments of the performance of the system.
- Keep a list of the cost of the spare parts from the manufacturer in order to be prepared for any future breakdowns or part replacement due to usage.

Annual Maintenance Contract

- Clinician must take the labor maintenance contract (LMC) or annual maintenance contract (AMC, which includes all parts and maintenance), after the warranty period is over.
- Annual maintenance contract is also essential for insurance purpose.

Insurance: Insurance coverage is a must following installation of the device:
- *Electronic insurance* that covers all the parts and electronics of the device. Many insurance companies offer electronic insurance that may be cheaper than the AMC offered by the laser companies after the warranty period is over. While taking insurance it is important to specify which parts are covered and mention it in the policy.
- *Fire and burglary insurance* and insurance for mobility from one clinic to another also need to be done.

Checklist for making a purchase contract is shown in Box 1. The exact format will vary according to the system, the company, the cost and payment terms and conditions.

Summary of important points to consider while buying a machine:
- Specifications of the laser, wavelength, spot size, pulse width, peak power, etc.
- Type of practice and patient profile
- Choice of laser, energy-based device
- Background check of the local company and parent company
- Costs of spares and consumables
- Warranty, maintenance contracts, service back-up, availability of spares

> **BOX 1:** Checklist for making a purchase contract.
> - Details of machine and handpieces
> - Full specifications of the system
> - Model name, number and year of manufacture
> - Expected date of delivery of system
> - Accessories included with the machine
> - Amount and mode of payment
> - Custom clearance—to be done by dealer
> - Transport insurance and transportation from airport to clinic—to be paid by the dealer
> - Installation of machine and checking the electrical system as per the laser requirement
> - Warranty or extended warranty
> - Annual maintenance contract (AMC) or annual service visit (ASV) comprehensive or service
> - Number of free visits and paid visits per year
> - Provision of standby system in case of delay in repairing machine
> - Any consumables and cost of these consumables

- Training provided and educational material offered
- Articles published on the system in journals

CONCLUSION

Prior to purchase of a machine or laser, it is imperative to access the practice profile, gauge the suitability of device in one's practice and cost-effectiveness of the system in consideration. Cross-checking with peers, rationalizing the purchase based on available evidence and scrutinizing the company in question regarding reliability will go a long way in ensuring peace of mind in the long run. Make a laser purchase contract signed by both the parties which will allow a healthy and hassle-free relationship between the buyer and seller.

ACKNOWLEDGMENTS

The author would like to acknowledge to Indian Association of Dermatologists, Venerologists and Leprologists (IADVL) Academy along with IADVL Special Interest Group (SIG) lasers and aesthetics for providing the template of consent forms for the laser procedures.

REFERENCES

1. Dhepe N. Minimum standard guidelines of care on requirements for setting up a laser room. Indian J Dermatol Venereol Leprol. 2009;75(Suppl S2):101-10.
2. Buddhadev RM. Standard guidelines of care: laser and IPL hair reduction. Indian J Dermatol Venereol Leprol. 2008;74 Suppl:S68-74.
3. Goel A, Krupashankar DS, Aurangabadkar S, et al. Fractional lasers in dermatology–current status and recommendations. Indian J Dermatol Venereol Leprol. 2011;77(3):369-79.
4. Krupashankar DS, IADVL Dermatosurgery Task Force. Standard guidelines of care: CO_2 laser for removal of benign skin lesions and resurfacing. Indian J Dermatol Venereol Leprol. 2008;74 Suppl:S61-7.
5. Aurangabadkar S, Mysore V. Standard guidelines of care: Lasers for tattoos and pigmented lesions. Indian J Dermatol Venereol Leprol. 2009;75(Suppl 2):111-26.
6. Srinivas CR, Kumaresan M. Lasers for vascular lesions: Standard guidelines of care. Indian J Dermatol Venereol Leprol. 2011;77(3):349-68.
7. Olson R. Continuous power to the OR and other critical care areas. Dimens Health Serv. 1975;52(2):29-30.
8. Kerr DR, Malhotra IV. Electrical design and safety in the operating room and intensive care unit. Int Anesthesiol Clin. 1981;19(2):27-48.
9. Alster TS. Getting started: setting up a laser practice. In: Alster TS, (Ed). Manual of Cutaneous Laser Techniques, 2nd edition. Philadelphia: Lippincott, Williams and Wilkins; 2000. pp. 2-4.
10. Mackety CJ. Purchasing lasers and related accessories. Hosp Purch Manage. 1985;10(11):7-10.
11. Christensen GJ, Child P Jr. New technology: mandatory, elective, or hype? Dent Today. 2011;30(2):134, 136, 138 passim.
12. Aurangabadkar SJ, Mysore V, Ahmed E S. Buying a laser–tips and pearls. J Cutan Aesthet Surg. 2014;7(2):124-30.

APPENDIX 1: INFORMED CONSENT FOR LASER HAIR REMOVAL

Mr/Mrs/Miss ....

Age ....

Address .... City ....

Phone Numbers ....

Name of procedure and indication ....

Laser system to be used ....

The purpose of laser hair removal is to diminish or reduce unwanted hair.

This procedure requires more than one treatment session.

Even after multiple sittings, 100% reduction (hair free skin) is not possible. The hairs will reduce treatment in numbers and thickness.

I have been explained about maintenance treatments that may be required after completion of treatment.

The total number of treatment sessions may vary among individuals. Exact number of session cannot be predicted. Patients with darker skin may require more number of treatment sessions and may be more prone to adverse effects.

No guarantee, warranty, or assurance has been made to me as to the results that may be obtained. On rare occasion there may be a patient who does not respond to treatment.

I understand that there are several alternatives to laser hair removal treatment including but not limited to electrolysis, shaving, waxing, and plucking or no treatment at all and that I have the right to refuse treatment.

Hair shafts may be expelled out during the 2–3 weeks following treatment and may mimic the appearance of regrown hair. These may be left to fall out, or they may simply be shaved.

If a patient develops growth in areas in distant regions other than the region treated, it could be due to underlying detectable or undetectable hormonal problem and if those areas are also to be covered by treatment, patient will have to bear the cost of treatment.

I understand that laser hair removal is an FDA-approved treatment method for removing unwanted hair. I have been advised of the possible adverse reactions which are as follows but not limited to:

- *Short-term effects* may include reddening, swelling, bumps, mild burning, temporary bruising or blistering. Hyperpigmentation (browning of skin) and Hypopigmentation (lightening of skin), although rare, may occur. These conditions usually resolve within 3–6 months, but permanent color change is a rare risk, less than 1%. Avoiding sun exposure before and after treatment reduces the risk of color change.
- *Infection* following treatment is quite unusual, but bacterial, fungal and viral infections can occur. Should any type of skin infections occur, additional skin treatments or medical antibiotics may be necessary.

- *Allergic reactions*, although very rare, may occur. Local skin allergies to topical preparations, tape, or preservatives used in cosmetics can occur.
- However slight, there is a *risk of scarring*.
- *Increased hair growth in or around the treated area* is a very rare consequence of laser hair removal. The scientific reason of this paradoxical regrowth is not known. However, these hairs can also be reduced with same laser.

I agree that any pictures taken of my treatment site may be used for publication or teaching purposes; however, my name or identity will not be disclosed and complete confidentiality will be maintained.

By signing below, I acknowledge that I have read the adverse reactions above and I feel that I have been adequately informed of the risks of laser hair removal treatments.

Before each treatment, I will inform the laser technician or doctor if I have taken any new medications since my last treatment or if I have tanned the areas to be treated.

I also agree to comply with the recommended aftercare instructions.

I hereby release Dr and its designated staff from liability associated with the above procedure.

My questions regarding the laser hair removal procedures have been answered satisfactorily.

I authorize Dr and his/her designated staff to perform laser hair removal on my body.

The payment and fee structure is informed to me. I am ready to pay per sitting or package basis. (Package if opted for includes minimum number of sittings and I have to pay accordingly if more sittings are required).

Signature of Patient/Thumb Impression

Signature of Parents/Guardian (For Minors)   Date:

....
Name and Relationship if Signed by other than Parent

Witness: ....   Date: ....
Name .... Signature ....
Date ....
Signature of Doctor .... Date ....
Translated in Patient's Language by ....

APPENDIX 2: CONSENT FORM FOR LASER FOR PIGMENTED LESIONS

Mr/Mrs/Miss ....

Age ....

Address .... City ....

Phone Numbers ...., ..., Mobile ....

Name of Procedure ....

Type of laser to be used: ....

I Mr/Mrs/Miss have been explained regarding above said procedure in my regional language.

I have been told that my skin will not look good for the first few days after the procedure. There will be some pain, swelling, redness, scabbing and crusting which usually recovers by 7–15 days.

I am fully aware of the possible side effects and risks involved in this procedure. I am also aware that this particular procedure may not always be successful and no guarantee can be made for successful outcome of such procedure.

The possible risks of the procedure include but are not limited to pain, purpura, swelling, redness, bruising, blistering, crusting or scab formation, infection, and unforeseen complications which can last up to many months, years or permanently.

There is a risk of scarring, textual and/or color changes in the skin, which can be permanent.

I have been explained that multiple sessions may be required for satisfactory results and even after final results, maintenance treatments may be essential.

Some of the pigmented lesions are sensitive to sunlight and there are chances of recurrence of the lesions even after complete clearance.

Some lesions cannot be removed completely and there is no way one can predict the final outcome and number of sittings.

Topical, local or general anesthesia is required in few patients. I am ready to take the appropriate form of anesthesia.

I also know that this procedure will be performed by Dr _____ or his/her staff.

I also give my consent that during this procedure, if any complication arises, I may be given any emergency treatment best suitable to me without asking my prior permission.

I further state that I have carefully read and understood the all information provided in this form and I under fully conscious mind hereby give my written consent for the said procedure with its risks involved.

I consent to being photographed before and after sessions and that the photos may be used for academic and educational purposes without compromising my identity in public.

The payment and fee structure is informed to me. I am ready to pay per sitting or package basis. (Package if opted for includes minimum number of sittings and I have to pay accordingly if more sittings are required).

Signature of Patient/Thumb Impression

Signature of Parents/Guardian (For Minors)   Date: ....

....
Name and Relationship if Signed by other than Parent

Witness: ....   Date: ....
Name .... Signature ....
Date ....
Signature of Doctor .... Date ....
Translated in Patient's Language by ....

APPENDIX 3: FRACTIONAL CO_2 LASER RESURFACING: INFORMED CONSENT

Mr/Mrs/Miss ....

Age ....

Address .... City ....

Phone Numbers ...., ..., Mobile ....

Name of Procedure ....

Type of laser to be used: ....

I Mr/Mrs/Miss have been explained regarding above said procedure in my regional language.

I consent to the use of the fractional CO_2 laser in an effort to improve:

Acne scar/other scars/Discoloration/Photoaging/Skin texture/Wrinkles/fine lines/Other ......
....

I have been told that results from laser resurfacing may be variable from patient to patient and from treatment to treatment.

I understand that more than one treatment session is needed in order to obtain the improvement.

It has been explained to me that, although ablative fractional laser resurfacing is effective in most cases, no guarantees can be made that I will benefit from treatment.

I have also been told that the improvement may not be immediate. Skin usually keeps on improving for a period of 3 months to 1 year after a laser session.

There will be a downtime of 5–15 days postfractional laser. During this time my skin will not look good.

I understand that *side effects and complications* of ablative fractional CO_2 laser resurfacing include, but are not limited to:

- *Pain.* The stinging or burning sensation from the laser can produce a moderate amount of discomfort. An anesthetic cream, oral and injectable pain relievers and antianxiety medications will typically be used to minimize discomfort.
- *Redness:* Redness resembling sunburn can occur in treated area. The redness will typically subside in 1–6 weeks, but could last longer.
- *Swelling:* Treatment may cause swelling which subsides in 1–2 weeks and can be minimized with application of cool water compresses.
- *Skin darkening:* Darkening of the skin rarely occurs in the treated areas and will usually fade within 1–6 months. This reaction is more common when treated areas are exposed to the sun. It is extremely important to protect the treated area from sun exposure with a hat and sunscreen for 6 weeks after treatment and carefully adhere to all post-treatment instructions.
- *Skin lightening:* Laser treatment can result in loss of pigmentation where the treated area becomes a lighter color than the surrounding skin. It usually repigment in 1–6 months, but in rare cases could be permanent.

- *Blisters or scabs:* Blistering is uncommon but can develop with treatment. Blisters will go away within 2–5 days and may be followed by a scab. The scab will disappear during the natural wound healing process of the skin. During this time, the area should not be manipulated or picked, which can lead to scarring.
- *Infection:* Swelling, crusting, pain, or fever could indicate an infection or reactivation of cold sores or fever blisters. This may require use of topical or oral antibiotics and/or antiviral agents.
- *Acneiform eruptions:* Breakouts from acne have been reported to occur after treatment with laser resurfacing. If this occurs, topical or oral antibiotics may be required.
- *Scarring:* There is a risk of skin scarring, including abnormal raised and/or depressed scars with any resurfacing procedure. Careful adherence to all advised postoperative instructions will help reduce the possibility of this occurrence.
- *Lesion persistence or failure to respond:* Some skin conditions may not improve or go away completely despite the best efforts made by the doctor. No guarantees can be made regarding any individual's response to treatment with laser resurfacing.
- *Additional side effects:* There are risks associated with any procedure. Since it is impossible to state every risk or complication that may occur as a result of treatment, the possible risks and complications listed here may be incomplete. There may be risks or complications associated with this treatment that are not yet reported in the literature.

Pregnancy and Nursing Mothers: Laser treatment is not recommended for pregnant women or nursing mothers. By signing below I indicate that I am not pregnant. Furthermore, I agree to keep the staff informed should I become pregnant during the course of treatment.

I understand that treatment is contraindicated in patients currently taking anticoagulants, active skin infection, compromised immune system, impaired healing (e.g. keloid scar formers) pregnancy, and pacemaker.

Alternatives: Ablative fractional CO_2 laser resurfacing is a strictly voluntary cosmetic procedure. No treatment is necessary or required. Alternative treatments, which vary in side effects, duration and results, include other laser treatments, intense pulsed light therapy, dermabrasion, chemical peels, tissue filler products, botulinum toxin (Botox and others), topical bleaching agents, topical retinoid therapy, surgical acne scar treatment, etc.

I have read and understand the information on this consent form.

I have had the opportunity to ask questions. My questions have been answered to my satisfaction.

I have read the pre- and postoperative fractional CO_2 laser instructions and agree to comply with them. I understand that failure to comply may result in a greater likelihood of unwanted side effects.

I consent to the administration of topical, oral or injectable medications considered necessary or advisable.

I understand that all forms of anesthesia involve risks and the possibility of complication, injury, allergic reaction and even death.

Section 2: Dermatology

Consent for Photography: For the purpose of documenting my progress and response to treatment, I give permission to take photographs that will be kept in my medical record.

I give permission for the use of my photographs for medical teaching or patient information without my name being used and without compromising my identity.

Cost and Payment Policy: I have been explained about the cost of each laser session which is INR (rupees)................

I am going to pay per session or package basis. Package if opted for includes minimum number of sessions and I have to pay accordingly if any additional sessions or treatments are required.

I agree that this constitutes full disclosure, and that it supersedes any previous verbal or written disclosures. I certify that I have read, and fully understand the above paragraphs and that I have had sufficient opportunity for discussion to have any questions answered.

Signature of Patient/Thumb Impression

Signature of Parents/Guardian (For Minors)   Date: ....

....
Name and Relationship if Signed by other than Parent

Witness: ....   Date: ....
Name .... Signature ....
Date ....
Signature of Doctor .... Date ....
Translated in Patient's Language by ....

APPENDIX 4: CONSENT FORM FOR LASER FOR VASCULAR LESIONS

Mr/Mrs/Miss ....

Age ....

Address .... City ....

Phone Numbers ...., ..., Mobile ....

Name of Procedure ....

I Mr/Mrs/Miss have been explained regarding above said procedure in my regional language.

The laser system to be used is ....

Vascular lesion laser is used to treat abnormal blood vessels that are seen in conditions such as port-wine stain birthmarks, strawberry hemangiomas, telangiectasia (broken capillaries of spider veins), leg veins, rosacea, other ....

I have been told that my skin will not look good for the first few days after the procedure. There will be some pain, swelling, redness, scabbing, crusting and bruising which usually recovers by 7–15 days.

I am fully aware of the possible side effects and risks involved in this procedure. I am also aware that this particular procedure may not always be successful and no guarantee can be made for successful outcome of such procedure.

The possible risks of the procedure include but are not limited to pain, purpura, swelling, redness, bruising, blistering, crusting or scab formation, infection, and unforeseen complications which can last up to many months, years or permanently.

There is a risk of scarring, textual and/or color changes in the skin, which can be permanent.

I have been explained that multiple sessions may be required for satisfactory results and even after final results, maintenance treatments may be essential.

Some lesions cannot be removed completely and there is no way one can predict the final outcome and number of sittings.

Topical, local or general anesthesia is required in few patients. I am ready to take the appropriate form of anesthesia.

I have also been advised post-laser procedure sun protection and not adhering to it may increase the chance of complications.

I acknowledge that I must not be pregnant when I am receiving laser treatments.

I also know that this procedure will be performed by Dr _____ or his/her staff.

I also give my consent that during this procedure, if any complication arises, I may be given any emergency treatment best suitable to me without asking my prior permission.

I further state that I have carefully read and understood the all information provided in this form and I under fully conscious mind hereby give my written consent for the said procedure with its risks involved.

Section 2: Dermatology

I consent to being photographed before and after sessions and that the photos may be used for academic and educational purposes without compromising my identity in public.

The payment and fee structure is informed to me. I am ready to pay per sitting or package basis. (Package if opted for includes minimum number of sittings and I have to pay according if more sittings are required)

Signature of Patient/Thumb Impression

Signature of Parents/Guardian (For Minors)   Date: ....

....
Name and Relationship if Signed by other than Parent

Witness: ....   Date: ....
Name .... Signature ....
Date ....
Signature of Doctor .... Date ....
Translated in Patient's Language by ....

APPENDIX 5: CONSENT FOR TARGETED PHOTOTHERAPY: EXCIMER LASER/ EXCIMER LAMP

Mr/Mrs/Miss ....
Age ....
Address .... City ....
Phone Numbers ...., ..., Mobile ....
Name of procedure and indication ....

I Mr/Mrs/Miss have been explained regarding above said procedure in my regional language.

I understand that UVB (Ultraviolet-B light) is the most common form of phototherapy used to treat various skin diseases including vitiligo, psoriasis, eczema, itching, and disorders including striae alba and hypopigmented scars.

308-nm laser or lamp phototherapy or targeted phototherapy is an advanced form of UVB phototherapy that delivers targeted, high-dose, monochromatic or therapeutic light directly to affected tissue without exposing healthy skin.

By targeting only the affected tissue without exposing healthy skin, the laser delivers high-dose treatment that may promote faster clearing and longer remission than conventional UVB phototherapy.

While treatment times vary, most sessions for diseases last about 1–25 minutes.

It has been explained to me that this treatment is not a cure, but 308 nm UVB laser phototherapy or targeted phototherapy may effectively control or improve disease or disorder.

Maintenance treatments may be recommended to sustain disease clearing or repigmentation.

Each condition and patient will vary in the number of treatments needed and the time it will take to reach clearing.

Most patients initially require 2–3 treatments each week to clear their lesions. It may take 12–25 treatments to improve psoriasis and cosmetic conditions and 15–50 treatments to improve vitiligo. However, these numbers are indicative only and not sacrosanct.

Not all patients will clear completely. Many patients go into remission and may then stop needing treatments for varying periods, and thereafter need treatment with recurrence of the condition.

Some patients will not be benefited from the treatment at all and it has been explained to me that, although excimer laser or lamp or targeted phototherapy is effective in most cases, no guarantees can be made that I will benefit from treatment.

Additional medical treatment needs to be taken for effective control of the disease in addition to this modality of treatment.

Risks and side effects of phototherapy:
- The most common side effect of this therapy is UVB-induced sunburn, which tends to be mild- and short-lived. This may occur at any time during therapy. Certain drugs may also

cause you to get sunburn. Please let your doctor or nurse know of any medications you are taking, or any that you begin while undergoing therapy. If sunburns occur, steroid cream or any other appropriate medication may be used after treatment.

- Other possible but rare side effects include blistering and hyperpigmentation, which tend to be mild- and short-lived. If blistering occurs, antibiotic ointment or steroid creams may be used after treatment.
- It is possible with any form of UV light that an increased incidence of skin cancer may occur later in some patients, usually only with many UV light treatments over extended areas of skin. The targeted nature of 308 nm UVB laser phototherapy, short treatment time, and the low number of treatments may reduce this risk.
- Ultrasound treatments may cause dryness and itching.
- Ultrasound treatments age the skin over time and may increase freckles and pigmentation of the skin. The targeted nature of phototherapy, short-treatment time, and the low number of treatments may reduce this risk.
- Ultraviolet rays may damage the eyes and increase your risk of cataracts. This is preventable with protective eye goggles worn during treatment. These will be given to you and are required for treatment.
- Ultravoilet light may cause exacerbation of other medical conditions such as lupus erythematosus that have sensitivity to UV wavelength. All medical or other conditions must be disclosed to your doctor prior to starting therapy.

I have fully read and understand the above information regarding 308 nm UVB laser phototherapy.

I also understand that no one completely knows the long-term effects of UVB phototherapy including 308 nm UVB laser phototherapy.

I realize that these treatments do not cure my skin disorder and that I may need maintenance therapy.

My practitioner has explained the nature, purpose, and expected benefits of 308 nm UVB laser phototherapy, as well as the risks.

I have also been presented with the alternative treatments and their potential risk. My questions were answered regarding the procedure. I authorize my doctor (above) to prescribe light therapy.

This authorization extends to his or her associates, including other physicians and assistants selected by him or her, to carry out phototherapy. I understand that I am free to withdraw my consent and stop treatment at any time.

Additionally, I consent to be photographed before, during, and after the laser phototherapy; that these photographs shall be the property of the above doctors and may be used as they deem proper for scientific and educational purposes, without compromising my identity in public.

The payment and fee structure is explained to me.

Signature of Patient/Thumb Impression

Signature of Parents/Guardian (For Minors) Date: ....

....
Name and Relationship if Signed by other than Parent

Witness: .... Date: ....
Name .... Signature ....
Date ....
Signature of Doctor .... Date ....
Translated in Patient's Language by ....

CHAPTER 39

Consent in Procedures with Less Evidence and Off-label Indications

Maya Vedamurthy

UNDERSTANDING AESTHETIC PRACTICE

At present, a precise definition of aesthetic practice is lacking.[1] Esthetic practice is relatively in its infancy and there are many gray zones in esthetic practice, compared to medical dermatology practice. On the contrary, the growth of esthetic practice is manifold due to consumer demand driven by popularity and market type.

There is a serious need to follow evidence-based medicine (EBM) impending current medicolegal implications. Simultaneously, there is a compelling situation to treat our patients satisfactorily and effectively to avoid them drifting away to quacks, beauticians, and spas who are ever ready to try new technologies without any fear as they are not bound by medical laws.

As members of the medical profession, we are expected to offer procedures, which are backed by evidence of their safety and efficacy. Unlike nonmedical service providers, qualified physicians are expected to deliver results more effectively and safely failing which they are liable to prosecution. Performing procedures for an off-label indication or procedures with less evidence amounts to a deviation from the reasonable conduct of a competent practitioner and any complications arising, therefore, would mean malpractice.

For example, a 31-year-old male with patterned alopecia was treated with stem cell and Dermaroller procedures for 2 years by a firm, treating hair disorders. Since there was no satisfactory regrowth, the patient filed a case in the consumer forum seeking compensation. At the end of 4 years, a judgment was passed ordering the firm to refund the cost with interest. The weakness, in this case, was the use of stem cells, which according to the law was not evidence-based medicine and that the complainant was not made aware of this technology.

Esthetic dermatology is a rapidly evolving and progressing specialty, with new techniques and technologies being introduced. At the time of introduction, there may be little published evidence, apart from the certification from either Food and Drug Administration (FDA) or CE. The evidence is accumulated with experience, as the physicians keep using them. Botulinum toxin, Hyaluronic acid fillers and lasers for different indications have all evolved this way and reached the current level, where they are accepted as standard treatments with good quality of evidence. If evidence had been insisted at the time of their introduction, there would have been no progress at all.

On the contrary, newer technologies are hyped, promoted, and advertised aggressively, some of them without much logic and evidence about their safety or effectiveness.[2] Most often, studies are conducted later or not at all but the devices/drugs are freely available in the market for use. Many of such devices and treatments get introduced and disappear within a few years. Nonablative lasers, certain types of permanent fillers, some energy devices belong to these categories. Some treatments such as mesotherapy do not get adequate evidence despite years of being available. In such situations, the physician has a tough job to analyze and separate the grain from the chaff. Patients are demanding, and often push doctors in trying out new treatments. Experience, wisdom, and adherence to proper protocols are necessary in such situations.

GRADING THE QUALITY OF THE EVIDENCE

A useful grading in esthetic practice to judge the quality of evidence is the Grading of Recommendations Assessment, Development, and Evaluation (GRADE) working group.[3] GRADE working group definitions in grading the quality of the evidence are given in Table 1.

TABLE 1: GRADE working group definitions in grading the quality of the evidence.

High	Further research very unlikely to change our confidence in the estimated effect
Moderate	Further research is likely to have an important impact on our confidence in the estimate of effect and is likely to change the estimate
Low	Further research is very likely to have an important impact on our confidence in the estimate of effect and is likely to change the estimate
Very low	Any estimate of effect is very uncertain

(GRADE: Grading of Recommendations Assessment, Development, and Evaluation)

CLASSIFICATION OF AESTHETIC PROCEDURES BY THE SINGAPORE MEDICAL COUNCIL

In Singapore, the medical council has classified esthetic procedures based on currently available scientific evidence into List A and List B:
- *List A*: Where there is moderate-to-high level of evidence and/or with local medical expert consensus that the procedure is well established and acceptable.
- *List B*: Where, there is low or very low level of evidence and/or with local medical expert consensus that the procedure is neither well-established nor acceptable.

Aesthetic treatments that are currently regarded as having low/very low level of evidence are:
- Skin whitening injections
- Mesotherapy
- Stem cell therapy for hair regrowth
- Endermologic for cellulite treatment
- Platelet-rich plasma for facelift (vampire lift).

Clinical situations where a physician may seek to perform procedures, which are neither well-established nor acceptable currently, include:
- Failure of hair regrowth with conventional/evidence-based treatments
- When patients request repeatedly for treatments such as skin tightening for which there are no evidence based treatments
- Treatments with anecdotal evidence which are often marketed aggressively
- When cost-effectiveness of certain procedures with less evidence makes it affordable to a greater number of individuals
- Lack of clear standards of protocols by the healthcare system in our country.

Based on the above clinical situations, there are circumstances, which allow the use of low-evidence procedures on patients. Those circumstances that are considered eligible are as follows:
- When conventional and evidence-based treatments have been attempted yet not shown desirable outcomes.
- When the procedure selected has not been shown to carry any risk of significant adverse effects or harm to any patient.
- When the patient is fully aware of the status of the current treatment and given specific consent to this on a consent form.

When the above criteria are met, the physician is still liable to document the outcome of the procedure with scientific evidence and to terminate the practice of the procedure in case of adverse events.

The cost of the procedure of low evidence should be a bare minimum covering the cost of procedure and cost of providing them. These procedures of low evidence should not be marketed or advertised in any form.

THE POSITION OF BOLAM TEST

The so-called Bolam test, which determines a doctor's conduct supported by a responsible body of medical opinion, no longer applies to the issue of consent. The law now encourages a doctor to take "reasonable care to ensure that the patient is aware of any material risks involved in any recommended treatment and of any reasonable alternative or variant treatments".[4]

REMEDY AND PREVENTION

It is common for aesthetic physicians to use less evidenced medicine or off-label indications quite frequently. However, the legal requirement makes it mandatory to get a consent for such procedures with relevant information:
- The patient should be informed about the low level of evidence and about alternative procedures available.
- The material risk versus benefit ratio needs to be discussed. Treatments with significant risks should be avoided.
- Documentation of perceived outcomes both by patient and physician is recommended.
- A written informed consent is mandatory.
- For a clinical trial with procedures with less evidence, an ethical committee clearance should be obtained.

SUMMARY

It is well-known in esthetic practice that therapeutic guidelines are not necessarily the same as evidence-based medicine. There is a wide gap between evidence and consumer-driven practice by esthetic dermatologists that has led to a lot of misconstrued opinions in the field of esthetic medicine. At present, it is difficult to find higher levels of evidence for most of the common cutaneous and esthetic procedures. For such treatments, it is wise to consider the outcome of uncontrolled trials, anecdotal reports or interaction with colleagues.

Although the gold standard is to choose EBM, one cannot disregard the value of alternative therapies in certain situations. A careful analysis of the individual case and choice of well-known procedures based on personal experience as well as the experience of colleagues is essential. Routinely updating one's knowledge is essential to offering the best practices to our patients. Look out for the fate of procedures with low evidence with a scientific mind.

As Osler quotes:
"The philosophies of one age have become the absurdities of the next, and the foolishness of yesterday has become the wisdom of tomorrow."

So, we need to have an unbiased opinion on new and off-label indications as well as procedures with a low level of evidence.

KEY MESSAGES

Beware of medicolegal implications while choosing procedures with a low level of evidence or when using them for off-label indications. Now equipment and techniques need careful handling and training provided by the manufacturers.[5] Care of selection of the patient who understands the procedure in depth is recommended. We have to learn to play the game fair within safety to avoid medicolegal issues. Even better would be to avoid them, as it is better to be safe than sorry.[6]

"Be not the first by whom the new are tried, nor yet the last to lay the old aside."
—**Alexander Pope**

REFERENCES

1. Goh CL. The need for evidence based aesthetic dermatology practice. J Cutan Aesthet Surg. 2009;2: 65-71.
2. Sarkar R, Santhalia S, Gupta T, et al. Chapter 132: Evidence-based medicine in cutaneous and Aesthetic surgery. In: Venkatram M (Ed). ACS (I) Textbook of Cutaneous & Aesthetic Surgery, 2nd edition. New Delhi: Jaypee Brothers Medical Publisher (P) Ltd. 2017. pp. 1342-7.
3. GRADE Working Group. Grading quality of evidence and strength of recommendations. BMJ. 2004;328:1490.
4. Dyer C. Doctors should not cherry pick what information to give patients, court rules. BMJ. 2015;350:h1414.
5. Rao KHS. Chapter 134: Medicolegal issues in aesthetic surgery. In: Venkatram M (Ed). ACS (I) Textbook of Cutaneous & Aesthetic Surgery, 2nd edition. New Delhi: Jaypee Brothers Medical Publisher (P) Ltd. 2017. pp. 1353-9.
6. Kapoor L. Informed consent in aesthetic surgery. J Cutan Aesthet Surg. 2015;8:173-4.

SECTION 3

Plastic Surgery

- Changing Face of Plastic Surgery: An Overview
- How can a Plastic Surgeon Avoid Getting into Trouble or Litigation?
- How to Identify an Unsuitable Patient for Plastic (Aesthetic) Surgery
- Revision Surgery in Aesthetic Plastic Surgery
- Esthetic Procedures and Surgery in Minors
- Legal Issues in Medical Tourism
- Delivering Bad News after Plastic Surgery
- Photography and the Issue of Patient Confidentiality
- Medicolegal Issues in Burns
- Medical Negligence in Plastic, Aesthetic and Reconstructive Surgery
- Medicolegal Issues in Setting-up a Plastic Surgery Day Care Surgery Set-up
- Medicolegal Issues in Liposuction
- Tips and Pearls for Medicolegal Situations

CHAPTER 40

Changing Face of Plastic Surgery: An Overview

Milind S Wagh

INTRODUCTION

Plastic surgery is a vast specialty comprising of multiple subspecialties, which taken together treat and manage conditions related to the entire human body, from head to toe. It involves the repair, reconstruction, and refining of all tissues from skin to bone for congenital, acquired and post-traumatic deformities and defects as well as their aesthetic considerations. The results of the surgeries and procedures that Plastic Surgeons undertake are usually apparent on the body surface in terms of scars, shapes, and contours, often in areas which are visible not only to the patient but to society at large. Furthermore, leaving aside emergency surgery in cases of trauma and cases of cancer reconstruction, plastic surgery is one of those rare specialties, which electively treats patients who are otherwise healthy and well and seeks to improve both function and appearance in these normal individuals. On the other hand, most other specialties treat a sick patient and try to make him/her better.

Advances in technology and techniques, availability and ever-increasing influence of social media, globalization and the change in socioeconomic standards have also meant the patients are more discerning and critical of their results, have greater choice of nonsurgical versus surgical treatment and ready access to all kinds of scientific and nonscientific information. Lastly, the medical field in general and ours in particular is squarely placed within the sphere of consumer protection; even if medicine and surgery are still a far from perfect science and the human body is not a machine but a flesh and blood entity with endless variables and vagaries, we are service providers to the patients; we are professionals with specialty-specific knowledge and qualifications practicing in an "open market" environment, who it is assumed and implicitly understood will provide a high-standard of care.

A failure of accepted Standard of Care may be defined as "Failure of the treating surgeon to willfully exercise a reasonable degree of skill, care, and level of treatment that might be normally expected from his qualified colleagues in the same specialty, keeping up with the advances in the field".

It is therefore imperative that all Plastic Surgeons be aware and beware of the law and its implications as applicable to our practice. Knowing our medicolegal responsibilities as well as anticipating and dealing with the possibility of litigation should be part and parcel of our knowledge base and practice protocol.

Due care and diligence in this respect as much as what we exercise in the surgical management of our patients, should be the norm, not the exception.

COMMUNICATION WITH PATIENT

In the great majority of cases of patients who contemplate litigation against their Plastic Surgeon, poor and ineffective communication and inadequate rapport between the two is the overriding issue. This rapport, this building of a doctor–patient relationship strengthens over time but it starts right from the time of the first consultation. In fact, just as a surgeon reaches a diagnosis about the patient's disease or condition after history taking and examination, the patient reaches a decision about his/her comfort level and confidence in the Doctor sitting across, within the first few minutes of that initial interaction. There are multiple factors involved in this complex issue, some tangible, others imponderable.

Completely nonclinical issues unrelated to the doctor's surgical ability, such as how well the Doctor appears to be listening to the patient's concerns *as perceived by him/her*, the doctor's sartorial elegance, sitting stance, eye contact, warmth, and sensitivity are important to the patient and play a great role in the patient's decision-making in choosing his/her surgeon.

A surgeon who is perceived as caring and cordial with a good sense of humor will score as much with a patient as a surgeon with known surgical skill, vast experience, and sterling reputation. On the other hand, irrespective of the surgeon's clinical abilities, someone perceived as cold, aloof, arrogant, or insensitive will score poorly. Similarly, the surgeon who will give the patient enough time at the consultation, who puts the patient at comfort, who offers a lot of relevant and up-to-date information, who openly and transparently discusses the pros and cons of the treatment to be undertaken, who is happy to discuss alternative treatments and even suggest colleagues who might be better and more experienced, will always be trusted more by the patient right there and in the future. Establishing this communication, rapport, and level of trust with the patient is, more often than not, the difference between an angry, sullen, and resentful patient leading to a potential malpractice or negligence suit versus the patient's understanding and acceptance of a less than satisfactory result.

It is critical for the surgeon to be aware and understand that as laypersons, patients and their family or relatives feel a sense of disappointment and shock when the procedure undertaken does not go as smoothly as expected or assured. Bewilderment and uncertainty slowly transform to anxiety and finally to anger, which is directed at the surgeon who is perceived as the root cause of their predicament. Everyone knows that there are complex variables and uncertainties related to treating the human body. However, at that juncture, any sequelae and complications in spite of the best standard of surgical and postoperative care are not taken into account by an angry patient. At that point, it is mandatory that the concerned surgeon be calm, hold hands and patiently explain the reasons for the present situation, assume responsibility, and re-establish trust and confidence and assure and reassure the patient that *together*, the problem can be overcome and corrected. The level of the patient's confidence, trust, and belief that the surgeon understands his/her fear and anxiety, that he empathizes and will be there through the journey to its satisfactory final outcome, can well be the deciding factor in the patient and relatives taking a legal recourse.

One issue that is often overlooked is comments and criticism of one's colleagues. Patients "shop" around a lot and it is their prerogative. It is unethical one-upmanship and crass to criticize a colleague's opinion, put him/her down as junior, uninformed, or wrong while extolling one's own virtues. It is true for both patients who are unoperated but have visited other colleagues before they came to you, as well as in cases of postoperative sequelae and complications at your colleague's hands. Unsatisfied patients often try to gauge your response, find vindication in it vis-à-vis their own anger and resentment and will attempt to use that against your colleague. It is wise to remember that it could happen to you as well and the shoe could very well be on the other foot. A polite but firm "no comment" or even elaborating that it is ethically poor form and unfair to make any comments on someone else's work should suffice to clearly let the patient know where you stand.

In summary, faulty and poor communication is the root cause of the vicious cycle of resentment, anger, and hostility from the patient that the surgeon is confronted with, in the face of an unsatisfactory outcome (Box 1).

> **BOX 1:** Tips on communication: How much is enough?
> - Do disclose the identity of the treating surgeon, if he/she differs from the attending surgeon
> - Do discuss risk of death or serious harm, if applicable
> - Do not inform patient that the procedure is simple and that no complications will occur
> - Do not perform procedures in addition to the principal procedure without specific consent unless an emergency situation develops
> - Do not expect to obtain informed consent by merely answering questions that the patient asks, volunteer the appropriate information
> - Do provide the patient with an opportunity to ask questions

PATIENT SELECTION

In the present era of surgical practice, particularly in Plastic Surgery, where we deal with normal healthy patients in whom we seek to improve function and aesthetics, it is critical that every surgeon acquires a modicum of intuition and perception in being able to pick and choose the correct patients for treatment. It is just as much if not more important than understanding and accepting the boundaries of one's own skill-sets, surgical comfort zones, and areas of core competence. It is more important to know when not to accept and treat a particular patient than it is to actually go ahead with the treatment.

Many patients have no comprehension whatsoever that surgery involves dealing with human flesh and blood, not a machine or material. It is not akin to modifying in two dimensions (or even three) on Adobe Photoshop or with sophisticated morphing software sitting at a computer terminal. They do not know the realities of the surgery, the variables of the postoperative healing process, the flexibility in the results, and the margins of error related even to a good or excellent overall result.

As the surgeon listens to and observes the patient at the time of consultation, it is important to pick-up signals and cues from the patient (and his/her relatives) as regards their suitability to undergo treatment under *your* care. The indications and contraindications for the treatment to be undertaken based on physical examination findings and patient's general fitness and even the surgeon's surgical abilities are sometimes secondary to the importance of listening to these "signals".

- Patients with unrealistic expectations and those with a utopian idea of what the procedure is likely to do. Often patients anticipate and assume that the result of the planned surgery will transform and improve their lives, their social standing, and their attractiveness to spouse, partner, or society well beyond the gamut of the actual result. Those who set that much store merely by the result of the procedure itself without making any other change in their lifestyles, personalities, and environment are likely to be disappointed and resentful.
- Patients with a vague idea of what they want and who leave it to the surgeon to decide on their behalf as to what will improve their function and appearance. These patients are intrinsically indecisive and will never be happy with the result.
- Patients with excessive demands, especially those who bring in photographs of celebrities and models, those who come in with extremely specific calculations of inches and kilograms and those who come with nonscientific articles and information from internet sites. They have no clue whether their own age, sex, individual body type, genetics, and metabolism lend to such likely results; they are merely fixated on what seems to them their personal idea of perfection.
- Patients who appear to be emotionally labile or immature. Their intrinsic psychological instability does not permit these patients to accept anything less than what their preconceived notion of the result should be and even there they may continually change their ideas. These patients can be a real threat to the Plastic Surgeon even outside the gamut of litigation.
- Patients who come on their own and insist that they do not want to reveal their surgery to spouses, partner, or families because of fear of disapproval and not being permitted to undergo the procedure. It is sometimes possible that if the result is not to the patient's expectations and the family member has disapproved or refused permission, the guilt, resentment, and anger that the patient feels is multiplied and directed at the surgeon. While adult patients can legally consent to their own procedure, many hospitals insist on kin being present at the time of admission as well as during the procedure to take medicolegal responsibility for the patient.
- Patients and relatives whom the surgeon does not like or trust intuitively are also risks for surgery. This mistrust and dislike can subconsciously affect and cloud the surgeon's judgment and behavior with the patient and relatives.
- Patients who want to keep their procedure secret and request more than normal precautions to hide their identities or even request falsifications in documentation. I would also include a warning against patients who request the surgeon to fraudulently modify the procedure they wish to undergo, on all official notations, in order to claim insurance benefits or cashless/TPA (Third Party Administrator).

These patients can be more trouble than they are worth, live aside the implications of insurance fraud on the reputation of the surgeon.

- Patients with conditions outside the sphere of the surgeon's core competence, surgical comfort zones and skill-sets. This is no longer an era for general plastic surgery where every surgeon will operate everything from head to toe. In this era of superspecialization and highly specific subspecialties, each surgeon with time in practice gravitates to a particular area where he develops additional skill and finesse, which directly reflect on the superior quality of his results. Occasional surgery on a condition or procedure outside this area of frequent practice can only yield suboptimal results, with all except the rare supremely skilled surgeon. An averagely skilled surgeon is well advised to seek help from or refer to colleagues who are better or more experienced than him for a particular procedure. Being junior and in need of experience and exposure across the spectrum of subspecialties and/or financial reasons are no excuse for such profligacy in the eye of the law.
- Minor patients below the age of personal consent (usually below 18 years of age) must have adult family members present at the time of consultation and throughout their treatment period. Apart from congenital, acquired and post-traumatic conditions that require reconstructive treatment in children and minors, there are anatomical, physiological, and psychological issues involved in treating minors before physical and emotional growth is complete and these must be carefully considered on a case-to-case basis. Cases of gender reassignment surgery pose a specific and different challenge as well.
- Last but definitely not the least, the Plastic Surgery "junkie" patient and the patient with body dysmorphic disorder (BDD). These patients, in spite of being essentially physical normal have a very poor body self-image and inferior self-worth and believe that plastic surgery, often repeated and unending, can improve their psychological and physical well-being and self-worth. They are patients to be avoided at all costs or at least be very careful about in the interests of the plastic surgeon's own personal well-being!!! They are unlikely to be satisfied with one, two, or even three procedures and will demand more and more, even when those areas are perfectly normal.

In general, it is prudent and smart to carefully and dispassionately weigh what is known as the risk-to-benefit ratio in the case of every single patient. The wise and experienced plastic surgeon refuses as many patients as he accepts, having considered all the implications related to his/her treatment. As a senior surgeon and medicolegal consultant in Mumbai has put it, it is always *better to be safe than sorry*.

INFORMED CONSENT

It is estimated that problems with informed consent are responsible for more than 15% of all medical malpractice cases in the USA. The statistics for India are as yet unknown. However, in the case of plastic surgery, it is logical to expect this figure to be higher, especially in cosmetic or aesthetic surgery (Box 2).

The singular basis for informed consent prior to a procedure is that any patient has the absolute right to be informed, fully know and consent to exactly what procedure is to be undertaken on him/her, while being in

> **BOX 2:** Elements of informed consent.
>
> Discuss the following six elements of a valid informed consent with patients and their families:
> 1. The diagnosis or suspected diagnosis
> 2. The nature and purpose of the proposed treatment or procedure and its anticipated benefits
> 3. The risks, complications, and side effects
> 4. The probability of success, based on the patient's condition
> 5. Reasonable available alternatives
> 6. Possible consequences, if advice is not followed

full command of his/her mental faculties, in a language that he/she completely understands. Not only is this related to the actual procedure itself, its pros and cons, its risks and benefits, possible common sequelae and complications well beforehand, the patient is also entitled to be fully informed about the alternatives available based on routine accepted standard of care, including the pros and cons of no treatment at all. It is not incumbent on the patient to ask for this information; it must be volunteered by the treating surgeon. All this must also be documented and signed by the patient and a witness (preferably patient's family member or adult friend) as well as by the treating surgeon with date and time mentioned therein, *prior* to the procedure itself.

As far as possible, informed consent should not be generalized but must be specific to the procedure to be undertaken. A blanket consent form of the hospital or clinic signed by the patient is not adequate in the court of law, it must be supplemented with personalized operation-specific forms. The consent form must specifically mention all the procedures to be performed, their risks and benefits, commonly anticipated sequelae, and the alternative treatments informed to the patient including the pros and cons of not undergoing that specific treatment. Any site marking done by the surgeon and the patient's consent or refusal for the same must be included. Consent for any photographs taken by the surgeon prior to surgery and in the course of postoperative follow-up meetings including specific consent for their use on websites, social media, presentations, and publications outside the gamut of surgeon–patient confidentiality are mandatory and separate.

While intraoperative modification of the procedure being consented for and being performed by the surgeon, based on possible unanticipated intraoperative findings is a gray area in law, the law explicitly, and clearly does not permit the surgeon to intraoperatively *add* any other elective procedure that the patient has not been explained and consented for in writing, while in full command of her mental faculties, if it is not a standard part of the actual procedure in toto. Apart from the exceptional emergency situation, where the closest present family member or spouse can consent on the patient's behalf in the event of an unforeseen intraoperative issue to save the life of the patient, the surgeon's hands are tied with respect to the procedure to be performed. He *must* adhere to only those procedures for which an informed consent has been taken from the patient himself/herself.

Informed consent must be taken by the surgeon who will perform the procedure. Any assistant or co-surgeons who will be part of the procedure should ideally be informed and consented to by the patient. It is not legally acceptable for the surgeon to give the patient the impression that he will perform the surgery personally and then have a trainee or qualified colleague perform the surgeon once the patient is under anesthesia. The phenomenon of "Ghost Surgeons" falls within the purview of this area of medicolegal quicksand.

Informed consent should include diagnosis, mention of relatively common minor sequelae, and complications, which would be considered associated with that procedure on peer-review and prognosis with the treatment and without it. The rare but well-known serious complication must be disclosed and included. The Supreme Court has decided in a particular case that every conceivable problem need not be informed. Information of rare complications, which will deter a patient from undergoing an absolutely necessary surgery, or an extremely rare complication of an ailment, which will scare a patient into undergoing the procedure, need not be informed.

The acceptable legal standard would perhaps be everything that a reasonable patient needs to be told and informed in writing about to make a rational decision to consent to the procedure.

DOCUMENTATION

Apart from the informed consent related to the procedure itself, there is other documentation that is important from the legal point of view. In our field, this includes photographs in different views taken preoperatively and then serially postoperatively in the course of the patient's postoperative follow-up. Consent for these photographs has already been mentioned. A questionnaire given to each patient, to fill in and sign with personal and medical/surgical details while they wait to see you, can be advantageous to keep in your records. It can be referred to while talking to the patient and any additional information given by the patient in the course of the consultation added by you and countersigned by the patient. Consultation notes with specific notations about patient's history, comorbid conditions, addictions, current medications, etc. are very important. So are any and all prescriptions and preoperative/postoperative advice given on your letterhead or prescription pad. A scanned copy or photocopy of the same for your office records should ideally be maintained.

Operation/procedure notes should ideally be written in your own handwriting or dictated to an assistant but countersigned by you. This is best done immediately after surgery while your memory of the procedure is fresh or at least the same evening. It should mention all the salient steps of the procedure including any additional steps undertaken due to intraoperative findings. Labels of any implants put in the patient's body, with the information related to the same, should be part of this operative note. A copy of the labels must be kept by you and also placed on the patient's discharge note.

All your postoperative visits to assess the patient's recovery during the patient's stay in hospital must be recorded with details of the patient's condition and important parameters related to his/her recovery at that time. These notations must have the date and time as well as your signature. Documents related to the patient's treatment must be kept as long as possible, as hard copies and soft copies or at least the latter. In the eyes of the law, if it is not in the records and is not documented, *it does not exist.*

PROFESSIONAL INDEMNITY INSURANCE

Plastic Surgery is broadly divided into reconstructive and aesthetic surgery. While reconstructive surgery has historically been covered by indemnity insurance, the same firms used to balk at covering aesthetic surgery fearing they may be inundated by claims from unsatisfied patients. The scenario is now changed with some insurance companies offering indemnity insurance covering aesthetic surgery as well, albeit at the cost of a much higher premium.

Our specialty is under the umbrella of consumer protection and we are deemed as service providers. The majority of suits and claims filed by patients are malafide, frivolous, and mischievous. The courts, however, have not been consistent in judging and deciding on these claims and there has been no clear-cut limitation or ceiling on the quantum of awards given to the patient in the case of established negligence or malpractice. It is therefore wise to invest in Professional Indemnity cover (of at least ₹ 50 lakhs for surgeons who do reconstructive work and at least ₹ 1 Crore for surgeons whose predominant field of work is aesthetic surgery).

THE PHENOMENON OF "GHOST" SURGEONS

Plastic Surgery and its subspecialties, particularly aesthetic surgery, have recently been under criticism and debate with respect to the issue of Ghost Surgeons. The perceived huge lure of the lucre associated with this branch has unfortunately meant that practitioners from allied specialties and even unrelated specialties have earnestly tried to jump onto the bandwagon, in an effort to retain and not lose any patient that primarily comes to them, whether or not the patient's ailment is related to their specialty.

The usual modus operandi for the primary referring Doctor is to consult with the said patient, already discuss and plan the surgical procedure to be done, encourage the patient to pay up the costs related to the procedure in advance and then "invite" a plastic surgeon, qualified or otherwise, only to perform the actual said procedure. Often the operating surgeon has had no interaction whatsoever with the patient till immediately prior to the procedure and meets him/her only fleetingly. Sometimes, even this is sought to be avoided and the surgeon enters the picture with the patient already under anesthesia, completes the procedure, and goes away, without once having seen or interacted with the patient. Even his name does not appear on the operative notes, which mention the primary referring doctor only. All postoperative care is given by this worthy and the actual surgeon has no further role in treatment. The patient has no clue—who performed the actual surgical procedure. The surgeon is paid his surgical fees, which are a small percentage of the overall bill paid by the patient.

More often than not, young surgeons fresh or still not established in their own practice but eager to "keep the money meter running" acquiesce to this condemnable phenomenon, little realizing that they are putting the patient at the grave risk of suboptimal postoperative care at the hands of an untrained and uninformed colleague (the eye does not see what the mind does not know) and also putting themselves in a virtually untenable position medicolegally should complications arise.

This is one of the truly regrettable offshoots of the burgeoning of "Cosmetic Clinics" in many urban and semiurban set-ups by nonmedical personnel with money to spare and invest, where the young and impressionable surgeon is exploited; his training, his qualifications, and often his desperation are used unscrupulously by a person to whom the patient is merely a via-media to make money without any regard to ethics, safety, and practice guidelines of any kind. The susceptible surgeon would do well to keep away from this temptation, which literally constitutes a betrayal of what the Hippocratic Oath stands for.

SUMMARY

Plastic surgical practice has undergone a seachange in the last two decades or so. As our so-called noble profession has slowly metamorphosed in keeping with societal changes, it is now clearly driven by market forces and commerce. Much as we would like to deny it, it is well-nigh time that we realize, recognize, and accept that though we are still "doctors" with "patients", we are now also categorized as service providers to consumers, like other professions. It is therefore imperative that all of us plastic surgeons get down from our egotistical high horse as practitioners of what we have traditionally been considered "a unique surgical specialty", *which is part art and part science*, and therefore in our eyes often subject to variables in results beyond our control. Be that as it may, the fact of the matter is that we are now firmly and unequivocally within the ambit of the Consumer Protection Act and therefore legally as liable as any of our colleagues in any other specialty for a failure to provide a "standard of care". In fact being deemed as highly qualified superspecialists, our liability extends further than most.

As such, we can no longer afford to be ostriches with our heads in the sand, believing that our responsibility and accountability begin and end with merely treating our patients to the best of our ability and knowledge. It is of course still our ethical responsibility to protect the sanctity of the doctor–patient relationship but we would be well advised to learn at the same time to be fully aware of our medicolegal obligations and liabilities as well. It is imperative that we exercise discretion and wisdom in carefully choosing patients for surgery and that we understand the vital importance of communicating with them promptly, clearly, and transparently not just in advance of the procedure but throughout the recovery phase. Similarly, the onus of taking a well-crafted and fully informed specific consent for every procedure and ensuring that the documentation related to every interaction with the patient is prompt, detailed and precise, and is entirely our own.

To successfully and safely practice in the scenario of the present and the foreseeable future, the continued evolution of our profession and our specialty will undoubtedly demand from each of us not just professional competence, surgical skill, and regularly updated knowledge, but equally a maintenance of high-ethical standards and medicolegal accountability.

SUGGESTED READING

1. Mathes SJ. Liability Issues in Plastic Surgery. Plastic Surgery, 2nd edition. Philadelphia: Elsevier; 2007. pp. 147.
2. Mad Mimi. (2016). Medical Malpractice Insights. Learning from Lawsuits. April 2016. [online] Available from: https://madmimi.com/p/ad4f87. [Accessed December, 2018].
3. Sharma RK. Medicolegal aspects of Patient Care, 3rd edition. New Delhi: Peepee Publishers; 2008.

CHAPTER 41

How can a Plastic Surgeon Avoid Getting into Trouble or Litigation?

Sanjay Parashar

KEY POINTS

- Introduction
- Ethical and medicolegal Hurdles
- Potential Problems for Litigation
- Documentation
- Role of Informed Consent
- Information Booklet
- Postoperative management
- Good Clinical Practice (GCP) Guidelines

INTRODUCTION

Cosmetic surgeons are more liable than conventional plastic and reconstructive surgeons to face a medicolegal situation. The elective nature of cosmetic surgery has risk of more malpractice claims; at the same time it is not easy for patients to bring legal claims successfully as he or she has chosen to do it on her Own accord, despite knowing the risks and benefit. Hence the key is to keep them informed and made aware of the risks and benefits realistically. While on one hand there are significant scientific and technological advances in our field but there have been negative changes such as unregulated commercialization, unethical practice, deterioration of moral values, employment of unskilled staff, cost cutting efforts compromising quality of care in cosmetic surgery (Box 1).

The doctor-patient relationship has undergone a vast change over the years. Patient often seeks multiple opinions from different doctors. Difference in opinion often causes confusion in the mind of the patient. And if the opinion is contradictory and or critical for various true or incorrect reasons the patient without having true knowledge moves the court to seek compensation. A promise to correct someone else's alleged mistake and provocative moves to motivate patient to claim for financial benefit are some of unethical practice performed by some doctors.

Use of marketing tools to lure the patient by enticing them, giving them unrealistic expectations have also played significant role

> **BOX 1:** Hurdles for successful plastic surgical practice: All U's for easy recall.
> - U: Unregulated commercialization of latest aesthetic surgeries
> - U: Unskilled staff and junior surgeons (cost cutting by hospital)
> - U: Undue expectations of patient
> - U: Unhappy patient (before elective surgery)
> - U: Uncooperative patient (child/mentally-ill/elderly Alzheimer's)
> - U: Unsuitable patient–SIMON stands for S-Single, I-Immature, M-Male, O-Overexpectations, N-Narcissistic
> - U: Undertaking inadequate consent
> - U: Unnecessary surgery (nose job for improving beauty)
> - U: Unethical practice for fee splitting among surgeons
> - U: Unavoidable medical errors (same named patients in OT list)
> - U: Unretrieved device fragments or sponges
> - U: Unstable clinical status of patient (on anticoagulants)
> - U: Unsteady hand of surgeon during surgery (postparty hangover)
> - U: Undesirable outcome of recovery (prolonged stay)
> - U: Unexpected outcomes of surgery (hypertrophied scar/keloid)
> - U: Ugly scar after surgery
> - U: Unseen leftover foreign body (gossypiboma)
> - U: Unsettled hospital bills by patient's coming for next surgery.

in malpractice suits. Marketing materials containing words as best, only, first, may be misleading to patients and should not be used in any communicating tools.

Potential Problems for Litigation in Cosmetic Surgery Practice

There are two problems patient come up with:
1. Dissatisfaction
2. Complications or side effects.

Dissatisfaction with Result is Due to Following Reasons

- Over expectations or unrealistic expectations
- Substandard results delivered by surgeon.

Dissatisfaction leads to psychological distress or morbidity and if proven by a psychiatrist, can be a concern for cosmetic surgeons. So screening of patient by psychological assessment before conducting aesthetic surgery is good preventive step for avoiding malpractice litigation.

Complications are Due to

- Usual known complications that are part of any surgery
- Unusual complications caused iatrogenically.

And complications may lead to pain, physical limitation, deformity and long-term morbidity.

According to statistical research, plastic surgery patients expressed dissatisfaction with their results in nearly three out of every ten claims made over a 10-year period. Problems such as infection, emotional distress, and scar deformities accounted for 14% of case each. The remainder of claims included burns, asymmetry, and death at 5% each, and account for the vast majority of claims made against plastic surgeons.

It appears that patient dissatisfaction with the results of plastic surgery is the driving force behind many plastic surgery claims, as opposed to physical harm from procedures. Contributing factors include unrealistic patient expectations and the patient's failure to comply with the plastic surgeon's instructions due to communication issues. It would appear that plastic surgeons might reduce their risk of being sued for plastic surgery malpractice if they more effectively communicate with their patients regarding the results they may expect as well as the instructions they must follow.[1]

Body contouring procedures were analyzed for medical malpractice. The most common injuries sustained were disfigurement and necessitation of a revision procedure. The most cause of action cited was negligence. The study emphasizes the need for adequate communication with the patient explaining realistic aesthetic results and risks of the procedure. In addition, iatrogenic organ injury must be handled expeditiously. Inappropriate delays can cause fatal complications and morbidity and hence is surgeon's liability. Incorporating these recommendations into clinical practice may promote an improved physician-patient relationship while reducing litigations.[2]

Face lift related risks: Common factors cited by plaintiffs for pursuing litigation included dissatisfaction with cosmetic outcomes and perceived deficits in informed consent. These factors reinforce the importance of a comprehensive, preoperative informed consent process in which the specific potential risks and outcomes are presented by the surgeon to the patient to limit or avoid postsurgical allegations. Intraoperative negligence and facial nerve injury were significantly more likely to result in poor defendant outcomes. The most common allegations raised in litigation were intraoperative negligence, 69% poor cosmesis or disfigurement, 64%; inadequate informed consent, 34%; additional procedures required, 16%; postoperative negligence, 14%; and facial nerve injury (11%).[3]

Finally, it is important to stress that physicians may be held liable for procedures performed by nonphysician ancillary staff.[4]

Retained Surgical Instruments and Unretrieved Device Fragments

Gossypiboma, textiloma or more broadly Retained foreign object (RFO) is the technical term for a surgical complications resulting from foreign materials, such as a surgical sponge, accidentally left inside a patient's body. The term "gossypiboma" is derived from the Latin *Gossypium* ("cotton wool, cotton") and the suffix—oma,[8,9] meaning a tumor or growth, and describes a mass within a patient's body comprising a cotton matrix surrounded by a foreign body granuloma. "Textiloma" is derived from textile (surgical sponges have historically been made of cloth), and is used in place of gossypiboma due to the increasing use of synthetic materials in place of cotton. To prevent gossypiboma, sponges are counted by hand before and after surgeries. The Association of Perioperative Registered Nurses (AORN) codified this method into recommended guidelines in the 1970s. Four separate counts are recommended: the first when instruments and sponges are first unpackaged and set up, a second before the beginning of the surgical procedure, a third as closure begins, and a final count during final skin closure. In most countries, surgical sponges contain radiopaque material that can be readily identified in radiographic and computed tomography (CT) images, facilitating detection. Some surgeons recommend routine postoperative X-ray films after surgery to reduce the likelihood of foreign body inclusion.

A retained surgical instrument is any item inadvertently left behind in a patient's body in the course of surgery. There are few books about it and it is arguably under reported.

As a preventable medical error, it occurs more frequently than "wrong site" surgery. The consequences of retained surgical tools include injury, repeated surgery, excess monetary cost, and loss of hospital credibility and in some cases death of patient.

Documentation in Cosmetic Surgery Practice

A structure of consultation involves:

General Consultation and Counseling

This is primarily done by plastic surgeons, but key information can be provided by other staff that has interacted with patients either on phone or emails or first encounter at the reception. The process of conversation, filling of patient information sheet, etc. helps to understand the psychic of patient, their temperament and attitude towards the medical practice. A red flag is indicated when patient are angry, annoyed, impatient and complaining-types without significant reason.

During consultation the surgeon listens to patient and records the detail in terms of primary concerns, expectations and medical background. All the details need to be entered either in manual or electronic record.

The surgeon that examines the patient and records all the details in brief. Then the process of explanation starts. It is recommended that surgeon explain the patient on a piece of paper along with illustrations (documented). The explanation should include following:
- What are the deformities, asymmetries, disproportions patient have?
- Procedure options including no treatment at all
- Details of each procedure with pros and cons of each
- Doctors recommendation to patient as per his or her expectations
- Limitations of the procedure recommended
- Specific complications or side effects if any.

At the end of consultation, patient is handed over a written document, which covers the details (Appendix 1).

Patient is then explained about the costs involved covering following information:
- What does the cost cover?
- What is excluded and additional cost of those exclusions?
- What happens when additional procedure or consumables are required?

Second Consultation

After providing complete information, patient has time to "cool off". Some treatment or surgeries may not require cooling off period. Or in case the patient has already consulted other doctors and merely waiting to make a final decision. Specific procedures that require second consultations include:
- Rhinoplasty
- Face lift
- Breast surgery
- Tummy tuck or body lift
- Hair transplantation (HT).

The second consultation involves questionnaires by patient, any doubts, etc. The surgeon then explains detail of pre-, intra- and postsurgery protocols, follow-up requirements, after care, etc.

This visit may require showing some photographs and videos of best and not so good results. Pictures of scars etc. also help the patent to make a well-informed decision.

Preoperative Checkup and Planning

This is after patient has decided to undergo surgery and requires medical checkup, etc. At this time a proper physical evaluation with documentation of the areas of concerns are recorded by the operating surgeon. A structured worksheet and prewritten instructions allows uniformity and standardization based on individual protocol. Photographic documentation is mandatory at this stage.

Informed Consent

It is a voluntary agreement made by a well-advised and mentally competent patient to be treated. The information must be explained in comprehensible nonmedical terms preferably in local language about the:

- *Diagnosis:* Primary concerns and bodily changes
- *Nature of treatment:* Surgery, procedures, etc.
- Alternative methods of treatment
- Risk and benefit of both proposed and alternative treatments
- Prognosis if procedure not performed
- Relative chances of success or failure, scars, potential deformities, need for secondary surgeries, etc.

The above needs to be explained by surgeon in presence of witness preferably one on behalf of each patient and surgeon, and all parties sign the consent forms at the same time.

Consent cannot be taken to be a valid defense where the complainant is able to show that there was negligence and carelessness on the part of the opposite parties at the time of surgery.[5]

Written Instructions

A complete written instruction with dates of follow-up care is helpful. Many times patient forget and it is hard to prove that surgeons have given all instructions required. An acknowledgement form that states that patient have received the documents is also essential as patient may forget or deny.

In email consultations, these need to be posted to the patient before surgery, particularly if a patient is visiting from another place, e.g. postop facial edema after HT may affect a patients' travel by flight and hence should be told to the patient.

Postoperative Management (Appendix 2)

This is the key to patient satisfaction. A regular preplanned schedule with close follow-up given personally by the surgeon will help relax the patient and relieve their apprehension. An early detection and action of complications will prevent disasters. Communication with patient about what is happening and with their relatives will also help maintain the trust. The attitude should be to help the patient.

Discharge protocol with details of contact and basic instructions to follow in case of need or emergency is a useful tool to maintain trust and confidence.

Medical Negligence can be avoided by following basic principles of Good Clinical Practice (GCP) guidelines for clinical management, clinical information, accurate documentation, clinical analysis and appropriate communication with the patient (Box 2).[6]

Scars

Scar is a big issue in aesthetic plastic surgery. Patient needs to be aware of the possible scars, its exact location, and possible length of scars and what could be the fate of the scars. Explain patient following things about scar:

- *Type of scars:* Fine line, discolored line, stretched scar, hypertrophic scars, keloids, etc.
- What protocols will be followed to minimize scars?

> **BOX 2:** All D's Mnemonic: Easy recall of avoiding the vicious circle of sequence of events during malpractice lawsuit.
>
> - D: Doctor patient relationship during first visit
> - D: Drawback in documenting informed consent
> - D: Defensive clinical practice: unnecessary investigations
> - D: Delay in diagnosis of disease/deformity/disfigured/damaged due to trauma
> - D: Duty of care
> - D: Dereliction of duty: negligence
> - D: Deviation from standard of care: Wrong site/side
> - D: Damage during surgery: Negligence/error
> - D: Deficiency in services: Forget to remove gauze piece
> - D: Deleterious complication: Infection/ugly scar/sepsis/
> - D: Defaulter (patient stops antibiotic before its due course)
> - D: Deficit developed after surgery
> - D: Death of patient on operation table
> - D: Direct causation (res ipsa loquitur)
> - D: Dissatisfaction in patient and attendants
> - D: Drama of threat to sue in court and refusing to pay the bills
> - D: Discharge and take second opinion
> - D: Documentation of diagnosed negligence
> - D: Drafting of legal notice by lawyer
> - D: Defend and deny approach of surgeon
> - D: Demand compensation for damages caused by duty doctor
> - D: Defamation of doctor/hospital by media trial
> - D: Defeat of doctor in proving himself right
> - D: Deduction of salary of doctor by hospital
> - D: Downfall in career of doctor
> - D: Death of profession: Penal erasure of Doctor's License to practice from registered medical council

- What possible treatment necessary to treat the scars, e.g. lasers, silicone sheets, revision etc? and what will be the cost implications?

Scars are not well accepted by younger patients as compared to older. A young patient male or female would be more critical about scars. They need clear vision about type of scars they can form. Scars on the face and breasts are most worrying. So make a careful decision and planning on younger patients.

Scars other than standard surgical scars caused due to iatrogenic trauma, e.g. burns, accidental cuts, unplanned scars, secondary scars after infection causes a lot of distress in the patient. The best way is to avoid such scars and in worst scenario be upfront and accept responsibility.

Psychosocial Analysis

Psychological analysis of patient allows us to identify and predict the behavior of the patient. A patient who is obsessed may be hard to please.

Perfectionist patients expect results with perfect symmetry and angles. They need to be given realistic expectations. Under promising and over delivering in terms of result will lead to a satisfied patient.

Body dysmorphic disorder is defined as preoccupation with an imagined or exaggerated defect in physical appearance. The diagnostic criteria include not only preoccupation, but also preoccupation causing clinically significant distress or impairment in social, occupational and other important areas of functioning.

It is observed in 5–15% of cosmetic surgery patients. These patients are usually not satisfied with their cosmetic results; some may seek legal action or become violent towards their treating surgeon.

Similarly some personality disorders are also worth identifying in your assessment such as narcissistic behavior (25% of cosmetic surgery patients) and histrionic disorders (9.5%).[7]

Social history–the reason for getting surgery needs to be carefully evaluated. A patient who is saving money to do a cosmetic surgery may not be a good candidate as his or her expectations are very high for the value of the money. And if they were not completely satisfied they would want their money back and would find ways to do that. Other reasons such as marital, divorce, jobs, etc. may also have associated psychosocial issues. Any result of the cosmetic surgery may or may not improve the psychosocial problems.

CASE EXAMPLES

CASE REPORT 1

Case facts: A 65-year-old female patient requested facial rejuvenation and eyelid rejuvenation. She had undergone face-lift surgery and some filler injections in past with the same surgeon (author). On physical examination patient had volume loss leading to deep nasolabial (NL) folds, labiomental (LM) depression, marionette lines and puckered chin. She also had lax skin with wrinkles and bags in lower eyelid.

A fat grafting procedure along with lower blepharoplasty was proposed. Patient was medically fit but was chronic smoker and she claimed to stop it. Procedure was done under local anesthesia and sedation in a day care facility. Closed system was used to perform microfat grafting to the required areas and lower blepharoplasty was performed to near perfection. The next day patient came back with mild swelling and pain. After 48 hours she came with severe redness, pain and swelling in the NL and LM areas. She was in hypotension; she was admitted in hospital and infused with fluid and antibiotics. The blood pressure did not improve so she was transferred to intensive care unit (ICU). Throughout she was alert and cooperative. Her white blood cell (WBC) count and C-reactive protein (CRP) were significantly elevated. On 4th day, she had abscess formation in NL and LM areas, while her lower eyelid healed well. All abscesses were drained and with 72 hours she recovered and was discharged.
Patient claims were:
- Fat grafting was not a recommend procedure for her and surgeon convinced her to do it.
- Being a nurse, patient identified and alleged breach in infection control policy.
- Cost that was involved in the hospital and potential lethal risks.

How was it managed?
Throughout the period, surgeon paid regular visit to patient and was available to help the patient. He took appropriate care and timely management. The patient was overall satisfied and had made no formal complaint. She demanded the reimbursement of hospital costs, which was paid out to the patient.

CASE REPORT 2

Case facts: A 54-year-old patient presented with significant weight loss resulting into facial sagging, brow ptosis, arms ptosis and axillary ptosis. Another surgeon in an institute operated her. A face-lift, endoscopic brow lift, brachioplasty and lateral thoracoplasty were performed. A thorough discussion and documentation was done and patient was consented well. However, she was unhappy immediately postoperatively and behaved very aggressively with the surgeon and staff. After few months she insisted that a revision be done by senior surgeon of same institute. Overall outcome was good but some of her concerns were not dealt with and she noticed asymmetries. A revision surgery was performed without additional cost to patient. A lateral brow lift was performed; revision brachioplasty and lateral thoracoplasty was done. Again immediate postoperatively she was not happy. She healed well without complications and had a good outcome. But she still seemed unhappy. Surgeon had an argument with the patient, as she would not understand surgeon's explanation and reassurance. Finally surgeon told patient that he cannot help and she can seek any other surgeon's second opinion from another institute. She decided to meet a very senior surgeon from a different hospital who assured her that he would "correct" all the "errors" made by previous surgeons and quoted her a hefty amount. Patient ultimately filed a malpractice lawsuit against the surgeons of previous institute to claim compensation for the damages.

Result: After thorough enquiry by medical health authority and medical board opinion presented to the court. Court acquitted the surgeon and warned the patient for frivolous complaint.

CONCLUSION

Do's and Don'ts for doctors:
- Be truthful about your qualifications, training, experience and designation
- Listen patient carefully–answering telephone calls during consultation can be an issue
- Examine thoroughly
- Document all the details precisely
- If after completing the examination the patient or attendant feels that something has been left out or wants something to be re-examined, oblige him or her
- Give instructions to the patient preferably in written form in comprehensible terms
- Specifically mention review–self-referral of symptoms (SOS) or follow-up schedule, if patient misses appointment, send a reminder and document it
- Mention all contacts including emergency contact details.

Patient may be illiterate but not unintelligent. Hence one must not deny them right to information.

REFERENCES

1. Paik AM, Mady LJ, Sood A, et al. A look inside the courtroom: an analysis of 292 cosmetic breast surgery medical malpractice cases. Aesthet Surg J. 2014;34(1):79-86.
2. Paik AM, Mady LJ, Sood A, et al. Beyond the operating room: a look at legal liability in body contouring procedures. Aesthet Surg J. 2014;34(1):106-13.
3. Kandinov A, Mutchnick S, Nangia V, et al. Analysis of factors associated with rhytidectomy malpractice litigation cases. GF Facial Plast Surg. 2017;19(4):255-9.
4. Svider PF, Jiron J, Zuliani G, et al. Unattractive consequences: litigation from facial dermabrasion and chemical peels. Aesthet Surg J. 2014;34(8):1244-9.
5. Singh J, Bhushan V. Medical Negligence and Compensation, 4th edition. Jaipur: Bharat Law Publications; 2017.
6. Koley TK. Medical Negligence and the Law in India: Duties, Responsibilities, Rights. London: Oxford University Press; 2010.
7. Malick F, Howard J, Koo J. Understanding the psychology of the cosmetic patients, Dermatol Ther. 2008;21(1):47-53.
8. Gibbs VC, Coakley FD, Reines HD. Preventable errors in the operating room: retained foreign bodies after surgery–Part I. Curr Probl Surg. 2007;44(5):281-337.
9. Shyung LR, Chang WH, Lin SC, et al. Report of gossypiboma from the standpoint in medicine and law. World J Gastroenterol. 2005;11(8):1248-9.

APPENDIX 1: PATIENT HANDBOOK

Chapter 1—Introduction
Chapter 2—Procedure Information
Chapter 3—Patient Medical History (Please Fill and Return to Office)
Chapter 4—Booking Procedure
Chapter 5—Instructions Prior to Surgery
Chapter 6—List of Medications, Beverages and Tobacco to Avoid
Chapter 7—Preoperative Protocol
Chapter 8—Financial Agreement: Please Return Original to Office
Chapter 9—Surgical Facility
Chapter 10—Operation Day Protocol
Chapter 11—Postoperative Instructions
Chapter 12—Consent for Clinical Photographs and Documentation: Signature Required and Return to Office
Chapter 13—Informed Consent Pregnancy Disclosure Consent (Female Only) Signature Required and Return to Office
Chapter 14— Acknowledgment Form for Information. Signature Required and Return to Office

APPENDIX 2: POSTOPERATIVE PROTOCOL

Duration	Potential Problems	Parameters and Management
1st Postoperative day—1st 24 hours	Nausea, vomiting, pain, dizziness, fainting attacks, breathlessness, bleeding	Body temperature, pulse rate, respiratory rate (TPR), blood pressure (BP), general condition, pain control physical movement treatment
2nd postoperative day	Pain, discomfort, physical limitations, wound drains, plaster irritation, dressing spillage	Pain control Physical movement wound check—for irritation, allergy, blood collection, skin vascularity, sensibility
5th postoperative day	Pain, physical limitation, wound problems	Pain control, physical movement wound care
7th postoperative day	Discomfort, physical limitation, allergies, swelling	Suture removal, dressing advice, garment advice, traveling advice, work-related advice, scar management
Overseas patient		Written instructions, email or telephone follow-up, arrangement to see local medical center if necessary
1 month	Swelling, scar itching, tenderness	Scar examination, swelling, assess skin redraping
3 months	Swelling, scar, lumpiness	Result assessment
6 months	Optional	
1 year	Residual issues	Result
3 years onwards		Long-term result

CHAPTER 42

How to Identify an Unsuitable Patient for Plastic (Aesthetic) Surgery

Lakshyajit D Dhami

INTRODUCTION

Cosmetic surgery is almost always an elective surgery, unlike other surgical specialties, which have both elective and emergency cases (Exceptions are when the patient has a social emergency for an upcoming important a social event for self or any other member in the family). So the surgeon gets enough time to choose a suitable patient for performing elective esthetic surgery, just like the patient who does window shopping before undergoing cosmetic surgeries, and has the right to choose his surgeon.

Unlike other traditional surgeries, the demand for esthetic surgery will keep on increasing despite the increasing price of the surgery due to addition of digital technological advances and improvement in precision of microscopic surgery. However, esthetic surgery is also uniquely, exposed to a considerably high risk of malpractice claims in India, So it is essential for the surgeons to choose their patients carefully, and avoid operating on patients who have high chances of being unhappy with the result and increased potential for suing the surgeon later.

The "Esthetic" word is derived from New Latin *aestheticus* and the Greek *aisthetikos*, both mean *sense of perception*. The terms *Esthetic Surgery and Cosmetic Surgery* is now a days used interchangeably. It therefore tends to mean surgery which has *only* to do with alteration of the external appearance or to *beautify* and is not related to *restoration of function*.

What do we mean by *function*? Is it merely to be able to use different body parts satisfactorily, to carry out or perform the work necessary for everyday living?

Body functions are the physiological or psychological functions of the body systems. Survival is the body's most important business. Survival depends on the body's maintaining or restoring homeostasis, a state of relative constancy of its *internal* and *external* environment. It is equally important to be able to function in the society with normal "self-esteem",

How to Identify an Unsuitable Patient for Plastic (Esthetic) Surgery

> **BOX 1:** Mnemonic for easy recall to identify an unsuitable patient for plastic (esthetic) surgery.
>
> Mnemonic for easy recall to identify an unsuitable patient for plastic (esthetic) surgery. The classic "SIMON" patient should be avoided as well as patients with body dysmorphic disorder. SIMON stands for:
> - S—Single
> - I—Immature
> - M—Male
> - O—Overexpectations
> - N—Narcissistic (egoistic admiration of one's idealized self-image and attributes).

with one's head held high and regarding oneself as an equal. We live in a society, which marks us by our external appearance. Every single interaction within the society is first based on our external appearance. We admire and look up to an individual with pleasing features and sculpted body and consider them as our role model. Our society is conditioned to reward beauty.

Finding beautiful and symmetric human bodies and figures attractive is inbuilt into our mind, and it is not necessarily what we imbibed during our growing up years under the influence of social and cultural behavior of our social circle. An infant of just 3–6 months of age is more attentive towards attractive faces. Scorpion flies have attraction towards symmetrical featured mates. The female zebra prefers symmetrically banded legged males. The list is unending, confirming our inherent desire to prefer good looking and attractive individuals.

Beauty-like happiness is a relative term and is primarily based on the desires and expectations of the person seeking it. It cannot be denied that esthetic surgery is indeed related to the external appearance, but it also cannot be denied that *"perception of self or body image"* plays an important role in an individual's existence. The concept of beauty varies not only at different ages, sex and social status of the client, but also from one generation to another and from one race to another.

Person who seeks esthetic or cosmetic surgery may have increased dissatisfaction with their body image, while the one who very little dissatisfaction with their body, are less likely to seek cosmetic surgery (Box 1).

As per the consumer court's data there is a special category of patients in Indian subcontinent, who have maximum chances to sue the surgeon, that include lawyer's family, NRI patient, Doctor's family, retired government servants, journalists or police officer (Box 2).

In olden, times, about two-third decades ago, the world over and more so in the Indian subcontinent, esthetic surgery was considered as surgery for the rich and elite class, since it was considered more for appearance and looks rather than the function of the body. In the current scenario, we have more and more people seeking esthetic surgery or cosmetic procedures due to innumerable reasons, the important ones being:

- Job pressure (organizations hiring prefer fit or younger looking individuals)
- Marriage prospects (in an arranged marriage, boys and girls always give preference to good looking life partner)
- Awareness of availability and popularity of various cosmetic surgery and its expected results

> **BOX 2:** Pathogenesis of medical malpractice litigation.
>
> *Pathogenesis of Medical Malpractice Litigation:*
> - First consultation: Establishes doctor-patient relationship
> - Patient feels injured due to wrong surgery, wrong anesthetic or postoperative infection or from bad or prolonged stay
> - Dissatisfaction of patient or attendants with surgeon or hospital
> - "Deny-and-defend" approach by doctor
> - Loss of faith and trust on doctor—doctor-patient conflict
> - Threat of Allegation—"warning signs"
> - "High-risk patients"—lawyer family/NRI/Doctor family/retired/journalist/police officer
> - Switching doctors (second opinion—proof of negligence)
> - Incubation period (2 years)
>   (RTI for MRD records–lawyer draft case allegations–complaint to police/consumer court –Govt. H medical board analysis—case filed)
> - Court notice/summon /warrant—"symptoms"
> - Doctor's visits to court on every date for hearing—"investigations"
> - Facing the charges of allegation—suffering
> - Medical Malpractice Stress Syndrome—"disease"
> - Punishment/Paying the compensation—"complications"
>   Even with proved innocence, it leads to trauma, anguish, loss of practice and social status.

- Wider social acceptance, tolerance and favorable attitude to these procedures.
- Advancement and safety in the surgical procedures and anesthesia techniques.
- Higher disposable income making cosmetic surgery affordable, as these procedures are not covered under medical insurance.

The key to a success but esthetic surgery is based on the plastic surgeon's responsibility of proper selection of patient (client). The core value of the surgical outcome does not only depend on the actual visible and desired result, but also on the patient's opinion, their interaction and interpretation of the outcome, along with other's opinion and response to the surgery, which in-turn results in positive personality changes.

Every surgical procedure has a definable risk benefit ratio. This is a very important consideration, especially while opting for esthetic plastic surgery. Surgical procedures other than cosmetic surgery are needed either to cure or control the disease or to correct the deformity and disability when there are not many nonsurgical options available. While in esthetic plastic surgery, an otherwise healthy person is temporarily made unwell, so as to again make her or him healthy and a better shaped individual.

When an individual (he or she is not a patient yet) seeks Cosmetic surgery, the Plastic Surgeon, after careful examination and counselling determines that the person's desires and expectations warrants the procedure. This patient, despite the inherent risks involved, is now motivated to undergo the Surgery; that is when a positive risk benefit ratio is said to exist.

MANAGING EXPECTATIONS OF PATIENT

The queries in the mind of the patient have been described in Box 3.

An inquisitive and indecisive patient may ask to meet and interview patients previously operated by the same surgeon.

> **BOX 3:** Queries in mind of patient.
> - Are you qualified and certified in cosmetic surgery?
> - What type of anesthesia will I receive, and who will provide my anesthesia?
> - How frequently do you (surgeon) perform the surgical procedure(s) I want?
> - What will my recovery be like?
> - What will be the total cost of my procedure?
>
> Source: https://safari-extensions.apple.com/details/?id=io.github.boazh3-6M8TBX46SU.

> **BOX 4:** Medicolegal case discussion: Ilizarov technique for improving height.
>
> *Medicolegal case discussion: Ilizarov technique for improving height:*
>
> *Facts of case:* In 2017, there was a big uproar in Hyderabad at a Corporate Hospital by the parents and relatives of a young software engineer aged around 23 years, height 5 feet 7 inches who underwent surgery (Ilizarov) for lengthening of limbs in his passion to get to 6 feet height, without consent of parents. Police registered a case against establishment and surgeon. Media trial ran, blamed surgeon's community with punch line scrolling throughout day!
>
> *Plaintiff:* Parents and relatives of patient alleged that surgeon cannot operate on patient, without consent of his parents. Ilizarov technique is not to be used for cosmetic purposes.
>
> *Defense:* Patient himself signed before operating surgeon and underwent surgery in preplanned manner, by taking 6 months leave from his job for undergoing surgery. Patient is major, aged around 23 years, independent, working as software engineer, and took loan from his bank for height lengthening surgery. Ilizarov technique can be used for cosmetic purposes.
>
> *Result:* Any person above 18 years of age, if competent can give consent to any operation or procedure that can even cost his life. Patient signing on his own for any major surgery like above is valid in the court of law. No need of approval or consent from anyone including parents.
>
> *Takeaways:* Media is irresponsible as always, it looks for sensational news to extort money from private hospitals. Surgeon should not worry as they are on right side of law, once informed consent from patient himself is taken before surgery. Private hospitals should hire better media handlers and qualified lawyers to defend doctors for such false allegations of medical malpractice.

This must be refused at the outset.

The reasoning the surgeon can offer is that "almost all esthetic surgery patients (including the new patient undergoing counseling) insist that identity should not their be revealed to any one, not even their close relative or friends. Hence as a policy, the surgeon cannot concede to one-to-one interaction amongst their clients (patients)."

The Plastic Surgeon must Ask their Client or Patient—Why does he or she wants to Undergo Plastic or Cosmetic Surgery?

It is very important for the patient to be honest with herself or himself about why she or he wants to correct or improve a certain part of her or his body. She or he may be doing it for reconstructive purposes, either because of congenital defect, disease, or a result of trauma, or merely for esthetic reasons to either slow or reverse the metabolic or aging process. In any case, here are some questions that should be answered honestly by the client (Box 4).

- What is your motivation? Do you think your spouse or your boyfriend or girlfriend would love you more after the surgery? Or, are you doing this for yourself?
- *Ask yourself:* What is it, about that flawed part of your body that you want to correct and why? When did you start thinking

about cosmetic surgery? Was it because you always wanted to do something about it? Or was it following remark made by someone else?
- What are your expectations from cosmetic surgery? Are they realistic? That is, are there just slight contour or shape irregularities that you seek to correct, or is this a way to make up for some not so obvious deeper (other than esthetic) issues?

Tell your patient: Cosmetic surgery is a significant investment in time, effort, and emotion. It probably will not change your social life or your outlook on life. Take a minute to assess why you really want cosmetic surgery, and whether you have realistic expectations.

Plastic surgeon should assess how much impairment is associated with the patient's perceived problem with his or her appearance. Patients with body dysmorphic disorder (BDD) often spend an inordinate amount of time looking in the mirror and thinking about their defect. It may be hampering their social life or their work life. Other indicators can include running from surgeon to surgeon, having undergone multiple procedures in the past, never being satisfied with results of the procedures, and having very unrealistic expectations about the cosmetic procedure and how it will affect their life.

Managing Unhappy and Demanding Patient

The patient, whom you carefully and gently took from a productive initial consultation through satisfactory surgery and the delicate postoperative recovery period, now sits in front of you in anger. Her or his demeanor has changed from all smiles to all frowns. What went wrong?

Angry, difficult or demanding patient pose one of the biggest challenge for a plastic surgeon. When a patient is angry about a bad or unhappy outcome, whether or not medical accident was a possibility, there are many ways in which a plastic surgeon can tackle the situation. How does one deal with the disgruntled patient and "reel them back in" and revive a good patient-physician relationship?

First, I think it is important to establish an excellent rapport with the patient before the surgery. The general unhappiness/dissatisfaction of the patient needs to be understood in terms of concrete issue that can be actually addressed. It is of a great significance, to never to disagree with the patient in the first place. If they see/feel something is wrong, you agree with them right away because the last thing we want to do is make then feel like we are discrediting them.

Not all unhappy patient are difficult. A surgeon can help by offering constructive solutions.

Third try to reason with the patient that the result will improve over a couple of months during the recovery process and in an eventuality, as and when any secondary corrective procedure is needed, reassure them that you are not only competent, but compassionate enough to do so. If feasible the surgeon must try to carry out this without any additional financial burden to the patient.

The problem is when you are faced with an unreasonable, on top of being unhappy. This is where your surgical skills does not matter anymore—it is all about your interpersonal expertise.

We all have them at some point, even the very best surgeons have dealt with this.

These are some of the tips described below which are learnt from senior and junior colleagues and also from personal experiences.

Preoperative Stage

- Slightly downplay expectations.
- Talk in numbers and give percentages whenever possible, e.g. "20% of patients may need a touch-up or an adjustment with this procedure."
- Stress the time required to heal.
- Beware of a patient who abuses your staff time and again. If so, tell her, "I am sorry, the staff and I cannot meet your expectations." You may want to refer them to another physician and then call that physician to apologize for the difficult patient referral.
- If a patient seems uneasy and difficult, encourage them not to undergo surgery. The money you collect from a difficult patient will not be worth your time.

Postoperative Stage

- Never disagree with what a patient sees is wrong, even if you do not see it at all.
- Remind the patient that healing can take from 6 months to a year.
- Take action—if the patient does not like the look of their scar, inject a small amount of steroid or make an appointment 4-6 months later for a touch-up. In our experience, most patients will be happy by then and will not even want the touch-up.
- See the patient with increased frequency and show that you care. Call them frequently and hand hold them throughout the recovery phase. A physical examination in the postoperative phase is advisable to put the patient's mind at ease. The worst thing a physician can do is to send the patient away for a month and hope that they will cool down. Even if it is stressful for you, ensure that the patient will returns frequently.
- A happy patient will tell two friends, and an unhappy patient will inform everyone on the planet via the Internet. As unethical and inaccurate as we know these Websites can be, they are here to stay. If a disgruntled patient posts a negative comment on a Website, contact five of your happy patients and encourage them to post positive comments to counter the negative comment.
- Consider doing touch-up surgery either for free or for a nominal fee—but set limits. Do not give free toxins or fillers touch-ups. These patients will want free touch-ups every time. They will "doctor shop" the entire medical community to locate the practices willing to give freebies.
- Maintain positive interactions with your colleagues so that you can refer patients for second opinions. Ask them in some cases to see your patients with worrisome outcomes.

Dealing with another Physician's Unhappy Patient

- Never say anything bad about another physician. The patient will naturally seek the physician with a higher level of self-confidence and who does not speak poorly about colleagues. Negative comments about colleagues will usually come back to bite you.
- Disgruntled patients who come to you from other practices will probably be unhappy with whoever treats them, even if you dramatically improve their situation. You may want to encourage that patient to return to the physician who did the original surgery.
- Consider giving a friendly call to the physician who did the original surgery

to let them know you have seen the patient. Mention that you supported that physician's original work. This helps establish healthy relations with colleagues.
- Never return a patient's money. Most lawyers advise that patients will view this as an admission of guilt, and is usually an excuse for them to complain some more.

INDECISIVE PATIENT

Cosmetic surgery focuses on improving morphologic traits of patients unsatisfied with their self-image. Self-image is highly influenced by public opinion, norms and esthetic trends in the society at a specific time era. Cosmetic surgery candidates share a defective body image and are not satisfied with their self-perception. Body image is a significant part of self-conceptualization and has two domains namely ideal self-conceptualization and perceived self-conceptualization.

The terms self-conceptualization and self-esteem are usually used interchangeably. However, there are fundamental and conceptual differences between these two terms. Self-conceptualization refers to an individual's perception of one's "self" in relation to the physical and behavioral characteristics and emotional qualities.

Self-esteem reflects a person's overall evaluation or appraisal of his or her own value based on their social experiences (or social status).

The difference between self-conceptualization and self-esteem relate to the beliefs, emotions, qualitative judgments and evaluations of one's self. Positive or negative self-evaluation of the individual is based on the social value felt and accepted by that person.

Ideal self-conceptualization is a collection of ideal mental pictures that are borne in mind, that the person seeks to achieve.

Perceived self-conceptualization results from how the individual sees himself or herself. Both ideal conceptualization and perceived self-conceptualization have been formed abnormally in subjects obsessed with their appearance. Ideal self-conceptualization is too idealistic while perceived self-conceptualization is unfavorably too negative. The greater the discrepancy between these two body images, the greater the confusion of the individual. Therefore, in order to overcome such negative feelings the subjects may change their perceived self-concept towards achieving an ideal one. This is what cosmetic surgery patients seek to pursue.

Impaired self-conceptualization and low self-esteem are among the main mental issues prompting patients to seek cosmetic surgery.

There exist 3 subgroups of cosmetic surgery candidates:
1. Pessimistic, shy, and insecure subjects with fragile and immature personality and poor self-esteem
2. Individuals concerned about the way they look and who spend more time thinking about persons who are more confident with stronger personality and greater self-esteem
3. A less differentiated group include more impulsive subjects who spend a moderate amount of time thinking about the way they look (Pecorari et al. 2010).

This classification is especially important for screening patients seeking cosmetic surgery because postoperative satisfaction may be affected by these factors.

Subjects with identity diffusion usually act immaturely. They usually do not follow specific principles and are not bound to their goals or values. They do not try to achieve any goals and are usually not satisfied with their lives. They are mostly lonely since they are not capable of establishing a close and sincere relationship with others. Such people usually do not know what they want to do with their lives and thus they cannot decide whether they like or need cosmetic surgery. That is why they are mostly not satisfied with the result.

Those with identity moratorium although are in "crisis," still continue to search and explore. They are indecisive and live in hesitation and uncertainty. They are competitive and undecided and do a lot of search for cosmetic surgery. Since they are determined to explore their identity, they accept the changes caused by the cosmetic surgery in a positive way. These patients usually have a lively spirit and are interested in making friends and get close to others. This spirit helps in accepting the changes following cosmetic surgery.

BODY DYSMORPHIC DISORDER

- In what situations would a plastic surgeon think that the patient is not suitable? What are the warning signs?

The eight danger signs that surgeons should be vigilant while dealing with patients are:
- A patient's preoccupation with an imagined defect
- Excessive concern over a minor blemish or flaw
- A perceived flaw causing significant distress and impaired social or professional functioning
- When their preoccupation is not accounted for by another mental disorder
- Multiple consultations for surgery
- Multiple surgical procedures
- Unrealistic expectations about the outcome of the surgery, such as wanting to look like a particular movie star
- Lack of clarity about their goals for the procedure.

The guidelines also ask surgeons to stop and think before approving someone for surgery. "Surgeons may spend a long time in consultation with a patient and it may feel easier to accede to their demands. But if the patient is not suitable, the outcome will only cause regret."

To make a diagnosis of body dysmorphic disorder (BDD) look at the extent of impairment it is causing, and that indicates how severe the disease is. Those who may not like their appearance but still have the confidence to go out and socialize might have a mild form of BDD. On the other hand, if you see patients who spend their whole day checking the mirror, fixing their appearance, limiting their social and occupational opportunities, which indicates they have a more severe form of the disorder.

Some people are almost psychotic—they have a fixed belief that something is wrong with themselves, even though doctors do not see anything wrong. Unfortunately, BDD can worsen over time if the doctor performs the requested procedure but the result does not meet the patient's expectation.

Doctors need to be aware of the fact that some of their patients do suffer from BDD. They have to consider the diagnosis and should not perform the procedure on patients with BDD. If they do perform the procedure, they probably would not make the patient better. In fact, they may make them worse. We go to medical school to help people, and we do not want to embark on a treatment that would not be helpful—especially an elective procedure. It is one thing if somebody has a life-saving procedure and a mistake occurs; it is a totally different situation, when you perform an elective procedure and it makes the patient worse in some way.

Body dysmorphic disorder patients can cause a lot of difficulties for physicians in terms of disruption of their office practices. People will be angry, a surgeon's reputation in the community could be damaged, or a surgeon could be sued. We all have heard some surgeons express concerns about violence from patients, and even murder threats. Doctors need to try to make an accurate diagnosis of BDD. Many surgeons have a screening questionnaire they routinely hand to prospective patients. Other doctors interview a family member to discuss how this perceived defect is affecting the patient. It can be helpful to contact previous surgeons who have operated on the patient. There are many different ways for doctors to protect themselves from operating on a patient with BDD, but the key step is getting to know your patient before embarking on surgery.

Take a careful history. Try to establish rapport. Walk into the room and appropriately introduce yourself making good eye contact-this help patients feel like you have plenty of time to listen. Do a detailed history taking in terms of what is bothering them, how they think it is affecting their life, what they have done to try to correct it, how often they look in the mirror. Try to get a handle on how this perceived deficit is affecting them. Ask what their expectations are for the procedure and how they expect their life to change; see if the expectations are realistic.

In clinical practice we know, how people with realistic expectations tend to do very well with cosmetic surgery and are very pleased with the results. People with unrealistic expectations tend to be disappointed. You want to sort those 2 groups out. Unrealistic expectations may be associated with a BDD; but they can also just be a consequence of naiveté, or confusion on the part of patient. Hence it is important to educate the patient about their condition, possible surgical options and their expected outcome.

With many psychiatric illnesses, lack of insight is one of the hallmarks of the disease. These patients do not self-refer to psychiatrists. They go to plastic surgeons with their perceived problem.

- If the plastic surgeon decides not to do the surgery, how would he counsel the BDD patient?

It is up to those doctors, who the patient consults first, to help him get to the right mental healthcare providers. It is difficult to convince them for psychiatric reference. These patients often do not feel that a mental health professional can help them and think they need plastic surgery. You need to be cautious to try to make appropriate referrals. We recommend try to establish rapport with patients—do not get rid of them at the first visit; but certainly do not operate at the first visit. If you suspect BDD, perhaps do one of the rating scales for BDD, and that will give you some data to talk to them about. Once you have established rapport, suggest that they consult a mental health professional.

I would like to add here that there are many patients who come back for repeat procedures who do not suffer from BDD. These are patients who come in for a procedure and are so happy with it they decide to try something else. They will say, "I feel really good; what do I want to do next? Next year, I will have some money and I will do something else." I am talking about people who have 2 or 3 operations over 5 years. They are not obsessed with plastic surgery and have a healthy attitude about it.

The Guidelines for Psychosocial Assessments for Sexual Reassignment Surgery or Gender Affirmation Surgery state that a Plastic surgeon needs a Psychiatrist's certificate (Box 5) before operating on transgender or patients with identity disorder or on hormonal therapy.

BOX 5: Psychiatrist's certificate: Letter of assessment by psychiatrist to surgeon for patient suffering body dysmorphic disorder (BDD) demanding gender change surgery.

Psychiatrist's certificate: Letter of assessment by psychiatrist to surgeon for patient suffering body dysmorphic disorder (BDD) demanding gender change surgery:
- It must be addressed to the surgeon or to the surgical team, if the actual surgeon is not known, for instance, to the Department of Plastic Surgery.
- Describe who you are, your experience with transgender clients and explain your relationship to the client and how long and in what capacity you know the person, e.g. "I am a psychiatrist in private practice working with the Private Provider Network. I have provided psychotherapy for several transgender people in the past year. I met to the XYZ once in July to assess the appropriateness of referral for hormones."
- The description of a typical patient and his current gender identity and a brief history of his gender evolution, e.g. "24-year-old Asian masculine appearing natal female who identifies as male and seeking a hystero-oophorectomy to decrease his gender dysphoria. He began social transition and cross dressing at the age of 14–18 years and began hormones at age 21, through medical center. He has responded well to hormones. He initially recognized his own gender when he went through puberty and had experienced body dysmorphia related to his developing breast.
- Any psychiatric diagnosis and medications that client is prescribed: The client has gender dysphoria and attention deficit disorder with hyperactivity. Dr A has prescribed 50 mg of lisdexamfetamine (Vyvanse) daily for attention-deficit *hyperactivity disorder* (ADHD) and Zolpidem (Ambien) which the client takes several times a week for sleep problems. The client has responded well to this medication:
- Any concerns about patient compliance. Client keeps appointments and has complied with treatment and the standards of care.
- Why the client wants this particular surgery; any research they did and what they understand, etc. Client wishes to have an oophorectomy in order to reduce her reliance on androgenic hormones. She is concerned about her long-term health and wants to be certain that her secondary sex characteristics never return. She does not want full SRS, preferring to have minimally invasive procedures. She does not want children and understand that she will not be able to have children of her own. She understands that her sexual drive and sexual function may change as a result of surgery.

Add to this your reasoning and assessment:
The client currently presents with a mixed gender presentation which puts him at risk for harassment and violence. He is very dysphoric about his breasts. He reports that he despises his breasts and that they feel like growths or tumors and he wished they were gone.
He would prefer scarring and a poor outcome to continuing to exist with breasts. He very likely will have decreased dysphoria following surgery.
- *Current and past substance abuse*:
  - The client is in recovery from opiate addiction.
  - The patient uses medical marijuana daily to manage her anxiety.
- *Aftercare plans and any unaddressed needs*: The client has a supportive relationship with her sister who will be with the client throughout surgery and for the following two weeks. The client has arranged to be off of work for four weeks and has saved money to pay for post-operative necessities.

She has arranged her apartment to easily get around and plans to freeze meals ahead of time. Her case manager will call her daily once she is ambulatory.
- You welcome a call for further information.

Name of psychiatrist

Signature

Date

AVOIDABLE MEDICOLEGAL ISSUES OF ESTHETIC SURGERY IN OPERATING ROOM AND COURTROOM (BOX 6)

In a study characterizing prevention of litigation related to facial plastic surgery procedures, Svider et al. (2013), reported 88 cases of which 62.5% were decided in the physician's favor, 9.1% were resolved with an out-of-court settlement, and 28.4% ended in a jury awarding damages for malpractice. The mean settlement was $577,437 and mean jury award was $352,341. The most litigated procedures were blepharoplasties and rhinoplasties. Alleged lack of informed consent was noted in 38.6% of cases; other common complaints were excessive scarring or disfigurement, functional considerations, and postoperative pain.

In another medicolegal study related to procedures using lasers represent a potential target for malpractice litigation, should an adverse event may occur. Svider et al. (2013) reported that, 82% included in this analysis involved female plaintiffs. Of 34 cases, 19 (56%) were resolved with a defendant verdict. The median indemnity was $150,000, and dermatologists, otolaryngologists, and plastic surgeons were the most commonly named defendants. The most common procedures were performed for age-related changes, acne scarring, hair removal, and vascular lesions, although there were also several rhinologic and airway cases. Of all cases, 25 (74%) involved cutaneous procedures, and common allegations were permanent injury (71%), disfigurement or scarring (68%), inadequate informed consent [17 (50%)], unnecessary or inappropriate procedure [15 (44%)], and burns [11 (32%)]. Noncutaneous procedures had higher trending median payments ($600,000 versus $103,000).

Facial dermabrasion and chemical peel are common cosmetic procedures for improving

---

BOX 6: Prevention of negligence is better than fighting the case in court of law.

19Cs to prevent negligence during aesthetic surgery:
- C-Continued training in safe surgical techniques regularly (CME)
- C-Consult with latest medical literature
- C-Choose your patient by screening him or her medically, psychologically, financially and social behavior.
- C-Correct Doctor (Have your colleague specializing in the technique to either operate or assist you)
- C-Correlate investigation reports with clinical findings
- C-Consent for surgery
- C-Communicate with patient or attendants about C-Complications before surgery
- C-Correct site of surgery on correct patient (Identification and site marking before surgery is must)
- C-Correct Doctor (Have standby anesthetist even for surgery under local anesthesia)
- C-Correct dose of anesthesia—via C-Correct route at C-Correct time to C-Correct patient
- C-Co-ordinate with duty nurse for counting of swabs before and after surgery
- C-Care about patient safety inside hospital—prevent fall from bed for elderly and children.
- C-Cooperate with colleague doctors for round the clock services to admitted patient
- C-Conduct of surgeon (maintain professional relationship with patient, but avoid personal relationship)
- C-Check up properly on every consult and ask for regular follow up the patient till complete recovery
- C-Condemn unfair trade practice
- C-Call legal helpline of hospital's lawyer in doubt or threat by patient or attendants.
- C-Complete documentation of surgical notes and adverse events before discharging patient
- C-Cross check medical audit during monthly morbidity and mortality (M&M) meet in hospital.

looks that are generally safe yet do possess inherent medicolegal risks. The patient's expectations, formed well in advance of treatment, strongly correlate with overall satisfaction. Out-of-court settlements and jury-awarded damages were considerable in cases where physicians practicing various (or multiple) specialties were named as defendants. These findings emphasize the need for physicians to thoroughly document potential complications prior to treatment, during the informed-consent process. Additionally, general considerations should be taken into account, such as patient expectations and the potential need for other procedures, which may enhance pretreatment communication and ultimately minimize liability. Finally, it is important to stress that physicians may be held liable for procedures performed by nonphysician ancillary staff. In analysis of medicolegal cases related to facial dermabrasion and chemical peel, Svider et al. (2013) reported that, 16 cases (64%) resulted in a decision for the defendant and 9 (36%) were resolved with payments. The median difference between out-of-court settlements (median, $940,000) and jury-awarded damages (median, $535,000) was not statistically significant. Factors raised in litigation included poor cosmetic outcome (80%), alleged intra-treatment negligence (68%), permanent injury (64%), informed-consent deficits (60%), emotional/psychological injury (44%), post-treatment negligence (32%), and the need for additional treatment or surgery (32%).

Study of various cases across the world suggest that malpractice litigation against esthetic surgery may be "plateauing." Defensive medical practices are pervasive and make up a considerable proportion of the "indirect" costs due to medicolegal issues, which contribute toward our healthcare system. Accordingly, these trends have spurred considerable interest in characterizing factors that play a role in alleged medical negligence, along with outcomes and jackpot awards of compensation by courts and jury to patients. These analyses characterize factors, in determining financial burden on surgeons in facial cosmetic surgery cases, for paying higher premiums for professional indemnity insurance as compared to surgeons in other specialties.

Many factors are found as potential targets for minimizing liability. Informed consent was the foremost argued entity in these malpractice suits. This finding emphasizes the importance of open communication between physicians and their patients concerning expectations, in addition to documentation of specific risks, benefits, and available alternatives.

Qualified surgeon with efficient training and good experience, carefully utilizing digital imaging techniques in association with the adoption of straightforward precautions and pointers of adequate communication alongside a completed patient's consent form, are vital necessities in defense of medical malpractice lawsuit.

CONCLUSION

Most malpractice claims in cosmetic esthetic surgery do not seem to be the consequence of actual medical negligence, instead lawsuits result due to improper patient selection criteria and lack of adequate communication between the patient and the operating surgeon. Prevention of litigation by avoiding unsuitable patients with high risk of suing in court, is better than fighting the malpractice lawsuit for proving self-righteousness, as it wastes surgeon's precious time, while punctually parading in court regularly for years before the dispute resolves, losing precious years of clinical practice in court cases. More important is loss of social prestige and status for professionals like plastic surgeons.

SUGGESTED READING

1. Aston, Sherrell. Aesthetic Plastic surgery, 1st edition. United States: Elsevier Publishers; 2009.
2. Gorney M. Recognition of the patient unsuitable for aesthetic surgery. Aesthet Surg J. 2007;27(6):626-9.
3. Mavroforou A, Giannoukas A, Michalodimitrakis E. Medical litigation in cosmetic plastic surgery. Med Law. 2004;23(3):479-88.
4. Menon M, Gopalakrishnan B, Ray K, et al. Legal aspects of Healthcare and Hospital Administration, 1st edition. United Kingdom: Bloomsbury; 2016.
5. Shah AK. Newer implications of medicolegal and consent issues in plastic surgery. Indian J Plast Surg. 2014;47(2):199-202.
6. Singh VP. Legal issues in Medical Practice—Medicolegal Guidelines of Safe Practice. 1st edition. New Delhi: Jaypee Brother Medical Publishers; 2016.
7. Svider PF, Carron MA, Zuliani GF, et al. Lasers and losers in the eyes of the law: liability for head and neck procedures. JAMA Facial Plast Surg. 2014;16(4):277-83.
8. Svider PF, Jiron J, Zuliani G, et al. Unattractive consequences: litigation from facial dermabrasion and chemical peels. Aesthet Surg J. 2014;34(8):1244-9.
9. Svider PF, Keeley BR, Zumba O, et al. From the operating room to the courtroom: a comprehensive characterization of litigation related to facial plastic surgery procedures. Laryngoscope. 2013;123(8):1849-53.
10. Tiwari, Satish. Chapter 21. Medicolegal issues in surgery. Textbook on Medicolegal issues related to various Medical Specialties, 2nd edition. New Delhi: Jaypee Brothers Medical Publishers; 2018. New Delhi. pp. 285-93.
11. Wildgoose P, Scott A, Pusic AL, et al. Psychological screening measures for cosmetic plastic surgery patients: a systematic review. Aesthet Surg J. 2013;33(1):152-9.

CHAPTER 43

Revision Surgery in Aesthetic Plastic Surgery

Shrirang Pandit

INTRODUCTION

Revision surgery is a discomforting situation. The surgeon is working in an anatomical environment that is no more virgin. Scarring, fibrosis, reduced tissue elasticity, and violated surgical planes make resurgery difficult. It is not easy to imagine the effect of changes that you plan to achieve. There can be more bleeding, more scarring, longer time for resolution, more noticeable scars, and so on. The surgeon feels responsible and a little guilty. That he has wasted the best chance of primary result, weighs on his mind. Reflexly he goes in the defensive mode. There is a tendency to do less and less and get out quickly.

Revision in any surgery is an unpleasant task and more so in aesthetic plastic surgery. A patient is not prepared to undergo another surgery and take on additional financial and "off time" burden. There are very few true statistics available to know the true incidence of revision surgery.

The surgeon and the patient both are very unprepared for this eventuality. It is also true that the number of patients who undergo revisions is pretty sizeable. Revision surgery is inevitable and must be accepted as an educator of sorts. You may have to revise your own surgery or the patient may have had surgery elsewhere, is unhappy and comes to you as second surgeon. He hopes that you will do better than the first one. We all know that the tissues change shape over time, get ptotic, can get displaced and hence modification is the rule. What looked good a few years ago may not look as good few years down the line. The patient needs to understand that there is nothing permanent or one hundred percent. Change is the rule! hence revision surgery falls into two broad categories—(1) cases where revision is to be expected over years, like a facelift, blepharoplasty, mastopexy, facial volumization, hair restoration, liposuction, rhinoplasty, vitiligo surgery, etc. and (2) the second group is where immediately after surgery patient needs revision; rhinoplasty, ptosis of the eyelid, abdominoplasty, breast augmentation, etc. The second group is where the patient's unhappiness is crucial factor (Box 1).

> **BOX 1:** Case law on malpractice in scar revision surgery.
>
> *Case:* Multiple scars all over the face of patient, despite surgery, scars increased leading to disfigurement of face, alleged to be due to negligence, and deficiency in services of the plastic surgeon.
>
> *Defense:* Surgeon is a skilled person and possessing requisite qualifications for conducting the plastic surgery and scar revision method. Surgery was performed after informed consent of the patient, explaining the risks, and benefits of the treatment. Treatment by cross hatching given—scar revision undertaken in three levels and stitching done with ultrafine suture materials, and patient followed up regularly and was advised for a cream massage on healed stitches of the scar. Patient never turned up for the further review. Disfiguration on the face was due to not following the surgery instructions of the patient.
>
> *Court decision:* Plastic surgeon adopted the right course of treatment best suited to the patient. Hence no negligence or deficiency in service.
>
> *Discussion:* As to the allegation of further disfigurement of the face of patient has produced photographs before and after surgery. According to the experts, the photographs themselves show a definite improvement in the scar. Scar revision surgery is neither plastic nor cosmetic surgery, and a scar cannot be removed but can only be revised to the best. While no scar can be removed completely, plastic surgeons can often improve the appearance of a scar, making it less obvious through the injection or application of certain steroid medications or through surgical procedures known as scar revisions.
>
> *Source:* SK Gupta(Dr) (Deceased) vs Neeta Tyagi, 2015 (5) Andh LD 44: 2015 (2) CPJ 686 (NCDRC)

THE PROBLEM

We as surgeons must accept it for a fact that every single case, we do, is not going to be a perfect result. Like no two patients are same, even no two results are going to be similar too. Exceptional results are exactly that, exceptional! Obviously very few. These are the results that find their way in the conference presentations and masterclasses. The common results are rarely put up for discussion. In our endeavor to project our skills and attract more patients to our practice, we show our best results to our patients during consulting. I will show a beautiful girl having a rhinoplasty and the postoperative makes her look prettier. What is not brought out is that she was very pretty without the rhinoplasty too!

What this conveys to my potential client is that "she" will look as beautiful after she gets the nose job done. Nothing can be further from the truth.

Rhinoplasty performed for an ugly nose on an ugly face has limited impact. I have inadvertently sown the seeds of unhappiness. When the patient looks at herself after surgery, she does not see a beautiful woman she perceived, but the same ugly face; with a little better nose stares at her. Now you have a very unhappy patient. Dissecting "the anatomy of ugliness" is a very vital exercise. I need to understand what makes the patient look ugly. If it can be defined as an anatomical excess or deficit or distortion, I may be in a position to correct it. I am very pleased as I use Vectra three-dimensional (3D) camera for counseling the patients. The patient gets a very real idea of her level of ugliness. She sees her face in every conceivable view and she also knows that the nose is not the only ugly part of her face. The 3D image modification is carried out on the face of the patient herself. She gets a fairly good idea what to expect after surgery. It is her face that she sees and not of someone else. I can recollect at least two occasions when patients expressed their frustration. One said I have come to you with a lot of hope. I thought I will look beautiful after nose surgery, what you have shown is not acceptable. I told her I can do only this much,

I can only work with what I have. It is good if someone goes away at this time.

Need for revision surgery can arise from many reasons—(1) a complication necessitating surgical treatment. Wound breakdown, excessive scarring, implant exposure, infection, etc. (2) Patient or surgeon unsatisfied with the outcome of primary surgery. (3) Modification in the shape of treated organ over few months or years. Development of asymmetry, tissue distortion, late implant exposure in nasal, or facial implants. This is common in hair transplantation as the process of baldness continues. It is also common in vitiligo surgery, where the autoimmune process can affect stability (4) ugly and unsightly scars. The patient takes the decision of aesthetic plastic surgery after a long deliberation. He will have few, or at times many consultations to zero in on a plastic surgeon who gives him enough confidence to entrust the job of aesthetic transformation to him. The decision is not easy. Cost considerations play an important role. Experience comes with a price tag. Seasoned and expert practitioners of this craft expect high fees. The patient may opt for a less experienced surgeon because he offers less expensive package to him.

Experience brings with it a host of considerations. Correct patient selection, appropriate choice of procedure, skill and practice in execution of the procedure, ability to manage surprises during surgery, minimize complications, and help the patient through recovery are issues that are part of the experience package.

It goes without saying that generally a well-experienced plastic surgeon will take a correct call on all these issues. It is also true that aesthetic surgery is an art and a young less experienced colleague may produce a brilliant result. The patient expects you to produce the best result, without knowing what it is (Box 2)!

BOX 2: Malpractice in revision procedures in rhinoplasty of nagging celebrity.

- *Case:* In the year 1986, while playing cricket, the patient met with an accident and hurt his nose, resulting in breathing complications. Subsequently, a septoplasty operation was performed removing most of the septum along with the tip support in the columella region. The patient felt sudden structural weakness in his nose, which was solved 3 years later, by plastic surgeon by grafting with the iliac crest bone. The patient averred that he was successful in his business and was also acting in TV serials and that in this profession the structure of his facial features is extremely important. During the year 2005, the patient again started feeling some functional disorder in his nose as the graft got dissolved giving rise to weakness in the support at the tip. Surgeon assured fixation of support at the tip by way of an L-shaped graft by multiple revision procedures of rhinoplasty, but failed and instead resulted in more disfiguration and disability.
- *Complaint:* The patient complained that after the operation, he found a much longer columella scar extending above the original tip position. There was further dumping of that portion of the skin below the nose, which was done to hide the scar and this resulted in aggravating his discomfort. Surgeon again operated his nose with vertical incision through columella and tip, on account of which a scar was caused extending from the base to the tip on the top of the nose and the doctor had tried to hide the scar and dispositioned the tip by bending it down. It is pleaded that only because of the negligence of the treating doctor that the patient found it difficult to breathe, as the Ala muscles of the nose were made dysfunctional. Due to nonclearance of the right passage properly, the patient was facing problems of suffocation during his sleep. The patient stated that he had suffered a lot on account of this scar which changed his looks affecting the beauty of his face, more so as he was a professional actor in TV serials and cinema. List of surgeries done:
    - *First surgery:* Revision rhinoplasty—tip implant done
    - *Second surgery:* Excision of offending nasal cartilage which was implanted previously

Contd...

Contd...

- *Third surgery*: Open rhinoplasty, debulking of spreader grafts done, costal cartilage relocated in the central plane
- *Fourth surgery:* Open rhinoplasty—removal of dorso laboratory and columella graft and silicon implant for dorsum and columella (L-shape)
- *Fifth surgery:* Reduction rhinoplasty

- *Defense:* Sebaceous cyst was the real cause for his subsequent nasal discomfort, for which the surgeon cannot be held negligent. 20 years ago, he suffered injury while playing cricket and 3 years later, the problem was solved by a plastic surgeon by grafting with the iliac crest bone from the waist. The surgeon pleaded that he had refused to operate on the patient on two previous occasions as the patient had shown nagging behavior and only due to the continuous insistence from the patient's side, he had finally agreed to conduct the surgery only after explaining to the patient clearly the prognosis and the expected risks. It is pleaded that the patient was obsessive with the shape of his nose and, therefore, he had started handling and fiddling with his nose too much. Later, patient had an infected collection of pus on the dorsum of the nose and immediately the surgeon attended to him and aspirated the pus. He was also advised to have proper drainage and washout under general anesthesia but the patient had refused to comply and decided to continue with the antibiotics. He was advised to get admitted for surgical drainage of pus. The patient had refused to get admitted due to financial constraints and the treating doctor arranged for drainage of the infected pus in the minor operation theatre (OT). Surgeon argued that the patient suffered from body dysmorphophobia, i.e. body image disorder, which is a psychiatric condition in which the patient is not happy with his looks.
- *Decision*: Patient underwent for multiple surgeries and paid for it, to improve his looks. The treating surgeon and the nursing home are jointly and severally liable to pay the compensation amount of ₹ 500,000 and the medical expenses of ₹ 100,000.
- *Discussion:* The surgeries dated 4/9/2007, 8/3/2008, 4/11/2008, 21/7/2010, and 1/12/2011, evidence that the patient had undergone open rhinoplasty and reduction rhinoplasty subsequent to the rhinoplasty in which the treating doctor, had not done the grafting as per standards of medical parlance, on account of which the patient had suffered structural and cosmetic complications namely deep scar and alignment of nose, functional complications like breathing problems, sleeping disorder, causing pain, tension, and mental agony. Patient had undergone rhinoplasty at surgeon, there was infection in the nose, which caused subsequent trouble. But from the treatment sheet issued by the surgeon on different dates, it appears that there was no endorsement about any infection in the nose. For these reasons, we find the treating doctor negligent in the manner and the line of treatment rendered to the patient, for which the patient deserves to be compensated.

Source: National Consumer Disputes Redressal. Mrinmoy Dutta vs Dr Anupam Golash Pvt. Ltd. & Anr. on 11 May, 2016. [online] Available from: https://indiankanoon.org/doc/16711588/ [Accessed December, 2018]

INTRODUCING THE IDEA OF REVISION SURGERY AT FIRST CONSULT FOR AESTHETIC SURGERY

Revision when needed after a proper consultation, thorough understanding of the patients' needs, proper selection of patient and surgical procedure, adequate support during the healing procedure, is not a very bad experience. If I expect a less than best result I find it a sensible idea to give a gentle hint to the patient that the result is looking "little different" than expected. I do it at the time of first dressing with a caveat that we will watch as it heals and decide what to do about it. It is a good idea to prepare the patients mind for the same as revision surgery is a rude shock to them. The best time to prepare their mind is during the first consultation. I never promise a 100% result, for the simple reason I do not know what is 100%. I discuss with the patient, the number of tissues that needs modification. In rhinoplasty, I explain that I am trying to modify the shape of the bones, cartilages, skin, mucosa, etc. and I have only limited control over how they will shape over next few months. Patient is told, in no uncertain terms, about the limited predictability of tissue behavior, tissue response to new location and stress generation by new alignments. It is very important to stress on the patients mind that "unpredictable" is a real possibility. I do take help of surgical intraoperative photographs to discuss the tissues and what we plan to do with them.

The common question that follows is what if we do not get the desired result? Can the undesired problem be corrected? I think every aesthetic surgery consultation should come to a point where we discuss an unfavorable result and its management. I have at times told the patient that some tissues like bone or cartilage may need treatment more than once as they need to be watched during the healing process. Revision surgery should be a part of primary consultation and must be done tactfully but fearlessly. We truly have limited control over tissue behavior and the patient must know it. The second and very pertinent question is, doctor what is the likelihood that in my case a revision will be necessary? This is a question you must be able to answer to yourself. Surgical inexperience, poor knowledge, and inadequate hands on, never done it before, are issues you need to comprehend. It is good to be honest. "I honestly do not know" is my answer, I add, we will do everything needed to see that such chances are negligible. It should reassure the patient and not frighten him or her. Be honest but not "frighteningly" honest.

Revision Surgery may be needed in following procedures:

Abdominoplasty, Rhinoplasty, Face lift, Breast augmentation, Breast reduction, Blepharoplasty, Liposuction, Hair Restoration, and fat grafting may require revision surgery.

How to handle problem of revision surgery? We need to answer the following questions before we contemplate revision surgery.

- Is revision surgery needed?
- Is it going to help the patient?
- Are your goals clear? Have you identified the cause of patient dissatisfaction?
- Have you decided the tissues you plan to modify? Are the tissues soft and supple to conform to new surgical needs?
- Have you made an accurate assessment of the anatomical anomaly?
- Is it the correct time to perform the procedure, or you want to wait more?
- Are you forced by the patient to perform surgery earlier than what you would have wanted to wait?
- Are you willing to seek help of a more experienced colleague?
- Economics of the surgery, are you doing it free? Who will bear the hospital costs, anesthesia fees, and medications?
- Have you done the primary surgery, or he has been operated "elsewhere"?
- Are there other specialists involved in the management?
- Is the patient in a confronting mood, talking in terms of compensation?

Handling a Revision Surgery when your own Patient comes to you, being Unhappy after the Initial Surgery

Revision surgery when you are the primary surgeon and revision for somebody else's patient is a whole different ball game. In the first case, it is an obligation while in the second instance your mind is free, you are not bogged down by your previous acts of omission and commission. If you were the primary surgeon, you may want to do the smallest, simplest, and least aggressive procedure when a more complex, thorough surgery may be required. A trusted senior colleague will be of great help. The responsibility is shared, good ideas will come up, and out of the box solutions are commonplace. I generally arrange a consultation with the surgeon whom I want to assist me. Honesty and transparency will calm your patient and help you provide good care for him. It is important to be compassionate and kind to patients seeking revision. As a policy, I do not charge them for the surgery, dressings, follow-up visits for almost a year or may be longer too. One can have a different take in these matters. It is vital not to allow a "trust deficit" to creep in. I am happy that my patient is confident and giving me a second chance to address his problem, for which I am partly responsible. A trusting patient who believes you are doing your best to help him is invaluable.

The types of patients who fall in the category of body dysmorphism need special mention. These will keep on seeking multiple revisions and never be satisfied. Their unstable mental status needs psychiatric help for many years. Identification of patients with dysmorphic problem is very crucial. One patient was referred to me by my psychiatrist friend, was extremely displeased with her nose and thought that her nose is responsible for all wrong things happening to her. She did have a reasonably good nose and some improvements would have made it look really nice. I dissuaded her for several months from getting any surgery. She came back with two more referrals from psychiatrists. Their argument was that the rhinoplasty can have some impact on her mental status and it may help her. It was to be done as a therapeutic procedure to help her mind. So, I agreed to help her. I established grounds for surgery with exhaustive documentation, consents, photos, stenciled images, and what not. She insisted that it must be done under local anesthesia. When I was to inject local, she jumped from the table and ran away! It never felt so good when a patient runs away from the operation theatre. I thought good riddance. But, my joy of losing a patient was short lived. She came back for sure, with profuse apologies, stronger, and more determined. This time I made her to have general anesthesia. Surgery was smooth, the nose looked very pretty and she was overjoyed. I saw her many years later. She did pretty well for few years and now was back again saying her face looks old and the nose much younger. I must say her observation was very apt. However, I am in no mood the take her up once again.

Example: I had operated on one such patient. She had a rhinoplasty several years ago from another surgeon and came to me for removal of a small lesion on the nose. She got it removed, all was well suddenly, I got a call from the previous surgeon that he received a mail from her that I have spoiled her rhinoplasty result and she is on the verge of committing suicide. I was shocked, but reported the matter to police inspector formally. Nothing happened but I learned my lesson (Box 3).

Handling a Situation when a Dissatisfied Patient comes to you for Revision Surgery when you are not the Primary Surgeon

Agitated patients seeking revision need to be handled with kid gloves. They are angry, unhappy, disillusioned, and in revenge mode. I make it a point "not" to ask the name of the first surgeon. I stick to only clinically relevant discussions. I do not ask how much it cost them. I do not ask why did they chose XYZ. This is not a time for loose talk. You will get enough opportunity to get the relevant information. Please do not make any loose comments on quality of surgery or patient management. I stick to absolute professional behavior. Full clinical examination, 3D photography, and proper documentation are done. I enquire if they have records of previous

> **BOX 3:** Case law on malpractice in facial reconstruction surgery and scar revision failure.
>
> - *Case*: A female patient aged 49 years with old history of cancer cheek with mandible and she was operated for that in Tata Cancer Hospital few years back on left side. She received chemo- and radiotherapy. Cancer disease of the complainant was fully cured, but due to operation, some deformity was found in left side of her lower jaw. Now she came to plastic surgeon for correction of deformity due to hemimandibulectomy on left side with node dissection along with soft tissue excision.
> - *Complaint:* Patient (a professor by job), underwent multiple facial surgeries by plastic surgeon, who promised to remove the deformed jaw bone on patient's face by fibular flap for functional mandibular microvascular reconstruction, but instead developed complications—flap failure in microvascular surgery, infected scar and suffered lower motor neurone (LMN) facial palsy due to nerve injury during negligent surgery, resulting in inability to close one eye even during sleep, causing corneal opacity and blindness—permanent disability.
> - *Defense:* Surgeon is qualified cosmetic surgeon, having obtained degree of Master of Surgery (MS), MCH, and Diplomate in National Board (DNB) in plastic surgery and has experience of 28 years in the treatment of such patients. There was deformity in the face of the complainant prior to operation. Due to treatment of disease of cancer whatever weakness comes, the rate of success of scar repair surgery decreased. The possibility regarding the postoperation was explained to the complainant prior to the operation.
> - *Decision*: Looking to the facts, circumstances and age of the complainant, it is just and proper to award a lump sum amount of ₹ 1,000,000 (Rupees Ten Lakhs) to the complainant, which is payable by the surgeon.
> - *Discussion*: In the instant case, in the discharge summary, no details were given by the surgeon, whereas it is essential for the surgeon that after listening the patient, to clinically examine the patient and the surgeon is duty bound to record full medical history of the patient. It is the professional duty of the medical practitioner to examine a patient thoroughly to find out the cause for which complications arose. To prescribe medicines mechanically without application of mind is certainly a deficiency in service. After first operation, there was pus formation and the pus was oozing out from the wound and thereafter the complainant again got admitted in the surgeon's hospital for treatment. According to the surgeon, the complainant had not followed the instructions given by the surgeon. The above defense of the surgeon, is not acceptable. There is no evidence that pus was oozing out due to negligent act of the complainant.
>   - After perusal of principal's certificate of patient's teaching job performance, it appears that before surgeries of the complainant conducted by the surgeon, the complainant was completely competent to speak properly and she had worked as Assistant Professor in various colleges and had given lectures in the classes. If the complaint was unable to speak properly, then it was not possible for her that she would have been continuously appointed as Assistant Professor in various colleges from year 2009 to 2016 to give lectures, therefore, the defense taken by the surgeon that the complainant was initially unable to speak and her eye lids were not closing is not acceptable. It shows that the problem to the complainant was occurred due to operation done by the surgeon.
>   - The surgeon filed all consent forms for three surgeries done, which bears signature, but it is not established that whose signature was obtained by the surgeon in the said consent letter. So, it was established that consent form was not signed by the patient herself, so incomplete consent form is not a valid ground of defense. The above consent is not proper and valid consent. It appears that the surgeon had not obtained valid consent form the complainant or her relatives prior to conducting her operation, which comes in the category of medical negligence and deficiency in service.
>
> *Source:* State Consumer Disputes Redressal Commission. Smt Purnima Mishra vs Kalda Cosmetic Surgery Institute on 2 August, 2018. [online] Available from: https://indiankanoon.org/doc/57893984/ [Accessed December, 2018].

surgery, discharge cards, etc. It is good practice to know, if there were any intraoperative or postoperative problems such as swelling, bleeding, infection, etc. We do not know why the problem happened, so we should not blame anyone. You are hearing patient's side of the story. I sometimes call up the surgeon and politely ask what is his take on the result and what could have gone wrong. I think we must extend basic professional courtesy to our fellow colleague. Most consumer litigation is result of loose talk and one-upmanship. Very important, you may be at the receiving end of it someday!

Timing of Revision Surgery

Patient wants earliest correction of his deformity. He has one unpleasant experience and is circumspect. Patient may be doubting your credentials and is unsure what is going to happen to him. I will want to wait as long as it takes for the tissues to become soft and supple. It may take 3 months, 6 months or may be a year. I generally make the patient feel the induration, skin adherence, and tightness of the tissues by his own hands and explain that unless this becomes normal like other nonoperated areas, it will not be wise to revise. Explaining the healing response is of great help.

It is important to buy as much time as possible without being blamed for procrastination. The hard indurated; operated tissues make decision making very difficult. Surgery becomes complex due to bleeding, scarring, and hard immobile structures. Sutures do not hold well and may cut through.

Time is of essence. I prescribe a number of creams and gels for massage, silicone gels, mild steroid creams on the scars to help them soften up. The patient is asked to massage several times a day. Patient feels he is participating in the treatment and feels included in the process. He also notices the changes in the tissues, sees them improve, becomes supple, and becomes aware of his own progress. Golden rule is, patiently wait, wait and wait. Patient wait, wait, and wait!

A very important thing happens during this phase. Tissues start changing shape, they regain sensation, soreness goes away and things look different and better! The patient in many instances starts to accept his new image, is not overly upset and is coming to terms with his problem. Number of times, he may not want any more surgery as his level of satisfaction stands modified.

Example: I had a patient who lost nasal mucosal sensation after open rhinoplasty and could not perceive air passing through his nostrils. He was terrified that he cannot breathe and got admitted in hospital. It took a few weeks for him to get back his sensations and he was happy. *The Gillies principle, what you can do today, do it tomorrow, what you can do tomorrow do after a week and what you can do after a week do after one month!* During this patient wait, I tell them I will see you every 4 weeks, but if you have a problem you can come anytime. Psychological support is crucial to establish your credibility and patient's confidence. It also indicates that you are not chasing his wallet, which is a big thing for the patient. Once, it is decided that revision is called for, a plan in consultation with the patient is finalized. Complications possible and surgical limitations are once more reiterated. I personally prefer general anesthesia as it offers freedom to discuss your concerns and technical issues with a colleague, if one is there, during the surgery. Difference of opinion can be freely aired without raising anxiety level of the patient. Preoperative photography is meticulously undertaken for important records. The value of documenting the discussions is manifold and imperative. I have experienced that talking to the patient when he is coming out of anesthesia has an effect of hypnotic suggestion. Me or my anesthetist speaks to the patient during this phase to reassure that things have gone well, as planned and we expect a good outcome. I have found this very useful way to modify the patient's reaction to the result.

I generally pay the assisting surgeon and the anesthesiologist from my pocket. If the later outcome is good and the patient is happy, they do volunteer to bear the cost and I let them do it. I must admit it does not happen very often. I do not charge them any fees. I work from my private clinic so I decide what to charge, in corporate or big hospital you may have to adopt a different strategy.

Many revision procedures are of such nature that a second procedure or revision is a part of treatment plan. Fat grafting to face, breast, or any area needs to be done several times. All grafted fat does not survive and repeated grafting has to be done to get to the final outcome. The result demands multiple interventions. We need to wait for 3 months to know what has happened to the fat injected earlier. How much needs to be filled again? At times, you may get almost total loss of injected fat. I tell the patients that we will do the grafting till the desired result is obtained. It may be one or it may be five times. In this way, we can do the best for our patient without being pressurized by the number of surgeries needed. When donor sites are limited reharvesting from same area needs to be done. It can be difficult. The areas tend to bleed more and graft yield is bloody and of poor quality. It can be difficult to inject fat as the previous surgery may have caused local fibrosis. Longer waiting between procedures and good massage for several weeks can be helpful.

Revision Surgery in Liposuction

The main issue here is under resection or over resection. Liposuction revision is very complex and difficult procedure. If it is simple additional debulking, it can be done. If there are contour problems, they are really tough to solve. Surface irregularities, depressions, excessive resections, skin burns, loss or damage, and skin pigmentations are extremely difficult to correct. Liposuction revisions should not be taken lightly. Repeated fat grafts will be required to fill in over resected areas. The graft survival in these vascular compromised areas is poor. We also need a good source for fat harvest. In absence of such store, we are unable to help the patient. Never over resect, under resection can be corrected by redo procedure but over resection is very very difficult. Special equipment like Vaser ultrasonic lipolysis may be needed to handle such issues.

I treat multiple lipomatosis with Vaser liposuction. Precise accurate fat lysis can be done and many lipomas can be treated this way through a small 5-mm incision. There is, however, a catch. The disease can have multiple small seedlings and they may grow later. This is not recurrence but growth of pre-existent lesions. Previous liposuction can induce extensive fibrosis in the treated area making a subsequent resurgery extremely difficult. We must wait for longtime for the resolution. Good massage and radiofrequency treatments to resolve fibrosis are needed. Even then, it is indeed a tough endeavor. Another problem which needs mention is occurrence of skin wrinkling. If lot of superficial fat is resected then the skin loses its support and can show gross surface wrinkling so much so that a skin excision may have to be done to address the skin wrinkles and skin excess. Your first chance is the best chance, things are never the same again!

Additional support is needed with well-fitting corsets and compression garments. Manual lymphatic drainage and radiofrequency skin therapy can be a useful adjuvant.

Revision Rhinoplasty

The nose is probably most revised structure in aesthetic surgery. Its prominent location on the face and the need to keep it exposed makes it most accessible for inspection by anybody and everybody. It is common to hear four revisions and five revisions in rhinoplasty. Contour of the nose is modified in the ageing process and a significant contour change over the years is the rule. It may contribute to high revision rates. In the cleft lip nose, several revisions are done as it is an evolving deformity and shape changes need to be corrected appropriate for the age. We have discussed the value of first consult. I have been using a 3D camera for discussing rhinoplasty with my patient. Patients are very happy to see the possible transformation on their own face. Photographs of other patients help, but do not really come close to a 3D consultation. Each aspect of rhinoplasty is discussed with the patient. The incision location, plan of structural modification, and possible outcome add immense value to the consult. This is a tricky issue. The patient imagines that she is going to look beautiful after the surgery and that is why she has come to you. It is her perception, that her nose makes her look ugly. The nose is a very small though important part of the face. Changing the nose does not change the way the eyes, forehead, and chin ears skin look like. When a modified image is shown the patient realizes the falsity of her perception. The improvement becomes insignificant in her mind. The changes are not so interesting anymore. It is good to stop at this time and avoid intense displeasure.

The nose comes with an intense network of blood vessels. It allows us to do these multiple revisions with ease. Skin loss is a very rare problem in rhinoplasty. Plastic surgeons do have a messiah complex. The ability to change anatomy makes them feel like Gods angels. It is important to know when to stop revising. It is always possible to make it a little better. We have to see the quantum of benefit to the patient. It should not be an ego issue and a holistic and rational view is in order. We should be able to say "this far and no more", and stand your ground against all temptations.

Scar Revision Surgery

A surgical scar is a surgeon's signature on the patient's body. It must look good. A scar is a tissue of repair, based on fibrous tissue. It is not primary regenerative tissue. Hence, it is always going to be seen as different tissue. When the wound heals, the skin does not regenerate. The gap is filled by fibrous tissue. There is a lot of difference between a good-looking scar and a bad-looking scar. We as plastic surgeons make good-looking scars. Scars require revision when they are broad and stretched, pigmented, raised and hypertrophic, contracted, and look ugly. Our job is to produce a thin, supple, matt finish, flat, and skin colored scar. Scars go through a process of maturation and at times, it takes almost 1 year for the scars to mature. In the healing response, scars go through certain phases. They look good initially, then they show signs of hypertrophy, become red, raised, and itchy. This stage can last for up to 3 months. Later gradually, the scars start to mature and over a year continue to improve. Crucial to know and realize that even the revised scar is going to go through the same stages of healing. Revising a scar before 3 months is bad surgery. We need to give enough time for scar to show spontaneous resolution. Every surgery adds a quantum of fibrous tissue to the area. Repeated revisions are undesirable and should be carefully avoided.

Scar is enemy number one of plastic surgeons. We want to do anything and everything possible to improve the quality and appearance of the scars. *I have been in laser practice since 1998 and have fairly extensive experience of using fractional carbon dioxide (CO_2), Erbium-doped yttrium aluminum garnet (YAG), invasive and noninvasive radiofrequency, needle radiofrequency, intense pulsed light, neodymium (Nd):YAG, vitamin C iontophoresis, and sonophoresis. I am sure all of them help scars. Scar modulation by modifying the quality and quantity of collagen can be very helpful in treating scars.*

I will want to put to rest some issues about these devices. Their main use is to improve the quality of scar, pigmentation in the scar, reduce the gloss and shine, and reduce scar hypertrophy. Some scars are due to an anatomical irregularity and they need to be identified clearly as no laser can ever make them better. Tissue distortion, steps in the scar, widely stretched scar, scars running across lines of skin relaxation, trap door scars, etc. There is a clear line that separates where lasers and where surgery is required. It is mixing these indications that creates confusion.

One word of caution, lasers do need local, topical, or general anesthesia. The treatment can be very painful. Large areas of scarring mean severe pain. Every single so called noninvasive modality needs a minimum of four to six sessions. The treatment can run up to several months or year to complete. Not to forget that waiting for a year may be responsible for some of the benefits attributed to the modalities. CO_2 causes significant wounding on the skin surface. Serous discharge, scab formation, intense redness, photosensitivity, and postinflammatory pigmentation are very real sequel of laser treatments.

There is a difference in the mindset of surgeons and physicians. Each has a way of looking at scars. Ointments, topical steroids, *Gels, oils, creams, lotions, and sprays will work on some scars while surgery will be necessary for some. We must select an appropriate treatment for a particular scar.*

If the scar continues to remain bad after such time, we can consider revising it. We have to establish why did it not resolve? Tension, infection, bad and rough surgery, and skin propensity to scarring are the reasons for bad scars. In effect, we need to do scar revision—reduce tension on wound edges, use nonabsorbable fine dermal sutures, and do a layered closure. Prolonged support, compression garments, topical silicone gel cream, and sheets will go a long way in getting good scars. A warning - A scar is a scar, is a scar! Once a scar, always a scar.

Revision in Breast Augmentation

Surgery for breast augmentation is possibly the most rewarding of aesthetic surgery. It may be comparable to a cleft lip repair where a dramatic transformation is the rule. The common reasons for revision are to get a larger implant, correct ptosis due to a heavy implant, remove the implants for fear of malignancy, treatment of capsular contracture, replace damaged or expired implants, and relocation to improve cleavage. I have experience couple of odd requests. One patient after implants shifted to Japan. Common bathing is usual in Japan. She had a fairly large implant and had firm breasts with nipples thrusting out. She requested explantation as her erect nipples were sending wrong sexual signals to her co bathers.

Another woman came with breast implants done about eight years ago, perfect shape, perfect scar, and great looks. On touch, they were stony hardball of tissue. She had extremely severe capsular contracture. Her capsulectomy was done and implants replaced with cohesive gel textured surface implants. Capsule was completely excised giving the breasts their inherent soft feel. The capsule excised weighed about 300 g. Leaving the capsule behind in only incision is not a good idea as a large lumpy feel remains for years.

Capsular contracture is always there, but is seldom discussed with the emphasis needed. It is grossed over. It is good idea to educate the patients about it. When very strong the capsule can crease the implants and may rupture them.

SUMMARY

Revision surgery is a part of aesthetic surgery. Every plastic surgeon worth his salt is going to face the prospect of revising his surgical outcomes for a variety of reasons. The value of the first exhaustive, detailed consultation must be well understood. Please do not promise what you cannot do. Underpromise and overdeliver should be the plan. Keep an excellent rapport with the patient. Keep them informed of what good or bad is happening. Take out the "shock" element. Help the patient to get through this phase with psychological support. Some hand holding, honest discussions, and genuine concern will see you through most situations.

Revision surgery is not crime. It is a part and parcel of what the patient has been seeking. We have so little control over how the wounds heal. There is still a lot of what we do not understand completely. Always be there for your patient who has put his life in your hands.

It is a good practice to involve the patient in all kinds of decision making. It gives him a sense of honesty and fairness on part of the surgeon. Builds excellent rapport and helps him understand that revision surgery is a rarity, but an expected fallout of the primary procedure.

Remember, if something can go wrong, it will!

CHAPTER 44

Esthetic Procedures and Surgery in Minors

K Ramachandran, Charan JC

INTRODUCTION

There is an increased incidence in esthetic surgery, also called as cosmetic surgery, especially in the younger population in recent years. This can be attributed to:
- Cultural attitudes about the benefits of physical attractiveness.
- Promoting the ideals of beauty, self-improvement, and competition.
- Exposure from the media to adolescents to esthetic surgery unlike ever before. Requests for cosmetic surgery in adolescents are emotionally or psychologically motivated, with peer pressure playing a major role.
- Esthetic procedures and surgery are safe and accessible, when done by a qualified dermatologist and plastic surgeon.

The most common esthetic procedures in patients younger than 18 years old include rhinoplasty, otoplasty, breast augmentation and breast reduction. In males, gynecomastia is the most common problem. Among dermatosurgical indications, acne scarring, pigmentation, laser hair removal, lasers for other conditions such as Becker's nevus, nevus of ota, hemangiomas, vitiligo surgery, and improvement in color are sought in this age group. Occasionally, children with large number of warts, molluscum may also need esthetic surgery (Box 1). Quite often it is the parents who complain, while the child himself/herself may be least bothered about it.

With increasing number of cosmetic surgeries in adolescent patients, there are also increasing number of concerns related to what are the main indications for surgery, the consent and need for counseling in such cases.

This is a brief overview of the most common procedures performed and some tips to avoid difficult situations. Following these Guidelines will ensure that the plastic surgeon keeps chances of facing litigation to the minimum.

OTOPLASTY

- The ideal age to operate on the ear is around 5–8 years of age.
- The child may be aware of the problem or the parents notice it and bring the child for consultation.

> **BOX 1:** Case study: Consider the "best interests test".
>
> - Parents of a boy, 5 years of age (legally incompetent), request a referral for otoplasty from their general practitioner because they fear that the child will be subject to teasing on starting school. The problem being Protruding Ears. The child also has a history of moderate-to-severe asthma. The asthma had required hospitalization with pediatric intensive care unit admission in the past. There is a positive family history in the form of the *child's mother*, who had prominent ears and had been subject to teasing as a child until otoplasty. This has been the stimulus behind the enthusiasm of the parents about having the child's ears "fixed". The child is not aware of the protuberant ears.
> - The best interests test dictates that the needs of each child must be addressed individually, independently and irrespective of the desires of parents or treating surgeons. While the majority of surgeons, parents and psychologists will only consider otoplasty after a child has voiced concerns, but, prophylactic otoplasty is not an uncommon request.
> - A subgroup of children exists in whom marked preoperative social isolation and distress is unimproved despite objective improvement in prominence of ears.
> - So, while it may appear that most children will psychologically benefit from such surgery, this cannot be guaranteed for all children.
> - Consideration must also be given to the complications which can happen in case of any general anesthesia or surgical procedure. Hematoma and infection which can lead to perichondritis, cartilage necrosis, and poor cosmetic results.
> - It is vital that when an incompetent child is presented for an otoplasty, an individualized assessment of the child's interests is conducted.
> - The best interests test is likely to be more easily satisfied where children are aware of their prominent ears and request that something can be done; however, underlying psychological issues should be investigated and addressed.
> - Despite current practice, it appears more difficult to legally justify preemptive otoplasty on children who are not aware of, or suffer no distress from their physical appearance.
> - In this case study, exposing this child to the risks of a general anesthetic and surgical procedure for no tangible benefits in the child's perspective does not seem to be in his best interests based on the available evidence.

- The main objective would be to elicit if the child is aware of the problem and disturbed by the deformity.
- In cases where the child is not affected, the parents must be counseled about the treatment options and also to wait until school going age.
- If the child is disturbed and also wants it to be corrected, the surgery may be planned after informed consent from the parents.

RHINOPLASTY

- The ideal age to operate on nose is around 15–16 years when the bony platform is well formed.
- Gross deformity is the usual complaint, and the child can be embarrassed about the body image which warrants treatment.
- Detailed counseling involving explanation of the risks, foreign materials (implants), need for autogenous material, postoperative complications (edema, redness, etc.), time taken for the final result, discomfort or difficulty in breathing.
- Even when done with the highest standards of safety, every surgery has an element of risk which should to be communicated to the patient and their attenders, both of whom need to be in concurrence.

GYNECOMASTIA

- One of the most common issues of the young adolescent boys.
- Usually presents at 12–13 years of age. Children experience a growth spurt which changes their body composition. This,

> **BOX 2:** Malpractice case insight: Breast reduction surgery in male of teen age.
> - *Facts*: A 17-year-old boy was taken up for liposuction for gynecomastia under general anesthesia. There was an anesthetic error during surgery which resulted in the death of the patient.
> - *Plaintiff*: There was a huge furore in the media, as to why surgery was necessary.
> - *Defense*: Parents pointed out that the boy was refusing to go to school because of the need for surgery.
> - *Result*: While no negligence was made out on the part of the doctors, the case highlighted the need for proper counseling and if necessary involving a psychiatrist in evaluation.

combined with sedentary lifestyle and increased incidence of childhood obesity, can lead to gynecomastia.
- The child faces ridicule from the peers at school. This can demoralize the child and leading to timid, shy, increasingly conscious, depressed child who finds it difficult to express the situation.
- They may suffer silently or can express it to the parents.
- The severity of the gynecomastia has to be evaluated, and detailed discussion about the treatment options, presence of scars, possible mismatch in the size, complications and if necessary a psychiatric counseling should be done with the parents and the child before deciding on surgical procedure (Box 2).

BREAST SURGERY

Breast Reduction

- Usually the patients for breast reduction present about 15–18 years of age.
- This can be presented with just increase in size of the breast which causes psychological discomfort to the girl or with associated medical symptoms like back pain, and neck pain.
- Counseling has to be done to the patient and the attenders in a detailed manner about:
  - The possible increase in size of the breast after pregnancy and lactation
  - Scars on the face of the breast, pictures of similar scars should be shown to the patient and attenders
  - Postsurgical difficulties in breastfeeding
  - Permanence of the scars especially if the girl is unmarried.
- The patient and the attenders need to understand all the pros and cons of the procedure.
- In severe cases with associated symptoms and the patient, attenders are compliant and willing, the breast reduction surgery can be planned.
- If the attenders are reluctant because of the scars which can cause cultural issues, better to wait until the girl can take an independent call on the surgery at a later date.

Breast Augmentation

- The main objective is to identify the patient's need for the surgery.
- If it is an impulsive decision, counseling should be done, not prudent to operate on this age group unless it is warranted.
- Presence of Poland's syndrome or other chest wall or breast abnormalities are good indications for this procedure.
- The patient and the attenders should be disclosed about the scars, complications, life of the implant, possible need for more surgical procedures in future, anaplastic large cell lymphoma, capsular contracture, possible loss of nipple sensation so that they can make an informed decision.

- Other alternatives like fat grafting to the breast can be explained to the patient. Fat grafting usually requires multiple sessions subject to availability of fat.

In dermatology, the following questions can arise in different procedures (Box 3):

- *Laser hair removal*: With early menarche, obesity and polycystic ovarian disease (PCOD) young girls start developing hirsutism. There is often a demand for laser hair removal in such young girls both by the girl and the mother (Box 4). The procedure is minor, and hence is tolerated well. But, starting a repetitive procedure in very young children, this may mean a very large number of sessions by the time when patient reaches 16–18 years of age. While there is no ideal age or starting laser hair removal, it is generally advisable to avoid it before 16 years of age, though patient at earlier age can be considered depending on discretion of the doctor after proper discussion with the parents.
- *Treatment of nevoid conditions*: These conditions, such as nevus of ota, beckers nevus, café-au-lait macules, lentigens are located on face and hence patients/parents may demand early intervention by lasers. However, they are often progressive, recurrence is common and hence is always preferable to wait till at least 16 years of age to avoid recurrence.
- *Vitiligo surgery*: Vitiligo causes much stigma and a child with vitiligo is often subjected to psychological trauma. Hence, parents often demand treatment for vitiligo early. Surgery may also be sought for nevoid depigmentations, when located on face. While vitiligo in young patients responds better to surgery as most lesions are segmental, young patients may not cooperate under local anesthesia, and general anesthesia for such a surgery in a child may be difficult to justify. Moreover, success of many surgical procedures depends upon the postoperative immobility of the operated part, which becomes difficult to maintain in young children. Older children and adolescents may be counseled about the procedure and the possible outcome of the surgery to achieve their cooperation. All children with vitiligo, especially among dark races, require thorough counseling as they may be the victims of peer-teasing

---

BOX 3: Possible medicolegal issues in dermatology.

- Was the procedure really necessary at that age?
- Could the primary condition have progressed? Should the surgery have waited till the progression is over? For example, Nevoid conditions?
- Psychological issues? Did the patient suffer sufficiently due to the condition? Or was it the pressure by the parents?

BOX 4: Malpractice lawsuit insight: Laser hair removal.

- *Facts*: A dermatologist performed laser hair removal in a patient of 15 years, who developed pigmentation. The matter was raised in a consumer court.
- *Plaintiff*: what is the justification for doing the procedure at that tender age.
- *Defense*: When asked, what is the justification for doing the procedure at that age, the dermatologist referred to IADVL guidelines which stated that a patient can be taken up at earlier age than 16 years, at the discretion of the treating physician.
- *Result*: The court dismissed the case, and acquitted the dermatologist.

and avoidance at schools. This may lead to anxiety, introvert personality and childhood depression. Hence again a balanced view has to be taken after consideration of all aspects.

A well-counseled child with vitiligo may render full cooperation to the treating physician, making his job easier. Mulekar et al. have observed that all the children with vitiligo in their series, treated by noncultured cellular grafting technique, accepted the treatment procedure willingly, even if it was a repeat session.

The age of the patient for vitiligo surgery: As such, no uniformly accepted opinion exists concerning the minimum age for surgery. However, studies have suggested that results of transplantation procedures were better in younger individuals than in older ones. Thus, no consensus exists in this aspect and physicians should exercise their judgment after taking all aspects of the individual patient into consideration.

- *Capillary malformations and vascular tumors*: Hemangioma may improve with time, but it is perhaps one condition in which early intervention is justified in some situations. Portwine stain often extends into nasal tract, or eye and can lead to obstruction. Capillary malformations when giving rise to hemorrhage, ulceration, necrosis or causing functional disability merit the use of dermatosurgical interventions.
- *Botulinum toxin, fillers*: It is generally agreed that these are not advised in young age.

It should be appreciated that any side effect or harm out of a procedure in a child or young patient would be viewed seriously in a court of law. Hence utmost caution is advised. Whenever in doubt, a psychiatrist opinion may be taken to assess the possible implications both of the condition and the treatment on the child.

How to asses adolescents/minor patients for esthetic surgery?

[Based on inputs from guidelines from General Medical Council (GMC), British Association of Aesthetic Plastic Surgeons (BAAPS), British Association of Plastic, Reconstructive and Aesthetic Surgeons (BAPRAS), Canadian Association of Plastic Surgery]

- If the surgeon feels that any proposed procedure is not prudent for that age or the timing of the procedure is not right, do not proceed even when subjected to compelling emotional pressure that might be brought from the patients, parents or the attenders—Trusting your first instincts on whether to continue will usually lead to correct decision making.
- Remember that those with parental responsibility could bring an action on behalf of the child and therefore you are exposed to both the young persons' interpretation at any stage of the process and also those holding parental responsibility.
- Involve the child in the decision-making process as much as possible. A parent can give consent for a surgical procedure for a child/young person when they are deemed to not possess the maturity and capacity needed to make the decision. *Do not perform a procedure or operate on a child who does not want it.*
- Marketing activities must not target children or young people, through either their content or placement.
- *Cooling off period*: Usually a 3-month cooling off period is recommended for all patients under the age of 18 years who are considering major cosmetic medical and surgical procedures.

The guidelines define major procedures as involving cutting beneath the skin. Examples include: breast augmentation, breast reduction, rhinoplasty and liposuction. Psychological evaluation by a qualified and registered psychologist or psychiatrist is also deemed compulsory for these patients before any major cosmetic surgery.
- *Cooling off period for minor procedures*: A 7-day cooling off period is recommended for all patients under the age of 18 years before minor (nonsurgical) cosmetic medical procedures. In accordance with the guidelines, minor procedures are those that do not involve cutting beneath the skin, but may involve piercing the skin. Examples include: nonsurgical cosmetic varicose vein treatment, laser skin treatments, use of CO_2 lasers to cut the skin, mole removal for purposes of appearance, laser hair removal, dermabrasion, chemical peels, injections, microsclerotherapy and hair replacement therapy.
- *Identify the motivation or the driving desire for surgery*: Teasing and ridicule at school from peers, and body dysmorphic disorder are powerful motivating factors, etc.
- *Adolescents must have realistic, logical goals and understand the benefits and risks*. Those individuals who state a specific concern and a logical goal are more likely to be happy with postoperative outcomes compared to those with vaguer concerns and unclear goals.
- The teen individual may take more time to articulate specific concerns and desired outcomes. To have a complete discussion, it is often necessary to have multiple meetings with the patient and parents to ensure that everyone is clear on expectations and risks, and that all questions have been answered.
- The adolescents tend to see situations in more black-and-white terms compared with adults, with outcomes viewed as either perfect or catastrophic. *Thus, it is important to be certain that the patient, surgeon, and parents are in agreement before surgery.*
- *Adolescents must be sufficiently balanced to tolerate temporary discomfort and possible negative outcomes.*
- An essential component in an adolescent's preoperative assessment is judging the maturity of the individual's response to difficult situations. Surgeons can help the patient to develop mature coping strategies by asking the patient directly about difficult postoperative situations. Such questions as, "How would you deal with this complication?" or "Have you thought about what you will tell your peers if they notice that you look different?" encourage the teen to think about these issues ahead of time, and also allow the physician to assess the maturity of the patient's response.

INFORMED CONSENT

In India, informed consent has to be obtained after thoroughly explaining the risks, complications, long-term effects and changes due to a particular procedure to the patient and the relatives and consent obtained from the "adolescent" or "minor" patient and also the legal guardians (Box 5):
- Assent is a formal consent of children above 12 years of age, without which proceeding with surgery is not recommended. This is besides the consent of "parent/guardian".
- Procedure is deferred if the "minor" does not approve for the procedure.
- Unaccompanied minors will need to bring the parents or guardians for the discussion.

Esthetic Procedures and Surgery in Minors

> **BOX 5:** Mental fitness of minors and consent for esthetic surgery.
> - It is strongly recommended that the child is found to be sufficiently mentally competent enough to fully comprehend any risks associated with undergoing a cosmetic surgery procedure.
> - A mental health assessment test should be administered to the child for the purpose of determining competency.
> - Suggested factors to take into consideration when administering the competency assessment include the child's age, any emotional and/or mental health issues or concerns, and any other issues or concerns that may have detrimental long-term effects on the child.
> - If the child is found to be incompetent to make decisions of a surgical nature for himself, a parent may act on behalf of their child, providing that they are truly acting in the child's best interests.
> - Acting in a child's best interests is generally recognized as acting in a way that benefits or improves a child's physical, mental, and emotional health.

> **BOX 6:** Malpractice case: Congenital defects.
> - *Facts*: Prenatal anomaly scans missed out amelia (absence of one limb) and unilateral renal agenesis (absence of one kidney) in intrauterine growth restriction (IUGR) fetus by two radiologists—they have reported "fetal spine, trunk and limbs are normal".
> - *Analysis*: The principle of Res-ipsa-loqiutor (the thing speaks for itself) is squarely applicable in this case—Radiologists to pay ₹1,500,000 jointly and severally to the parents—No negligence by gynecologist.
> - *Insight*: The act of radiologists, it was medical negligence and deficiency in service.
> - *Discussion*: The USG was performed at 21 weeks of gestation; it is unfortunate that, even if it was diagnosed, there was no treatment or any cure except the termination of pregnancy (MTP). But, MTP Act 1971 prohibits, MTP at 21st week of pregnancy. Hence, the patient has to continue the pregnancy till its delivery.
> - *Citation*: NCDRC judgment in case of Anil Dutt and Anr. vs Vishesh Hospital and Ors. on 16 May, 2016.

- Do not operate on an unwilling patient even if there is pressure from the parents or guardians.

Parents' and physicians' perceptions of facial plastic surgery in children with congenital defects (Box 6): Although the practice of attempting to normalize children with congenital defects (e.g. Down's syndrome) by subjecting them to major facial plastic surgery has no therapeutic benefit, and should be seen as mutilating surgery comparable to female circumcision. Both parents' and physicians' attitudes and perceptions concerning facial plastic surgery in persons with Down's syndrome vary. In a study by Pueschel SM et al., more physicians (63%) than parents (28%) feel that the children's facial features negatively affect their social development; most parents (85%) see their children well accepted by society whereas only 4% of physicians do so; approximately half of the physicians (51%) and parents (41%) thought that after hypothetical facial plastic surgery a child with Down's syndrome may accomplish more socially; the majority of the parents (92%) and physicians (76%) were concerned with the risk of the operation; and only 13% of parents but 44% of physicians indicated that facial plastic surgery should be done on children with Down's syndrome.

Latest legal role of esthetic surgery in correcting permanent disability due to genetic, congenital disorders, trauma (acid attack) and infectious diseases (leprosy) causing facial deformity in children: After the enactment of "Rights of Persons with Disabilities (Equal Opportunities, Protection of Rights and Full Participation) Act", 2016 (RPWD): Let us see provisions of RPWD act 2016 in detail:

Disability includes:
- "Dwarfism" means a medical or genetic condition resulting in an adult height of 4 feet 10 inches (147 centimeters) or less
- "Muscular dystrophy" means a group of hereditary genetic muscle disease that weakens the muscles that move the human body and persons with multiple dystrophy have incorrect and missing information in their genes, which prevents them from making the proteins they need for healthy muscles. It is characterized by progressive skeletal muscle weakness, defects in muscle proteins, and the death of muscle cells and tissue.
- "Acid attack victims" means a person disfigured due to violent assaults by throwing of acid or similar corrosive substance.
- "Leprosy cured person".
- "Cerebral palsy" means a group of nonprogressive neurological condition affecting body movements and muscle coordination, caused by damage to one or more specific areas of the brain, usually occurring before, during or shortly after birth.

As per provisions of RPWD Act 2016 (Box 7), the appropriate Government and the Local Authorities shall take necessary measures for the persons with disabilities to provide:
- Free healthcare in the vicinity especially in rural area subject to such family income as may be notified.
- Barrier-free access in all parts of government and private hospitals and other healthcare institutions and centers.
- Priority in attendance and treatment.
- Essential medical facilities for life-saving emergency treatment and procedures.
- Take measures for prenatal, perinatal and postnatal care of mother and child.
- Sexual and reproductive healthcare especially for women with disability.
- Provisions of aids and appliances, medicine and diagnostic services and corrective surgery free of cost to persons with disabilities.

Punishment shall be punishable with imprisonment for a term which shall not be less than 6 months but which may extend to 5 years and with fine, whosoever:
- Intentionally insults or intimidates with intent to humiliate a person with disability in any place within public view.
- Assaults or uses force to any person with disability with intent to dishonor him or outrage the modesty of a woman with disability.
- Having the actual charge or control over a person with disability voluntarily or knowingly denies food or fluids to him or her.
- Voluntarily injures, damages or interferes with the use of any limb or sense or any supporting device of a person with disability.

So after going through the above provisions, it is clear that esthetic surgery for correcting

---

BOX 7: RPWD Act, 2016: Possible medicolegal queries in future unanswered.
- Does viable fetus with congenitally futile disorder (anencephaly) qualify as a handicapped and disabled person in need of surgical repair in the eye of Indian law after the RPWD act 2016?
- Can children with congenital disorders and diseases claim for free treatment as disabled person as per RPWD act?
- Can doctors and hospitals be penalized for delay or denial of surgical measures to child, who is congenitally malformed (anencephalic), or develops deformity due to burns, acid attack or leprosy: because they can be covered as physically disabled person under RPWD act in court of law?

congenital defects does not fall into life-saving surgery, so it will not be covered under RPWD Act for free surgery.

But multiple sittings of plastic surgery for cosmetic correction of deformity of face due to facial burns after acid attack in pediatric victims, comes under provisions of 166B of IPC—free treatment to the victims of sexual assault and acid attack victims, which includes not only the first-aid but complete recovery from the injury occurred, as per the new 2013 amendments in criminal law in India. IPC Section 166B—Punishment for nontreatment of victim. All government and private hospitals have to provide immediate first-aid or medical treatment, free of cost, to victims of sexual assault and acid attack as mandated by laws.

Under IPC Section 166B, whoever being in-charge of a hospital, public or private, whether run by the Central Government, the State Government, local bodies or any other person, if denies victims of any treatment would contravene the provisions. The person would be punished with imprisonment of 1 year or fine or with both. This is still a debatable issue for private hospitals to provide free treatment under corporate social responsibility, as the Supreme Court of India has emphasized that the State Government should bear the expenses of treatment of these victims, without any delay.

Compensation for acid attack: In India, often incidences of acid attacks on schoolgirls due to love affair grab the headlines of Indian media. The offence is registered as grievous hurt under Section 326A. The punishment for acid attack is defined in Section 326B of IPC, which states—Whoever throws or attempts to throw acid on any person or attempts to administer acid to any person, or attempts to use any other means, with the intention of causing permanent or partial damage or deformity or burns or maiming or disfigurement or disability or grievous hurt to that person, shall be punished with imprisonment of either description for a term which shall not be less than 5 years but which may extend to 7 years, and shall also be liable to fine.

Section 357B has been newly inserted in CRPC which reads as: "The compensation payable by the State Government under section 357A shall be in addition to the payment of fine to the victim under section 326A or section 376D of the Indian Penal Code."

Free medical treatment: Section 357C has been newly inserted whereby all hospitals, public or private are required to provide first-aid or medical treatment free of cost. The section reads as "All hospitals, public or private, whether run by the Central Government, the State Government, local bodies or any other person, shall immediately, provide the first-aid or medical treatment, free of cost, to the victims of any offence covered under section 326A, 376, 376A, 376B, 376C, 376D or section 376E of the Indian Penal Code and shall immediately inform the police of such incident."

CONCLUSION

Plastic surgeons can expect to encounter increasing demands for referral and surgery from the pediatric population from India and abroad with prior consent and financial support from their parents, due to rise of medical tourism and selfie culture of looking good. Currently, the inconsistent legal approach and the lack of clear guidance on how to apply the legal test of best interests of the child, mean that more professional guidelines are needed. Dermatologists also need to understand that their current professional and legal obligations require them to undertake individualized assessments of children, before any procedure.

When attending a child victim of acid attack, hospitals are bound by the Indian laws to provide free first-aid and treatment without any delay, otherwise they can be penalized.

SUGGESTED READING

1. Buddhadev RM. Standard guidelines of care: Laser and IPL hair reduction. Indian J Dermatol Venereol Leprol. 2008;74:S68-74.
2. College of surgeons and physicians of Ontario. (2011). Surgical cosmetic procedures. [online] Avialable from: https://www.cpso.on.ca/uploadedFiles/policies/.../expectations-cosmetic-surgery(1).pdf [Accessed Jan., 2019].
3. General Medical Council. (2018). GMC ethical guidelines for doctors. [online] Available from: https://www.gmc-uk.org/ethical-guidance/ethical-guidance-for-doctors/0-18-years [Accessed Jan., 2019].
4. Gupta S, Kumar B. Epidermal grafting for vitiligo in adolescents. Pediatr Dermatol. 2002;19:159-62.
5. Gupta S, Kumar B. Epidermal grafting in vitiligo: Influence of age, site of lesion, and type of disease on outcome. J Am Acad Dermatol. 2003;49:99-104.
6. IPC Section 166B—Punishment for non-treatment of victim.
7. Kitipornchai L, Then SN. Cosmetic surgery on children—professional and legal obligations in Australia. Aust Fam Physician. 2011;40(7):513-6.
8. Mathews B. Children and consent to medical treatment. In: White B, McDonald F, Willmott L (Eds). Health law in Australia. Sydney: Thomson Reuters; 2010. pp. 113-47.
9. Parsad D, Gupta S. Standard guidelines of care for vitiligo surgery. Indian J Dermatol Venereol Leprol. 2008;74(Suppl S1):37-45.
10. Pueschel SM, Monteiro LA, Erickson M. Parents' and physicians' perceptions of facial plastic surgery in children with Down's syndrome. J Ment Defic Res. 1986;30 (Pt 1):71-9.
11. Rights of Persons with Disabilities (Equal Opportunities, Protection of Rights and Full Participation) Act, 2016.
12. Royal College of Surgeons. (2018). Good Surgical Practice. Royal College of Surgeons. [online] Available from: https://www.rcseng.ac.uk/-/media/files/rcs/standards-and.../gsp/gsp-2014-web.pdf [Accessed Jan., 2019].
13. Royal College of Surgeons. (2018). Professional guidelines for cosmetic practice. [online] Available from: https://www.rcseng.ac.uk/-/media/files/rcs/.../standards_for_cosmetic_practice.pdf [Accessed Jan., 2019].

CHAPTER 45

Legal Issues in Medical Tourism

Rakesh Kalra, Vivekanshu Verma

INTRODUCTION

Medical tourism or health tourism is defined as the practice of traveling across international borders to seek healthcare services. Usual reasons are the availability of treatments better than in home country, or more economical treatments in countries conceived to have standard facilities, or the possibility of enjoying a holiday simultaneously while recovering from a treatment.

Queries in mind of medical tourist visiting another country for plastic surgery:
- Is the surgery safe?
- Is the surgery of international standards?
- Does it save me a lot of money?
- Does it save me time in getting surgery earlier?

Queries in the mind of surgeon when a medical tourist is visiting from another country:
- What are the visa formalities? Should he have a medical visa or tourist visa?
- Should police be informed on arrival and on departure?
- What if he does not depart?
- What if he indulges in other activities? What is doctor's liability?
- When can he travel?
- Is he educated enough to understand postoperative care?

India has a great advantage in facilitating medical tourism because we have some world-class hospitals with state-of-the-art facilities, our doctors and nurses are well trained at a relatively young age, English is a widely spoken language, pharmaceutical products and services both are very economical as compared to the West, and the country has rich traditions, culture, history, monuments and natural attractions for tourists all combined together. Indian Medical professionals working abroad are great in numbers and have established the impression of doctors from India being good at their profession.

Surgical procedures sought by travelling patients for medical tourism in India:
- Cosmetic surgery for correction of scars and deformities, rhinoplasties, face lifts
- Bariatric surgery for weight reduction
- Cancer surgery for removal of tumor
- Dental surgery for implants
- Smile surgery for improving beauty
- Cardiac bypass surgery
- Knee and hip replacement
- Spine surgery
- Organ transplants—kidney, liver, and corneal
- Stem cell therapy for regeneration
- Surrogacy and infertility
- Breast augmentation/reduction/reconstruction
- Gender modification surgery
- Body contouring, liposuction, tummy tucks.

SOME SPECIAL ISSUES WITH RESPECT TO DERMATOLOGY

Dermatological surgeries for which assistance is sought are usually minor and minimally invasive. These include hair transplantation, botulinum toxin, fillers, and facial rejuvenation. Most of these can safely be performed as they are lunch time procedures.

However, rejuvenation, hair removal, tattoo removal, etc. are repetitive procedures needing multiple sessions. Often patients show keenness to do the procedure, because of lower cost, but are unable to continue their sessions when they go to their home country due to higher cost.

This should be made clear to the patient and specific consent obtained as to the level of improvement that can be obtained. This will prevent accusations of lack of results or exploitation. Facial features may also affect outcomes and this needs to be factored in consent. The temptation to do the procedure for a "foreign well paying patient" should be resisted.

It should also be recognized that even minor side effects such as bruising or erythema can be bothersome while on tour and patients may react adversely. Often these patients have little time and wish to do procedures in a hurry and then may end up blaming the doctors. Hence, it is important to be thorough during consent taking.

MEDICAL VISA VERSUS TOURIST VISA

For seeking treatments in India, the medical tourist should get a medical visa. This has now become mandatory.

Q. What if he comes on tourist visa and then decides to get a treatment?
The embassy usually issues a medical visa for up to the required or requested period of treatment, or up to 1 year maximum, with up to 3 times entry within the year.

The patient seeking the medical visa, can apply for treatment at hospitals of repute in India. While making their request, they can submit an advice issued by their own local doctors or hospitals.

Prospective patients may also submit a letter of invitation by the hospital where they are seeking treatment in India, which mentions that the required treatment is available at that hospital. It is important for the inviting hospital to mention that they are relying their tentative opinion or provisional diagnosis on information provided hitherto by the patient through email, and that the same may vary and shall be finalized after a personal consultation only, which shall happen upon the final arrival of the patient. Secondly, it is also important for the hospital to clarify in their invitation letter, that the patient is not personally known to anyone on the staff of the hospital, including the doctor.

Intimations to Local Authorities including Form

The hospital where a foreigner is admitted under a medical visa, needs to intimate the local Foreigner Regional Registration Office/ Foreigner Registration Office (FRRO/FRO) in person in the following conditions:
- Where the patient is admitted for treatment for a period of over 14 days
- Within 24 hours in case the patient is a Pakistani national
- Within 7 days in case the patient is an Afghanistan national, unless their visas are stamped "Exempt from Police Reporting".

This intimation is sent in Form C.

Extension of Medical Visa

The period may be further extended to more than 1 year, or to an additional visit by moving an application or special request to the FRRO/FRO. Up to two relatives or friends are allowed on a Medical Attendant Visa (Med X) as attendants with the patient.

Any further extension beyond 1 year is allowed only by moving the application on the recommendation of FRRO/FRO to the Home Ministry, on producing relevant documents, medical history, and certificates from established/recognized/specialized hospitals/treatment centers in India.

For Extension of Visa for Pakistan Nationals

The initial period of validity of medical visa/ Med X may be up to a period of 3 months or the period of treatment, whichever is less. This period can be extended by the Ministry of Home Affairs on the recommendations of the State Governments/FRRO supported by appropriate medical documents. Only one Medical Attendant is permitted with one patient.

For Extension of Visa for Bangladeshi Nationals

The initial period of validity of medical visa/ Med X may be up to a period of 1 year or for the period of treatment whichever is less. The medical visa and the Med X will be extendable by another 1 year subject to production of the required medical report. Up to three Medical Attendants are permitted with every patient.

TREATMENTS FOR A FOREIGNER ON NONMEDICAL (TOURIST) VISA

Tourist visa conversion is possible, in case a tourist falls sick and needs to be hospitalized. This is done by the FRRO/FRO after a certificate to the effect is issued by a government or Indian Council of Medical Research (ICMR) recognized hospital. In such a condition, the accompanying person's visa can also be converted into a Med X, coterminus with the medical visa of the patient.

Extension of such issued visas is possible by submission of relevant medical documents and certificates from established/recognized/ specialized hospitals/treatment centers in India.

RELATIONSHIP BETWEEN HOSPITALS AND FACILITATING AGENCIES

There are many agencies or brokering firms across the World that facilitates medical tourism. These agencies advertise heavily and promise out of the country medical treatments, besides providing travel facilities, sight-seeing and excursion trips, hotel stay, etc. Some charges an overall inclusive package, while others charges for the travel and accommodation facilitation only, leaving the medical fee to be charged independently by the hospital.

Hospitals and doctors providing medical tourists the medical facilities should keep the fee independent of an overall package always. Reasons are simple, as medical care has its uncertainties, and the patient may need extra procedures to overcome unexpected complications and longer than expected stay to allow for full healing, etc.

Thus, it is mandatory that the relationship between the facilitating agency and the hospital be formalized by a notified contract or legally binding document, clearly outlining the independent roles of either party.

The hospital must resist letting the agency speak on behalf of the doctor, and promising results, etc. The doctor must always speak to the patient before they book their travel and explain to the patient the full workup and expected procedure, the fee and complications, etc. A lack of proper preoperative communication, and worse than that a rosy picture painted by the travel facilitator can produce a legal mess.

"Better" offers promoted by hospitals to seek maximum medical tourism:
- Better access to medical technology
- Better pricing for specialized surgery
- Better quality of care
- Better qualified surgeons and staff
- Better food and accommodation facilities.

CONSENT OF FOREIGN PATIENT: LANGUAGE BARRIER IN COMMUNICATION

Informed consent is the document whereby the patient is informed of the risks, and likely shortfall in expected results so as to allow the patient to make an informed decision before opting for the procedure. Depending upon local regulations, the hospital informs and under witness gets the patient to document having been given the necessary information. For an out of the country patient, the doctor needs to ensure that the information is well understood by the patient, in his or her own language. Hence, a mutually understood language needs to be used, and if need be, services of an interpreter must be used as well.

A preliminary draft of the consent must be shared through emails as well, even before the patient takes any decision to make plans for the trip and does bookings, etc. This is to circumvent any issues of having made any expenses and undertaken a trip, and then discovering that the likely complications do not suit the patient. There should of course, not be any surprises on actual arrival of the patient. However, the final signing of the document has to be in the actual presence of the patient at the hospital.

A draft of postoperative care should also be shared with the patient—postoperative appearance may change after surgery on face which may lead to issues in immigration. It should also be clarified as to whether he can take further tour of the country after surgery.

Patients may not at times divulge their personal information to their relatives back home when they get some personal surgeries done. However, there has to be a decision maker, and next to kin that may need to be contacted in case of a disaster happening to the patient. Such a name with contact details must be mentioned by the patient as a mandatory inclusion in the consent form, though with the rider that the hospital shall not misuse the same, but fall back upon only in dire consequences situations. The consent should also include a clause mentioning that such a next of kin could be relied upon to give further consent for additional procedures in case of a life-threatening situation say during anesthesia or unconsciousness when consent may be required.

PAYMENT AND INSURANCE BENEFITS

The patient must be aware fully of whether or not insurance payment benefits are available when expensive health care procedures and treatment are involved and if at all applicable outside of the patient's home country borders. Medical tourists, their providers and insurers should understand how the local rules in the patient's and the provider's jurisdictions affect payment and claims processing. For health coverage benefits, it is more likely that the patient must bear the burden of paying all expenses out of pocket and submitting a claim to his or her insurer for reimbursement later. Providers and patients should know if there are auditing procedures after payment (postpayment review) that these require timely response and submission of supporting documentation.

MAINTAINING MEDICAL RECORDS FOR MEDICAL TOURISTS

With regard to sharing and providing medical records to the out of country providers in advance of treatment, and in return the supply of medical records by the provider to the patient, or insurers, or advocates, etc. must be clear beforehand and part of the understanding. Also, provision of sufficient records of the on-going treatment for the benefit of the patient for follow-up in the country of origin should all be settled well in advance between the provider and the patient.

PATIENT PRIVACY AND OTHER PATIENT RIGHTS

How the personal patient's data, treated as "individually identifiable health information" is protected by the provider must be understood by the medical tourist fully. This data can include financial and other very personal and private information beyond just the medical care and conditions.

Also, what rights are provided to patients under the laws of the provider's jurisdiction must also be made clear. These include the right to be informed and participate in their care decisions, the right to have advance notice of their payment obligations, the right to have visitors, and the right to access and have complete copies of their own medical records?

> **CASE STUDY 1:** Confidentiality in Medical Tourism
>
> A celebrity patient requires varicose vein removal, but she wants to have the procedure quickly and has decided to pay for it privately in Singapore hospital, to hide from Indian media coverage. You can think of no clinical reason why she should not go and would like to help her. The patient has asked you to complete a case summary setting out her medical history and clinical findings.
> If after a discussion with the patient, you think it appropriate to complete the form, you should appropriately write the reports and not omit any relevant information. As with any other confidential information, the patient's informed consent is necessary before disclosing these details.

DISPUTE RESOLUTION

Medical tourists should be informed about the range of optional and mandatory dispute resolution methods that are available. Disputes can vary, such as a payment dispute or a liability claim for a bad result. The claims can be limited to return or forgiveness of fees, or actual recovery of consequential damages, such as lost earnings. Also, if it is possible to recover monetary damages for claims of permanent harm or disfigurement.

Indian government should formulate specific laws for medical tourism so that the sense of safety to a patient shall encourage even greater medical tourism. Insurance covers for doctors should be adequate, so that the patient can be compensated properly. However, newer insurance products are available where the patient is directly covered for medical malpractice occurring overseas.

ONLINE CONSULTATION FOR PROMOTING MEDICAL TOURISM

The patient seeking consultation should be sincerely informed about the limited value of the online consultation, and also that the final opinion can be given only upon an examination in person. But short of that, the online consultation, online review of suggested investigations, and consideration of the extent of the problem by viewing still photographs, or functions by video are always helpful in making a "provisional diagnosis" as an intermediate step towards the final diagnosis.

However, the Indian courts have also opined that telephonic consultation is illegal. Owing to the possibility of something goes wrong as a result of the online consultation, or a telephonic advice, the provider should take care that sensitive, life-threatening matters are not opined upon in this manner.

SURGICAL PROCEDURES IN LONE PATIENTS WITHOUT ACCOMPANYING COMPANIONS

Surgical procedures should not be done on children who are not accompanied by at least one parent, or a guardian, unless it is a dire emergency.

Similarly, adults should not be discharged after day care surgery in a sedated condition.

The surgeon must make his decision on whether he is ready to undertake a life-threatening procedure without the presence of relatives or accompanying persons of a patient. Such risks must be avoided by the surgeon. Proper consent must be taken accordingly. Also, before sedating the patient, the contact details of the next of kin must be clearly disclosed by the patient and recorded.

POSTSURGICAL FOLLOW-UP

This issue is always of concern as to who shall do a late follow-up of the patient operated abroad. The patient should have access to getting some follow-up, and whether that is covered by insurance in their parent country or not should be looked into by the patient. Late complications, requiring a secondary procedure, are taken to be a burden by the health authorities in the parent country, and are taken care of depending upon the commitments of the authorities towards the health of their citizens.

Prescriptions from abroad may also not be serviced in the parent country easily, and this issue must be looked into.

The service provider should take into consideration all these aspects and safeguard him by adequate information given and consent recorded. The service provider should also be ready to continue at least some general support by advice online and promptly responding on the e-mails.

RISKS AND CONTROVERSIES IN MEDICAL TOURISM

Medical tourism is lucrative business for developing countries, but there are risks of postoperative infections due to lack of hygiene and humid environment creating fertile soil for bacterial and fungal infections. World Health Organization (WHO) has launched the program of World Alliance for Patient Safety in 2004, for improving the standards and hygiene in hospitals of developing countries like Africa, Malaysia, and south eastern countries including India.[1]

Economy class syndrome results in patients travelling long distances for medical tourism, developing complications like pulmonary embolism, stroke or acute myocardial infarction due to thromboembolism as a result of prolonged immobilization and lack of leg space in economy class seating in flights.[1]

FOREIGN EXCHANGE TRANSACTIONS

Payments from patients should always be preferred in the digital mode. Any amount of payment taken shall automatically be converted by the bank or the credit card company to the local currency into the provider's account.

However, if the payments are received in cash, then the provider must ensure the deposition of the foreign currency in his account within the shortest possible banking working time and a proper documentation should be kept as to the reason for the payments received.

THE DARK SIDE OF MEDICAL TOURISM, REPRODUCTIVE TOURISM AND SURROGACY

Unmarried pregnant females travel for seeking secret abortion (away from their residential city). Married pregnant females also travel for getting abortion on tourist visa, after determination of gender of unborn child through ultrasound or deoxyribonucleic acid (DNA) study of embryo, which is illegal and considered a crime under Pre-Conception and Pre-Natal Diagnostic Techniques (PCPNDT) Act, 1994. But some use the legal loophole of getting aborted unwanted gender (female feticide) pregnancy under Medical Termination of Pregnancy (MTP) Act 1971, under social indication of unplanned pregnancy, which is unethical for the medical professionals to do, but still practiced to make easy money. Infertile couples are travelling to India on tourist visa and fertility clinics plan for their surrogacy by hiring and exploiting Indian female from financially poor family, in want of money. As surrogacy bill is still pending in Indian parliament, so this unethical practice is going on making quick money.[1]

ORGAN TRANSPLANT TOURISM

Indian kidney and liver patients are travelling abroad to Nepal, Sri Lanka, and China for undergoing organ transplant in exchange of hefty amount of money under medical tourism, as it is illegal in India to buy organs for transplant.[2]

SUICIDE TOURISM

Cancer patients on palliative care are seek active euthanasia to die by administering sedatives in fatal doses by doctors practicing euthanasia in few countries like Australia, Netherlands, etc, and travel on medical visa where its legally permitted, since its illegal in most of the countries including India.[3]

ETHICAL ISSUES IN ADVERTISING FOR MEDICAL TOURISM

Recently, it has been observed that many private hospitals and practicing surgeons are getting published about the patient's positive experiences and feedbacks about their surgery by patients themselves, by ghost writing patient's biographies in formats of books and posts in newspapers in the patient's or their kin's name, for getting indirect publicity and advertisement at international level, by distributing the books/articles to future patients. Because direct advertising for medical services are considered unethical conduct under medical council rules and regulations.

DEALING WITH MORTALITY OF FOREIGNER PATIENT IN HOSPITAL DURING TREATMENT

This section deals with the most unfortunate part of the chapter, but a true possibility that the health provider should be prepared for. Information shall need to be given immediately to the next of kin, the embassy of the patient's parent country, the local police, the Chief Medical Officer, and the District Magistrate. The service provider should be ethically and morally prepared to bear any expenses that the state shall not bear but that may ensue, right up to transportation to the parent address.

CONCLUSION

The plastic surgeon must be careful when using patient information or photography in a commercial way, such as on a website, advertisement or patient outcome booklet, shown to prospective patients for promoting medical tourism. A breach of privacy is not covered by your malpractice insurance and any judgments as a result of this breach must come from you alone and not your insurance company.

REFERENCES

1. Tiwari S. Medical tourism. Textbook on Medicolegal Issues: Related to Various Medical Specialties, 2nd edition. New Delhi: Jaypee Brothers Medical Publishers (P) Ltd.; 2018. pp. 489-93.
2. Nundy S, Desiraju K, Nagral S. Healers or Predators: Healthcare Corruption in India, 1st edition; 2018. Oxford, United Kingdom: Oxford University Press.
3. Menon M, Gopalakrishnan B, Ray K, et al. Legal Aspects of Healthcare and Hospital Administration, 1st edition. London, United Kingdom: Bloomsbury Publishing; 2016. pp. 227-40.
4. BBC. (2017). India hospital builds new unit to operate on '500kg' Egyptian woman. [online] Available from https://www.bbc.com/news/world-asia-india-38594559 [Accessed December 2018].
5. BBC. (2017). '500kg' Egyptian woman's sister accuses Indian doctors of lying. [online] Available from https://www.bbc.com/news/world-asia-india-39702373 [Accessed December 2018].

CHAPTER 46

Delivering Bad News after Plastic Surgery

Medha A Bhave (Khair)

KEY OBJECTIVES

- What is bad news?
- Why is way of breaking bad news important?
- What is unique about bad news in plastic surgery?
- How does it affect healthcare delivery?
  - Patient reaction and effect on further treatment
  - Effect on doctors.
- Why is training essential? Summary of training methods.
- What are the protocols?
  - SPIKES
  - McPhee
  - BREAKS
  - ABCDE
- Epilog
- Pitfalls: Do's and don'ts
- Appendix—The Indian Plastic Surgeons Survey:
  - Questionnaire
  - Analysis

WHAT IS BAD NEWS?

Bad news in medical field was defined by Dr Buckman, a Canadian Oncologist in 1984.[1]

He defines bad news as any news that adversely and seriously affects the patient's perspective of future, i.e. news that drastically and negatively alters his/her view of his or her future.[2]

Ptatek in 1996 provides more comprehensive definition as follows—Bad news is defined as one which is pertaining to situation where there is a feeling of no hope, a threat to a person's mental or physical wellbeing, a risk of upsetting an established lifestyle or where a message is given which conveys to an individual fewer choices in life.[3]

In the current days of enhanced patient awareness and sensitivity and particularly in cosmetic practice, the definition of bad news can be expanded to include: any side effect, complication, or inadequate result or extended hospital stay or even increased hospital costs.

The medical field has traditionally concentrated on improving clinical and technological skills. In older days, whether to deliver bad news to the patient and/or relatives used to be the prerogative of the treating doctor. Over last few decades, the changing equations of doctor–patient relationship, patients' human rights, Right to privacy and decision-making, and Consumer Protection Act have shifted the paradigm. Addition of good communication skills to core competence requirements of graduate accreditation program in first world countries is enough indication of its importance.[4]

Figure 1—core skills needed for graduate program.

Nevertheless, emphasis on how to deliver bad news is still missing in curricula; except Oxford Graduate Training Program.[5]

WHY IS THE WAY OF BREAKING BAD NEWS IMPORTANT?

The way of bad news is delivered to the patient changes not only the patient's reaction and long-term adjustment to the news; it is also the most common cause of litigation and a spoiled doctor-patient relationship. Communication issues are a more common trigger in medical negligence suits rather than actual negligence.[6]

Communication issues do not necessarily mean lack of skill on doctor's side. Communication is two way tool. The receptors, i.e. the patient and kin; are equally important variables.

Badly delivered news can lead to:
- Altered perception by patient and family of outcome of the disease
- Increased probability of litigation due to inappropriate communication
- Deviation of further course of treatment from best possible scientific course in given situation—treatment or raising false hopes
- Increased stress on doctor.

Two eminently preventable disasters, namely negligence claims and wrong choice of further course of treatment can be avoided with use of strategic approach and training in delivery of bad news.

WHAT IS UNIQUE ABOUT BAD NEWS IN PLASTIC SURGERY?

Bad news in plastic and cosmetic surgery can be:
- An unexpected death—due to allergy, bleeding, embolism, etc.
- Common and uncommon surgical complications
- Patient's expectations not met with
- Prolonged postoperative course
- Unfavorable results that would need more tests, surgeries, and extra financial provisions.

Plastic and cosmetic surgery is unique in that except for trauma, most cases are elective with a predictable outcome. The surgeons are trained and geared for it. The patients may be conditioned by advertisements and media news and may be inclined to believe more in success and ignore the complications and failures, which have been explained during preoperative visits (differential listening). Preoperative counseling assumes paramount importance in assessing whether patient has realistic expectations and to ensure that all possible eventualities are conveyed to the patient. It is important to include patient's kin

	(Outcome)
IV.A.5.c).(8)	Participate in the education of patients, families, students, residents and other health professionals. (Outcome)
IV.A.5.d)	**Interpersonal and Communication Skills**
	Residents must demonstrate interpersonal and communication skills that result in the effective exchange of information and collaboration with patients, their families, and health professionals. (Outcome)
	Residents are expected to:
IV.A.5.d).(1)	Communicate effectively with patients, families, and the public, as appropriate, across a broad range of socioeconomic and cultural backgrounds; (Outcome)
IV.A.5.d).(2)	Communicate effectively with physicians, other health professionals, and health related agencies; (Outcome)
IV.A.5.d).(3)	Work effectively as a member or leader of a health care team or other professional group; (Outcome)
IV.A.5.d).(4)	Act in a consultative role to other physicians and health professionals; and, (Outcome)
IV.A.5.d).(5)	Maintain comprehensive, timely, and legible medical records, if applicable. (Outcome)
IV.A.5.e)	**Professionalism**
	Residents must demonstrate a commitment to carrying out professional responsibilities and an adherence to ethical principles. (Outcome)
	Residents are expected to demonstrate:
IV.A.5.e).(1)	Compassion, integrity, and respect for others; (Outcome)
IV.A.5.e).(2)	Responsiveness to patient needs that supersedes self-interest; (Outcome)
IV.A.5.e).(3)	Respect for patient privacy and autonomy; (Outcome)
IV.A.5.e).(4)	Accountability to patients, society and the profession; and, (Outcome)
IV.A.5.e).(5)	Sensitivity and responsiveness to a diverse patient population, including but not limited to diversity in

Fig. 1: Accreditation program.

in this session as they may be the ones to face the bad news before the patient. Often, such counseling may have been done on email as patients move to another city or even country for surgery. The patient may even decide to get operated while on tour in another town. Thus, the relatives may not be aware of the facts mentioned during counseling. Sometimes, new kin hitherto totally unaware may suddenly take over responsibilities. It thus makes sense to record the details of the kin during counseling. Even in medical tourism patients, it is very important to confirm presence of legitimate kin or at least contact with one.

According to American Consent requirements,[7,8] various available alternatives need to be conveyed as well. Documentation of all these aspects amounts to informed consent, in the language that the patient understands. The documentation plays a very important role as usually patients may not remember or understand everything that was said. Standard consent formats should be created by associations to protect their members in a court of law as this establishes a peer practice. The consent should include all complications with their incidence as well as alternatives to the procedure. This is in interest of the patient ultimately by allowing them to take informed decision after considering available options. It helps doctors by eliminating inhibition in mentioning dreadful but uncommon complications that would dissuade a needy patient. A good example would be blepharoplasty where most of colleagues would shudder to mention blindness in the list of possible complications unless it is an integral part of every practitioner's standard format. Even patients would be desensitized then.

HOW DOES DELIVERY OF BAD NEWS AFFECT THE HEALTHCARE DELIVERY?

Patient Reaction and Effect on Further Treatment

In India, kin are important factors in affecting patient's reaction to any news—good or bad. Related and unrelated kin constitute a mob, which has a completely different psyche and reaction. Increasing attacks on doctors bear enough testimony to this. There is no doubt that any negative outcome has immense repercussions on patient's life and future. At the same time, both the patient and doctor tend to forget that the doctor is not the *cause* for the original malady even in cases of negligence.[1] 90% doctors are absolved by courts;[9] which speaks volumes about need to handle communications rationally and effectively.

It is natural for the patient to go through response of denial, anger, shock, disbelief, despair, anxiety. They often forget what was said during preoperative counseling. This peak of emotion is difficult for the doctor to handle unless he/she is trained specifically for it. The doctor's peak of stress is when the incident occurs.[10] It is over much before the patient's, which may lead the patient to feel a lack of empathy. The patient in distress will try to identify a target to blame. The doctor who has been authoritatively dictating investigations, treatment, and surgery so far is easily available as ready "cause" of what has been happening. The patient quickly forgets that the origin of his ailment was not the fault of the doctor. The doctor was merely fighting the ailment along with him.[1]

Effect on Doctors

Little attention has been given to effects on surgeon; as it has been given to all aspects of patient's care. Primary focus being patient, the stress on the surgeon has been always underestimated. Equal importance should be given to latter because at the end of the day, the outcome and patient treatment would suffer at the hands of a stressed and psychologically burdened surgeon.

According to Survey of Speech-Language Pathologists in Israel, the doctor suffers lot of negative emotions while breaking bad news.[11]

The spectrum of negative emotions suffered by surgeon has been studied by Tesser et al. in various experiments.[12]

They showed that deliverer of bad news feels the burden of responsibility and is worried about negative evaluation; which brings on reluctance to carry out the task. This was coined as MUM effect. It is a challenge for the surgeon to be honest and still not shatter the patient's hopes. Even though most of the doctors in his survey had no problem in finding time for the patient, dealing with their emotions was a major stress factor.

Fears of the surgeon:[1,10,13]

- Being blamed:
  - Fear of litigation
  - Fear of being manhandled
  - Peer reaction
  - Defamation
- Not knowing answers to all queries of relatives
- Fears of facing negative emotional outbreak
- Personal fear of dealing with illness, death, litigation, expressing own emotions
- Fears of unknown and untaught—shame/guilt.[14]

It is interesting to note that doctors are trained to maintain a cool and composed image and hide emotions while discharging their duty. In the novel "The Cry and the Covenant", the protagonist, Dr Ignaz Philip Semmelweiss, is a medical student who gets attached to the babies he is supposed to treat. His teacher asks him to consider patient's disease in scientific spirit and overcome emotions—lest the overflow of emotion may ruin his judgment. Paradoxically, this very attitude may also lead to impression of lack of empathy.

WHY IS TRAINING ESSENTIAL? SUMMARY OF TRAINING METHODS[2,15]

Importance of training cannot be overemphasized in current scenario of compromised doctor-patient relationship, litigation, and violence. Many a times, the operations in plastic surgery are vulnerable for malpractice suits because patient's expectations were not met with rather than due to genuine medical negligence.[10] Communication skills can turn the winds in favor of a genuine plastic surgeon. Lack of the same can tip the balance toward litigation with long, tenacious course, consuming better part of one's professional as well as private life, in the Indian legal system. Proper training can help to reduce stress and emotional burden on the surgeon to large extent and improve patient's satisfaction.

All over the world, the need for training in communication skills has been recognized only recently. In developed countries, communication skill is considered essential core competence in graduate accreditation program. Still, delivery of bad news is not particularly included as a training module. The untrained surgeon not only alters the patient's psychological balance but suffers him/herself. Thus, special training can potentially benefit both—surgeon and the patient.

Various training modules have been described depending on level of experience of the doctor seeking the training.

- Classroom lectures do not require excessive faculty time and can deliver the concepts to large number of trainees at different level and type of experience. But there is no assessment of individual skill, improvement in the level after the session and eliminations of personal errors.

Small group discussions with role play are very useful especially in recognizing error patterns and corrective measures but are demanding on the faculty time. Training and updating of faculty is mandatory back end for such programs.
- Interactive lectures with trigger videotapes showing example situations may provide best of both worlds but fail to recognize inefficient ways of interaction. Peer role play with doctor entering patient's role, use of multiple scenarios to broaden the experience, self-rating before and after the course improve the affectivity of interactive lectures.

The points of learning are:
- Timing of delivery of bad news
- Rate of delivery—abrupt, gradual or very slow, and graduated
- Choice of words and emotions by the doctor
- Handling patient's reaction
- Creating positive outlook
- Closing the encounter appropriately with tentative outline of remedial measures.

WHAT ARE THE PROTOCOLS FOR BREAKING BAD NEWS?

Various protocols have been described to deliver bad news effectively.
1. **SPIKES**[2]
   SPIKES is perhaps the best known and well-studied protocol; with respect to its affectivity.[2,14] Outlined by Baile and Buckman, the protocol was originally designed for oncology patients but has found application in many clinical fields. The premise of the protocol is that perception of bad news is discrepancy between patients' expectations and the medical reality. The detailed description is out of scope of this chapter, but salient points as adapted to plastic surgery by the author would go as follows:
   - *S—Setting*: Privacy—close door, minimize distraction, sit down directly in front of patient/kin without barriers, look calm but receptive, keep eye contact, allow touch if needed, listen, repeat as much as needed. Questions to bring out and acknowledge patient's emotions.
   - *P—Perception*: Usually patients forget the preoperative counseling and enter denial mode. This is natural mechanism to cope with the stress. Do not focus too much on it in eagerness to get rid of "blame". Initial target is inevitably the doctor as he/she is seen in the driver's seat. Note patient's language and reaction. A verbal duel at this stage can land you in an antagonistic relationship with the patient or increase his/her anxiety and stress excessively.
   - *I—Invitation*: Ask patient how much he would like to know details of the problems. Some patients/relatives are interested in detail, like to see the wound or flap. Others may decline and leave everything to you. You can document the patient's decision. Further sessions should keep this choice open every time. Most like to see an improvement when it takes place. You should warn the relative that he/she must walk out if feels giddy. It is useful to have help handy to take care of collapsing relatives lest they incur injury—to add fuel to fire on hand. Privacy issues must be respected.
   - *K—Knowledge*: Warn the patient in language the patient understands about the bad news. It gives them time to prepare for the same and eases

your task. For example—"Mrs XY, there is some problem in the expected outcome". Provide information in nontechnical language—in small chunks. Intersperse sentences like—"Did you get that?", "are you on same page as me?" This will help you alter the rate of delivery according to the response you get. Acknowledge patient's reaction and emotions with a little pat on the back or a brief hand holding.

- *E—Empathy*: Too much empathy deters truthful delivery of all the information. You have been identifying and addressing patient's emotions. Now find out their source. For example—is financial consideration bothering him the most or the protracted course would be interruption in some major errand like parent or child care expected of the patient? Show that you realize nonclinical implications of the situation that would adversely affect the patient. For example—"you need to take antibiotics and rest longer than expected. It might be problem at home, but you need to arrange help". Adding—"I completely understand how you feel" will validate emotions of a patient who needs amputation in face of failed salvage.

How to explain complications/ perception of lack of results—with specific examples?

It is very common to see a cosmetic surgery patient dissatisfied with initial result as edema is yet to subside or scars are visible. It is better to begin with scientific truth that each body is different. Tell that the books also mention initial dissatisfaction in many patients but this invariably resolves and improves with time. Remind the patient of preoperative counseling and assure that final result will improve to some extent at least. This way the doctor prepares the patient for less than optimum outcome. Massage and physiotherapy work on body as well as mind. Most important gesture is being available, answerable, and non-evasive. If the outcome is indeed not desirable, it is better to admit that the result was not desirable despite full efforts. One can recruit help from capable seniors. It is important not to have played god beforehand and empathize with the patient. Most normal patients do understand human limitations. For those who are willful aggressors, legal help, second opinion from senior must be sought without delay. A good indemnity insurance helps as they provide legal help and timely out of court settlement when indicated.

- *S—Strategy and summary*: Present a short review with clear action plan at the end. Allow patient to voice concerns. Ensure availability. Document!! Use videos, proformas, and special hand-written communications. Obtain patient's signatures as proof of receipt. Effectivity of training in SPIKES protocol has been well-studied and documented.[15]

The others like Fine, Breaks, McPhee are based on similar premise with a few added points.[13,15,16]

2. **ABCDE**
   - *A—Advance preparation*
     - Find out what patient and relatives already know
     - Find private, quiet place without disturbance

- Doctor's own preparation—emotions and choice of words.
- B—*Building therapeutic relationship and environment*
    - Sit down and seat everyone
    - Do not take pages and phone calls
    - Appropriate touching the patient or relative
    - Adequate reassurance and detailed discussion of options.
- C—*Communicate well*
    - Be direct
    - Avoid medical jargon and short forms
    - Allow time for information to percolate in.
- D—*Deal with patient and family reactions*
    - Listen to the patient
    - Find out intermittently how much and what they are understanding.
- E—*Encourage and validate emotions, evaluate the news*
    - Address further needs of the patient
    - What are the patient's immediate and long-term plans?
    - Appropriate medical referrals, opinions, and social help as needed.

3. **BREAKS**[16]
    - B—*Background*: Beware of Google-habituated relatives. Keep all data and expected questions in mind.
    - R—*Rapport*: A good rapport with positive regard but avoid patronizing.
    - E—*Exploring*: With good preoperative counseling, much exploring of patient understanding is not needed. One need not "burst a bomb"; rather, merely recall the already discussed possible negative outcome and confirm the same.
    - A—*Announce*: At the first opportunity when the disaster is imminent. When flap or replanted finger has sluggish circulation—do not hide it. Include patient and relatives in progress so that when the gangrene sets in, patient and relatives are nearly prepared for it.
    - K—*Kindling*: Allow the patient to react in own way—be it silence, tears, or retraction. Make sure later that patient has listened to you and understood. Interruption like—"Are we on the same page"? Help. Patient should clearly understand the complications, the gravity and proposed realistic treatment. False hope should not be raised by giving unrealistic options.
    - S—*Summarize*: The situation, treatment options should be presented in a nutshell at the end of the session. Written summary is legally safe and available to the patient to go over again later; after overcoming first outburst of emotions. Availability of consultant in case of need, assurance that care is being taken and finding out the kin with whom the patient is sharing the news are important aspects. Assessment of psychological status to ensure that patient does not develop suicidal tendency is significant consideration in summarizing.

Few common scenarios:
- How to handle aggressive patients who make direct accusations? E.g. How could you do this?
You did not take care, otherwise this would not have happened.
You have not used the right technique.
We want another opinion.
In all the above situations, a second opinion is priceless. Senior colleagues need to be trained in how to give a balanced second opinion to limit damage. Most importantly, one must review one's qualification and

experience before undertaking any surgery. Unfortunately, training in India is not uniform, the practice rights are not defined according to qualifications. Those who are not trained in surgical operations and conduct in operation theater in correct discipline undertake major surgeries presuming that one is guilty only if caught. They should always keep in mind the legal risk they are taking and should not expect fellow qualified colleagues to save them in case of mishap.

How to break bad news when negligence has indeed happened?
When negligence has happened, it is most important to seek legal help. The definition of negligence is breach in "average" care. Best policy in such situations is by containing the damage. Aim should be to prevent mob violence in order to protect already admitted patients. The author has seen that nothing less than police and political intervention can save the situation. Usually medical professionals undermine the role of local leaders but they have their hand on the pulse of the mob. It is best policy to identify a reasonable group leader, explain to him first and then take the situation ahead. Help from colleagues can be a double-edged sword. If the colleagues are trained in legal aspects, they can alleviate the situation while careless comments from casual colleagues can escalate the matter.

A specific mention of instances of what has happened earlier:
For example, a patient who sustained a burn on her legs, because electrocautery plate or hot-water bottle was not shielded properly by the nurse.

In such a situation, it is better to own up, show that action is being taken against the nurse. It is important to call an expert and treat the burns as clinically indicated. Hospitals should cooperate as far as charges are concerned. Hospitals should take indemnity insurance for all the employees with extra premium for untrained ones. It is important to have all machines under maintenance contract in writing and regular service must be documented.

A patient who sustained an arrhythmia due to nurse mixing wrong amount of xylocaine in tumescent solution for liposuction:
In this situation, you need to call on an expert in the field, a Cardiologist and find out whether the arrhythmia was indeed due to xylocaine. If yes, you need to write appropriate notes and get legal and police help to contain the damage.

The recent example of a large private hospital in Delhi when an extremely premature baby (the fetus at 18 weeks) upon delivery was declared dead and was handed over to the kin. A few moments later, after the family left to dispose of what they believed was the dead body, the neonate was found to be moving body parts, which caused a furore. What should they have done differently?

The above tragedy was merely due to callous attitude and lack of empathy toward the family that lost the 18-week "baby" while the staff merely thought of it as "products of conception" for disposal. It should have been checked before handing over that the baby was actually dead. The relatives should have been explained that such premature babies never make it. The medical profession should not become a mechanical, assembly-line factory. Personalization of care and compassion must be extended to every patient irrespective of our own work load. The doctors should set an example of the same before the staff.

Video recording of these sessions:
This has been suggested but the author is not sure of the huge data management load that would fall on the short-staffed medical field. It may be useful to identify potential problems and selectively record videos with prior intimation to the patient.

EPILOG

Plastic surgery has been philosophized by many legendary surgeons. Indian philosophy has some golden advice for every mortal human, which is perfectly applicable to all practicing doctors. The mentality of "non-doer ship" would not only protect from damage due to failure of a case but also will prevent mishaps due to overconfidence of success. This concept of non-doer ship—as explained in Gita—means detachment from effects of action while putting in 100% effort in the action—should reflect in all conversations with the patient and relatives right from preoperative counseling. This would help surgeons be realistically truthful to patients instead of trying to convince him/her for surgery. Surgeon's emotional damage in case of a mishap can thus be minimized. A patient-centric balanced approach to guide the patient on best possible path with patient's consent can then be adopted.

PITFALLS: DO'S AND DON'TS

Do's:
1. Ask before you tell
2. Deliver information at first opportunity—counseling is the best time
3. Document consent with—treating physician as primary counselor:
   a. All complications and risks divulged—general and specific
   b. Alternative options given and understood by patient
   c. Full document in language that patient understands
4. Provide ample time and more sessions as needed
5. Select quiet place
6. Be seated and comfortable yourself
7. Ensure privacy and full attention. Listen to the patient
8. Involve kin as per wish of the patient
9. Be forthcoming and honest. Remember you are not cause of patient's malady to start with
10. Use simple language
11. Understand patient's perspective, nonverbal communication such as tears, silence, and aggression
12. Show enough empathy, essential eye and hand contact help
13. Create positive outlook
14. Encourage second opinions and seek help of relevant specialties
15. Video record consent and counseling sessions
16. Summarize with documentation and signatures. Assess the patient's understanding at the end. Assure availability
17. Address financial issues and arrange help legitimately

Most of common bad news for patient improves with time in plastic surgery. Patients just forget this part of counseling.

Don'ts:
1. Delay or delegate delivery of bad news
2. Allow external disturbance with mobile, pagers, etc.
3. Use scientific jargon or lay analogies
4. Shatter hope and create false hope
5. Hide or suitably modify truth
6. Appear callous and unconcerned as well as trying to brush off blame
7. Shower excessive positive or negative emotions
8. Get emotionally involved, be critical or judgmental
9. Ignore patient's wishes and choice
10. Forget to inform your lawyer immediately
11. Dismiss plea for more visits, more explanation, and more kin joining in
12. Gossip in public places with other colleagues
13. Provide direct financial help as it may be seen as admission of guilt in the court of law

Failure of full disclosure and documentation is seen as negligent, unethical, and improper behavior.

APPENDIX—INDIAN PLASTIC SURGEON SURVEY: QUESTIONNAIRE ANALYSIS

Questionnaire

1. Describe the type of your practice.
   (a) Private—small and medium set-ups   (b) Corporate
   (c) Government
2. How many years have you been working?

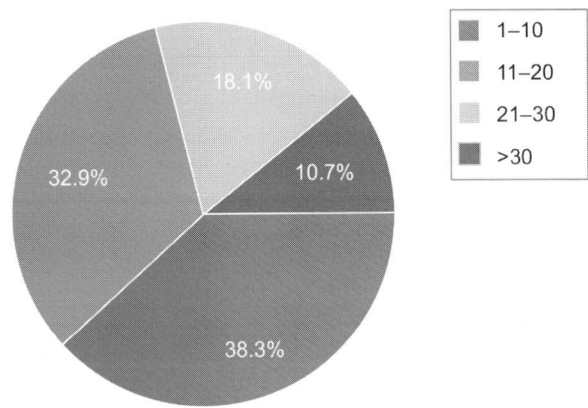

   (a) 1–10   (b) 10–20
   (c) 21–30   (d) More than 30
3. Which of the following best describes the type of patients you have?

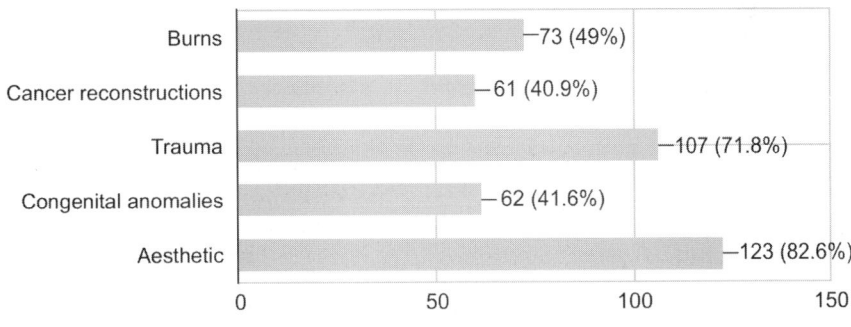

   (a) Burns   (b) Cancer reconstructions
   (c) Trauma   (d) Congenital anomalies
   (e) Aesthetic   (f) Mixed

4. Do you have "SOP" (standard operating procedure) for various procedures?

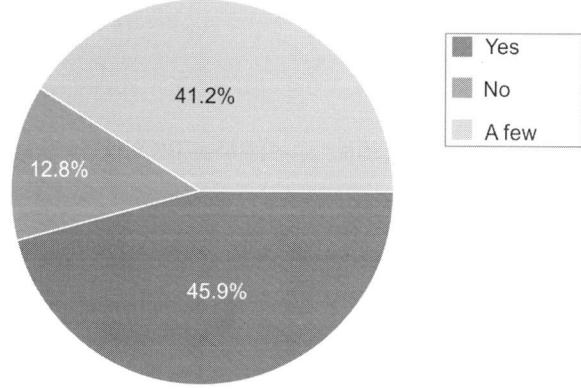

Yes/No for some

5. Do you use website to counsel the patient?

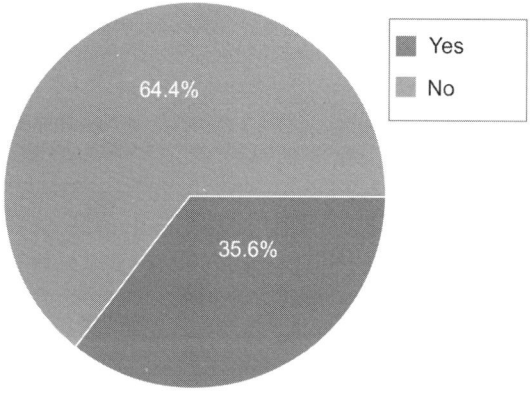

Yes/No

6. Do you use brochures to counsel?

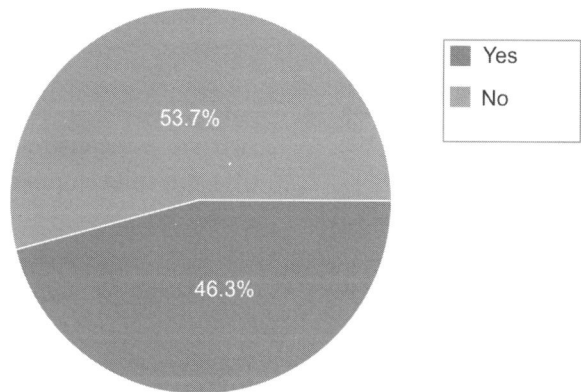

Yes/No

7. Do brochures and website mention possible complications of surgery?

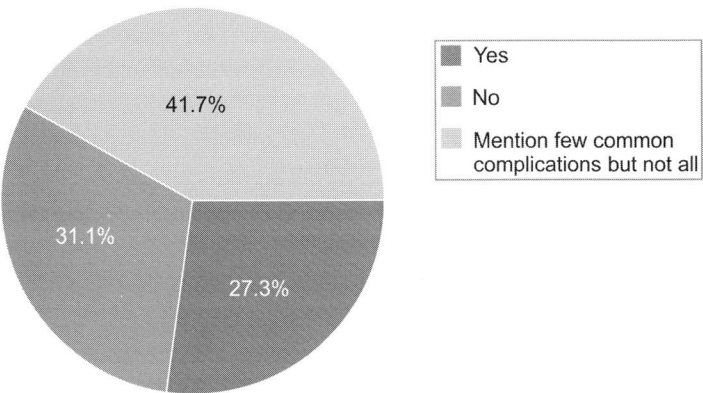

Yes/No/Mention few common complications but not all

8. Do you explain all possible complications and expected outcome to the patient and family?

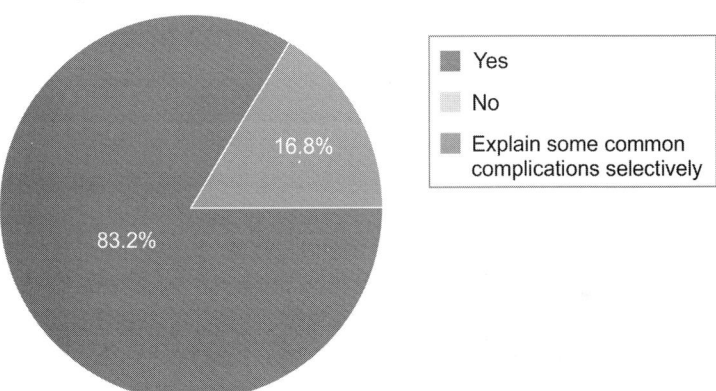

9. Do you use language that patient understands for documentation of counseling and consent?

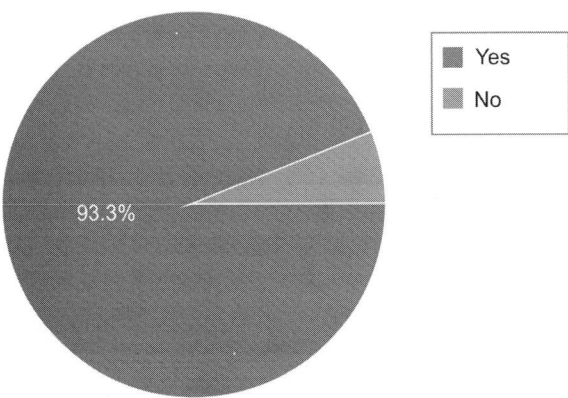

10. Will you refuse to operate a patient coming without a kin for surgery under local anesthesia/general anesthesia (LA/GA)?

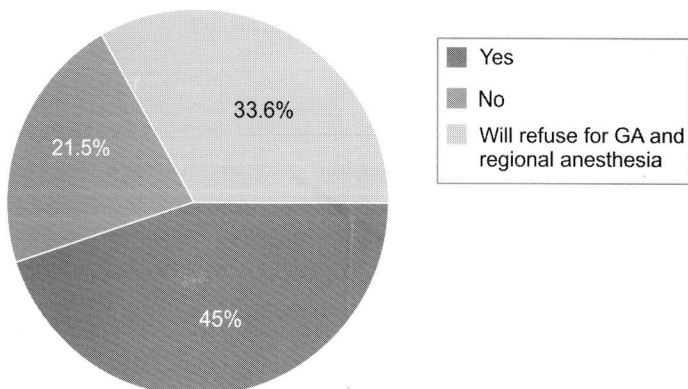

Yes/No/Will refuse for GA and regional anesthesia

11. How many times a year do you have to break bad news after surgery?

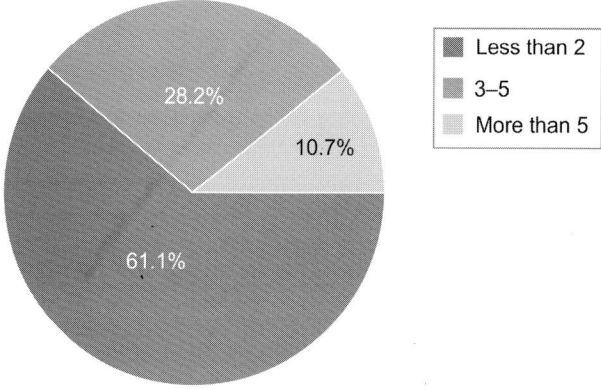

(a) Less than 2
(b) 3–5
(c) More than 5

12. Which of the following fears do you experience while breaking a bad news?
    (a) Possibility of being blamed
    (b) Fear of litigation
    (c) Shame/guilt
    (d) Fear of being manhandled
    (e) Peer reaction
    (f) Defamation

13. Do you give adequate time for the patient and relatives to discuss after delivery of bad news?

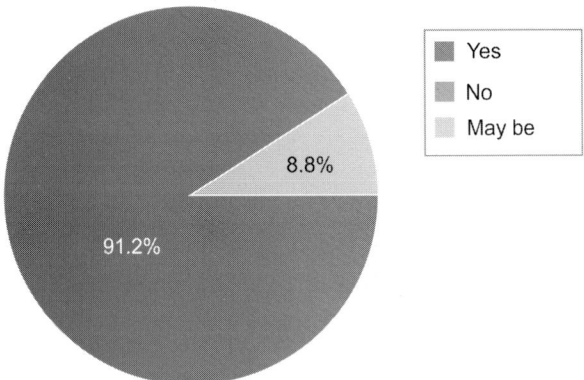

Yes/No/May be

14. Do you allow a second consultation a while later with new set of kin?

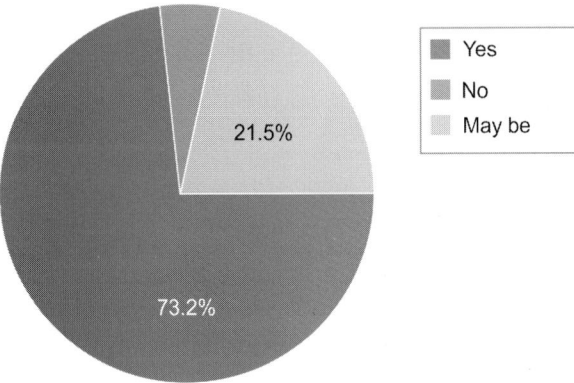

Yes/No/May be

15. Which of the following is the biggest challenge for you?

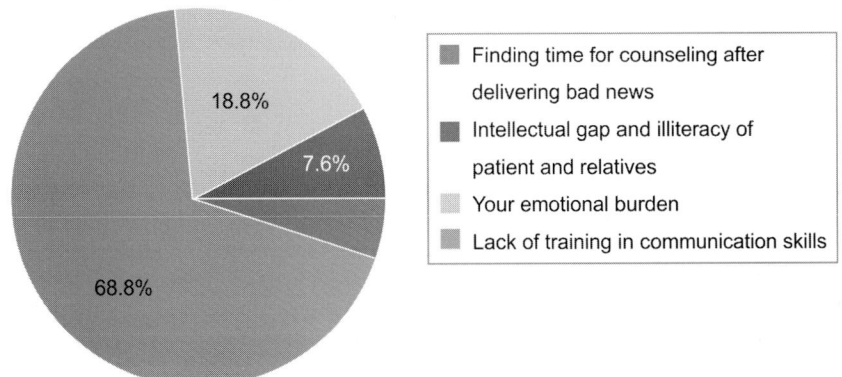

(a) Finding time for counseling after delivering bad news
(b) Intellectual gap and illiteracy of patient and relatives
(c) Your emotional burden
(d) Lack of training in communication skills

16. Do you think communication training would help?

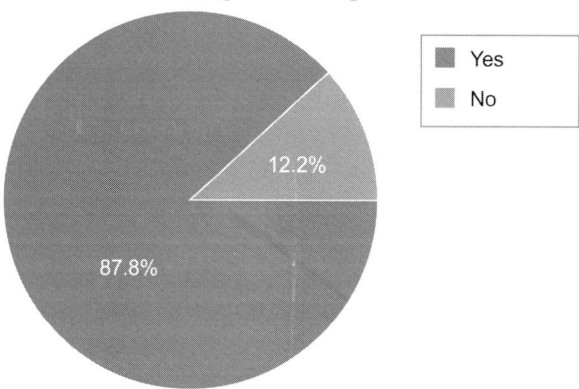

Yes/No

17. Are you aware of international protocols and training modules?

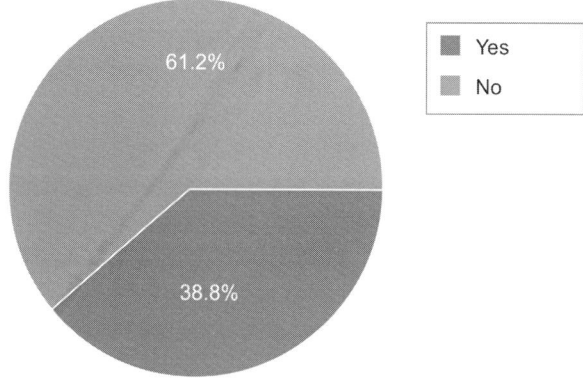

(Do not Google now ☒)—Yes/No

18. Please share your strategy in short if any in tackling a situation when bad news has to be delivered.
19. Will you provide monitory help to patient?

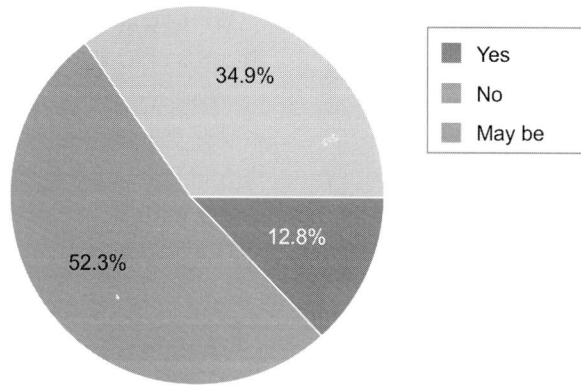

Yes/No/Sometimes

20. How important is it to show empathy to patients?

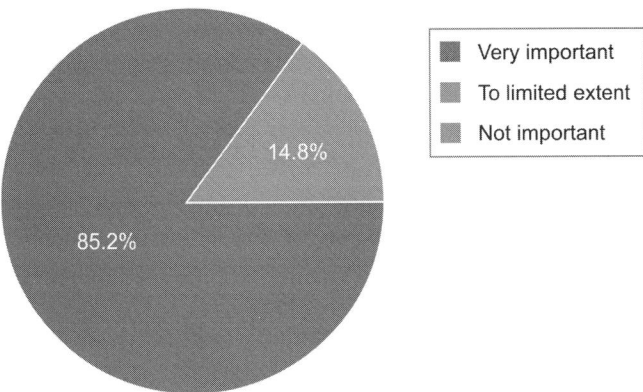

Very important/To limited extent/Not important

Summary of Survey

This is summary of strategies used by Indian Plastic Surgeons, not in particular order of priority.

- Take second opinion
- Compassion
- Patience
- Referring back to the original consultation sheet and pointing out possible complications that were mentioned in pre-operative counseling session
- Honesty
- Good communication
- Point out that best of precautions had been taken
- Offer correction at concessional rate, explain problem in stages to prepare ground for acceptance of bad news
- Recording communication and consent on video
- Explain to patient and close relative only. Respect privacy of the patient
- Have colleagues with you
- Inform police in advance
- Call upon a doctor known to the patient
- Confidence needed. Do not have guilty feeling
- Empathy
- Being available physically and/or phone
- Explain that biology cannot be predicted
- Frank explanation
- Do not delay
- Eye contact
- Prayer
- Record keeping/precise preoperative counseling and consent
- Meet relatives daily, address by name focus on the meeting without distractions
- All doctors to meet the relatives together (Differences in opinion, some would be blunt while some prefer to break the news gradually)

Author's comment: The Indian doctors manage the situations intuitively based on their day-to-day experiences and have understanding about slat of the recipe to handle such events. An indigenous program that channelizes these perceptions is needed to consolidate and validate the strategies.

REFERENCES

1. Breaking bad news: why is it still so difficult? Robert Buckman Br Med J (Clin Res Ed) 1984;288:1597.
2. SPIKES—A Six-Step Protocol for Delivering Bad News: Application to the Patient with Cancer Walter F. Baile, Robert Buckman, Renato Lenzi, Gary Glober, Estela A Beale, Andrzej P Kudelka. The Oncologist August 2000 vol. 5 no. 4 302-311. doi: 10.1634/theoncologist. 5-4-302.
3. Ptacek JT, Eberhardt TL. Breaking bad news. A review of the literature. JAMA 1996;276:496-502.
4. http://www.acgme.org/Portals/0/PFAssets/ProgramRequirements/360_plastic_surgery_2017-07-01.pdf?ver=2017-08.
5. http://www.oxfordmedicaleducation.com/palliative-care/breaking-bad-news/.
6. Am association of ophthalm https://www.aao.org/eyenet/young-ophthalmologist/tips-delivering-bad-news.
7. http://advrohiterande.blogpot.com/2017/07/why-informed-consent-is-of-utmost.html.
8. https://bmj.com/content/350/bmj.h1796/rr-0 BMJ 2015;350 Letter New UK law on consent https://doi.org/10.1136/bmj.h1796---7/apr/2015.
9. https;//www.hindustantimes.com/the-wait-never-ends-complaints-of-medical-negligence-increase-but-justice-eludes-victims/story-eFDpT6vKYQSVhN0ovgCUBN.html.
10. Dealing with bad outcomes in aesthetic surgery,Delivering bad news. Alberto Rancati, M.D. Feb 25, 2010 https://www.researchgate.net/publication/293958987.
11. Delivering Bad News: Attitudes, Feelings, and Practice Characteristics Among Speech-Language Pathologists. Gold R1, Gold A2. Am J Speech Lang Pathol. 2018 Feb 6;27(1):108-122. doi: 10.1044/2017_AJSLP-17-0045.
12. On the reluctance to communicate undesirable messages (the MUM effect). A field study. Tesser A, Rosen S, Tesser M. Psychol Rep 1971;29:651-4.
13. Breaking bad news in clinical setting: a systematic review. Dr Madhav Madhusudan Singh,Dr Rajiv Kumar Agarwal, Indian Journal of Applied Research, Volume-7 | Issue-12 | December-2017 | ISSN - 2249-555X | IF : 4.894 | IC Value : 86.18.
14. Delivering bad news to patients. Kimberley R. Monden, PhD, Lonnie Gentry, MTh, and Thomas R. Cox, PsyD. Baylor University Medical Center Proceedings Volume 29, Number 1.
15. Teaching Medical Students and Residents Skills for Delivering Bad News: A Review of Strategies. Marcy E. Rosenbaum, PhD, Kristi J. Ferguson, PhD, and Jeffrey G. Lobas, MD academic medicine, vol. 79, no. 2/February 2004.
16. BREAKS' Protocol for Breaking Bad News Vijayakumar Narayanan, Bibek Bista, Cheriyan Koshy DOI: 10.4103/0973-1075.68401 www.jpalliativecare.com.

CHAPTER 47

Photography and the Issue of Patient Confidentiality

Mukund Jagannathan, Amarnath Munoli

INTRODUCTION

A picture is worth a thousand words. Nowhere is it more applicable than the specialty of plastic surgery. Ours is a very "visual" specialty where seeing is believing. Without going into issues of image manipulation and honesty in reporting results, this chapter attempts to discuss certain vital aspects of patient confidentiality with respect to use of clinical photographs for medical reporting, presentations, and publishing (both in print and social media platforms). The issue of revealing of identity is also interwoven with this.

INFORMED CONSENT FOR CLINICAL PHOTOGRAPHY

All patients have the right to take well-informed and voluntary decisions regarding their own health and any planned interventions—surgical or otherwise. This necessitates a full and frank discussion about possible lines of treatment and their outcomes, adverse effects, and dangers. The integral role of photographs in this process cannot be underestimated; suffice it to say, it is absolutely vital in plastic surgery.

However, this asks a very important question. What are the photos for? To begin with, they serve as a common medium for real time discussion, one on one (or through emails, etc.) with patients regarding specific "deformities" (lumps and bumps) they might perceive and possible corrective options. They also reveal nuances not immediately observable to the naked eye, but which need to be documented and pointed out to the patients nonetheless, before any planned intervention. They serve as an integral part of patient records, which is mandatory. Comparing before and after images provides to some extent, an objective measure of therapeutic efficacy in an otherwise highly subjective patient population and helps temporal evaluation of scars and longevity of surgical results.

Let us now turn to the less discussed role of clinical photographs, other than the primary objectives already mentioned. Photographs can serve as discussion points for several purposes.
- As part of medical presentations which can include presentations in closed forums or publication in an open forum.
- Use in social media and nonmedical forums, which basically means open to all for viewing.

The Hippocratic oath[1] mentions clearly, the right to confidentiality *"And whatsoever I shall see or hear in the course of my profession, as well as outside my profession in my intercourse with men, if it be what should not be published abroad, I will never divulge, holding such things to be holy secrets".* Were this to be followed literally, nobody would ever be able to display a single photograph! However, we accept the fact that medical reporting is vital and a part of continuing education. The issue at hand relates to the willingness/consent of patients to have their pictures revealed to persons other than the immediate circle of physicians responsible for their treatment.

There are also some unanswered questions. Does revealing of images of a "good" result carry more weight, if the person is a celebrity? Does it constitute a subtle or an overt form of advertising, irrespective of whether it is displayed in a medical forum or a social one? Unfortunately, it seems that the answer to both these questions is "yes".

The next related issue is the revealing of identity, whether by showing the face or some identifying mark like a tattoo or a birthmark. If we accept the fact that any display of images of a "celebrity" constitutes, at the very least, a subtle form of advertising, we have to first look at the law of the land. In several western countries, advertising is legal.

The American Society of Plastic Surgeons permits photographs to be used even on social media and has a separate consent form for this purpose. Dr Surajit Bhattacharya in his editorial[2] in the Indian Journal of Plastic Surgery clearly states the moral responsibilities of the physician regarding the storage and use of clinical photographs, whether or not identity is revealed.

However, apart from the moral and ethical dimensions, lawsuits regarding display of photos in the western world are mostly related to revealing of identity and not related to the quality of the results.[3,4] In our country, complaints regarding display of patient profile and identity are more related to the concept of "advertising", which as per the law of the land and is not permitted.[5]

ISSUES RELATED TO ETHICAL DISPLAY OF PHOTOGRAPHS[6-12]

We now come to the crux of the matter:
1. Should we have different guidelines for "celebrities" as opposed to the common man?
2. Is the issue of identity relevant, or merely a moral dimension?
3. Should we differentiate between medical and nonmedical forums for display of photographs?
4. How do we safeguard ourselves at the same time be fair to our patients?

Should we have different guidelines for "celebrities"?

Ethically the answer is "No". Practically speaking, one has to discriminate and play safe. People who are in the limelight may have different reasons for not wanting the public to know. As a matter of fact, a lot depends on the culture and attitudes of the people undergoing cosmetic surgery. In the West, many people

> **BOX 1:** Freedom of Expression versus Right to Confidentiality.
>
> *Case facts*: The daily mirror magazine published photograph of the actress leaving her meeting of narcotic anonymous, accompanied by article giving details about her treatment.
>
> *Plaintiff*: Actress patient sued the publisher and author for breach of confidentiality of the patient, by taking photograph and intruding privacy of the individual by publishing the story in magazine.
>
> *Defense*: We as media personnel, under right of media, to impart information to public. In public interest, Publisher published the photograph accompanied by article praising the actress's battle with her drug addiction, for public education. Actress has herself made various public statements to the effect that she (unlike many other models) did not take drugs, by doing so, patient had herself made her drug taking a public matter, and so no longer, confidential. Her statements created sufficient public interest to justify the press correcting the misleading impression she had created.
>
> *Decision*: UK Court found the publisher guilty for causing breach of confidence by taking photograph and intruding privacy of the individual by publishing the story in magazine. Someone receiving treatment for drug de-addiction would be confidential information. Even if patient has given video statement in media about drugs, but it does not mean that every aspect of her drug taking and treatment was now public information. The time, place, and form of drug therapy were still confidential. Judge emphasized the right to respect for private and family life under international convention of human rights. Protection of confidential information is about respecting the autonomy and dignity of individual. Recovering drug addict is in vulnerable position, needing all support she can get. The publication of information about her treatment was likely to distress her at what might a particularly vulnerable time. There was little public interest in the story and therefore the right of privacy trumped the right of freedom of expression.
>
> *Result*: Actress patient won monetary compensation of 2,500 pounds damages plus 1,000 pounds for aggravated damages from the publisher and author of story.[7]

accept that aesthetic surgery, especially for aging is inevitable and therefore necessary. It is assumed that people, aespecially women, have undergone some aesthetic procedure by the time they are in their 40s. Not so in several other countries and populations. For these people, it is a highly confidential process, and they would be loath to having it being discussed in a public forum, even an academic one (Box 1).

There is one more issue, when posting pictures of celebrities (on public forums especially). The common man may not realize that most screen celebrities are fairly good looking to begin with, and may have undergone a minor facial procedure, for example. The lay public then firmly believes that the celebrity's good looks are solely because of surgery, which can cause a total misconception in their eyes.

To sum up, morally and ethically, there should be no difference in maintaining the confidentiality and privacy of all patients, irrespective of whether they are recognizable in the public domain or not. However, if it is public figure, the adverse implications can be far greater, as obvious in the above discussed case.

Is the issue of identity relevant, or merely a moral dimension?

There are some situations where the identity is clearly revealed:

- When it is a facial photograph, even if the eyes are "blacked out"
- When clearly visible tattoos, or birthmarks are present in the photo.

However, there is more to this. I am citing three examples.

Someone in the surgical room filmed a cesarean section[6] and shared the video on social media. There was no question of identity being revealed. However, the patient came to know and instituted legal proceedings against the doctor(s) who is/are responsible. Disciplinary action was taken against the concerned doctor.

An editor of a reputed Plastic Surgery Journal received a letter from a patient, stating that the patient's photograph was displayed in an article without expressed consent. Further investigation revealed the photograph in question was an extremely limited view of a particular deformity, with the rest of the areas cropped off. It is extremely unlikely that anyone would recognize the person from the photograph. The point was that the patient recognized it and that was enough. At the time of publication, it must have been assumed (erroneously) that since identity could not be established, it was permissible. The article had to be retracted.

Even if there are no identification marks, the nature of the deformity may be such that it may be recognizable by another physician who had been consulted for the same issue. There is scope for trouble to occur, especially if the patient or relative were to meet the other physician.

A colleague of mine had a patient who was a well-known actress, who consulted him for some facial procedures. When he explained the need for pre- and postoperative photographs, she consented, but made it clear that he would have to sign a legal undertaking never to display these photographs to anyone on any platform. She eventually did not get operated, but the point is moot.

In short, whether a photograph carries identifiable features or not, it is ethically and legally incumbent on the treating physician to ensure that the concerned patient has given his/her express consent for utilizing their pictures for the said purpose.

Should we differentiate between medical and nonmedical forums for display of photographs?

The display of photographs in a medical setting is ostensibly for the purpose of continuing medical education. However, there are some additional issues:
- Is the cross-section of delegates restricted to people from the same specialty?
- Can it be ensured that the display is not being recorded or photographed?
- The organizing committee has a key role in ensuring that the presentations are erased (ideally) after the event, and that no copies are made.
- Do the conference, organizers ensure that the presenters have taken express consent from their patients for the display of pictures?
- There is a trend to convert the proceedings of the conference into videos, which are then made available to members of the fraternity. Whether it is a commercial venture or not, the fact remains that these images are now no longer in the control of the primary surgeon. There is scope for misuse. To what extent is the onus of responsibility on the organizers? On the primary presenter? This can be argued endlessly. Even multiple consents may not protect the multiple parties involved.
- Medical books and journals are being increasingly accessed by patients and even by lawyers in their search for relevant data. Since in this case, the entire article and its contents including photographs become the exclusive property of the publishers, the onus of ensuring adequate consent falls in the purview of the editorial board. Ethical reporting demands that the authors be fully aware of their responsibilities.

Nonmedical forums include anything outside the purview of a closed conference. In short, anywhere in cyberspace. If patient images are used without detailed consent, it violates patient confidentiality and also serves as a means of advertising. The law of the land will prevail in these situations. While in our country, there is no specific legal provision governing the topic of clinical photography in particular, Clause 6.1 of the Indian Medical Council (Professional Conduct, Etiquette and Ethics) Regulations specifically deals with this issue: *"A physician shall not make use of his/her name as subject of any form or manner of advertising or publicity through any mode.... which is of such a character as to invite attention to him or to his professional position, skill, qualification, achievements, attainments, specialties, appointments, associations, affiliations or honors and/or of such character as would ordinarily result in his self-aggrandizement...... nor shall he boast of cases, operations, cures or remedies or permit the publication of report thereof through any mode."* This would indicate that any use of photographs for the purpose of soliciting patients or advertising, through any mode, constitutes unethical conduct. The Medical Council of India (MCI) and State Medical Councils have been empowered to adjudicate and prescribe appropriate penalties and disciplinary action in such cases.

All in all, use of patient photographs even in academic presentations for the furthering of medical knowledge should be subject to prior consent of the patient and with the caveat that these images be displayed with the utmost respect for privacy to avoid recirculation and misuse. The ultimate burden of responsibility may well fall on the treating physicians, since it is to them that the patients have entrusted their private information and records, including digital facsimiles. As far as nonmedical forums and advertising are concerned, the MCI guidelines make it pretty unambiguous: any form of advertising/self-promotion/soliciting of patients through any mode is unethical and needs to be discouraged.

How do we safeguard ourselves, at the same time be fair to our patients?
It should start with respecting the rights of patients. They have a right to confidentiality and privacy. This should not be compromised, except for very specific purposes, and that too with clear and informed consent taken.

Adhering to the precise tenets of the Hippocratic oath,[1] we would not even be able to discuss these cases! However, we accept that in the larger interests of medical education, and patient information, we need to be able to display patient photographs.

Keeping in mind all that has been discussed, the following are some recommendations for daily practice:
- At the start, it is best to recognize that patient confidentiality comes first, and that is the overwhelming consideration.
- It needs to be explained to the patient, that photographs are an essential requirement and part of the whole process. Notes can express only so much. Many fine points of symmetry and unevenness may be discernible only in photographs. Pre-existing miscellaneous deformities or lesions will be documented. For medicolegal purposes and protection too, they are a must.
- A special and informed consent must be taken, apart from the procedural consent, with respect to the use of the photographs. It must be emphasized that they can be used in medical forums, on public forums, and for journal publication. The patient should be given the option of denying the use of these photographs in any or all of these aspects, without affecting his/her treatment. Of course, photographic documentation is an absolute must, just that the images will not be displayed anywhere.

INTERMEDIARY LIABILITY OF MEDICAL FORUM/BOOK/JOURNAL EDITOR/PUBLISHER IN INDIA

Intermediaries, such as hosts, transitory communication systems, information location tools, etc., are widely recognized as essential cogs in the wheel of exercising the right to freedom of expression on the Internet. If the liability of an intermediary is not limited then an intermediary would be required to prescreen all content, which would render its services impractical or technically infeasible. Under the rules,[8] limitation of intermediary liability has been made contingent to a privately administered takedown mechanism. The intermediary, on whose computer system the information is stored or hosted or published, upon obtaining knowledge by itself or been brought to actual knowledge by an affected person in writing or through email signed with electronic signature about any such information, shall act within 36 hours and where applicable, work with user or owner of such information to disable such information that is offensive/obscene/vulgar.

- If consent is given only for use in medical forums, great efforts must be taken by the surgeon to prevent any unauthorized reproduction or use of these photographs. The conference organizers must also be made aware of this, and a request must be made to them in writing, and acknowledged. Needless to say, these may not be part of the conference proceedings, as a permanent record.
- Conference organizers must get in writing from the presenter, that all images which are being displayed have the specific consent of the patient(s). The organizers should ensure that the presentation is not surreptitiously recorded. A request can be made to the presenter to give handouts of important but nonphotographic material. The ethical standards must be as stringent as for publications.
- The conference organizers or other organizations may wish to use the proceeds of the meeting as educational videos. Whether there is a commercial interest or not, it is advisable to take consent from the presenter, who is the absolute owner of the video/presentation, that the required consent has been taken in writing from the patient. At the present moment, this is a relatively recent concept, and safeguards must be taken by all the concerned parties.
- If it is a facial photograph, the patient must be counseled that the identity will be revealed, and they must accept that. In body pictures, if there are any identifying signs, such as tattoos, scars, or birthmarks, again, the possibility of identity being revealed must be mentioned.
- Use on social media is a little controversial. It looks like a form of advertising or self-promotion. These may invite action from the regulating medical council, either state or national. However, if something noteworthy or laudable has been achieved, it makes infinite sense to have the patient put this up on his/her social media sites. Even the name of the concerned surgeon can be shared. This is safe, and may not invite any disciplinary action.
- Watermarking of images, which are going into any sort of public presentation, is a very good idea, thus ensuring that these images cannot be misused.
- In the event that some images have been uploaded without the knowledge or consent of the primary surgeon, cybercrime investigations may pinpoint the source of the material, and may go a long way in protecting the surgeon.

IMAGING IN MINOR PATIENTS

Plastic surgeons and dermatologists should be very careful in clicking and sharing clinical photographs of private parts of minors below 18 years (both male or female patients) on WhatsApp, Facebook, or other mobile applications with their colleagues or seniors for getting second opinion or showing improvements/results of their treatment, because they may face allegations of criminal offence under POCSO.

As per Section 13 of POCSO (Protection of Child against Sexual Offences) Act, 2012, Whosoever uses a child in any form of media (including electronic/printed form) for the purposes of sexual gratification, which includes representation of the sexual organs of child or indecent/obscene representation of child, shall be guilty of offence under POCSO Act, 2012.[13]

SHARING PHOTOGRAPH WITH OTHER PATIENTS/COLLEAGUES/MEDIA

Plastic surgeons and dermatologists should be very careful in clicking and sharing clinical photographs of private parts of female patients on WhatsApp, Facebook, or other mobile applications with their colleagues or seniors for getting second opinion or showing improvements/results of their treatment, because they may face the allegations of criminal offence to outrage modesty of female:

354A IPC (Indian Penal Code): Sexual harassment of nature of unwelcome physical contact and advances or demand or request of sexual favors showing pornography to other females is cognizable criminal offence, punishable for 3 years imprisonment and fine.[14]

This can happen when the surgeons/dermatologists share photos of private parts of their treated female patients for promoting their effective treatment results to other future patients/fellow female doctors/nurses.

CONCLUSION

To summarize, patient rights and physician responsibilities vis-a-vis clinical photographs is an increasingly complex issue with the omnipotent and ever intrusive digital presence in our lives. The guiding principles laid down by our ancient teachers and reiterated by generations of practitioners, however, continue to hold true even today. The need of the hour is to recognize patients' right to privacy as all important in today's litigious world and to ensure a comprehensive and informed photography consent in every single case while continuing to have regular discourse on this fascinating yet (slightly) vexing topic.

REFERENCES

1. Wikipedia (2018). Hippocratic Oath. [online] Available from: https://en.wikipedia.org/wiki/Hippocratic_Oath. [Accessed December, 2018].
2. Bhattacharya S. Clinical photography and our responsibilities. Indian J Plast Surg. 2014;47:277-80.
3. Masnick M (2013). Woman Sues Plastic Surgeon For $23 Million Because He Put Before/After Pictures Of Her On The Web. [online] Available from: https://www.techdirt.com/articles/20130627/18004323644/woman-sues-plastic-surgeon-23-million-because-he-put-beforeafter-pictures-her-web.shtml. [Accessed December, 2018].
4. Daily Report Online (2018). Client sues clinic. [online] Available from: https://www.law.com/dailyreportonline/2018/07/12/plastic-surgery-client-sues-clinic-over-nude-pics-

posted-on-web/?slreturn=20180805004612. [Accessed December, 2018].
5. Medical Council of India (2002). Chapter 6: Unethical Acts; Clause 6.1: Advertising. Indian Medical Council (Professional Conduct, Etiquette and Ethics) Regulations, 2002, (published in Part III, Section 4 of the Gazette of India) amended upto 8th October 2016. [online] Available from: https://www.mciindia.org/documents/rulesAndRegulations/Ethics%20Regulations-2002.pdf. [Accessed December, 2018].
6. The Hindu. Video recording of delivery case. [online] Available from: https://www.thehindu.com/todays-paper/tp-national/tp-kerala/video-recording-of-delivery-case-registered/article6433485.ece. [Accessed December, 2018].
7. UK Court (House of Lords) (2004). Campbell v MGN (2004) UKHL 2. [online] Available from: https://publications.parliament.uk/pa/ld200304/ldjudgmt/jd040506/campbe-1.htm. [Accessed December, 2018].
8. Intermediaries not to be liable in certain cases: Section 79, Chapter XII of 'THE INFORMATION TECHNOLOGY (AMENDMENT) ACT, 2008'. Available from: http://meity.gov.in/writereaddata/files/it_amendment_act2008%20%281%29_0.pdf"
9. Primary Evidence: Section 62 of THE INDIAN EVIDENCE ACT, 1872. Available from: https://indiacode.nic.in/acts/5.%20Indian%20Evidence%20Act,%201872.pdf
10. National Human Rights Commission, India. NHRC Guidelines for video-filming and photography of post-mortem examination in case of death in police action. [online] Available from: http://nhrc.nic.in/Documents/Guidelines_for_video_photography_of_PME_death_in_police_action.pdf. [Accessed December, 2018].
11. UCPI, UK (2006). McKennit vs Ash (2006) Civ 1714. [online] Available from: https://www.ucpi.org.uk/wp-content/uploads/2017/11/McKennitt-v-Ash-2008-QB-73.pdf. [Accessed December, 2018].
12. Herring J. Photography. Oxford's Book of Medical Laws & Ethics, 4th edition. London: Oxford University Press; 2012. pp. 226-8.
13. Ministry of Law and Justice. (2012). POCSO (Protection of Child against Sexual Offences) Act, 2012. [online] Available from: https://childlineindia.org.in/pdf/POCSO-ACT-Gazette.pdf. [Accessed December, 2018].
14. PRS Legislative Research (2013). Indian Penal Code with Criminal Law Amendment, 2013. [online] Available from: https://www.prsindia.org/uploads/media/Criminal%20Law,%202013/Criminal%20Law%20Amendment%20Bill%20as%20passed%20by%20LS.pdf. [Accessed December, 2018].

CHAPTER 48

Medicolegal Issues in Burns

Sunil Keswani, Vivekanshu Verma

KEY MEDICOLEGAL QUESTIONS IN ANY BURNS CASE

Q. Are burns classified as simple or grievous hurt?

Burns of first and second degree are simple injury if they are not extensive. Deep burns are grievous as they produce permanent scars. If the person goes into shock after burns, they may be classified as grievous. If burns cause deformity or impairment of movement of joint, they may be classified as grievous. Even extensive first- and second-degree burns can be classified as grievous if it endangers life or puts the person in severe body pain or if he is unable to carryout daily pursuits of life for more than 20 days (Fig. 1).

Q. Are burn suicidal, homicidal or accidental?

Accidental burns are quite common in women and children. Women may sustain burns while working in kitchen. Children may unknowingly touch hot liquids or solids. Suicidal burns are rare in men, but common in women. Due to the prevalent dowry tradition, there may be harassment of brides in their in-laws house. Many cases have been reported where brides have committed suicide by pouring kerosene oil on themselves and later igniting it. In such cases, severe burns may be seen on head, chest, and abdomen. Legs and feet are spared. Presence of a large amount of soot particles in respiratory passage may be seen.

MEDICOLEGAL APPROACH TO "ACUTE BURNS" PATIENTS

The description ahead is meant to highlight the specific points that are relevant to the legal safety of both the burn victim and the treating surgeon, during burns care.

To see patient in the ambulance—to see the stability of patient—if patient alive or dead at the time of arrival in emergency. If alive admitted and if brought dead, than to examine and assess for antemortem burns or postmortem (PM) burns and rule out foul play of murder or sexual assault, and burned to destroy the evidence of crime.

MEDICOLEGAL CASE TO NEARBY POLICE STATION: OLD MEDICOLEGAL CASE NUMBER (FIG. 2)

Medicolegal Case (Section 39)

- All major burns when received
- Unexplained severity, not matching with the history or circumstances
- Patients received after several days of burns
- Patients received without proper treatment
- Patients likely to succumb to the injury
- Patient received dead
- Mass casualties.

Q. Why is burn injury considered a dangerous weapon or means to cause an act endangering life?

Dangerous weapon is defined under section 324 and 326 of Indian Penal Code (IPC), as any instrument or means, used for shooting,

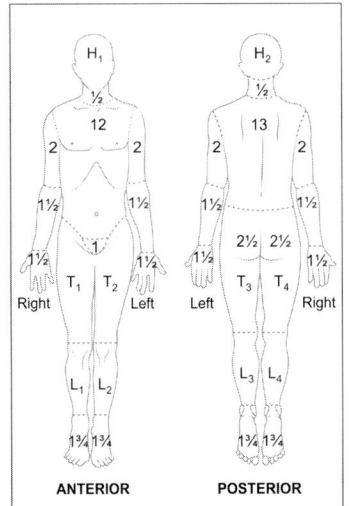

Contd...

Contd...

GENERAL INFORMATION:

1.1 **MATRIMONIAL STATUS:**
☐ Child N/A,   ☐ Married,   ☐ Unmarried,   ☐ Widowed,
☐ Divorced,   ☐ Separated,   ☐ Other (specify) _____

1.2 **No. OF CHILDREN:**
☐ Child N/A.   ☐ None,   ☐ Yes,   Total _____ Sons _____ Daughters

1.3 **SIZE OF THE FAMILY**
Adults _____, Children _____, Servants _____, Total _____

2.1 **OCCUPATION - FATHER / HUSBAND***
☐ Unemployed.   ☐ Manual labourer.   ☐ Factory worker.   ☐ Technical,   ☐ Clerical,   ☐ Executive,
☐ Business. (specify)   ☐ Professional, (specify)   ☐ Other. (specify) _____

2.2 **OCCUPATION MOTHER/ WIFE***
☐ Housewife ☐ Manual labourer. ☐ Factory worker, ☐ Technical, ☐ Clerical ☐ Executive, ☐ Business. (specify) _____
☐ Professional. (specify) _____   ☐ Other, (specify) _____

2.3 **OCCUPATION - PATIENT :**
☐ Infant N/A. ☐ Student, ☐ Unemployed, ☐ Housewife, ☐ Manual labourer, ☐ Technical, ☐ Clerical
☐ Executive ☐ Business. (specify)   ☐ Professional (specify)   ☐ Other. (specify) _____

2.4 **PATIENT'S INCOME PER MONTH**
☐ Low ☐ Average   ☐ High.   ☐ Child N/A

2.5 **FAMILY INCOME. PER MONTH :**
☐ Low ☐ Average ☐ High   ☐ Unknown

3.1 **EDUCATION - PATIENT :**   ☐ Infant N/A. ☐ Illiterate   ☐ Primary.   ☐ Secondary ☐ University
3.2 **EDUCATION - MOTHER /WIFE***   ☐ Illiterate   ☐ Primary   ☐ Secondary ☐ University
3.3 **EDUCATION - FATHER/HUSBAND ***   ☐ Illiterate   ☐ Primary   ☐ Secondary ☐ University

TRANSPORT

4.1 **METHOD OF TRANSPORT TO THE HOSPITAL (AFTER ACUTE BURNS)**
☐ Walking   ☐ Bullock cart   ☐ Taxi   ☐ Car   ☐ BUS,
☐ Ambulance   ☐ Train   ☐ Air   ☐ Other, (specify) _____

ACCIDENT

5.1 **TIME OF - ACCIDENT**
☐ Early Morning (5 a.m. to 8 a.m.) ☐ Late Morning (5 a.m. to 11 a.m.) ☐ Mid-day (11 a.m., to 2 p.m.)
☐ Afternoon (2 p.m. to 5p.m.).   ☐ Early evening (5 p.m. to 8 p.m.) ☐ Late evening (8 p.m. to 11 p.m.)

5.2 **PLACE OF ACCIDENT:** ☐ At home, ☐ At work, ☐ In the School ☐ In transit, ☐ Other, (specify) _____

5.3 **IF ACCIDENT TOOK PLACE AT HOME - SPECIFY THE AREA**
☐ Kitchen (cooking area), ☐ Bedroom (sleeping area),   ☐ Dining place,   ☐ Drawing room (living area),
☐ Bath room,   ☐ Store room.   ☐ Around the house,   ☐ Other (specify) _____

6.1 **ACTIVITY - PATIENT :** What was patient doing at the time of accident _____
6.2 **DESCRIBE THE ACCIDENT:** _____

6.3 **CAUSE OF ACCIDENT**
☐ Personal (Patient) ☐ Personal, (other person) ☐ Impersonal. ☐ Combined,
☐ Can't say   ☐ Any other. (specify) _____

6.4 **ANY PRECAUTIONS TAKEN TO PREVENT FURTHER ACCIDENT?**
☐ No,   ☐ If yes, Describe

6.5 **WHO ELSE WAS PRESENT AT THE TIME OF ACCIDENT?**
☐ Mother.   ☐ Father.   ☐ Siblings, (specify) _____   ☐ co-workers,   ☐ Relative, (specify) _____
☐ Neighbour   ☐ Teacher,   ☐ Other, (specify) _____

7.1 **PREVIOUS BURN ACCIDENTS TO THE PATIENT (WHICH REQUIRED DOCTOR'S VISIT):**
☐ Nil   ☐ One   ☐ Two   ☐ More (specify) _____

7.2 **PREVIOUS BURN ACCIDENT IN THE FAMILY :**
☐ Nil ☐ One ☐ Two ☐ More. (specify) _____

7.3 **HOW MANY PERSONS WERE INJURED IN THE PRESENT ACCIDENT (INCLUDING PATIENT)?**
☐ Nil ☐ One ☐ Two ☐ Three ☐ Four ☐ Five ☐ More (specify) _____

Contd...

Section 3: Plastic Surgery

Contd...

8.1 **WHAT DID THEY DO TO EXTINGUISH THE FIRE?**
 ☐ Not a flame burn ☐ Poured water ☐ Used blanket ☐ Used bare hands ☐ Drop and roll
 ☐ Indifferent ☐ N/A ☐ called fire authorities ☐ Other. (specify) _____

8.2 **FIRST AID:**
 ☐ Poured water, ☐ Applied ice, ☐ Applied ointment, ☐ Indifferent, ☐ Blanket, ☐ Other (specify) _____

DESCRIPTION OF BURN INJURY:

9.1 **DEPTH**: Epidermal_____ %, Dermal_____ %, Sub dermal_____ %

9.2 **DESCRIPTION OF POST BURN DISABILITY AT ADMISSION - IF ANY:**
 ☐ Nil, ☐ Hypertrophic scars, ☐ Hypopigmentation, ☐ Depigmentation, ☐ Hyperpigmentation, ☐ Itching and scratching,
 ☐ Mild disfigurement, ☐ Mild deformity, ☐ Severe disfigurement, ☐ Severe deformity

9.3 **NUTRITIONAL STATUS:**
 ☐ Excellent, ☐ Good, ☐ Fair, ☐ Poor, ☐ Gross Hypoproteinemia,

9.4 **PREVIOUS TREATMENT (OF PRESENT ACCIDENT):**
 ☐ No, ☐ If Yes, Describe ☐ Hospital, ☐ Burn Unit, ☐ Domestic, ☐ Other

9.5 **PREVIOUS OPERATIONS:** ☐ No, ☐ If Yes, describe _____

CAUSE OF INJURY:

10.1 **HISTORY OF INJURY:** ☐ Not known, ☐ Accident, ☐ Suicide, ☐ Homicide.

10.2 **NATURE OF INJURY:**
 ☐ Flame, ☐ Scalds, ☐ Chemical, ☐ Electrical, ☐ Radiation, ☐ Tar, ☐ Hot Plate,
 ☐ Hot Jaggary, ☐ Other. (specify)_____ ☐ Unknown.

10.3 **FLAME BURNS:**
 ☐ Open fire, ☐ Choola/Segree, ☐ Pressure stove, ☐ Wick stove, ☐ Gas stove, ☐ Petrol, ☐ Oil lamps.
 ☐ Kerosene lamps, ☐ Crackers, ☐ Other inflammable material, (specify)

10.4 **SCALDS:** ☐ Hot milk, ☐ Hot beverages, ☐ Hot water, ☐ Hot food, ☐ Hot bath water
 ☐ Hot soap solution, ☐ Steam, ☐ Other hot liquids. (specify) _____

10.5 **CHEMICAL CORROSION:**
 ☐ Strong acid, ☐ Strong Alkali, ☐ Phosphorus, ☐ Other chemical, (specify)

10.6 **ELECTRICAL:** ☐ Electrical contact-open wire, ☐ Electric flash, ☐ Defective plug/switch,
 ☐ Electrical appliance, ☐ High tension cable _____ volts, ☐ Other, (specify)_____

10.7 **RADIATION:** ☐ Radiation (Ionising), ☐ Radiation (heat), ☐ Any other. (specify) _____

10.8 **MISCELLANEOUS:**
 ☐ Molten metal, ☐ Hot Oil, ☐ Hut jaggery, ☐ Hot tar, ☐ Other. (specify) _____

10.9 **OTHER INJURIES:** _____

AGENT

11.1 **WAS THE AGENT DEFECTIVE?** ☐ No, ☐ Yes, ☐ Partially, ☐ Can't say

11.2 **IF THE AGENT WAS DEFECTIVE DESCRIBE THE DEFECTS:** _____

11.3 **DID THE VICTIM KNOW OF THE DEFECTS?** ☐ N/A, ☐ No, ☐ Yes

11.4 **DID THE FAMILY KNOW OF THE DEFECTS?** ☐ N/A, ☐ No, ☐ Yes

CLOTHING

12.1 **CLOTHING - MATERIAL:**
 ☐ Cotton, ☐ Silk, ☐ Wool, ☐ Synthetic, ☐ Blended fabric, ☐ Other, (specify) _____

13.1 **TYPE OF CLOTHING (MALE - UPPER GARMENTS)**
 ☐ No clothes, ☐ Banian, ☐ Shirt full/half sleeves, ☐ Sweater full / half sleeves, ☐ Coat,
 ☐ Other. (specify) _____

13.2 **TYPE OF CLOTHING (MALE - LOWER GARMENTS):**
 ☐ No clothes, ☐ Trousers, ☐ Pyjama, ☐ Lungi, ☐ Shorts, ☐ Dhoti, ☐ Underwear.
 ☐ Other, (specify) _____

13.3 **TYPE OF THE CLOTHING (FEMALE - UPPER GARMENTS):**
 ☐ No clothes, ☐ Blouse, ☐ Frock, ☐ Khamees, ☐ Top/Kurta, ☐ Coat, ☐ Sweater
 ☐ Brassiere, ☐ Other. (specify) _____

13.4 **TYPE OF CLOTHING (FEMALE - LOWER GARMENTS):**
 ☐ No clothes, ☐ Underwear, ☐ Petticoat, ☐ Saree, ☐ Skirt (short/long), ☐ Salwar, ☐ Shorts,
 ☐ Trousers, ☐ Maxi, ☐ Other, (specify) _____

WHERE DID THE ACCIDENT TAKE PLACE.?

14.1 ☐ Metropolitan city : ☐ Large city, ☐ Town, ☐ Rural area, ☐ Other. (specify) _____

Contd...

Contd...

15.1 **DESCRIPTION OF THE HOUSE WHERE THE ACCIDENT OCCURED:**
☐ Pavement house, ☐ Cloth zopada, ☐ Wooden hut, ☐ Mud hut, ☐ Tin or Asbestos shed,
☐ Brick and Mortar chawl, ☐ Brick and RCC construction, ☐ Other (specify) _____

15.2 **NUMBER OF ROOMS:**
☐ One, ☐ Two, ☐ Three, ☐ Four, ☐ Five, ☐ Six, ☐ More. (specify) _____

15.3 **KITCHEN (COOKING AREA) :** ☐ Floor level, ☐ Raised platform, ☐ Both

15.4 **HEATING DEVICE:** ☐ Open fire, ☐ Choola/Segree, ☐ Pressure stove, ☐ Wick stove, ☐ Gas stove.
☐ Electric Stove ☐ Other (specify) _____

15.5 **HOW LONG WAS FAMILY USED TO IT?** ☐ Not used to cooking ☐ 0-1 year. ☐ 1-5 years. ☐ >5 years

15.6 **STORAGE IN KITCHEN :** ☐ Above cooking place. ☐ Across cooking place, ☐ Side of cooking place,
☐ Below cooking place, ☐ No storage shelves

FINAL DISABILITY

16.1 **RESIDUAL DISABILITY (AT FINAL DISCHARGE FROM TREATMENT):** ☐ Nil, ☐ Hyper-ophic scam.
☐ Hypopigmentation, ☐ Depiginentation, ☐ Hyperpigmentation, ☐ Itching and scratching.
☐ Mild disfigurement, ☐ Mild deformity, ☐ Severe deformity, ☐ Severe disfigurement

16.2 **DESCRIBE THE DISABILITY:** _____

16.3 **IS DISABILITY LIKELY TO AFFECT:**
☐ No effect, ☐ School life, ☐ Social life, ☐ Family life, ☐ Economic life, ☐ Mind

16.4 **HAS PATIENT SOUGHT CORRECTIVE SURGERY?** ☐ Not required, ☐ Yes, ☐ No.

16.5 **NUMBER OF OPERATIONS PERFORMED:**
☐ One, ☐ Two, ☐ Three, ☐ Four, ☐ Five, ☐ Six or more, Describe (with dates) _____

17.1 **PAST MEDICAL HISTORY (SPECIFY)**
1. _____
2. _____
3. _____

17.2 **STATE OF HEALTH (AT THE TIME OF BURN)**
☐ Recent illness, ☐ Chronic illness, ☐ Mental disease, ☐ Alcoholic, ☐ Drug addict, ☐ Leprosy, ☐ Impaired vision.
☐ Impaired, ☐ Epilepsy, ☐ Acute illness, ☐ Other. (specify) _____

SOCIAL. HISTORY

18.1 **WAS THE PATIENT ABSENT FROM SCHOOLWORK DUE TO ACCIDENT?**
☐ N/A, ☐ No, ☐ If yes. (specify) _____ days.

18.2 **DID THE PATIENT RETURN TO SCHOOL?** ☐ N/A, ☐ Yes - same school,
☐ Yes - different school, ☐ Placed in the specialised school for the handicapped. (specify) _____

18.3 **DID THE PATIENT RETURN TO WORK?** ☐ N/A, ☐ Same place, ☐ Different place,
☐ Same department, ☐ Different department, ☐ Same work, ☐ Different work, ☐ Required to he placed in the specialised training centre for the handicapped, ☐ Any other. (specify) _____

RELATIONSHIP OF PATIENT WITH OTHERS

19.1 Before the accident : ☐ Nil, ☐ Cordial, ☐ Strained.
19.2 After the accident : ☐ Nil, ☐ Cordial, ☐ Strained.
19.3 **ATTITUDE OF FAMILY MEMBERS AFTER THE ACCIDENT:**
☐ Indifferent, ☐ Sympathetic, ☐ Helpful, ☐ Emotional, ☐ Other (Specify) _____
19.4 **ATTITUDE OF CO-WORKERS/CO-STUDENTS AFTER THE ACCIDENT :**
☐ Indifferent, ☐ Sympathetic, ☐ Helpful, ☐ Hostile, ☐ Other (Specify) _____
19.5 **ATTITUDE OF TEACHER/EMPLOYER AFTER THE ACCIDENT:**
☐ Indifferent, ☐ Sympathetic, ☐ Helpful, ☐ Hostile, ☐ Other (Specify) _____

20.1 **REMARKS:** _____

Resident doctor Incharge   Signature _____
Name Dr. _____
Designation _____

Unit Incharge _____

Fig. 1: WHO assessment forms for burn severity.

stabbing or cutting, or any instrument which, when used as weapon of offence, is likely to cause death, or by means of fire or any heated substance, or by means of any poison or any corrosive substance, or by means of any explosive substance, or by means of any substance which it is deleterious to human body to inhale, to swallow or to receive into the blood, or by means of any animal.

When police comes for the statement after—if patient is in shock then need to give endorsement to the police that patient is not able to give verbal statement for 48 hours still he/she is in shock.

In surgical management, informed consent for surgical procedure and anesthesia is mandatory. Need to take consent for photography of burn wounds from patient or their relative.

AMPUTATION IN GANGRENOUS LIMB AND ELECTRIC BURN

To dispose amputated part, fill up Form No. 2 (Fig. 3) and for fetus fill up Form No. 3 stillbirth record (Fig. 4) and dispose according to Biomedical Waste Act 2018.

In case of *death* occurs hospitalized burn victim:
- To inform the close relatives by treating doctor
- To inform the nearby police station about the death of the patient
- To write the *death* summary

Date:

To,

Sr. Inspector of Police,
   Police Station,

Sub.: Information of admission of Shri/Smt/Kum_____ a case of Burns.

Sir,

This is to inform you that a male/female aged_____years named_____

_____Residence at_____

_____

_____is admitted in   Hospital on_____at_____am/pm

with_____% burns injuries.

This is for your information and necessary a from.

Yours faithfully.

Date

Time

Fig. 2: Police notification form at the time of admission.

FORM NO. 2   **DEATH REPORT**

Legal information
This part to be added to the Death Register

To be filled by the informant
1. Date of Death:(Enter the exact day, month and year the death took place e.g. 1-1-2000) _____
2. Name of the Deceased:
 (Full name as usually written) _____
 Aadhar/UID No. deceased (if any) _____
 ☐☐☐☐☐☐☐☐☐☐☐☐
3. Sex of the deceased: (Enter "male", "female") do not use abbreviation _____
4. Name of Mother _____
 Aadhar/UID No. Mother (if any)
 ☐☐☐☐☐☐☐☐☐☐☐☐
5. Name of Father _____
 Aadhar/UID No. Father (if any)
 ☐☐☐☐☐☐☐☐☐☐☐☐
5a. Name of husband/wife _____
 Aadhar/UID No. husband/wife (if any)
 ☐☐☐☐☐☐☐☐☐☐☐☐
6. Age of the deceased: _____

7. Address of the deceased at the time of death:

8. Permanent address of the deceased:

9. Place of death: (Tick the appropriate entry 1, 2 or 3 below and give the name of the Hospital/Institution of the address of the house where the death took place, if other place, give location)
 1. Hospital/Institution Name:
 2. House Address:
 3. Other Place:
10. Informant's name:
 Address:
After completing all columns 1 to 21,
Informant will put date and signature here)
Date: Signature or left thumb mark of the informant

To be filled by the Registrar

Registration No.:   Registration Date:
Registration Unit:
Town/Village: District:
Remarks: (If any)
      Name and Signature of the Registrar

Fig. 3: Form 2 (Death report).

- To fill up the Form No. 2 for death report for registration at municipality along with death Police Notification Form (Fig. 5) and PM Notification Form (Fig. 6).

AADHAAR CARD HELPFUL IN SUDDEN DEATH DUE TO BURN, FOUND AS UNKNOWN/DISPUTED IDENTITY

The Ministry of Home Affairs, Government of India, and the Registrar of Births and Deaths, have made it mandatory to mention the following in Form No. 2, Death Report. Aadhaar card number becomes very useful to establish identity for life insurance claims, as identity of burned victim remains obscured due to facial burns and burn of fingerprints, recorded in Aadhaar directory and destruction of deoxyribonucleic acid (DNA) due to exposure to extreme heat in fatal burn cases. It can be very helpful in future litigation for reappearance of victim after his/her claimed deaths due to burns (Fig. 7).

Name of patients with Aadhaar No.	Father name with Aadhaar No.	Mother name with Aadhaar No.	Husband/wife name with Aadhaar No. and age and contact details
Mandatory	Mandatory	Mandatory	Mandatory

- After police *panchanama*, to remove all catheters [central line, Foleys catheter, endotracheal (ET) tube, nasogastric tube (NGT), and vein flow) and to wrap the body in white sheet
- Shift the body to the mortuary till further process
- To hand over the dead body to the police for PM in presence of the close relatives and after PM the body handed over to the relatives
- If the relatives denied for PM then police needs to give no objection certificate (NOC)
- We cannot hold back the body for the outstanding payment of the hospital.

POSTMORTEM IS MANDATORY FOR ALL MEDICOLEGAL CASES

Every burn patient, if dies unnatural death shortly after registering MLC, needs PM examination to establish cause of death, so that the culprit can be punished. If body needs to cross the boundary of the municipal corporation/state then they need separate police NOC.

Q. When is PM done without any antemortem MLC?

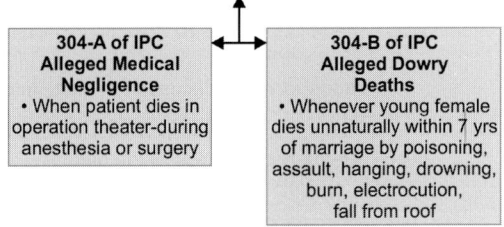

Q. Why PM is done in every burn case victim?
- To find out the actual cause of death.
- To find out the time passed since death to corroborate the day of crime.
- To identity of the deceased, in cases where it is unknown unclaimed (Nitish Katara murder case—blunt injury head by hammer—road traffic accident (RTA)—burn cannot identify).
- To find out the burn injury on body before death/after death.
- To collect relevant information to assist the investigating officers to arrive at a conclusion whether death is accidental, suicidal or homicidal.
- In case of infants born in burned pregnant, whether it is live born/stillborn/deadborn

Fig. 4: Form 3 (Still birth reports).

and if live born the period of survival and the cause of death.
- To collect evidence—pieces of vital organs and samples of blood and body fluids and foreign bodies—gunshot bullets—to establish the weapon of crime.
- To opine as to whether medical attendance following burn injury was given or not

Section 3: Plastic Surgery

THE MUNICIPAL CORPORATION OF THE CITY OF
PUBLIC HEALTH DEPARTMENT, NAVI MUMBAI
FORM NO. 4

(See Rule 7 of the Maharashtra Registration Of Birth and Deaths – Rules 2000)
MEDICAL CERTIFICATE OF CAUSE OF DEATH
(Hospital in patients not to be used for still births)
To be sent to Registrar along with Form No. 2 (Death Report)

Name of the Hospital _____ I hereby certify that the person whose particulars are given below died in the hospital in ward No. _____

_____ on _____ at _____ A.M. /P.M.

NAME OF DECEASED					For Use of Statistical Office
Sex	Age of Death				
	If 1 Year or more, age in years	If less than 1 Year, age in Months	If less than one Month, age in Days	If less than one day, age in Hours	
1. Male 2. Female					

CAUSE OF DEATH		Interval between onset and death approx.	
I Immediate Cause State the disease, Injury or complication which caused death not the mode of dying such as heart failure, asthenia etc.	(a) _____ Due to (or as a consequences of) (b) _____ Due to (or as a consequences of)		
Antecedent Cause Morbid conditions if any, giving rise to the above Cause, Stating underlying conditions last	(c) _____		
II Other significant conditions contributing to the death but not related to the disease or conditions causing it	_____ _____		

How did the injury Occur ?

Manner of Death
1. Natural 2. Accident 3. Suicide
4. Homicide 5. Pending investigation

If deceased was a female, was the death associated with pregnancy ? 1, Yes   2. No.
If yes, was there a delivery ? 1. Yes   2. No.

Name and signature of the Medical Attendant Certifying the cause of death
Date of verification _____

(To be detached and handed over to the relatives of the deceased)

Certified that Shri/Smt. /Kum. _____ S/W/D/of

Shri _____ R/o _____ was

admitted to this hospital on _____ and expired on _____ at _____ A.M./P.M.

Doctor _____
(Medical Supdt. Name of Hospital)

Fig. 5: Form 4 (Cause of death).

Date :

The Civil Surgeon,

Dear Sir,

This is to state that Shri/Smt/Kum/Master_____

_____

_____Years old patient admitted on date_____has died on

Date_____at_____a.m. / p.m._____

Cause of death is_____

_____

_____

Doctor-in-charge

Please Note : Details of death are attached

Fig. 6: Postmortem notification form

(Kennedy phenomenon)—in VIP cases, e.g. John F Kennedy's murder and Indira Gandhi's murder—suturing and repair of wound vanished the track of gunshot wound, but still culprit was found guilty.
- To ascertain the period of survival following receipt of burn injury.
- To find out the time passed since death since last meal (poisoned before burn).
- Whether the position of the dead body was changed or dragged after death.
- To opine as to the place and circumstances of death—basing on detection of modified forms of putrefaction.
- In presence of multiple injuries—what was the number of assailants (Nirbhaya case of Delhi).
- To connect the accused with the offence (Priyadarshini Mattoo case).
- To collect samples for chemical analysis, histological exam (Sunanda Pushkar case—polonium or alprax poisoning).
- To opine as to whether medical attendance following injury was beneficial or deleterious, thus causing death due to medical negligence.

Case Law: Tandoor Murder Case

Case facts: Burned Charred body of young married female—Discrepancy in two medical opinions during repeat postmortem—importance of X-ray in Burn case—Lead bullets found impregnated in Skull—Trial judge doubted competency of first doctor—Postmortem burn and antemortem gunshot injuries.

Discrepancy in postmortem report: The first postmortem was conducted at LHMC

Date:

To,

Sr. Inspector of Police,

_____

_____

_____

Sir,

This is to inform you about the death of our in-patient mentioned below,

Name :_____

Male/Female:_____ Age :_____

Date :_____ Time :_____

This is for your information and further action.

Thanking you,

Yours faithfully,

Doctor-in-charge

Fig. 7: Death Notification to Police.

Delhi, the cause of death was opined to be burn injuries. The second postmortem was conducted by team of three doctors from three different hospitals, they detected two bullets in head and neck region, opined cause of death due to firearm injuries, with that the course of investigation changed and the actual story came to light, this case is a landmark citation for fruitful second autopsy. Limbs of the unfortunate female were chopped off and bevelling was also noticed. In fact, even as per the report of Board of Doctors, it was not possible to give the exact location of entry wounds in view of extensive burns. In these circumstances, the remarks of the learned trial Judge against first doctor that he had 'obstructed the administration of justice.' or that 'His conduct does not seem to be above board' were unjustified. Blood stained articles seized from the barbecue restaurant on the day of the incident, those recovered from the victim's home and the dried blood lifted from the dickey of accused's car were also sent to Forensic Science Laboratory whereon examination it was found that human blood found on all these articles was of B' group, which was the blood group of the female whose body was being burnt on the tandoor and who later on was identified. The case involved the use of DNA evidence to establish the identity of the victim.

Result: After 22 years, accused was found guilty of murder, and was sentenced to death and restaurant manager, was given seven years rigorous imprisonment.

Citation: Delhi High Court decision in infamous Naina Sahni murder case: State vs Sushil Sharma. 2007 CriLJ 4008. https://indiankanoon.org/doc/504254/

Death Certificate

- Form No. 4 (Fig. 5) can issue if the patient is elderly or child.

- *Autonomous decision*: A person is free to decide that someone else may make decisions on his/her behalf. This remains an autonomous decision provided that it was made freely and without coercion.

CASE LAW: Burn after roadside trauma or murder by assault: Can orthopedic surgeon give opinion on head injury (domain of neurosurgeon) and severity of burn (domain of plastic surgeon)

Case facts: Honor killing of victim by his girlfriend's brothers after kidnapping him from Haryana, assaulted him physically with hammer—head injury—died on spot—thrown on roadside in Noida (another state to hide crime)—burned the dead body of victim by pouring kerosene, to simulate accident—head on collision while driving and burning of vehicle due to accidental leakage of petrol tank of car. Accused burned the dead body of victim and charred dead body was found as unknown by roadside attendants after 2 days of crime—PM done as unknown—doctor reported to police and did PM—found communicated fracture skull—victim was identified by his parents by recognizing his unburned hands (which were typically small, genetic trait of the family)—confirmed by DNA analysis.

Plaintiff: Homicidal physical assault by blunt weapon—comminuted depressed skull fracture of frontal bone by hammer, victim was thrown on roadside, and burned after his death (PM burn)—to hide the identity of victim and destroy the evidence of crime.

Defense: Defense lawyer proposed that it was a case of high-speed RTA as victim was found by police in the bushes near roadside. During court evidence, most common question of defense lawyer to a doctor (who made MLC) in injury/burn/assault/roadside trauma case—can this injury be caused by falling of victim by self, on hard and blunt surface? Now defense lawyer asked first question—can skull fracture be caused by falling on hard and blunt surface?

Doctor replied—No. Wound of this nature could be caused only when a moving person hits a stationary hard surface—results in "contrecoup injury" and will result in a lesion in an area opposite to the point of impact. But no countercoup lesions found in victim's head.

Result: Defense lawyer lost the case. Victim got justice after his death. Both accused found guilty of heinous crime of honor killing: rarest of rare offences, and convicted for imprisonment for whole life.

Discussion: Accused' lawyer tried to prove that the murder was an accident. Accused act kills the victim—accused plea to judge in court that his act was just an accident. Accused plea guilty under section 304-A IPC, death by accident. It has lesser punishment and is bailable offence, unlike murder under section 302 IPC, nonbailable offence.

Citation: Infamous case of honor killing of Nitish Katara. Delhi High court judgment in Vishal Yadav versus state of UP on 2 April, 2014. https://indiankanoon.org/doc/34613760/.

MEDICAL RECORDS IN BURN CASE

Medical records are acceptable as per section 3 of the Indian Evidence Act (IEA), 1872 amended in 1961 in a court of law. These are considered useful evidence by the courts as it is accepted that documentation of facts during the course of treatment of a patient. The patient or their legal heirs can ask for copies of the treatment records that have to be provided within 72 hours.

Q. How long medical records should be preserved?

Under the provisions of the Limitation Act, 1963 and section 24A of the Consumer Protection Act, 1986, which dictates the time within which a complaint has to be filed, it is advisable to maintain records for 2 years for outpatient records and 3 years for inpatient and surgical cases (Medical Council of India Regulations 2002 guidelines). MLCs should be maintained until the final disposal of the case even though only a complaint or notice is received.

Questions asked to treating doctor by police/lawyer/judge in court of law in burn case

1. Whether the smell of inflammable material (petrol/kerosene) was appreciated at the time of arrival in hospital?
2. Whether the burnt clothes were on the body of the victim at the time of admission? If yes, did doctor preserved the burnt clothes in sealed packet for forensic science laboratory for

identification of inflammable petroleum substance, if any? If not, it comes under destruction of evidence of crime by duty doctor.
3. What is the mode of burn, as per history and examination?
4. What are the lesions found due to burning or scalding or corrosives?
5. What was the percentage of total body surface area involved with burn?
6. Is there any spared area of the body not affected by burn? E.g. thumbs, fingers, palms, and soles. Thumb impression and mark of identification written in MLC are difficult to get in burn cases.
7. Was the burn victim pregnant at the time of incidence? What was the impact of burn on pregnancy, did burn injury resulted in abortion?
8. If the burn is an accident at workplace, what is the percentage of permanent disability caused to claim monetary compensation under Employees' Compensation Act for death on whether it was in the course of employment or suicidal attempt by the employed person?
9. Can this injury be caused by fall on hard and blunt surface? Brush burn
10. Was it antemortem or PM burn in victim brought dead in emergency?

DYING DECLARATION IN BURN VICTIMS

Dying declaration (DD) is a statement made by a person who is conscious and knows that death is imminent, declares cause of his death or as to any of the circumstances of the transaction, which resulted in his death when the cause of his death is in question. DD is a kind of hearsay evidence, but it is admissible as an exception to the general rule that hearsay evidence is not admissible. A three-judge bench of the honorable Supreme Court of India in 1984, laid down guidelines in landmark case of Sharad Birdhichand Sarda versus state of Maharashtra, regarding admissibility of DD in evidence under section 32 (1) of the IEA.

CASE LAW: Verbal dying declaration

Supreme Court of India observed: A statement was made by the victim of rape and murder. She died of burns. She made the statement to one of the witnesses while she was under severe pain due to grievous burns. It was alleged that the accused had committed rape on her and later by pouring kerosene on her, burnt her alive. The Court found the DD to be truthful and reliable and thus, admissible. The honorable Court held that the conviction could be based on the DD which is found to be truthful and reliable.

Citation: State of Assam versus Muhim Barakataki, 1986 SCR (3)1038.

Dying declaration should be recorded by the executive magistrate and police officer to record the DD, only if condition of the victim was so precarious that no other alternative was left. Certificate of the doctor should mention that victim was in a fit state of mind. Magistrate recording his own satisfaction about the fit mental condition of the victim was not acceptable, especially if the doctor was available. DD can be recorded by the attending doctor, who is the best person to opine about the fitness of the deceased to make the statement and when the doctor finds no time to call the police or magistrate, in such situation, the doctor is justified indeed duty bound to record DD, which is admissible in law. If the victim succumbed to the injuries, the statement can be used as a DD as to his cause of death. A suicidal note written, found in the clothes of the deceased, it is in the nature of DD, and is admissible in evidence under section 32 of IEA.

Dying Declaration Format as Prescribed by MOHFW (2014)

In critically ill survivors on death-bed in dowry-related violence, aggravated sexual assault, severe burn, and fatal homicidal poisoning. [Recorded on format by magistrate/

police officer/compos mentis certified by registered medical practitioner as per section 176 of Criminal Procedure Code (CrPC)]
- Is survivor mentally fit for statement: Yes/No (to be certified by RMP)
- Is survivor under influence of sedatives/hypnotics/narcotics: Yes/No
- Description of incidence of assault:
- Name of accused causing assault:
- Address of accused:
- Relation of survivor with the accused:
- Place of assault:
- Time of assault:
- Mode of injury: Homicidal/abetment of suicide
- Survivor brought by whom:
- Name and address of eye witness of assault:
- Any suicide note/written statement found: Yes/No
- Police intimated on 100 number helpline: Yes/No
- Details of RMP treating survivor:
  – RMP name and signature:
  – RMP council registration number:
  – RMP address:
- Signature or thumb impression of the survivor:
- Name and signature of the witness/female nurse attending survivor:
- Signature and name of magistrate/police officer
- Date, time, and place of recording DD.

CASE LAW ON COMPOS MENTIS: Burned rape victim in severe pain, sedated by morphine for pain relief—fit for statement for DD or not

Case facts: Burned rape victim in severe pain, sedated by morphine for pain relief—fit for statement for DD or not.
The honorable Supreme Court held that the High Court has erred in finding the accused not guilty of murder. Even if the evidence of the eye witness is eschewed, there is convincing and satisfactory evidence to prove that the accused was responsible for the murder of the deceased victim. Sessions Judge disbelieved the DD on flimsy grounds based on irrelevant considerations. Whether the Executive Magistrate reached the hospital in a scooter or any other conveyance or whether the Magistrate had noted the percentage of burn injuries on the body of the deceased are irrelevant matters, which should not have weighed with the Sessions Judge in disbelieving the DD. The honorable Court held that if the DD is truthful and reliable, conviction can be based solely.

Result: Accused and his wife were found guilty and imprisoned for life.

Citation: Shambhu versus State of Madhya Pradesh, 2002 SCR. https://indiankanoon.org/doc/1592889/.

FREE MEDICAL TREATMENT

Section 357A governs payment of fines to victims of crimes. Section 357C has been newly inserted whereby all hospitals, public or private are required to provide first aid or medical treatment free of cost. The section reads as: Section 357C of Cr PC—All hospitals, public or private, whether run by the Central Government, the State Government, local bodies or any other person, shall immediately, provide the first aid or medical treatment, free of cost, to the victims of any offence covered under section 326A, 376, 376A, 376AB, 376B, 376C, 376D, 376DA, 376DB of the IPC and shall immediately inform the police of such incident. In section 357C of the Code of Criminal Procedure, for the figures and letters "376A, 376B, 376C, 376D", the figures and letters "376A, 376AB, 376B, 376C, 376D, 376DA, 376DB" shall be substituted.[2]

In view of the increasing number of dowry deaths, guidelines have been laid down by the Government of India for examination of such cases, and the law in respect thereof has been suitably amended. The IPC, CrPC, and IEA are amended as per the Criminal Law (Second Amendment) Act, 1983 and was approved by

President of India to deal effectively with cases of dowry deaths and also the cases of cruelty to married women by their in-laws.

ACID ATTACKS BURNS (VITRIOLAGE)

Evolution of Law on Acid Attack in World

Since 1996, the number of cases of "acid violence" reported to the police annually has risen to 338 in 2001.[3] In 2002, in response to the epidemic, the Bangladeshi Government passed one law controlling the production, importation, storage, and use of acid and another providing the death penalty for convicted acid attackers.[4] The court battle in a case of this nature ought to have been simple since cases of acid attack are gruesome, and the easy availability of acid is a known fact. It was also accepted that corrective surgeries are extremely expensive. The first material order came only in 2011 when the Supreme Court passed an order directing all the state governments to indicate what steps they had taken to allocate resources for providing compensation to victims of acid attack under the amendment made to the CrPC by way of insertion of section 357A in 2009. The same order also asked the state governments to file their responses about banning of sale of acid. Even though this order was passed in 2011, as it would be seen below, it took over 3 years for the governments to finally come up with a proposal on the manner in which acid sale could be banned. In the meantime, in early 2012, the government of India filed in the Supreme Court an amendment to the Penal Code that was proposed but could not be passed in the parliament since the opposition parties were not allowing the parliament to function. This proposed amendment which had been approved by the cabinet, but to be passed by the parliament, had introduced two sections 326A and 326B to the Penal Code specifically dealing with acid attack. This was the first success in the case. This section eventually came to be passed in 2013 in the Criminal Law Amendment Act, 2013.

In spite of these strict laws, years 2011, 2012, and 2013 witnessed 83, 85, and 66 cases being reported respectively, but this number shot up to 309 in 2014—almost four times the average number of acid attack cases in the preceding years.[5] Uttar Pradesh topped the list with 185 cases till November 2014, followed by Madhya Pradesh with 53 cases. The most common reasons for acid attacks are usually revenge or jealousy, disputes over rejected sexual advances or marital disputes (41%); land and family disputes (32%), and dowry dissatisfaction (13%).[6]

Landmark case law for monetary compensation for medical treatment to acid attack survivor

Case facts: An acid attack survivor from New Delhi filed this Supreme Court Public Interest Litigation (PIL) to control the sale of acid, to ensure compensation for survivors, and to guarantee access to medical care for survivors.

Case: A young girl with big dreams, chirpy, confident, and beautiful was walking to her workplace from her home which is a mile away. As she reaches halfway, she hears her name being called out, and turns to see who the caller was. She looks at two people on a motorbike and walks towards them. The girl on the pillion is familiar and the man riding the bike is known to her. He wanted to marry her and she had declined. As she reaches them, the girl hurls some liquid on her. She experiences excruciating pain, a burning sensation, and falls on the street. She experienced a gruesome acid attack. Her face, her chest, and arms were burnt beyond recognition and she was in tremendous pain. It has taken many painful corrective surgeries for her to partially heal and she would never look the same again.

Result: A criminal case of attempt to murder was registered and those two persons on the bike have been convicted by a court in Delhi. When the man went in appeal in the Delhi High Court, the High Court ordered that she should be ordered a compensation of INR 300,000 which has now been paid to her.

Supreme Court drafted guidelines for private hospitals in this case: First aid must be administered to the victim and after stabilization; the victim/patient could be shifted to a specialized facility for further treatment, wherever required. Action may be taken against hospital/clinic for refusal to treat victims of acid attacks. We, therefore, issue a direction that the State Governments/Union Territories should seriously discuss and take up the matter with all the private hospitals in their respective State/Union Territory to the effect that the private hospitals should not refuse treatment to victims of acid attack and that full treatment should be provided to such victims including medicines, food, bedding, and reconstructive surgeries. We also issue a direction that the hospital, where the victim of an acid attack is first treated, should give a certificate that the individual is a victim of an acid attack. This certificate may be utilized by the victim for treatment and reconstructive surgeries or any other scheme that the victim may be entitled to with the State Government or the Union Territory, as the case may be. In the event of any specific complaint against any private hospital or government hospital, the acid attack victim will, of course, be at liberty to take further action.

Supreme Court drafted guidelines for monetary compensation from state by Criminal Injuries Compensation Board.

Citation: Laxmi versus Union Of India and Ors. (WP (CRIM) 129/2006)(SC).

Medicolegal Issues of Vitriolage in India

There was no separate statistics for acid violence cases in India till early 2013, because the Indian criminal law did not recognize it as a separate offence. With the amendment in IPC in February 2013, incidents of acid attack are now being recorded as a separate offence under section 326A and 326B of IPC. Earlier only permanent disfiguration of the face due to acid attack was considered as grievous hurt.

But now, after amendments under criminal law (amendments) 2013, even disfiguration of any other part of the body by throwing or administering acid is considered as grievous hurt. The damage or deformity shall not be required to be irreversible. The punishments have been enhanced and may extend to life imprisonment and a fine, which may extend to INR 1,000,000. Even an attempt to throw or administer acid on any person is punishable. Offences under section 326A and 326B of IPC are cognizable and nonbailable.

The IPC was amended by the Criminal Law (Amendment) Act, 2013, to include the offence of acid attack within its ambit

Section 100: When the right to private defense of the body extends to causing death. An act of throwing acid or administering acid, or an attempt to throw or administer acid which reasonably causes the apprehension that grievous hurt will be the consequence of such an attack. Thus, acid attack has been included under the list of grievous crimes under which the right to private defense extends to causing death. This means that an acid attack is so grave that a survivor may be justified in killing the perpetrator to defend herself from the attack.

Section 326A: Whoever causes permanent or partial damage, deformity, burns, maims, disfigures or disables any part or parts of the body of a person with the intention of causing or knowing that it is likely to cause such injury or hurt, shall be punished with either simple or rigorous imprisonment for a term of at least 10 years, which may extend to imprisonment for life and a fine. The fine shall be paid to the victim, and shall be just and reasonable to meet the medical expenses of the victim.

Section 326B: Attempting to throw or administer acid with the intention of causing permanent or partial damage, deformity, burns, maim, disfigure, disable, grievous hurt shall be imprisoned with either simple or rigorous imprisonment for at least 5 years, up to 7 years, and a fine. Acid includes any substance of acidic, corrosive or burning character that is capable of causing bodily injury which leads to scars, disfigurement, temporary or permanent disability. For the purposes of both these sections, the damage or deformity need not have to be irreversible.

Section 166A: A public servant who refuses to record any information in relation to an offence under section 326A and 326B (as well as some other sections), shall be imprisoned with rigorous imprisonment for a term of at least 6 months which may extend up to 2 years, and be liable to pay a fine.

Section 166B: Whoever is in charge of any hospital, whether public or private, run by the Central or State Government, a local body, or any person, and who contravenes section 357A of the Code of Criminal Procedure, shall be imprisoned for a term which may extend to 1 year, or with fine, or both.

The state must ensure medical treatment and free ambulance services to survivors. The state is also obligated to identify private hospitals that can provide treatment to survivors. Denial of treatment by hospital to survivors of physical assault with acid vitriolage and sexual assault survivors is punishable under section 166 B IPC with imprisonment for a term which may extend to 1 year or with fine or with both.

While "victim" may be the accurate legal term, many women prefer the word survivor because it reflects their postattack reality of undergoing surgeries, attending court hearings, speaking at awareness meetings, and moving forward with their lives.

The Code of Criminal Procedure was amended twice (2013 and 2018) in relation to free treatment of acid attack victims and further judicial proceedings in increasing punishment to deter the crime, by rigorous punishment of the criminal who did the heinous act. It was called as Criminal Law (Amendment) Act, 2018.

Section 154: When the information is given by the woman victim of a crime under section 326A and 326B which are the sections dealing with acid attacks (and other sections of the IPC), the information will be recorded by a woman police officer or any woman officer.

Section 154(a) provides for special provisions for survivors of offences under sections 354, 354A, 354B, 354C, 354D, 376, 376A, 376B, 376C, 376D, 376E, or section 509 of the IPC (sexual harassment, criminal force to a woman with intent to disrobe, watching a woman in a private act, stalking, rape, and aggravated rape). In section 154 of the Code of Criminal Procedure, for the figures and letters "376A, 376B, 376C, 376D", the figures and letters "376A, 376AB, 376B, 376C, 376D, 376DA, 376DB" shall be substituted. (Criminal Law -Amendment Act, 2018.). When an offence under the sections has been committed and the victim has been permanently or temporarily mentally or physically disabled, then the police officer shall, in the presence of a special educator or interpreter record information from the victim at the victim's residence of any place of the victim's choosing. The recording of such information may be videographed if needed. Section 154(a) seems to have overlooked acid attack victims as section 326A and 326B has not been included. This might be particularly problematic as in most cases acid attack victims suffer from significant physical disability following the attack.

Section 164 (5A)(a) makes similar provisions as section 154(a), for a Judicial Magistrate to record the statement taking the assistance of a special educator or interpreter in cases wherein the victim is temporarily or permanently mentally or physically disabled, and for the statement to be videographed. This statement shall be considered in lieu of examination in chief under the IEA.

DOWRY DEATH AND LEGAL PROTECTION OF WOMEN IN INDIA

Domestic violence by burn on married women and legal protection of women in India

D—Domestic Violence Protection Act. 2005
D—Dowry Prohibition Act, 1961
D—Deceased's—Sati (Prevention) Act, 1987—Sati means the act of burning or burying alive any widow with the body of her Deceased husband, irrespective of whether such burning is claimed to be voluntary on the part of widow
D—Dowry Death—304B IPC—nonbailable offence—within 7 years of marriage—7 years punishment—killing by in-laws and simulating it accident—D—Dry heat fame burn while cooking in kitchen stove of kerosene.
D—Domestic cruelty—498A IPC—physical by burn/chemical torture by acid burn.

IPC section 304-B deals with dowry death. When the death of a married woman is caused by any burns or bodily injury or occurs under abnormal or suspicious circumstances within 7 years of her marriage duration and it is clearly shown that soon before her death she was subjected to cruelty or harassment or torture by her husband or any relative of her husband or in-laws for, or in connection with, any demand for dowry, such death shall be called as "dowry death", and such husband or relative or in-laws deemed to have caused her death. Whoever commits dowry death shall be punished with imprisonment for a term minimum of 7 years, which may extend to imprisonment for life.[7]

IPC section 498-A deals with husband or relative of husband of the subjecting her to cruelty. Whoever being the husband or the relative of the husband or in-law of a woman, subjects such woman to cruelty or harassment or torture shall be punished with imprisonment for a term which may extend up to 3 years and shall also liable to pay fine. The cruelty can be either mental or physical torture, which drives the women to commit suicide or to cause serious injury, or danger to life or health.

SCREENING FORM FOR DOMESTIC VIOLENCE (BY MOHFW GUIDELINES, 2014)

Please tick mark [✓] the column applicable by treating doctor in emergency.

Domestic violence: Yes/No
If domestic violence, then:
- Initial resuscitation/first aid given: Yes/No
- Information about available service: Yes/No
- Medicolegal certificate: Yes/No
- Safety assessment: Yes/No
- Informed protection officer: Yes/No
- Counseling done: Yes/No

Physical violence:
- Hitting, slapping, punching, pinching, pushing, throwing objects
- Painful bending and twisting of limbs
- Physical restrain by tying limbs with cord, handcuffs, locked in a room
- Keeping hungry: Not providing food and water for nutrition
- Electric shocks and burns
- Causing skin burns with flame of fire/cigarette butts/heated utensils/acid throwing
- Choking/strangulation/hanging
- Denying the victim needed medical care, depriving them of sleep or other necessary functions
- Forcing the victim to engage in drug or alcohol use against their will
- Attempted suicides by victim, often admitted in the hospitals as accidental consumption of poison.

Criminal Procedure Code section 176(1) provides inquest by executive magistrate and CrPC section 174(3) provides as follows:

When (1) The case involves suicide by a woman within 7 years of her marriage, (2) The case relates to the death of a woman within 7 years of her marriage in any circumstances raising a reasonable suspicion that some other person committed an offence in relation to such woman, or (3) The case relates to the death of a woman within 7 years of her marriage and any relative of the woman has made a request in this behalf, the police officer will forward the body for autopsy to the nearest medical officer for opinion.

CASE OF FALSE ALLEGATION BY BURNED VICTIM: Alleged dowry death, DD pointing towards husband, evidences not enough to convict the husband

Case facts: It is not the case of prosecution, which mainly relies on the two oral DDs in which the victim mentioned that her husband demanding money for buying motorcycle, just before the incidence of burning, cannot be termed as "cause of her death" or "circumstances of the transaction which resulted in her death". Since no police complaint was made before the incidence of burn, therefore the High Court cannot rely upon that evidence for bringing home the guilt under section 498A IPC.

Citation: Shivkumar Maruti versus State of Maharashtra, 2009 Cri LJ 2549 (Bom).

IEA Section 113-A deals with presumption as to abetment of suicide by a married woman. When the question is whether the commission of suicide by woman had been abetted by her husband or any relative of her husband and it is shown that she had committed suicide within a period of 7 years from the date of her marriage and her husband or such relative of her husband had subjected to cruelty, the court may presume, having regard to all the other circumstances of the case, that such suicide had been abetted by her husband or by such relative of her husband.

IPC section 304–A: Accidental death due to negligence while cooking (unintentional)
IPC section 304–B: Bridal Burning death in demand of dowry (intentional)
IEA section 113–A: Abetment of suicide (provocation by husband and in-laws)
IEA section 113–B: Bridal murder in demand of dowry

IEA section 113-B deals with presumption as to dowry death. When the question is whether a person has committed the dowry death of a woman and it is shown that soon before her death, such woman had been subjected by such person to cruelty or harassment for, or in connection with, any demand for dowry, the court shall presume that such person had caused the dowry death.

Case law on mentally ill burn victim

Case facts: Alleged dowry death, abetment of suicide pointing towards husband, medical evidence that deceased wife was mentally ill. Accused husband and his family acquitted.

Plaintiff: Victim committed suicide on 28-9-1985, when all the other family members had gone outside. Brother of the victim, filed a complaint dated 30-9-1985, against the accused, i.e. the husband and parents in-law of the deceased victim, alleging that they had been demanding dowry and had given ill treatment to the deceased, and that is why she committed suicide.

Defense: It was a clear cut case of suicide because of depression, as the deceased victim had been suffering from epilepsy and other mental disorders. The medical evidence, particularly, the deposition of psychiatrist made it clear that the deceased had been suffering from serious depression and such a patient often develops suicidal tendencies. He had examined the deceased and prescribed medicines for manic depressive psychosis. In past, she had gone out of the house, i.e. on the main road, half-naked and she had brought disrepute to the family of her in-laws. Love letters written after marriage, showed illicit relationship between the deceased and one family friend. The deceased had also made an attempt earlier to commit suicide in 1985 and she had been taken to the local hospital and received electroconvulsive therapy (ECT). Subsequently, she had also been treated at Kanpur. The findings of fact recorded by the Trial Court that there was neither any demand of gold ornaments or any kind of dowry, nor had the deceased been subjected to cruelty, could not be held to be perverse by the High Court to bring home the charges against the appellants under sections 306 or 498A IPC.

Decision: All accused are acquitted from the criminal charges. It is a clear cut case of gross abuse of the dowry laws. The deposition of psychiatrist reveals that ECT treatment is given only to mental patients, who have mental depression and tend to commit suicide; the ailment of epileptic fits is a neurological problem.

Citation: Sunil Kumar Shambudayal Gupta versus State of Maharashtra, 2011 Cri LJ 705 (SC).

Female Burn in Reproductive Age

All female burn patients of childbearing age should be tested for pregnancy unless the pregnancy is obvious.[8]

If it is known that a burned female is pregnant, it is important to establish as precisely as possible the exact stage of pregnancy at the time of the burn accident. This must be based upon the menstrual history and fetal ultrasound examination. (Burns center has to registered ultrasound machine and need to follow guideline of Pre-Conception and Pre-Natal Diagnostic Techniques (PCPNDT) Act, 1994).

In first and second trimester, best chance for fetal survival is to ensure maternal survival and in the last trimester fetal survival depends upon fetal maturity. Maternal survival is less likely if the burn wound exceeds 50% total body surface area. Thermal injury does increase the risk of spontaneous abortion and premature labor. Early obstetric intervention is indicated in patients with fatal burn and complications.[9]

According to Medical Termination of Pregnancy (MTP) Act 1971, medical practitioners can terminate the pregnancy when continuation of pregnancy is a risk to the life of a pregnant woman and child or could cause grave injury to her physical or mental health.[10] Death of fetus (in case of spontaneous abortion) registered under Rule 5 of the Maharashtra Registration of Birth and Death-Rules 2000 by medical officer.[11]

> **Q. What to write MLC to describe 90% antemortem burn caused by kerosene?**
>
> Indian law enquires burn severity—type of burn (dry heat/scald) depth of burn, nature of injury (simple/grievous/dangerous to life), location and percent of burn and its duration.
> It should be described superficial to deep burns with blackening and peeling of skin with singeing of hair with red line of demarcation over the following parts of the body. Head as whole with singeing of scalp hair, face as a whole with singeing of eyebrows and eyelashes, neck and chest as a whole, abdomen in its whole circumference, genitalia in patches and both buttocks in patches with singeing of pubic hair, both upper limbs and both lower at places, sparing the soles. Total burnt surface area is about 90%.
> Opinion of injury (grievousness, duration, type of burn, antemortem): Dry heat flame burn of fresh duration and antemortem burn, dangerous to life.

INTENTIONAL BURNING IN CHILDREN; CHILD ABUSE OR MUNCHAUSEN SYNDROME OF PROXY

All studies show associations between inflicted burns and both low family income and single parenthood (which is not to say that the wealthy do not abuse children by burning them, only that this form of child abuse is more commonly associated with low income families).[12-16] Children with inflicted burns were 9.6 times more likely to come from single parent families, while other studies show that over 70% came from single parent families,[17,18] and that up to 96% came from families with low income.[19] This may well be a reflection of the strong, common association between low educational attainment on the part of parent(s) and inflicted burns.[2]

> **CASE LAW:** Failure to detect child abuse by doctors results in $45 million verdict
>
> *Femur fracture missed; no follow-up system in place*
>
> *Facts*: A two-and-a-half-month-old infant is brought to the emergency department (ED) by his mother because he is not moving his right leg and cries every time it is touched. The ED physician orders an X-ray of the leg. It is read by a teleradiologist as normal. The child is discharged with conservative treatment and advised to follow-up as needed. The following morning the film is over-read and a possible femur fracture is reported. The ED is notified that further imaging is recommended, but

the family is not informed so it is never done. A month later, the child returns with seizures and altered mental status. Workup reveals a skull fracture, intracranial bleeding, and healing rib and right femur fractures. He is left with significant disability and requires long-term support. A lawsuit is filed against the radiologists, ED physicians and group, the hospital and the abusing father, who is later convicted of child abuse and sent to prison.

Plaintiff: You missed my son's broken femur and sent us home. You never called us when you were notified of the fracture the next morning. If you had done what the radiologist recommended, my son would be normal today.

Defense: Radiologists: We told the ED about this and recommended further imaging. ED: We never received any report from the radiologist. Hospital: The doctors are not our employees. We are not responsible. Even so, everyone met the standard of care. The first ED doctor properly managed as per standard of care managed your son based on the radiologist's original report.

Result: After a 4-week trial and 6 hours of deliberation, the jury rendered a plaintiff verdict for $45 million. This was attributed 60% to the abusing father, 35% to the ED physician responsible for notifying the family and 5% to the ED physician who first saw the patient.

Takeaways:
- Have a low threshold to suspect child abuse.
- Have a system in place to send, receive, and act upon lab and X-ray reports that are only available after patient discharge.
- Emergency department physicians should at least lay eyes on the actual imaging and use their knowledge of clinical context when ordering imaging.

Citation: Gloucester County Superior Court in Ethan Burgos-Bonilla versus SJ Health Care. South Jersey (USA) February 17, 2017.

In up to 70% of cases inflicted burns the assault is perpetrated by young women and 50% of these women are the children's mothers[5]—possibly reflecting only the predominant role of females in early age child rearing, toilet training, and discipline, which represent emotional flashpoints. A strong association has been noted between a past history of abuse (spousal or parental) suffered previously by an adult who then inflicts a burn on a child.[17,19]

Legal provisions for protection of children

The key federal legislation addressing child abuse and neglect is the Child Abuse Prevention and Treatment Act (CAPTA).

Section 317 of IPC: Exposure and Abandonment: Crime against children by parents or others to expose or to leave them with the intention of abandonment.

MISUSING BURNS, MISLEADING TERMS, AND CONFUSING WORDS BY LAWYERS/MEDIA TRIALS

Burning is misused to cause automobile fire to collect insurance money, to burn incriminating evidence, during domestic quarrel, and as a method of revenge/jealousy in acid attack. Some misleading terms are mentioned below:

- Brush burn slang medical term for roadside abrasion caused by scratching on hard and blunt surface found commonly in roadside trauma.
- Patient declared dead erroneously by doctor leading to wrongful cremation—attendants and relative alleged that patient was wrongly declared dead by the treating doctor, thus burning him alive, which lead to media trial of doctor. Police complaint was registered, and police constituted medical board for enquiry, but after doing PM, it was proved that patient died before cremation, and PM burns during cremation can result in muscle contractions of large limb and trunk muscles, cremation heat causes heat rigor and pugilistic movements, thus misleading impression of body movements even after death of deceased.

> **Case report of cremation (without postmortem) in sudden death of young married female**
>
> *Burned*: Cremation of married female after killing by poisoning by her husband (in demand of dowry), husband took deceased to doctor, who declared her brought dead, but did not informed police and handed over body without postmortem (PM). Later parents of victim filed First Information Report (FIR) and made doctor as culprit in helping the accused husband in disposing the dead body of victim. Doctor was arrested and imprisonment for 3 years for helping accused in destruction of evidence by burning the deceased without PM.

- *Chest wall burn*: Emergency medical treatment of direct current (DC) shock in cardiac arrest may cause rib injuries, contusions, and defibrillator marks on precordium. It may be mistaken for burns or injuries. It is most common defense of prisoner's death in custody during physical torture.
- *Burn blister*: Burn blisters may occur before or after death and it is often difficult or impossible to differentiate between them if they occur perimortally (at the time of death). This has important forensic importance, related to the possibility of a dead body being disposed of in a fire. Classical differentiation is said to be (1) a red margin to living blister and (2) fluid containing high concentration of protein if formed during life. In practice, these points may be of little help if death occurred soon after burning. "Barbiturate" blisters are a misnomer for those seen in any case of coma. The cause is obscure, but is due partly to gravitational accumulation of fluid due to immobility and partly due to oxygen lack in the skin. As well as drugs inducing long coma, like barbiturates, they may be seen in carbon monoxide poisoning, natural cerebral hemorrhage, etc. Often seen on dependent parts such as buttocks, thighs, calves, and loins. Many diseases give rise to blisters, usually from infections, for example, smallpox, chickenpox, etc. Also in skin diseases, such as pemphigus. The fluid from contagious diseases is often highly infectious.
- Sunburn due to overexposure of the unconscious intoxicated victim to direct sunlight after overconsumption of alcohol, left unattended for hours at isolated places, can confuse the cause of unconsciousness as burn, although its can be heat stroke. Alcohol appears to be the most important single contributing factor in the majority of deaths associated with sunburn.
- *Self-inflicted burn*: Criminals sometimes attempt to mutilate the patterns of fingerprints by inflicting wounds or burns, application of corrosives but they are not obliterated unless true skin is completely destroyed.

> **Case report of self-inflicted burn to blame her husband:** plastic surgeon's court evidence
>
> An 18-year-old woman filed a complaint at the City Magistrate's court at Lucknow that she was burnt by her husband with a pair of tongs, in demand of dowry. As per plastic surgeon's opinion on prescription, she had several small marks of superficial burns causing redness and vesication on the wrist, forearms, legs, and thighs. Some of these have the shape of the knob of the tongs. During the court trial, it was found that they have been self-inflicted, in as much as they are approachable by the woman herself. It was found that she had inflicted the burns to strengthen her case for divorce from her husband, as she was in love with her boyfriend.

IATROGENIC BURNS

"Iatrogenic burns" are burns caused due to medical negligence/error during treatment in hospital, e.g. electrocautery burns, laser burns, contact burns from recently autoclaved instruments, warm compresses, magnetic resonance imaging (MRI) interactions with

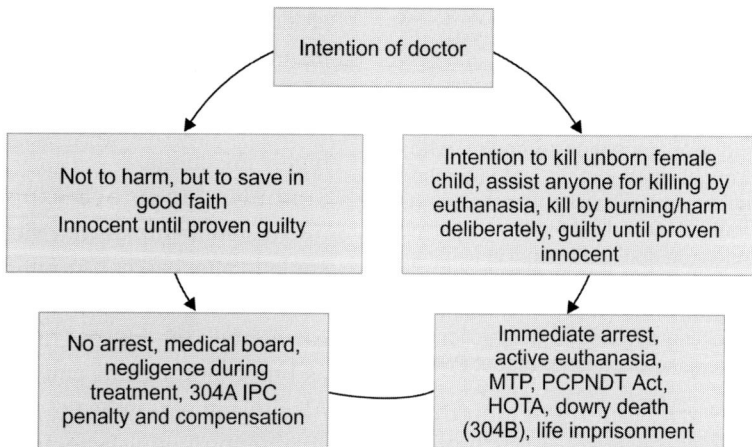

Fig. 8: Intention of doctor while deciding the case of medical negligence or wrongful act by doctor. (HOTA: Human Organ Transplant Act; IPC: Indian Penal Code; MTP: Medical Termination of Pregnancy; PCPNDT: Pre-Conception and Pre-Natal Diagnostic Techniques)

coiled electrodes or metallic transdermal drug patches or various other foreign bodies, thermal blankets, warming bottles, microwaved objects, alcohol or other substances put on skin, and radiation overdoses.

Burns is a three-dimensional injury. Burn injuries present challenging problems to the dermatologist and plastic surgeon, as dermatologists use lasers for dermal disorders, thus can cause iatrogenic burns on overexposure, thus requiring plastic surgery care. The principal issue usually is causation, particularly when a distinction is to be made between an accident and a deliberate act. Court of law judges the intention of doctor while deciding the case of medical negligence or wrongful act by doctor (Fig. 8).

Burn is a double-edged sword in which intention of doctor is differentiated by the law during investigation. Burn can be used to save a life as laser/radiation therapy to kill the unwanted tissue, e.g. cancerous tumor. But burn can be misused as dangerous means to harm/kill innocent victim by throwing acid, pouring kerosene, and overexposing with heated substance. Burn can be accidental (domestic—cooking and hot bath), industrial (working in glassblower factory), iatrogenic (laser burns), suicidal, homicidal, self-inflicted, intentional (physical torture), or by acid attack (corrosive burns) or an act of terrorism (incendiary bombs). It is important that electrical burns be looked for and recognized, especially in the absence of a good history suggesting electrocution. The principal additional issue with burn-related fatalities is establishing the cause of death, which usually is either "burn shock" or infection. Doctors need to be familiar with heat-related PM artifacts and their distinction from antemortem changes.

CASE OF FRIVOLOUS LAWSUIT: Surgeon burned patient's mouth during tonsillectomy

Facts: A 6-year-old female undergoes a tonsillectomy during which the blade of the Bovie surgical knife comes loose as the ear, nose, and throat (ENT) surgeon withdraws it, causing a "serious burn" (5 × 7.5 mm) to the inside of her mouth. Her mother sues the doctor, clinic, and hospital.

Plaintiff: You should have made sure the blade was properly attached to the device. My daughter has a lifelong scar on her face caused by your negligence. She might need plastic surgery. This should not have happened. You owe us $4,868.09 in expenses and even more for pain and suffering. Oh, and "res ipsa loquitur," so I do not need any expert witnesses.

Defense: The equipment was defective. I saw you four times in the next 4 months. The burn healed well and is hardly noticeable, as photographs of your daughter prove. I met the standard of care for an ENT surgeon, and both my ENT expert and plastic surgery expert agree. Oh, and "the thing does not speak for itself".

Result: 6 years after the incident, 3 years after the lawsuit was filed, and after a 3-day trial, a jury renders a defense verdict after only 1 hour of deliberation.

Citation: Padula V Dharia et al., Norfolk County Superior Court #NOCV2011-01126, Massachusetts.

Fire in operation theater can occur due to cautery. The "fire triad" has three components that must come together to ignite a fire: (1) heat or an ignition source, (2) fuel, and (3) an oxidizer.

BURN BY NEGLIGENCE IN SURGERY CAUSING BURNS OF SEVERE NATURE

An electrocautery burn is a medical error, which also has medicolegal and ethical implications. There is a long list of such errors, from simple misdiagnosis to more serious harm that may culminate in the patient's death. Such errors may emanate from negligence or system failure. Unfortunately, such errors continue to occur in every part of the world. Ideally the professional staff and hospital administration concerned should ensure patient safety by preventing such mishaps and compensate for the harm that ensues to the patients. Reporting such errors as adverse event is imperative as this will ensure safer management of future patients by sensitizing the professionals involved, leading to the adoption of preventive strategies.

CASE LAW: Tropical diabetic hand syndrome simulating iatrogenic burns during surgery

Case facts: A 65-year-old diabetic patient operated for cardiac bypass surgery—in postoperative period developed lesions on left hand palm simulating burn—plastic surgeon diagnosed it as tropical diabetic hand syndrome (TDHS) and did surgical debridement of gangrenous part. In start, patient sued the cardiac surgeon and hospital for causing burns on hands. Later during arguments (when he could not prove the burn caused), patient modified complaint and sued the plastic surgeon for TDHS mismanagement and negligently amputating the finger of hand, thus resulting in permanent disability.

Plaintiff: Patient got burns on hands in operation theater during cardiac surgery by overexposure to? operation theater (OT) heater? OT warm blankets? Cautery burns during surgery.

Defense: Patient was suffering from long-standing diabetic condition, which led to development of TDHS with blisters on palm, redness, and cellulitis. TDHS is a complication affecting patients with diabetes mellitus in the tropics. The syndrome encompasses a localized cellulitis with variable swelling and ulceration of the hands, to progressive, fulminant hand sepsis, and gangrene affecting the entire limb.

When heater was not in the OT, why fingers could have burnt and developed blisters. Histopathology diagnosis of the suspected burns of the palm is on record and it is taken to be final diagnosis of TDHS which is supported by the expert evidence by a well-known plastic surgeon, who followed approved protocol of treating burns due to gangrene and no deficiency was shown in treating the complainant-patient. Management of TDHS is not different from management of burnt hand. The cause of gangrene is insufficient blood supply to the affected part, which caused because of endarteritis known sequelae in long-standing diabetic case of complainant. Complainant fingers as alleged had never been amputated. Timely measures were promptly initiated for removal of phalanges as the patient developed gangrene in the left hand palm and not amputated the fingers of the complainant-patient as alleged in the complaint.

Decision: Hospital case paper record of the patient and documentary evidence placed on record by the opponents lead us to conclude that surgeons have exercised due care and caution to treat and operate the complainant-patient on two occasions, i.e. for open heart surgery and for removal of terminal phalange of the burn fingers without amputating the fingers of hand of the patient. The patient failed to establish negligence of the opponents for treating him as inpatient in the hospital and further, could not make out case of deficiency of service against the cardiac and plastic surgeon.

Citation: Maharashtra consumer commission: CC/06/95. Murlidhar R. Chhabria versus Breach Candy Hospital Trust and Ors. on 28 March, 2012. https://indiankanoon.org/doc/192706319/.

Electrocautery burns to patients are usually predictable and easily preventable and have been reported to result from insulation failure of the active electrode, direct coupling from the active electrode to another conducting instrument or capacitive leakage of current. Necessary information should be given to the healthcare staff about the installation and connections of the equipment, proper placement of the cautery plate, monitoring of the plate during the procedure, and aspects that need the attention of the user. The surgeon himself should have a proactive attitude and personally ensure that the grounding pad is adequately applied with firm contact to the skin over an adequate surface area.

Case report of electrocautery burn during cardiac surgery resulting in permanent disability later

Case facts: A 55-year-old patient who had acute chest pain due to rupture of aortic aneurysm. While he was being taken into operation, cardiopulmonary arrest developed. He was resuscitated intraoperatively and the operation was completed. After this operation burns on the anterior surface of the right hand, elbow, and the distal forearm were noticed, with second to third degree burn injuries, extending from his forearm to his fingers. He was treated with silver sulfadiazine dressings and fusidic acid. 2 years after the operation, he was referred to Department of Forensic Medicine for an expert report of his disability. He had a burn scar on the volar side and radial edge of his right forearm, and over the dorsum of his right thumb. There were atrophies on his right forearm, hand, and fingers and flexion contracture of his right elbow and hand, especially on his third finger. There were paresis of the plantar (2/5) and dorsal (1/5) flexion of the right elbow, and hand (3/5) and hypoesthesia on the whole of his right forearm and hand. The electromyography (EMG) revealed a total lesion of the right distal median nerve, severe lesion of the right radial nerve, moderate lesion of the ulnar nerve, and mild-moderate partial lesion of the right musculocutaneous nerve.

Opinion: He was right handed and there was a 57% loss of his complete ability, according to regulations determining impairment and loss of capacity to work and earn.

Citation: Demircin S, Aslan F, Karagoz YM, et al. Medicolegal aspects of surgical diathermy burns: a case report and review of the literature. Rom J Leg Med. 2013;21:173-6.

CASE LAW: Cautery burn during circumcision surgery (for nonmedical indication: cultural) resulted in loss of more than half of his genitalia

Case facts: A Muslim child underwent circumcision surgery under local anesthesia, and suffered cautery burns on the shaft of the penis with electric cautery to coagulate the bleeding while doing circumcision on 24-5-2001. On the next day, the child was again brought and discoloration and edema over the penis with signs of necrosis of the skin was noted. Entire shaft of penis was found denuded of epithelium with edges at the root of penis. The scrotum was red and edematous. Meatus was found covered with scab. There was no sensation of glans. Debridement was done on 8-6-2001 under anesthesia. Patient was referred to CMC, Vellore, where dead tissues were debrided on two occasions following which split thickness skin graft was applied to the skin and superficial tissues of the penis and a large superficial portion of the glans was sloughed off. The corpus spongiosum around the urethra was also sloughed off leaving a papery thin urethra exposed. Split thickness skin grafting over penile area was done under general anesthesia on 27-6-2001. The size of the penile shaft and the glans penis seems to have markedly shrunken in size to about half of the original size.

Plaintiff: After circumcision surgery, there was a lesion on the umbilicus and another on the back of right leg of the child. Child's father sought second opinion of plastic surgeon from another hospital, who documented that the burning and swelling was on account of electric cauterization done at the first hospital. On 2-6-2001 he was admitted at CMC, Vellore. He underwent skin drafting, taking the skin from the left thigh. The genital organ was reduced to half in size. He has also to apply some local aesthetic ointment and use a tube that has to be inserted for expelling urine. He could not attend classes. He still has to use the tube, etc. for removing urine. It is alleged that the entire consequences ensued was on account of the negligence on the part of the first surgeon. He had to spend about INR 40,000 for treatment at Vellore. He had also to spent amounts for travel, accommodation, etc. He has sought for a sum of INR 50,000 as compensation and INR 25,000 towards loss of 1 year of schooling. He has sought for INR 360,000 of the disability and altogether a sum of INR 500,000.

Defense: The pediatric surgeon contended that there is no negligence on the part of them. It is pointed out that the patient was having phimosis requiring urgent surgery, guardian's consent was taken before circumcision and risk of complications explained verbally. There was excessive bleeding at the site of circumcision, which could not be controlled. The bleeding was stopped by using electric cautery. It is denied that there was skin burn over the penis or burns and swelling over the umbilicus or the right lower limb. Necrosis may have resulted as adverse effect of Xylocaine injection used for anesthesia.

Discussion: No authority/literature has been produced to substantiate the contention that administration of Xylocaine can result in such consequences. We find that negligence on the part of the second opposite party is evident. Being a surgeon, a specialist he should have to done the procedure properly.

Decision: Negligence of pediatric surgeon was proved, hence a sum of 150,000 as monetary compensation with interest at 12% per annum from the date of complaint.

Take-home message: Negligent surgery done even for nonmedical indications can cost a fortune.

Citation: Noushad Rahman (Minor), versus City Hospital and Diagnostic Centre, on 9 November, 2010.

Scald burns to patients in the operating room (OR) can occur from dramatic events such as fire or relatively benign activities such as maintenance of normothermia. Burn injury in the OR is a significant source of morbidity for patients and a source of liability for anesthesiologists. The most common devices causing burns in the OR were intravenous (IV) bags or bottles.

CASE LAW: Iatrogenic burn due to placing hot water bag on legs of pediatric patient in operation theater

Case facts: An infant was undergoing surgery by pediatric surgeon for right inguinal hernia. During the operation, a hot water bottle was kept under baby's legs caused severe burns.

Plaintiff: The doctors kept an extremely hot water bag under the child's leg resulting in burns on both legs necessitating prolonged treatment and resulting in permanent scars.

Defense: Hot water bottle was required to prevent fall of body temperature during infant's surgery. Surgeon did his surgery well, but there was the possibility that the hot water bottle might have come into contact with steel plate attached with diathermy cautery machine and overheated the bottle.

Court decision: Expert evidence by plastic surgeon stated that there were scars on the legs of the child, resulting in permanent disability, requiring plastic surgery in future, to correct them. A compensation of INR 500,000 was awarded payable by pediatric surgeon, anesthetist, and the hospital jointly and severely.

Citation: Master PM. Ashwin and Others versus Manipal Hospital, Bangalore. 1997(1) CPR 393 (Karnataka).

BURN BY NEGLIGENCE AT DERMATOLOGY CLINICS CAUSING LASER BURNS OF SEVERE NATURE

Individuals who suffer an injury from a laser hair removal treatment may suffer second or third degree burns. Second degree burns penetrate past the top layer of skin, sometimes causing blisters, redness, and a sore sensation to the point of impact. This type of burn can cause the victim to suffer, possibly up to 3 weeks. Skin grafting is sometimes required to repair the damage of such burns. While individuals who are injured while receiving medical treatment or plastic surgery may sometimes file a medical malpractice lawsuit, this is not usually the cause of action for laser hair removal cases. This is because these procedures are usually not considered "medical treatment" but cosmetic enhancement for beautification at beauty parlors. Furthermore, they are often not required to be performed by a licensed doctor. Cosmetologists, technicians or other nonmedical personnel may be hired to complete these procedures.

CASE LAW ON ALLEGATION OF LASER BURNS: Who is permitted to practice laser assisted hair-removal? Only a dermatologist can do, or even a trained nurse can do?

Case facts: Patient, who had some unwanted hair on her face and neck, approached dermatologist clinic, for permanent removal of the same through laser technology, which was to be done in four sittings in 2007.

Plaintiff: It was alleged that patient was planning to arrange her marriage, but after laser burns, due to disfigurement of her face, her skin was burnt and scars appeared on her neck due to laser treatment, causing mental tension and psychological trauma after burn. Scars on the face and neck of patient were caused due to medical negligence and deficiency in service on the part of doctor's clinic, which ruined her personality and caused mental pain and agony besides financial loss. It was argued that the laser treatment should have been given by the doctor himself and could not be left to the technician. Fluency of 50J/cm² given to the complainant was on the higher side due to which scars appeared on her neck causing disfiguration.

Defense: Process of laser treatment was given by the technician who operated the laser machine and doctor had no role. It was mentioned that these machines such as X-ray, computed tomography (CT) scan, hair removal, and electrocardiogram (ECG), etc. are to be operated by the staff after proper training. There is no expert evidence produced by the complainant to prove that the scars are permanent in nature.

Decision: State Consumer Disputes Redressal Commission noted that suspicion of the patient having developed scars is not well founded and it is only hypopigmentation, which would fade away with the passage of time. Since this is a known side effect of the laser hair removal, the OPs could not hold liable for it and the complainants were expected have known the same and undertook the treatment within open mind that this hypopigmentation is likely to happen. There is therefore no deficiency in service by clinic.

Citation: Jitender Kumar Joshi. versus General Hospital on 13 September, 2011 https://indiankanoon.org/doc/7852787/.

Laser surgery has proliferated tremendously for the past 2 decades with regard to aesthetic and medical therapy for the skin. Common applications of lasers include depilation, removal of pigmented lesions, tattoo removal, treatment of vascular lesions, and facial rejuvenation, among multiple other applications. The most common procedure that ultimately results in litigation involves hair removal. Unsurprisingly, with the advent and increased use of laser technology in medicine has come a concomitant increase in lawsuits alleging malpractice arising out of the misuse of a laser device. This increase is partly attributable to the performance of laser surgery by untrained and nonphysician operators. Despite stringent regulatory requirements by the Food and Drug Administration regarding manufacturing and distribution, there is a lack of overarching federal regulation governing who can operate a laser, what procedures require physician supervision, and where the procedures are performed. A large number of physicians are offering laser skin treatments outside the scope of their specialty. Indemnity payments for medical malpractice historically have increased, and as more elective procedures are being performed, dermatologic surgeons as well as medical dermatologists performing procedural dermatology treatments are likely to face increasing claims. In an effort to identify common risk factors and errors, we sought to catalog common causes of action, allegations, injuries, and other trends associated with medical malpractice litigation secondary to cutaneous laser surgery. In a recent analysis of closed medical professional liability claims, improper performance of procedures was the most prevalent claim, with failure to supervise procedures and staff also included in this list.

From 1985 to 2012, Ray et al. (2013), identified 174 cases related to injury stemming from cutaneous laser surgery. Burns (47.0%), scars (38.8%), and pigmentary alterations (23.5%) were the most common alleged injuries. Burns included both second and third degree burns, as well as full-thickness necrosis. Of the 120 cases with public decisions, 61 (50.8%) resulted in decisions in favor of the plaintiff. The mean indemnity payment was $380,719.[20] The incidence of litigation related to laser surgery shows an increasing trend, with peak occurrence in 2010. Laser hair removal was the most common litigated procedure. Nonphysician operators accounted for a substantial subset of these cases, with their physician supervisors named as defendants, despite not performing the procedure. Plastic surgery was the specialty most frequently litigated against. Of the preventable causes of action, the most common was failure to obtain an informed consent.[20]

Specific allegations provide insight into how physicians could minimize their risk of litigation. First, physicians should ensure that their staff is trained and, if delegating a task, should supervise their staff to minimize the risk of injury or to truncate damage from injury should it occur. Second, laser operators should be careful when evaluating skin type and selecting the proper laser parameters for treatment. Finally, laser operators should bear in mind that in certain instances, it may be prudent to conduct a test spot before administering laser treatment, even though there are few data to support the utility of such practice.

Iatrogenic Radiation Burn

The person may also get electrocuted or sustain burn injuries by accidental exposure to X-rays or nuclear radiation in a hospital.

CONCLUSION

Save our career as doctors by proving accused's crime by timely meticulous medical documentation of burn in MLC and inform police in critically ill burned victims for DD. In current scenario of medicolegal litigation against doctors for extortion of money, as courts are giving hefty amounts in crores in medical negligence but gives meager amounts in thousands to victims of crime as per IPC. Example; a victim of acid burn will get fixed amount for covering treatment expenses from government, but if acid attack victim patient files negligence suit against doctor, who has treated his best facility, but scar will remain on face, and consumer court will find fault in medical documentation of consent or records and award hefty amounts to be paid by doctor to victim. Burn victims goes for out of court settlement with accused by taking money, and than files medical negligence case against doctor to claim compensation for alleged negligence in reporting crime, or for permanent damages due to injury. If the doctor reports crime and works for the law, doctor can safeguard his career and his reputation during false allegations.

REFERENCES

1. Section 357C of the Criminal Procedure Code. Available at https://www.kaanoon.com/indian-law/crpc-357c/
2. Criminal Law (Amendment) Act, 2018. Available at https://mha.gov.in/sites/default/files/CSdivTheCriminalLawAct_14082018_0.pdf

3. Acid Survivors Foundation at Bangladesh, Statistics, available at http://www.acidsurvivors.org/Statistics.
4. Acid Offence Control Act, 2002 and Acid Control Act,2002. Bangladesh Available at http://ncrb.gov.in/NCRB_Journal/NCRB_Journal_October_2018.pdf
5. Kumar P. Child abuse by thermal injury. Burns. 1984;10:344-8.
6. Morrison J. Statistical facts on acid attacks. Acid Survivors Foundation; 2003.
7. Singh G, Kumar A, Singh N. Dowry death and legal protection of women in India. Int J Appl Res. 2017;3(8):100-4.
8. Guo SS, Greenspoon JS, Kahn AM. Management of burn injuries during pregnancy. Burns. 2001;27:394-7.
9. Agrawal P. Thermal injury in pregnancy: predicting maternal and fetal outcome. Indian J Plast Surg. 2005;38(2):95-9.
10. Agarwal P, Kain R, Raina VK. Plastic surgery in rural area: a report. Indian J Plast Surg. 2005;38(1):30-3.
11. The Medical Termination of Pregnancy Act; 1971 (Act No. 34 of 1971).
12. The Registration of Births and Deaths Act; 1969 (Act No. 18 of 1969, Chapter III.
13. Ayoub C, Pfeifer D. Burns as a manifestation of child abuse and neglect. Am J Dis Child. 1979;133:910-4.
14. American Burn Association/ American College of Surgeons. Guidelines for the operation of burn centers. J Burn Care Res. 2007;28(1):134-41.
15. Directorate General of Health Services. (2017). National Programme for Prevention and Management of Burn Injuries. [online] Available from: dghs.gov.in/content/1357_3_NationalProgrammePreventionManagement.aspx [Accessed December 2018].
16. NPPMBI. Operational Guidelines for Establishment of Burns Units at Medical Colleges under National Programme for Prevention & Management of Burn Injuries (NPPMBI). [online] Available from: dghs.gov.in/WriteReadData/userfiles/file/Operational_Guidlines_Medical_College.pdf [Accessed December 2018].
17. Andronicus M, Oates RK, Peat J, et al. Non-accidental burns in children. Burns. 1998;24(6):552-8.
18. Hight DW, Bakalar HR, Lloyd JR. Inflicted burns in children. Recognition and treatment. JAMA. 1979;242(6):517-20.
19. Showers J, Garison KM. Burn abuse: a four-year study. J Trauma. 1988;28(11):1581-3.
20. Jalian HR, Jalian CA, Avram MM. Common causes of injury and legal action in laser surgery. JAMA Dermatol. 2013;149(2):188-93.

CHAPTER 49

Medical Negligence in Plastic, Aesthetic and Reconstructive Surgery

Rakesh Kumar Khazanchi

INTRODUCTION

With the introduction of consumer protection law, there has been a surge in litigation against doctors. Whereas majority of patients are satisfied with their care and outcome, in a small percentage of patients, things may go wrong and lead to medical negligence claims. In the current atmosphere where medical profession is seen more as a business venture rather than a service, this type of litigation is likely to increase. It is therefore imperative that one should have fundamental knowledge of medical negligence law in order avoid facing litigation and to have good defense, should such a situation arise.

A patient who has suffered harm through negligent conduct of a doctor has two avenues to bring action against the doctor:
- A civil action wherein the claimant files a case in the consumer court or a civil court and seeks financial compensation for damages.
- A criminal prosecution wherein a criminal charge of gross negligence brought against the doctor under criminal law for which the defendant may face imprisonment and fine.

There is a clear difference in the degree of negligence required in civil and criminal law.

CIVIL LAW

Majority of litigation following medical negligence is brought under the tort of negligence. In order to succeed, the claimant needs to prove the following three things:
- The doctor who is being sued owed him a duty of care
- The doctor was in breach of the duty of care
- The damage for which the clamant is seeking damages was caused by breach of this duty of care.

Duty of Care

The duty of care is easily established. Once a doctor sees a patient and starts treatment, he owes him a duty of care since his actions or lack of any action has the potential to cause injury. In certain situations the treating doctor may owe duty of care not only to the patient, but also to his family, where the family members may be at risk of getting the disease.

The Breach of Duty

Having established that the doctor owed a duty of care to the claimant, the claimant must prove that the doctor was negligent in discharge of his duty. In medical context it is difficult to define when an act by a doctor is negligent. The principle of finding a doctor negligent was laid down in a land mark British Case (*Bolam v Friern HMC*)[1] which held:

A doctor is not guilty of negligence if he has acted in accordance with a practice accepted as proper by a responsible body of medical men skilled in that particular art. There may be one or more perfectly proper standards and if the medical man conforms to one of those standards, he is not negligent even if there is a body of opinion that takes a contrary view.

This however does not mean that he can pursue any outdated or illogical technique, get some doctors to support it and escape liability. In a subsequent British Case (*Bolitho v City and Hackney Health Authority*)[2] it was held:

The court must be satisfied that the exponents of the body of opinion relied on should be able to demonstrate that such opinion has a logical basis.

Going deeper into the "*Bolam*" test, some noteworthy points are:
- The standard of care provided by doctor is to be judged against the average practitioner of the same specialty and not the highest expert in that field. A General Practitioner (GP) is to be judged against GP and a specialist against a specialist.
- A doctor is to be judged on the state of knowledge prevalent at the time of incident and not necessarily some treatment which has appeared in journals recently.

- The body of opinion in favor of the doctor does not need to be substantial body. Even if the number of experts in favor of the doctor are a fewer in comparison to those in favor of the claimant, the doctor likely to succeed.

In some cases, the doctrine of *res ipsa loquitur* (the thing speaks for itself) may be enough to prove negligence, e.g. leaving a sponge or an instrument inside a patient or operating on the wrong side.

Causation

Simply proving that the medical professional has been negligent in discharge of his or her duty does not mean that the claimant is entitled to damages claimed. It must also be shown that the negligence caused the damage for which compensation is claimed. The test that needs to be satisfied is the "but for" test, i.e. whether "but" for the doctor's negligence, the patient would not have suffered the injury. Many cases of medical negligence fail on the grounds of causation. A claimant will only succeed if he or she can show that on balance of probabilities, the injury was caused by the defendant's act or had the defendant not acted in negligent manner, the claimant would not have suffered the harm. In cases of complications postsurgery, if the claimant claims to have not been warned of the risk and it can be established that—if properly advised, he or she would not have undergone surgery, the claim can be established.

CRIMINAL NEGLIGENCE

Criminal negligence is the failure to exercise duty with reasonable and proper care and employing precautions guarding against injury to the public generally or to any individual in particular. It is, however, well settled that so far as the negligence alleged to have been caused by medical practitioner is concerned, to constitute negligence, simple lack of care or an error of judgment is not sufficient. Negligence must be of a gross or a very high degree to amount to criminal negligence.

There are two ways an aggrieved claimant may file a criminal complaint against a doctor. He may approach the police to file an FIR or in the event the police refuse to do this, he has an option of filing a private complaint in a court seeking the courts direction to the police to file an FIR.

Giving guidelines to the police in such cases, the Supreme Court in *Lalita Kumari v Government of UP*[3] (2014) held that in the case of allegations relating to medical negligence on the part of doctors, a preliminary inquiry is to be conducted by the police before registration of an FIR. This preliminary inquiry entails that the police has to mandatorily verify the allegations made in the complaint and cannot initiate proceedings on a mere complaint. While laying down guidelines in relation to prosecution of medical professionals the Court noted that once the criminal process is initiated, it subjects the medical professional to serious embarrassment and sometimes harassment. He has to seek bail to escape arrest, which may or may not be granted to him. At the end he may be exonerated by acquittal or discharge but the loss which he has suffered to his reputation cannot be compensated by any standards.

> Court issued guidelines in relation to prosecution of medical professionals and directed that:
> - A private complaint may not be entertained unless the complainant has produced *prima facie* evidence before the court in the form of a credible opinion given by another competent doctor to support the charge of rashness or negligence on the part of the accused doctor.
> - The investigating officer should, before proceeding against the doctor accused of rash or negligent act or omission, obtain an independent and competent medical opinion preferably from a doctor in government service, qualified in that branch of medical practice who can normally be expected to give an impartial and unbiased opinion applying the *Bolam test* to the facts collected in the investigation.
> - A doctor accused of rashness or negligence, may not be arrested in a routine manner (simply because a charge has been leveled against him). Unless his arrest is necessary for furthering the investigation or for collecting evidence or unless the investigating officer feels satisfied that the doctor proceeded against would not make himself available to face the prosecution unless arrested, the arrest may be withheld.

In *Martin F. D'Souza v Mohd. Ishfaq*,[4] (2009), it was directed that whenever a complaint is received against a doctor or hospital by the Consumer Forum (whether District, State or National) or by the criminal court, then before issuing notice to the doctor or hospital against whom the complaint was made the Consumer Forum or the criminal court should first refer the matter to a competent doctor or committee of doctors, specialized in the field relating to which the medical negligence is attributed, and only after that doctor or committee reports that there is a prima facie case of medical negligence should notice be then issued to the doctor or hospital concerned. This ruling was later partially overturned by the Supreme Court[5] which held that in the case of consumer court, expert opinion is required only when a case is complicated enough warranting expert opinion, or the facts of a case are such that forum cannot resolve the issue without expert assistance.

The level of negligence required to seek conviction of a medical professional under criminal law is of a much higher degree than in civil law. In the case of *Suresh Gupta (Dr)* versus *Government of NCT of Delhi*,[6] (2004), the Honorable Supreme Court, observed that for fixing criminal liability on a doctor or surgeon, the standard of negligence required to be proved should be so high as can be described as "gross negligence" or "recklessness." It is not merely lack of necessary care, attention and skill. It was further held that every careless act of the medical man cannot be termed as "criminal." It can be termed "criminal" only when the medical man exhibits a gross lack of competence or inaction and wanton indifference to his patient's safety and which is found to have arisen from gross ignorance or gross negligence. The Court came to the conclusion that where a patient's death results merely from error of judgment or an accident, no criminal liability should be attached to it.

In a landmark decision, the Supreme Court in *Jacob Mathew versus State of Punjab*,[7] (2005) upheld the earlier decision in *Suresh Gupta* and for the first time created a different standard of liability under criminal law for professionals such as doctors. The Court was cognizant that criminal law has invariably placed medical professionals on a pedestal different from ordinary mortals. Section 88[8] of the IPC provides exemption for acts not intended to cause death, done by consent in good faith for person's benefit. Section 92[9] provides for exemption for acts done in good faith for the benefit of a person without his consent even though the acts cause harm to a person and that person has not consented to suffer such harm.

The Court held that even though the word "gross" has not been used in Section 304-A IPC,[10] yet it is settled in criminal law that negligence or recklessness to be so held must be of such a high degree as to be "gross." The expression "rash or negligent act" as occurring in Section 304-A IPC[11] has to be read as qualified by the word "grossly." It further directed that to prosecute a medical professional for negligence under criminal law it must be shown that the accused did something or failed to do something which in the given facts and circumstances, no medical professional in his ordinary senses and prudence would have done or failed to do. The hazard taken by the accused doctor should be of such a nature that the injury which resulted was most likely imminent.

MEDICAL NEGLIGENCE IN PLASTIC SURGERY

Plastic and Reconstructive Surgeons are particularly vulnerable to malpractice claims because outcomes in their field are obvious on one hand and difficult to assess objectively on the other and these may not meet patient expectations. There are no data available in India as to the extent of malpractice claims against plastic surgeons in comparison with other specialties. In a study of malpractice claims between years 1985–2010 in the US, plastic surgery claims were 3.6% of the total closed claims and indemnity payment for plastic surgery procedure was 1.86% of total payments for all medical specialties combined.[12] These figures suggest that even in the US, claims associated with plastic surgery represent a small fraction of other specialties.

In an Online search of cases of medical negligence involving plastic surgeons which were decided by National or State Consumer Disputes Redressal Commission, all High Courts and Supreme Court of India, the author came across seven cases which went against the doctor. Of these, four were due to deficiency in treatment and three due to inability to support the defense with adequate records.

CASE I[13]

A patient presented with a swelling on the foot which was diagnosed to be a vascular malformation. It was excised, but the specimen was not subjected to histopathological examination. Biopsy of a recurrence after 6 months showed it to be a synovial sarcoma and the patient had to undergo above knee amputation. The State Commission found the hospital to be negligent. In appeal to the National Commission, the court again found the hospital to be negligent stating that had the excised tissue at the time of first operation been sent for histopathology, proper diagnosis would have been made at that time and a better or more effective line of treatment could have evolved. The order of the state commission was up held.

The lesson here is that any excised tissue must be submitted for histopathology.

CASE II[14]

A 15-year-old girl suffered crush injury of the leg. Surgery was done after a delay of 3 days. She died of septicemia and multiorgan failure. The complainant argued that undue delay lead to septicemia and death. The defense said that there was an overload of patients and no operating room could be made available and she had to wait for her turn. The state commission ruled in favor of the complainant. On appeal by the hospital, the National Commission dismissed the appeal and enhanced the compensation from 10 lakhs rupees to 20 lakhs rupees. It said that a prestigious institution should not work in a bureaucratic manner, i.e. treat the patient as per seniority in a queue but should do it in a professional manner.

The lesson here is that in such a situation, priorities of treatment should outweigh bureaucratic formalities and the hospital should have laid down standard operating procedures and guidelines to deal with such situations.

CASE III[15]

A patient with 50% TBSA burns received wrong blood transfusion resulting in complications. The patient died of septicemia 40 days later. The complainant argued that the patient's condition nosedived after wrong blood transfusions. The hospital argued that she had recovered from the complications caused by mismatched transfusion and later died of septicemia which was not connected to the transfusion. The State Commission found for the complainant and awarded compensation of 2 Lakhs. On appeal by the hospital, the National Consumer Dispute Redressal Commission (NCDRC) too held the doctors negligent stating that the mismatched transfusions materially contributed to patient's death and dismissed the appeal.

CASE IV[16]

The facts of case are as follows:
- Complainant suffered an injury to his foot after a fall from a motorbike.
- He took local treatment but developed severe pain, swelling, headache and vomiting, and was referred to the respondent 3 days later.
- He was admitted to the respondent's hospital with diagnosis of cellulitis, started on antibiotics, and magnesium sulfate dressing was done. No blood tests were advised and X-ray was done in the evening.
- Next day a black patch around the injury on the foot was noticed. As per records this patch was excised by the respondent in the ward and the process was painless.
- Next day, the complainant carried out a surgery, i.e. multiple incisions and drainage of edematous fluid with fasciotomy and decompression of leg.
- Patient's condition continued to worsen. Two days later another orthopedic surgeon was consulted who recorded his observations as necrosis of skin patches and sloughing of skin on the left leg (which the court concluded to be unmistakable symptoms of gangrene having set in and advanced to some parts of the leg). Next evening another plastic surgeon was consulted who recorded his observations of spreading gangrene involving the foot, ankle and 2/3rd of leg and advised debridement.
- Debridement was carried out the day after.
- The complainant left against medical advice next day and got himself admitted in another hospital where further debridement and fasciotomy was done. He eventually required skin grafting of multiple leg and foot wounds.

The State Commission found that there was no evidence against the doctor having committed any negligence or deficiency of service.

On appeal, the National Commission reversed the judgment and found for the complainant on the following grounds:
- This was a case of cellulitis progressing on to necrotizing fasciitis.
- While a correct diagnosis of cellulitis was made, no blood tests, cultures of pus or fluid or blood were done till just before the second

surgery. At no stage did the respondent make an explicit diagnosis of necrotizing fasciitis till it was in an advanced stage and other specialists were consulted.
- The surgery of debridement and fasciotomy done were inadequate as the same had to be repeated in another hospital.
- They further noted that there was no informed consent on record for the first surgery and the same for second surgery was signed by his mother while there was nothing to prevent the complainant from signing it.

The appeal was partly allowed and lump sum compensation of 100,000 rupees was awarded.

The lesson here is that the records must be complete and indicate the treating doctors thought process and reasoning of line of treatment chosen which could explain the reasons for delay in diagnosis. The author is not in agreement with court's observations that the surgery done was inadequate as the same surgery was repeated in another hospital. It should have been brought to court's notice with supporting evidence that very often multiple debridements are required in patients with necrotizing fasciitis.

CASE V[17]

Facts of the case are as follows:
- An 8-month-old child with cleft palate, who was having recurrent episodes of pneumonia, was taken for surgery 2 weeks after one such episode without any recorded preoperative tests and pre anesthetic check.
- On induction, the patient suffered severe bronchospasm for which resuscitation was immediately started and surgery was abandoned.
- The child went into persistent vegetative state which on subsequent consultation was diagnosed to be hypoxic brain damage.

The state commission found for the complainants on following grounds:
- Not conducting the required preoperative investigations and to performing an operation without these when there was no emergency.
- Not taking due care during administration of anesthesia and giving thiopentone which is known to be risky in patients with respiration tract infection.

A compensation of 3 lakh rupees was awarded. On appeal by the complainant to enhance the compensation and nursing home owners to absolve them of any wrong doing as the facilities provided by them were not found to be deficient, the National Commission observed that since the surgeon and anesthesiologist were on the pay roll of the nursing home and regardless of whether they were consultants or full time staff, the nursing home cannot be absolved of its responsibilities which they have to share with the others. They upheld the State Commissions decision and enhanced the compensation to 700,000 rupees.

CASE VI[18]

The facts of the case are as follows:
- A middle aged male sought liposuction to reduce obesity and overweight at the respondents hospital. He failed to disclose that he was suffering from hypothyroidism.
- Following anesthesia and after injection of tumescent fluid, the patient had a cardiac arrest, was given cardiopulmonary resuscitation (CPR) and revived within 3 minutes. Surgery was abandoned and patient shifted to ICU. Subsequently the patient was diagnosed to have hypoxic brain damage and after prolonged treatment in different hospitals, he died about 4 months later.

An expert opinion from AIIMS found many deficiencies in the management. While the respondents challenged the qualification and experience of the AIIMS medical board, the board's main argument was that there was no detailed tabular representation of vitals and SPO_2 in the records. Two senior anesthesiologist on behalf of respondents gave opinion that there was no negligence in anesthetic management of the patient in period leading up to bradycardia and cardiac arrest.

The court relied heavily on AIIMS opinion and opined that the patient had hypoxia which was not detected in time and the resuscitation was not proper and/or timely and resulted in brain damage. Based on this, they found both the surgeon and the anesthetist negligent and awarded a compensation of 25 lakhs rupees.

The main lesson here is the importance of maintaining detailed intraoperative records of vital signs and events if and when they happen. There should also be a detailed informed consent in all patients.

CASE VII[19]

Facts of the case are:
- In 2005 he consulted the defendant for a postseptoplasty nasal deformity and breathing difficulty. After examination and analysis the defendant gave him the option of L-shaped graft and surgery was done subsequently.
- The complainant was aggrieved that the doctor had given him a long scar, the tip was dispositioned, ala muscles were dysfunctional and he found it difficult to breath.
- The complainant later underwent operations in multiple other hospitals.

The State Commission did not find any merit in the case and found for the defendant. The complainant filed an appeal with the National Commission, his main complaint was that an L-shaped graft was not done and cartilage implanted obstructed his breathing. It was further admitted that the operation notes were not available and neither were these written in the discharge summary.

The court concluded that:
- L-shaped graft was essential to cure him in the first place.
- There are no operation notes available to substantiate what was done.
- Subsequent surgeries proved that L-shaped graft was not done.

The national commission found for the appellant and awarded a compensation of 5 Lakh rupees. The defendant has appealed in the Supreme Court against the decision of National Commission forum and appeal is pending.

Above case once again signifies the importance of good records.

CASE VIII[20]

In this case, a claim was made for a poor result after multiple scar revisions. The surgeon was held not liable as he gave proper treatment with due care and the court held that there can be no guarantee of a result.

CASE IX[21]

In this case, a patient claimed for a failed replant. The court found for the doctors on the grounds that there was no inordinate delay or defect in the surgery done. The court also made an important observation that unless a healthcare provider has given an explicit guarantee or warranty or assurance in writing, no action is maintainable against him for such a claim.

CONCLUSION

In the face of increasing threats of litigation by patients, the doctors must first ensure that their house is in order. Their practice must be ethical and evidence based, medical records must be meticulously maintained, and they must maintain proper and honest communication with the patient and family at all times. Good communication is the most important key to prevent litigation. Should one be confronted with a malpractice suit, the law offers enough protection to those whose practice is ethical and evidence based and is supported by proper documentation.

REFERENCES

1. Tort-Negligence-Standard of Care for Medical Professionals. Bolam v Friern Hospital Management Committee [1957] 1 WLR 583. [online] Available from https://www.lawteacher.net/cases/bolam-v-friern-hospital-management.php/. [Accessed December, 2018].
2. Tort-Negligence-Standard of Care for Medical Professionals-Causation. Bolitho v City and Hackney Health Authority [1998] AC 232. [online] Available from https://www.lawteacher.net/cases/bolitho-v-hackney.php/. [Accessed December, 2018].
3. Criminal Procedure Code, 1973. Lalita Kumari v. Govt. of U.P., (2014) 2 SCC 1. [online] Available from http://www.supremecourtcases.com/index2.php?do_pdf=1&id=44552&itemid=99999999&option=com_content/. [Accessed December, 2018].
4. M Katju. Martin F. D'Souza v. Mohd. Ishfaq, (2009) 3 SCC 1. [online] Available from https://indiankanoon.org/doc/1092676/. [Accessed December, 2018].
5. Ganguly. V Kishan Rao v Nikhil Super speciality Hospital and another, (2010) 5 SCC 513. [online] Available from https://indiankanoon.org/doc/1920027/. [Accessed December, 2018].
6. Dharmadhikari. Suresh Gupta (Dr.) v. Govt. of NCT of Delhi, (2004) 6 SCC 422. [online]

Available from https://indiankanoon.org/doc/650550/. [Accessed December, 2018].
7. R Lahoti. Jacob Mathew v. State of Punjab, (2005) 6 SCC 1. [online] Available from http://jajharkhand.in/wp/wp-content/judicial_updates_files/15_Motor_Vehicle_Act/05_Professional_Negligence/Jacob_Mathew_vs_State_Of_Punjab_&_Anr_on_5_August,_2005.PDF/. [Accessed December, 2018].
8. Central Government Act. Section 88 of the Indian Penal Code. [online] Available from https://indiankanoon.org/doc/862963/. [Accessed December, 2018].
9. Central Government Act. Section 92 of the Indian Penal Code. [online] Available from https://indiankanoon.org/doc/870189//. [Accessed December, 2018].
10. Central Government Act. Section 304 of the Indian Penal Code. [online] Available from https://indiankanoon.org/doc/409589/. [Accessed December, 2018].
11. Central Government Act. Section 304A of the Indian Penal Code. [online] Available from https://indiankanoon.org/doc/1371604/. [Accessed December, 2018].
12. Weng WW, Ford RS, Ford AR, et al. Medical malpractice risk assessment in Plastic Surgery. Plast Reconst Surg. 2012;130:1-65.
13. Case I (2017) NCDRC 32.
14. Case II (2015) NCDRC 13.
15. Case III (2009) 75 SCC 330.
16. Case IV (2009) NCDRC 202.
17. Case V (2012) NCDRC 512.
18. Case VI (2016) NCDRC 775.
19. Case VII (2016) NCDRC 1524.
20. Case VIII (2015) NCDRC 824.
21. Case IX (2016) NCDRC 74.

CHAPTER 50

Medicolegal Issues in Setting-up a Plastic Surgery Day Care Surgery Set-up

Milan Doshi, Rani Umul Khair Mulla

INTRODUCTION

India is a rapidly developing economy. Culture contact, Bollywood influence, increasing awareness, Internet and communication media, an increasing disposable income, and a one-to-one service-based industry have increased the demand and service front of cosmetic surgery in India.

In parallel with the clinic culture in dermatology, which has evolved including surgical procedures in clinical set-up, it has been realized that people opt for a clinic over hospital set-up to undergo cosmetic procedures as the overall cost of the procedure is quite economical. Clinical set-up is also more comfortable and convenient. Bearing this in mind, offering cosmetic surgical procedures at optimum safety and avoiding medicolegal litigations are of utmost importance. Over the last decade, a number of cosmetic surgery centers operated by independent doctors have increased. Government authorities consider Cosmetic Surgery Center/Clinic as a commercial enterprise and as a service provider comes under the Consumer Protection Act, 1986. Clinical establishments in the country are regulated by The Clinical Establishment (Registration and Regulation) Act, 2010. With the exception of clinical establishments run by the Armed Forces, this act is applicable to all types of clinical establishments.[1]

The lacunae in the medical training and its curriculum leave most of the doctors with insufficient knowledge in business/hospital management. However, owning a commercial enterprise has legal responsibilities and in this chapter, we will be emphasizing on the operation theater (OT) set-up in a day care center complying with the standards, as has been addressed in the chapter on Legal aspects in setting-up a clinic.

MINIMUM REQUIREMENTS TO SET-UP AN OPERATION THEATER IN PLASTIC SURGERY DAY CARE CENTER

Guidelines requirements (when we speak of day care surgery) are minimum standards that support the safety of both patients and staff, in the surgical and surgical support areas of the establishment.

Operation theater is a dynamic area of the day care center. Good designing of the surgical unit allows surgical procedures to be carried out efficiently and maximize safety and comfort of the patients. It also contributes to enhanced staff morale due to smooth flow of work. Hence, planning and execution are essential for the establishment and smooth operation of the OT.[2] The entire process needs an coordinated planning among the medical, engineering, electronic, and biomedical departments considering the safety of the patient and the need, preference, and safety of the medical staff.[2]

Surgical procedures that were previously performed in an inpatient hospital setting are now increasingly performed in outpatient facilities. Members of the Health Guidelines Revision Committee (HGRC) have recommended that the physical environment for surgery irrespective of inpatient or outpatient setting should meet the same standards. As the day care setting does not require a lot of equipment or staff, there is flexibility regarding the space requirements, however, without compromising asepsis.

Requirements to set-up an OT in plastic surgery day care center can be briefed as follows:

Infrastructure

Surgical room requirements usually include communications base/reception, admissions lounge with patient changing facilities, waiting area, interview examination room, staff support areas (changing room, toilets, team reporting station), storage (for instrument packs, fluids, consumables and disposables, fire hazard, medicines fridges/freezers, equipment, stationery, linen and specimens), disposal (dirty utility, disposal hold, domestics room), recovery, theater suites comprising of scrub room, preparation room, operating room and anesthetic rooms, and sometimes office and training areas.

Goal[3]

1. Ensure the safety of patients undergoing surgical procedures
2. Protection of the surgical team.

Objectives[3]

The main objectives are to ensure: (1) Appropriate preoperative assessment and preparation of the patient, (2) adequate preparation for anesthesia and surgical procedures, (3) observation of asepsis and the principles of sterile technique, and (4) appropriate postoperative care.

THEATER DESIGN: (KEY ASPECTS OF THEATER DESIGN) AND THEATER ROOM

Theater Complex

Operating departments have specialized ventilation requirements. OTs use positive-pressure ventilation of filtered air for four main functions:

1. To dilute airborne contamination.
2. To control air movement within the OT to minimize the transfer of airborne contaminants from less clean to cleaner areas.
3. To control the temperature and humidity of the space
4. To assist the removal of waste anesthetic gases.

Theater is the workstation of the surgeon and it encompasses the following essential areas:

Types of operating theaters:[4,5]
Based on the ventilation, there are two main types of OT's.

Ventilation should be based on the principle of unidirectional flow movement. The direction of air flow should be from the OT toward the main entrance.[6,7]

In the conventional OT, a mechanical ventilation duct delivers 20–24 air circulations per hour (ACH) into the room and exhaust evacuates it.

Laminar flow OT is a unidirectional airflow system that recirculates 80% of the air. Airflow can be up to 300 m/s (meters per second). This type of OT is recommended for highly sterile operations like implant surgery.

Air-conditioning units must be changed at regular intervals as the ducts are a source of microorganisms, which pass through their filters.[4,5]

Temperature and humidity:[3]
The temperature should be maintained at 21 ± 3°C inside the OT all the time with corresponding relative humidity between 50% and 60%. Sparks form more readily with low humidity with potential fire hazard. Ideally, temperature and humidity regulators and monitors should be installed in the OT.

Theater Room

Layout and Design[8]

The minimum square footage for an outpatient operating room included in the *2014 FGI Guidelines for Design and Construction of Hospitals and Outpatient Facilities* was determined by combining the square footage of the minimum number of people required in the OT and the minimum amount of equipment required. A space of approximately 4 feet (1.22 meters) on all four sides of the sterile field was recommended for safe traffic pathway. The sterile field includes the OT table width of 1.75 feet plus 2 feet for outstretched patient armrests on each side, which also accommodates scrubbed personnel.

The safe traffic pathway allows two people in the sterile field, to pass each other without contaminating their sterile attire by touching unsterile surfaces. Safe traffic pathway provides space for personnel to set up a sterile field, space for the stretcher for patient evacuation in case of an emergency, enough space to pass between the back table and the wall during the procedure, and to pass at the head end of the patient without interfering with the work of the anesthesiologist.[8]

Operation theater room should preferably be square (6 m × 6 m) with more than 4 m height of concrete ceiling for effective laminar flow.

There should be only one operation table per OT. Electromechanical tables are more convenient for intraoperative change of patient position and avoiding accidental contamination of sterile field.

The minimum equipment for a surgical procedure includes:
- *Equipment for anesthesia*: Anesthesia machine with the anesthesia supply cart, professional chair for the anesthesiologist, intravenous pole, equipment delivery system cart, portable documentation station with chair, trash container, and a sharps disposal receptacle.
- *Equipment for surgery*: Instrument trolley, two trash containers, hazardous waste receptacle, mayo stand, kick bucket, soiled linen container, surgical field suction attached to a wall, image viewers.

Sewage/drain pipe, fire pipe, and sprinkler should not be installed inside the OT. Theater lights ideally should be shadowless helium/LED (light-emitting diode) based. Anesthesia machine should be low-flow anesthesia circuit machine.[4,9]

Walls and Ceilings

The walls and ceiling must be solid and robust as they are used to mount essential equipment, which helps to reduce crowding of the floor area.

The walls must be fitted with outlets for oxygen, other medical gases, and vacuum. Anesthetic gas scavenging system should ideally be fitted at floor level. Multiple electric outlets should be fitted on the walls 2–3 feet height from the floor.

Floor edges should be curved up the wall to 2.5 cm for the ease of cleaning. Main door of the OT complex should be ideally 1.2–1.5 m wide. Ideally, sliding doors are recommended as with swing doors, every time doors swing open the microbial count in the air rises. The doors to the OT complex must remain closed unless indicated, particularly during an operation.

X-ray film illuminators should be preferably recessed into the wall.

Electrical Requirements

All electrical equipment in the OT needs proper grounding.

Following criteria are ideal with respect to electricity in OT complex:[4]
- Circuit interrupters are desirable, if there is an overload or ground fault.
- Power line should be 220 Volts
- Ceiling mounted equipment should have locking plugs to avoid accidental disconnection.
- Insulation around electrical power sources should withstand frequent bendings and flexings to prevent cracks.
- Wall outlets should be installed 2–3 feet above ground (as already mentioned).
- Use of explosion proof plugs.
- Avoid multiple outlets from single electrical source, multiple sources should be available.
- Electrical load calculation should be based on equipment likely to be used and appropriate current carrying capacity cords to be used.
- *Emergency power*: OT electrical networks need to be connected to the emergency generators with automatic two-way changeover facility.

SCRUB SPACE

Definition[3]

The surgical scrub is the process of mechanical and chemical antiseptics washing for the removal of possible dirt, natural skin oils, and microorganisms from the hands and forearm before participating in an operative procedure.

Scrub room should preferably be in-between OT or next to the OT. It should always be equipped with plumbing line and a drain line for supply and outflow of the water from scrubber respectively. Water supply should be at the rate of 400 liters per bed per day, with a separate reserve emergency overhead tank provided for OT.

Handwashing Facilities

Ideally, taps should be elbow or foot operated. The scrubber sink should have handsfree operation through infrared sensors or have manual foot operation mode.

The scrub sinks should be used only for scrubbing or handwashing and should not be used to clean or rinse contaminated instruments or equipment. The sink should be deep and wide enough to prevent splashing.

Procedural hand hygiene includes a full surgical scrub from the fingertips to the elbow using running water and 4% chlorhexidine scrub solution. Scrubbing should be performed for a minimum of 2–3 minutes.

A dedicated scrub and gowning room should be provided for the OT with sufficient space for a minimum of three people (minimum size: 11 m²).

DIRTY UTILITY[10]

Dirt utility should be large enough to enable cleaning of theater equipment, and disposal of human waste like the contents of bedpans, vomit bowls, etc. It consists of a deep sink and hopper with a concealed cistern. Mops and buckets used in theater are also stored here. It should necessarily have a handwashing facility.

Recovery[11]

The recovery room must be situated near the OT, as it should be easily accessible to the doctor in the event of a medical emergency.[3]

After the procedure is performed, the patient is shifted to the recovery room/PACU (post-anesthesia care unit); as this is usually managed by the anesthesiologist.

The recovery room should be equipped with an emergency trolley with different items, such as resuscitation medication, syringes, needles, intravenous infusions with different intravenous sets. A monitor with a defibrillator must be available in the recovery room at all times. Oxygen supply, masks, endotracheal tubes, and laryngoscope should be available. Suction apparatus should be in working condition.

Recovery is a continuous process and can be divided into three phases:
1. *Phase 1—Early recovery*: Awakening and recovery of vital reflexes
2. *Phase 2—Intermediate recovery*: Immediate clinical recovery as coordination and allowing ambulation/home readiness
3. *Phase 3—Late recovery*: Full recovery including its psychological recovery.

Recovery is usually achieved by using different scoring system. The Aldrete's and Keoulik scoring system was first described in 1970. With the advent of pulse oximetry as a more reliable indicator of oxygenation; the modified Aldrete's scoring system has been designed.

The Modified Aldrete's Scoring System

- *Activity*—Able to move voluntarily or on command:
  - 4 extremities 2
  - 2 extremities 1
  - 0 extremities 0
- *Respiration*:
  - Able to deep breath and cough freely 2
  - Dyspnea, shallow, or limited breathing 1
  - Apneic 0.
- *Circulation*:
  - BP ± 20 mm of preanesthesia level 2
  - BP ± 20–50 mm of preanesthesia level 1
  - BP ± 50 mm of preanesthesia level 0.
- *Consciousness*:
  - Fully awake 2
  - Arousable on calling 1
  - Not responding 0.
- *Oxygen saturation*:
  - Able to maintain oxygen saturation more than 92% on room air—2
  - Oxygen saturation less than 90% even with oxygen supplementation—1
  - Need oxygen inhalation to maintain saturation more than 90%—0

Discharge Criteria

Following criteria should be met by the patient prior to discharge:
- Patient should be accompanied by a responsible adult.
- The patient should be oriented to time, place, and person. He/she should be able to ambulate independently.
- Vital signs should be within acceptable ranges of preoperative levels (i.e. 20% above or below preoperative levels).

- There should be minimal bleeding or discharge from the operative site.
- Pain should be controlled, and at least 1 hour has passed since receiving a narcotic.
- Patient should have voided and is able to tolerate oral fluids. Nausea and vomiting are controlled.
- There should be return of sensory and motor abilities after regional anesthesia.

When the patient is ready for discharge or if criteria are not met prior to unit closing time, physician/designee should be notified. The physician will evaluate the patient and suggest discharge or advice admission and or assignment to observation status and document depending upon the circumstances.

There are also other guidelines like Wetchler's and Kortilla's guidelines for safe discharge after ambulatory surgery.[12,13]

Upon discharge, patient is provided with the information and education regarding analgesia, oral intake of food and fluids, postoperative instructions, and time to revisit is written on patient case paper.[11]

STAFF AREAS

Men and women change to OT attire before entering the OT in the designated changing rooms. Lockers and lavatory are essential to staff areas.

Sanitary facility for staff: One wash basin and one western closet (WC) should be provided for 8–10 persons. Showers are optional.[7]

LASER ADAPTATION

It is imperative that the laser room should not be integrated with the OT. However, depending upon the surgeon's preferences cases needing on table laser requirement for instance facial laser resurfacing with surgical face lift the laser machine can be moved to the theater.

THEATER EQUIPMENT: SURGICAL INSTRUMENTS, MISCELLANEOUS THEATER ROOM EQUIPMENT

All equipment shall be kept in good working condition through a process of periodic inspection, cleaning, and maintenance. An equipment log-book shall be maintained for all the major equipment.[14]

Clinical staff must check that the theater environment is fit for use prior to the day's surgery commencing. This includes checking that the ventilation provision to each theater suite is working. Some systems have integral alarms to alert staff to outage, this might be auditory or a warning light. It is imperative that teams are trained in the procedure to follow, if ventilation is prevented for any period of time.

ANESTHESIA AND RESUSCITATION

The procedure is performed, with close involvement of the anesthesiologist; his/her professional skill will greatly determine the success of day surgery.[15] At least one anesthesiologist should be in the team involved in planning an OT. It is imperative that certain mandatory considerations with respect to the anesthetic equipment and monitors be planned during the planning and design stage itself.[4]

Standard preoperative guidelines should be followed whether the patient is low-risk or high-risk or whether a procedure is performed under local or general anesthesia. Ideally, an anesthetist should always be available even when a procedure is performed under local anesthesia unless the surgeon/member of the available team in capable of managing untoward complications of local anesthetic medications. Where these procedures are performed outside a main theater complex, clear, agreed and regularly tested protocols and pathways must be in place to enable the patient to receive advanced medical care, including intensive care, in a timely manner.[16]

It is expected that only patients with an American Society of Anesthesiologists (ASA) 1 or ASA 2 score will be offered day care surgeries.[17]

Preoperative assessment is essential for the smooth running of surgery. The purpose of preoperative assessment is to ensure that the patient is fit for the planned procedure. This process should instill confidence in the patient, minimize unexpected problems, and prevent late cancellation. Preoperative assessment is increasingly undertaken at the initial consultation.[16]

No local anesthesia technique is totally free of the risk of serious systemic adverse events, which may occur irrespective of the choice of surgery or anesthetic technique. Contributing factors include pre-existing medical conditions, anxiety, and pain or stress reactions to the operation.[16]

Contraindications to Local Anesthesia[16]

These may include:
- Patient refusal after careful counseling
- Local sepsis
- Grossly abnormal coagulation
- Severe reaction, allergy, or other complication of local anesthesia (LA)
- Confusion, inability to communicate, or to comply with instructions
- Uncontrolled tremor
- Inability to adopt acceptable positioning.
  The alternative is general anesthesia or LA with sedation.

As per the ISA (Indian Society of Anaesthesia) Guidelines, a patient undergoing a procedure under local anesthesia need a minimum of complete blood count (CBC), urine routine, and chest X-ray as a baseline investigation. After the age of 35 years, an electrocardiography (ECG) and more than 50 years a 2D-ECHO are mandatory.

Test dose of local anesthesia should always be given preoperatively to check for sensitivity. Preoperative intravenous (IV) cannulation is mandatory. Detailed and complete documentation should be stressed upon. Monitors need to be in working condition and systemic parameters always recorded. In case of untoward event during the procedure under local anesthesia always call for help. He/she could be a paramedic, physician, and ideally an anesthetist/intensivist. And if need arises, patient should be transferred to the nearest hospital equipped to handle the situation after confirming their acceptance of the patient.

Surgeons and resuscitation team including the nurses should be trained in Basic Life Support and Adult Cardiac Life Support at regular intervals as per the recommendations of local bodies.

The routine and emergency drug box should be routinely checked and reported once a month for refill and check date of expiry.

Emergency Equipment Required[14]

Resuscitation equipment including laryngoscope, endotracheal tubes, suction equipment, xylocaine spray, oropharyngeal and nasopharyngeal airways, Ambu Bag—adult and pediatric (neonatal if indicated).

- Oxygen cylinders with flow meter/tubing/catheter/face mask/nasal prongs
- Suction apparatus
- Defibrillator with accessories
- Equipment for dressing/bandaging/suturing
- *Basic diagnostic equipment*: Blood pressure apparatus, stethoscope, weighing machine, thermometer
- ECG machine
- Pulse oximeter
- Nebulizer with accessories.

DRUGS AND THERAPEUTIC AGENTS

In resemblance to hospital set-up, a day care unit should have adequate drugs, medical devices and consumables commensurate with the scope of services. Emergency drugs and consumables should always be available. Drug storage shall be in a clean, well lit, and safe environment.

MINIMIZING RISK OF CONTAMINATION

Infection Control Measures in OT

It is essential that the clean to dirty workflow within theaters is maintained, and clean and dirty elements are kept separate.

Evidence-based infection control principles and practices include:[18]
- Sterilization
- Disinfection
- Adherence to universal precaution.

Cleaning of floors and other area should be done as specified in the housekeeping Standard Operating Procedure (SOP). The tables should be redraped with Macintosh and a cotton cloth after every case, and OT table should be cleaned periodically.[18]

Periodic swab culture and sensitivity test of OT (OT table/shadowless lamp/floor/OT trolley/shelf or platform over which sterilized drums are kept) have to be done. Register for swab culture and sensitivity should be maintained.[19,20]

FUMIGATION[20]

Objective

To prevent transmission of infection to the healthcare worker and patient.

Preparation for Fumigation

Clean the whole area, floor, and equipment. Close air incoming or outgoings like AC, ducting, exhaust.

Before putting the fumigation agent open all the drawers, trolleys, etc.

Procedure

- Take fumigation machine
- Add 200 mL formalin solution
- Keep the machine at the center of the area and set the desired time for fumigation
- Seal the door from outside
- Put a notice on the door: Stating "under fumigation"
- ....Date
- ....Time: started at and end at

Precautions to be taken
- Do not dilute formalin with water
- Do not open the door until the fumigation process gets over
- Do not come in contact with the formalin solution.

Fumigation records should be maintained with the date, time, and the person who performed the procedure.

Disinfection of Equipment

Reuse of instruments, endoscopes, etc. can only be performed after decontamination and sterilization. Equipment should never be handled with used/soiled gloves.

Spill cleanup: Spills of blood or body fluids should be covered with 1% of freshly prepared sodium hypochlorite for 10 minutes. This should be followed by mop drying. If necessary, a second decontamination may be performed. After the above process, the area is further cleaned with detergent and water.[20]

Linen Management[14,20]

Used linen must be placed in plastic bags taking care to prevent seepage of blood-body fluids. Where linen is contaminated, appropriate decontamination shall be carried prior to dispatch for washing. Appropriate cleaning agents should be used to wash the linen.

Universal Precautions[19-21]

It is an essential infection control measure. Features include:
- Use of personal protective equipment (PPE)
- Management of sharps
- Handwashing.

Personal Protective Equipment

The aim of theater attire is to:
- Minimize the transfer of microorganisms from the surgical team to the patient.
- Provide the surgical team with some protection from the patient.
- Instill a sense of discipline among the surgical team members and others working in the OT.

Components of attire:
Each component of OT attire is a specific means of protecting the patient from the sources of contamination and thereby the risk of infection.
- *Body cover*: Scrub suits and dresses
- Surgical mask
- Head cover
- *Eye protection*: (Goggles and face shields) should be used in any situation where splash injury to the eyes could occur.
- Appropriate operation room shoes and shoe covers
- Gown
- Gloves.

Management of Sharps

Sharps handling should be absolutely minimized. Surgical blades should be removed to and from a handle with an appropriate instrument. Intraoperatively, a kidney tray should be used by the scrub nurse to hand over the surgical blade/needle-mounted needle holder to the surgeon and vice-versa. At the end of the procedure, needles and sharps should be disposed safely in a disposable device.

Handwashing

Appropriate handwashing is an essential component of infection prevention and should be inculcated at appropriate levels.

CLEANING CENTRAL STERILE SERVICES DEPARTMENT (CSSD) PROCEDURES

Ethylene oxide (EtO) gas sterilization, moist heat sterilization, dry heat sterilization, and H_2O_2 gas plasma vapor sterilization are various sterilization modalities. Autoclaving is used most commonly. Most day care centers, these days, have both autoclave and EtO gas sterilization.

Autoclaving[20]

Objective

To sterilize the articles, dressing material, trays, drums, etc.

Procedure

The process includes:
- *Cleaning of articles*
- *Material preparation*
- *Loading autoclave*
- *Operating autoclave*
- *Unloading autoclave.*

Autoclave log must be maintained: These records are used for maintenance/service schedules and reporting of incidents, accidents, and/or faults. Entries should include: operator's name, date, time, and duration.

Maintenance and repair are to be monitored by the incharge. The autoclave should be serviced regularly.

BIOMEDICAL WASTE MANAGEMENT[20,22]

Objective: Prevent harm to workers, property, and general public and protect the environment.

Segregation, collection, transportation, storage, and disposal of biomedical waste shall be as per Biomedical Waste Handling Rules, and that of general waste shall be as per applicable local laws.

Every nursing station should have the biomedical waste management chart displayed on the wall. There should be a display on the bins as well. Every staff member should follow biomedical waste management policy and the infection control nurse will supervise this. The syringes should be cut and the needle should be burned before discarding. New staff should be trained by the nurse incharge.

PLANNED PREVENTIVE MAINTENANCE AND QUALITY CONTROL (TABLE 1)

Operation Theaters[5,23,24]

Culture swabs and air sampling plates are sent from OTs after fumigation every fortnightly.

Monitoring of Working OT

Air sampling of a working OT is done once a month. Sampling of in use disinfectants: 1 mL of sample of in-use disinfectants, hand-wash agents are sent to microbiology laboratory in

TABLE 1: Procedures and responsibilities for quality control of operation theater environment.[5,19]

Sr. No.	Procedures	Responsibility
1.	Before bringing the patient to the OT complex, the fitness of the patient for undergoing surgery should be checked	Surgeon
2.	PAC (preanesthesia checkup) should be done before surgery and the documents should be stored	Anesthetist
3.	All the happenings during the surgery should be properly documented for medicolegal purposes	Anesthetist
4.	Slipper stand should be stationed at the entrance of the OT complex and any entrance in outside slippers should be prohibited	OT incharge nurse
5.	OT store: Consumables and other supplies such as gloves, catheters, Ryle's tubes, infant feeding tubes, suction cannula, mucus extractors, etc. should be kept in buffer as per the load. OT store register should be maintained properly.	OT incharge nurse
6.	Consent form: • Consent form for the surgery should be obtained from the relatives of the patient. The relatives should always be counseled regarding the type of surgery and its pros and cons	Anesthetist
	• It should be clearly mentioned on the consent form that the jewelry and other valuables of the patients have been returned to the patient attendants. The list of valuables should be clearly mentioned	OT incharge nurse

(OT: operation theater)

a sterile container once a month or 6 month or annually depending upon the local policies.

Records are kept with OT incharge. In case of unacceptable results, decision on corrective measures is taken.

Central Sterile Supply Department

Swabs are sent for sterility check after cleaning weekly. Records kept by pathology department.

Managing Exposure to Potentially Infectious Body Fluid

Categories of exposure:
- Needlestick injuries
- Nonintact skin exposure
- Mucosal exposure, e.g. splash into eye.

DISASTER PREPAREDNESS AND MANAGEMENT

This includes preparedness and risk reduction in handling medical emergencies and fire disasters. All the OT staff should essentially be trained in BLS. Defibrillator is an essential parameter required as per law in every OT. Multiparameter monitor should be available in the OT and recovery. The unit must be designed to evacuate during a fire incident and the team trained to evacuate safely.

MONITORING QUALITY—USE OF AUDIT AND STANDARDS[15,25]

Clinical auditing is a process of improving the quality of medical care that involves identifying problems by collecting data, analyzing it, and implementing changes and quality measures to prevent future occurrences and ensure that the quality of care is not compromised. Audit and subsequent action are quintessential for successful day care surgery practice. Hence, it is essential to establish standards and implement satisfactory monitoring to ensure that problems experienced by patients are quickly identified and rectified by regular auditing. The move to ambulatory surgery is probably the biggest change in healthcare practice and requires effective monitoring of the quality of care.

TELEPHONE FOLLOW-UP SERVICE[15]

Telephone follow-up after day care surgery has been found to be very useful when developing ambulatory surgery. The purposes of such a service are twofold:
1. To provide postdischarge support for patients.
2. To gather specific data for audit purposes in this early postoperative period.

THE REGISTERS USED IN THE OPERATING THEATER

Different registers are used in the OT, namely:
- *Operation register*: It should record the following details of every operated case:
  - Date of operation
  - Full name and surname of patient/age/sex
  - Initials and surname of surgeon and assistant
  - Anesthetist—initials and surname and type of anesthetic administered
  - Operation done, amount of swabs used, drainage tubes, suturing material, and catheters used
  - Nurse who assisted during operations—initials and surname
  - Circulating (runner) nurse—initials and surname
  - Time—beginning to end of anesthesia
  - Remarks.

This report may be needed for medicolegal cases. It is therefore essential that it is at all times complete.

- *Autoclave register*: Name of the personnel handling the drum, date, and time of autoclaving. Formalin chamber is discontinued from practice.
- *Fumigation register*: Method of fumigation/ who does it/when is it done?
- *OT sterility register*: Name of the personal taking the swab, date and time of collection, swab sample/air sample (to be done twice a month).
- *Equipment maintenance register*: List of equipment, time-to-time service, name of the personnel involved in getting the service. Weekly check of equipment to be performed and any malfunctioning equipment timely serviced/repaired/ replaced.
- *Instrument maintenance register*: List of instrument, time-to-time service, name of the personnel involved in getting the service. Instrument should be oiled every 15 days and sharpening of sharp instruments as and when required. Structural and functional operations of the instruments need to be checked at intervals and entered in the register.
- *Medicine/suture material/surgical consumables register*: Opioid register/ schedule drugs/ketamine
- *Specimen register for biopsies*
- *Death register*.

CONSENT

It has five parts:
1. *Procedure-specific details*: The consent form clearly states:
   - The name of the patient
   - The type of operative procedure or surgical performance:
   - The date
   - Type of anesthetic
   - Alternative procedure
   - The proposed operation:
     - The purpose of the operation
     - The nature of the operation
     - The extent of the surgical procedure
     - Potential risks and complications
     - Expected outcome of the procedure proposed.
2. Anesthesia consent and related details
3. Photography consent
4. Financial consent
5. Visiting doctors/personnel consent.

RECORD MAINTENANCE

Meticulous recording of important data is mandatory, and is a prerequisite for communication, safe practice, clinical governance, and audit. As a minimum, the record should include details of:[16]
- Preoperative assessment
- Consent
- Use of the appropriate World Health Organization (WHO) surgical safety checklist
- Procedures performed, including side of surgery
- Monitoring with contemporaneous recording
- Anesthetic technique
- Safety/infection control measures taken
- Outcomes such as patient comfort.

This data recording is necessary, even if the most simple technique is chosen, e.g. local anesthesia.

Where possible, there should be standardized forms to record all components of the process.

PROCESS[17]

- The full requirements set out in the WHO publication "Guidelines for Safe Surgery,

2009" must be met in policy and practice within the unit.
- Preadmission and patient selection processes are of key importance to ensure patient safety in day surgical care. As well as the normal preadmission consultation with their surgeon a senior anesthetist must carry out a preadmission consultation to establish ASA score and ensure patient is appropriate for day care.
- The patient's situation postdischarge must be established, prior to admission, to ensure their domestic situation will support their postdischarge needs and that an attendant is available.
- Processes must be in place on day of admission to check the patient's current health status, vital signs, laboratory reports, informed consent, and fasting requirements have been followed, fulfillment of preoperative orders, and anesthetist reassessment.
- Formal written arrangements must be in place for patient transfer should their clinical condition deteriorate beyond a level which the day care provider can meet during their stay.
- Arrangements must be in place to meet the needs of patients who are not fit for discharge at their projected time. This will probably require a formal contract with a care provider who is registered to provide overnight stay.
- Arrangements must be in place to show advice given to patients, should they require advice or attention post discharge and the operator must provide an on-call service for patient advice.
- A follow-up call to all patients must be made within 48 hours of discharge to ensure all is well.

Day surgery is an expanding specialty due to economic benefits, patient preference, and modern minimally invasive surgical techniques. Effective, long-lasting postoperative analgesia, and stringent discharge criteria are essential in order to run a successful day-surgery facility. Designated lead clinicians incorporating anesthetists, surgeons, and nursing staff should work together in the development of local guidelines and the safe running of a day-surgery facility. Upon discharge, patients and their caretakers should be given a set of procedure-specific written instructions containing useful information and an emergency helpline. Regular audit is mandatory for the effective running of a day-surgery facility.[26]

REFERENCES

1. Ministry of Health and Family Welfare (2010). The Clinical Establishments (Registration and Regulation) ACT, 2010. [online] Available from: http://clinicalestablishments.gov.in/cms/Home.aspx. [Accessed December, 2018].
2. Royal College of Ophthalmologists (2018). Theatre facilities and equipment ARMS. [online] Available from: https://www.rcophth.ac.uk/wp-content/uploads/2018/12/Theatre-facilities-equipment.pdf. [Accessed December, 2018].
3. Ministry of Health and Social Services (2015) Ministry of Namibia. Operation Theatre Manual, 1st edition. [online] Available from: https://www.medbox.org/namibia-operation-theatre-manual/download.pdf. [Accessed December, 2018].
4. Harsoorl SS, Bhaskar SB. Designing an ideal operating room complex. Indian J Anaesth. 2007;51(3):193-9.
5. Arogyakeralam (2014). Guide Book to NABH Standards for Hospitals. [online] Available from: http://arogyakeralam.gov.in/docs/Quality/2014/Operation-Theatre-Guidelines.pdf. [Accessed December, 2018].
6. Gupta SK, Kant S, Chandrashekhar R. Operating unit—planning essentials and

design Considerations. J Acad Hosp Admin. 2005;17:01-12.
7. Bridgen RJ. Chapter: (1) The Operating department, (2) Organisation and Management, (3) Electricity & Electromedical Equipment, (4) Static Electricity. Operating Theatre Technique, 5th edition: Churchill Livingstone; 1988. pp. 09; 10; 13; 16-21; 27-31; 41; 43-45; 109.
8. Burlingame B; FGI Guidelines Update #3 (2014). Operating Room Requirements for 2014 and Beyond. [online] Available from: https://www.fgiguidelines.org/resource/operating-room-requirements-for-2014-and-beyond/. [Accessed December, 2018].
9. HSCC India Limited (2015). Specialized services. [online] Available from: http://hsccltd.in/other_report/Guideline%20for%20OT%20works_11Aug15.pdf. [Accessed December, 2018].
10. Ophthalmology Service Guidance. Theatre Procedures. The Royal College of Ophthalmologist. February 2018. Available from: https://www.rcophth.ac.uk/wp-content/uploads/2018/02/Theatre-procedures.pdf
11. Makwana1 DS, Parmar N, Prem K, et al. Discharge criteria and complications after day care surgery. Asian Pac J Health Sci. 2016;3(3):82-6.
12. Moemen ME. Recovery Characteristics. J Anaesth. 2004;20:449-57.
13. Utmb Health (2014). Institutional Handbook of Operating Procedures. [online] Available from: https://www.utmb.edu/policies_and_procedures/IHOP/Clinical/Admission_Discharge_and_Transfer/IHOP%20-%2009.01.24%20%20Admission%20Discharge%20Criteria%20for%20Day%20Surgery%20Unit%20(DSU).pdf. [Accessed December, 2018].
14. Karnataka State Physiotherapy Federation (2002). Clinical Establishment Act Standards for Hospital (LEVEL 2) Standard No. CEA/Hospital-002. [online] Available from: http://www.karnatakaphysio.org/pdfclinicalestablishmentact/885%20Hospital-%20002.pdf. [Accessed December, 2018].
15. International Association for Ambulatory Surgery (2014). Ambulatory Surgery Handbook, 2nd edition. Available from: http://www.iaas-med.com/files/2013/Day_Surgery_Manual.pdf
16. Royal College of Anaesthetists and Royal College of Ophthalmologists (2012). 2012-SCI-247-Local-Anaesthesia-in-Ophthalmic-Surgery-2012. [online] Available from: http://www.fpm.ac.uk/system/files/LA-Ophthalmic-surgery-2012.pdf. [Accessed December, 2018].
17. Ministry of Health. Day Care Surgery Guidelines and Requirements. [online] Available from: https://www.moh.gov.om/documents/18824/0/Day+Care+Surgery+Guidelines+and+Requirements/38dbec39-24e3-4a1c-9541-e0478965fc26.
18. MODEL CURRICULUM HANDBOOK OF OPERATION THEATRE TECHNOLOGY. Ministry of Health and Family Welfare Allied Health Section 2015-2016. Available from: https://mohfw.gov.in/sites/default/files/56325415236589_0.pdf
19. Indian Council of Medical Research. Hospital Infection Control Guideline. [online] Available from: https://icmr.nic.in/sites/default/files/guidelines/Hospital_Infection_control_guidelines.pdf. [Accessed December, 2018].
20. https://sites.google.com/a/hopehospitals.in/for-dot-in/hospital-infection-control
21. CDC (2007). Guideline for Isolation Precautions: Preventing Transmission of Infectious Agents in Healthcare Settings. [online] Available from: https://www.cdc.gov/infectioncontrol/guidelines/isolation/index.html. [Accessed December, 2018].
22. Ministry of Health and Family Welfare Allied Health Section (2015–2016). Model Curriculum Handbook of Operation Theatre Technology. [online] Available from: https://a2hp.mohfw.gov.in/StandardCurricula/Model_Curriculum_Handbook_Operat.pdf. [Accessed December, 2018].
23. CDC (2003). Guidelines for Environmental Infection Control in Health-Care Facilities. [online] Available from: https://www.cdc.gov/infectioncontrol/pdf/guidelines/environmental-guidelines.pdf. [Accessed December, 2018].
24. CDC (2008). Guideline for Disinfection and Sterilization in Healthcare Facilities, 2008. [online] Available from: https://www.cdc.gov/infectioncontrol/pdf/guidelines/disinfection-guidelines.pdf. [Accessed December, 2018].
25. https://sites.google.com/a/hopehospitals.in/for-dot-in/continuous-quality-improvement
26. Rastogi S, Vickers PV. Postoperative analgesia and discharge criteria for day surgery. Anaesth Intens Care. 2010;11(4):153-6.

CHAPTER 51

Medicolegal Issues in Liposuction

Shrirang Pandit

HOW IT BEGAN?

In the 80s, liposuction brought in a very significant change in plastic surgery. It transformed the way we looked at shaping the body. The prospect of modifying the form with a tiny incision of 5 mm was an unbelievable idea. The possibilities were mind boggling. The added benefit of losing few kilograms of weight and getting lighter on the weighing scale was the clincher.

Liposuction surgery has truly caught the imagination of people as a means of improving shape, but also with a misplaced hope of reducing weight. Improvement in techniques, machines, and anesthesia have brought about enhanced safety and easier acceptance of the procedure. However, several mishaps have happened during liposuction, and hence, the topic needs further consideration.

The demand for liposuction is growing up exponentially. Over years techniques got refined, and the equipment improved tremendously. Scientists got busy designing optimum cannulas, suction machines got better and better. The incisions found better locations, they became smaller.

One key step in enhancing safety in liposuction was the introduction of tumescent anesthesia by Jeffrey Klein. This made the surgery in to an outpatient procedure. Refinements in technique, equipment, energy-based devices, ultrasound, and lasers have added a new dimension to liposuction practice.

Blood loss is well controlled and now we expect 10 mL for 1,000 mL of aspirate.

Liposuction is all about shape. What is left behind is far more important than what is taken away. The "left over" is going to be with the patient. It better be good. What to remove, from where to remove and how much to remove, is what constitutes to artistry and science of liposuction. High-definition body sculpting has added an altogether new dimension to this form of visual art!

Several guidelines have established the safety of this procedure and the standards of care. These guidelines are useful tools in

PERSONAL EXAMPLE ONE

A senior surgeon witnessed some unfortunate outcomes with liposuction surgeries in Mumbai during his training four decades ago. The indications were misconstrued, equipment was poor and surgical skills did not exist. One was a major liposuction done by a gynecologist, who used a sharp MTP cannula and scraped fat from all over the body. The patient was a case of ovarian cancer. The aspirate was pure blood, very little fat. Patient had torrential primary hemorrhage and succumbed to the blood loss. The cannula was an 18 mm sharp MTP curette. It was a very frightening experience!

Since very few trained surgeons were doing the procedure, going overseas to learn was the only option. In 1992, this Plastic Surgeon had his first brush with liposuction, a live surgery workshop with Dr Illouz in Singapore. Pure white fat harvest was from the arms of a young woman. That was day he was initiated in this art and specialty of liposuction. Liposuction had come off age. Soon, journals and textbooks were soon flooded with scientific evidence of efficacy of the procedure. Refinements in technique, equipment, energy-based devices, ultrasound, and lasers have added a new dimension to liposuction practice. Lasers, ultrasound, radiofrequency-based devices have proved to be very effective in body sculpting procedures.

PATIENT CONCERNS AND QUERIES

Patients want to know a few things about surgeon, his credentials and his capability. Patient wants to understand the expected course or surgery and its consequences. He also wants clear advice on how to manage his time and other social commitments. Possibility of complications and their intensity if they do occur. Cost considerations are extremely important as money becomes the bone of contention once things go wrong.

- **About the Surgeon Credentials**
  - How many years you have done this surgery?
  - Have you done such a procedure before?
  - Do you know how to do it?
  - How many liposuctions you have done?
  - Have you had any complications?
  - Did any patient have pulmonary embolism?
  - What is the risk of such complication?
- **About their Own Case**
  - What is the age limit for liposuction? No age limit, avoid extremes of age.
  - How many kilograms of fat you can remove? Differs from case to case. Fat-specific gravity is 0.8. One liter of pure fat weighs 800 gm. Generally safe limit is about 10% of body weight, and it is surgeon's call on the table.
  - Is liposuction a weight loss surgery? No, it is used for shaping the body and not to lose weight.
  - Am I a good candidate for liposuction?
  - Am I fit to have liposuction?
  - What are the risks involved?
  - Can I die during liposuction?
  - Is it safe?
  - How much blood loss? Do I need blood transfusion?
  - How soon can I start exercising?
  - What is the downtime?
  - When can I resume work?
  - How many days I need to stay in the hospital?
  - What anesthesia will be used?
  - Why general anesthesia (GA) and not local?
  - Will I wake up after anesthesia?
  - How long will the surgery take?
  - Will I get a lot of swelling?
  - Will there be bruising?
  - Will it hurt?
  - How long will the pain last? Is it bad?
  - Do I need to diet?
  - How much weight I will lose?

practice. These are included under Suggested Reading.

- My girth will go down by how many inches?
- Will there be skin wrinkling?
- **Social Issue**
  - Where will you do the surgery? Hospital or clinic?
  - Can I go home on the same day?
  - Do I need assistance after surgery?
  - When can I start doing household work?
  - Is it OK if I do not tell my spouse that I am having this surgery?
  - Do I need someone to accompany me for and during surgery?
  - How many times I have to come for dressings?
  - I want to do it and go home immediately as I am not telling anyone about this, OK?
  - When can I buy new clothes?
  - I have my wedding in 15 days, is it OK to do liposuction as I want to look slim during my wedding?
  - When can we become intimate?
  - When can I plan my pregnancy?
  - Will insurance cover the costs of surgery and hospitalization? Can you word it in such a way that my claim gets passed?
  - I am fat and my marriage is not happening will liposuction help?
  - I am participating in a beauty pageant and need to lose some inches stat, can you help?
  - We three friends want to have liposuction can you give discount?

These and many more questions are asked by patients wanting to have liposuction. This is not an exhaustive list, as newer questions keep coming up. I will try and give a complete and comprehensive answer to most questions.

What they want is simple painless surgery, lose all the fat they have accumulated, have no incisions or cuts, no dressings, no follow-ups and they do not have to take care of diet for the rest of their life. I am afraid that no such treatment exists today.

What makes the patient unhappy and prospective litigant?

Is inadequate consultation:

PERSONAL EXAMPLE TWO: Answer to Patient Queries

The Author has described the advice given to patient seen below in first person singular. The idea is that the consultant must be able to communicate as "this is what I plan to do" and not that "I can do this or may be this or may be that". The author finds patients want the surgeon to lead the discussion and are happy when they see clarity of thinking.

Illustrative answer
- My surgical credits are as follows: I passed Master of Plastic Surgery M.Ch in the year .... and since then I am in active in plastic surgery practice. I did my first liposuction in .... I have had special training in Singapore and in Colombia.
- I have done close to .... liposuction surgeries. None of my patient has died due to this surgery. No patient suffered from pulmonary embolism.
- I did have some complications like severe pain for days, bruising, minor bleeding, and skin swelling for several weeks. Some patients had paresthesia, numbness, tingling, shooting pains for several weeks. No patient had a skin loss but it can happen.
- Liposuction needs some form of anesthesia. Regional, local, or GA is must. Patient needs to be fit to undergo surgery and anesthesia. You will be fully evaluated for fitness and suitability of anesthesia. Please get all your tests done as advised. They do not waste your money.
- The expected blood loss is 15–20 mL for 1,000 cc aspirate. It can vary form case to case and depends to an extent on surgical technique. Generally, blood transfusion is not required.
- Be prepared to spend one night in the clinic. If we find you are in good shape, stable and fully oriented, we will send you home. Please ask someone to take you home as you may be dizzy or tired and not in a position to drive by yourself.

- Avoid being home alone and it is good idea to have someone stay with you for the night or till you feel confident to be alone.
- We take all care to make your surgery as pain free as possible. However, some pain is inevitable. Surgery is totally painless as you will be under anesthesia. Medication intravenous (IV) and oral will help you to control pain. We use skin patches for pain control and they can be effective for as long as a week. You will be prescribed medication for pain to take at home.
- It is very difficult to predict the loss in inches as the skin does not respond immediately after surgery and may take a few months to take shape. Skin can become edematous and you may gain some weight due to accumulation of water in the space occupied by fat. Water is heavier than fat.
- Swelling, bruising, and pain happen to a varying degree in all patients. The intensity of these symptoms varies in a very wide range and is not easily predictable. Patients with thin and fair skin do show the bruise more.
- Effects of liposuction take few weeks to become fully manifest. I ask the patients to keep a gap of at least 8 to 12 weeks before any planned event. Weddings, parties, and social gatherings must be spaced about 3 months later. Never do this liposuction in a hurry unless it is a very small area.
- Patient is expected to get someone who he trusts, to the hospital on the day of surgery. We are using GA and patient will need some capable person to be with him during all the time.
- Catheterization is done to monitor your health and avoid frequent toilet visits in postoperative period. The catheter will be generally removed once your condition is stable. IV fluids and medicines are needed for a few hours. They will be discontinued before you leave the clinic.
- Patient is requested to follow-up after 48–72 hours for dressing change. The first dressing is removed and a much smaller one around the skin port will be placed. Patient may be allowed to bathe and shampoo hair. A compression garment or corset will be put on. Patient needs to wear this for about 3 months.
- If you are pregnant, it is not safe to have liposuction. If you are planning pregnancy, do it 6 months after the liposuction surgery. If you need a cesarean section delivery, the abdominal skin will have resolved by then and minimal scarring will be there.
- This surgery is not covered by any insurance cover. I cannot it any differently and I do not give false reports. This surgery attracts Goods and Service Tax (GST) and it is 18%. You need to pay this when you settle the bill.
- Patient is explained that he must notify someone that he is undergoing such surgery at a particular clinic or hospital. Leave the contact number on indoor records. It is very common to have patients undergoing cosmetic surgery under fake names. It is good practice to establish identity by some document such as Aadhaar, driving license, passport, etc.
- Controlled well-balanced diet, exercise, and healthy lifestyle are a must to keep up the good result. There are no shortcuts.
- Please do not feel guilty, if the patient does not get married or fails to top the beauty pageant or cannot get into size zero clothes. You are here to perform good liposuction surgery. If the patient fails to succeed in life or does not achieve his goals, it is not your fault. Never promise these goodies like marriage, girlfriends, beauty crown as the end result of surgery.

INITIAL CONSULTATION: POINTS TO EMPHASIZE

During the first visit, it is imperative to stress on the patient the following points:

- *Liposuction is proper surgery*: We consider that every surgery is major surgery and so is liposuction. Please do not trivialize the surgery as very simple, can be done in short time, a quick in out procedure. It makes the patient feel that everything is very easy. It may be a useful tactic to make the patient at ease, but can backfire when the patient undergoes surgery. Liposuction involves anesthesia, hospitalization, major surgery, significant discomfort, and pain. The patient needs to wear big dressings, weepy dressings. The clothes and bedsheets at home are going to be soiled. The patient needs to visit the clinic, has to get a few dressings done, and has to bear the costs for the same. It must be told clearly that patient will not be able to bathe and shampoo hair for few days. Forced to be at home, off work, and outcast from social life they feel miserable. Why was I not told before that all these things could happen? The gravity of surgery needs to be related without fear. Aesthetic surgery is subconsciously related with beauty parlor treatments and patients expect miraculous results without a sting of pain. A very clear explanation is mandatory. I tell the patient that this is proper surgery with its inherent risks and rewards! A patient may go away for your honesty but is very likely to come back that too in a better frame of mind.

It is the unexpected pain, and discomfort that irritates the patient. If the result after all this is not good then all agony is an unwelcome gift from the surgeon. Do not omit any possible issue related to pain.

Why are so many tests required?

The surgery is performed under GA. It is very vital to know that the patient is in good health to undergo anesthesia and surgery. The cardiac function, respiratory assessment is necessary. Please do not compromise on this aspect as the whole success of surgery may depend on the fitness or otherwise of the patient. Diabetes and cardiac problems call for thorough evaluation. Medications such as aspirin, clopidogrel, and garlic foods can cause severe bleeding episodes. Coagulation profile will be useful. Abundant caution can prevent many disasters. It will be difficult to defend your actions in absence of documented evidence that you have taken all measures to evaluate the patient preoperatively.

I generally make it a point to arrange a meeting with the anesthesiologist. Whatever more studies or consultations he wants are carried out. This is aesthetic surgery and we must try to make it 100% safe. Fatality or serious complication due to pre-existent disease is not acceptable.

- *Edema bruising and surface irregularities*: Liposuction involves extensive subcutaneous dissection. A large amount of fat is removed and it creates a huge dead space. This third space gets filled up soon with tissue fluid. The tissue edema sets in. It happens in every single liposuction. The quantum may vary. Surface irregularities are a rule. The skin looks bloated and bruised. A bruise results from accumulated blood in the subcutaneous areas. It is visible through the skin. It looks black, blue, and purple and changes colors over a week, eventually fading away. The abdomen and arms and thighs can look pretty ugly and the patient may have to cover herself to hide the bruise. It puts severe restriction on her wardrobe for almost 10 days. These restrictions are disliked by the patient, and they become a point for concern and reason for unhappiness. Such occurrence is the rule and patient needs to know beforehand.

- *We expect the patient is accompanied by some responsible person during surgery*: It is good practice to establish the identity of the patient and this accompanying person. We use a driving license, passport, or any other Government approved photo ID.

- Expected weight loss in kilograms (kg) and loss in inches is a very tricky situation. I refuse to commit at all. Patient wants to put words in my mouth in terms of fixed figures. I steadfastly refuse to get into this trap. Never mention any figure in kg or inches is my principle. It is highly unpredictable to make a guess. The response from patient will change over time and habits. It is futile to take a call on one encounter with weighing machine or tape. The skin retraction is a function of many factors and not simple mathematics.

- Liposuction is not a cure for obesity. This is an effort to reduce fat from resistant area of the body. It is not a way to lose weight. Weight loss is only incidental. When physically several liters of fat has been aspirated from the body and discarded, it is natural to expect some loss of weight on the weighing scale. Somehow, I do not find a consistent relationship on these parameters. Weight loss may take several months to manifest on the scale. I recommend that no promise should be made to a patient as to how much and when will it happen.
- Time-dictated surgery should be avoided. I have my marriage in 15 days and I want liposuction done and I do not want to tell anyone even my fiancée is a sure trap. I suggest a minimum period of 6 weeks between the surgery and the planned event, longer the better. I tell them I do not want to be responsible for spoiling your very important day.
- Patients want their whole body treated in one go. I strongly recommend not to do it. Patients are very unhappy during recovery. There is pain everywhere. It is very difficult to get proper sleep as everything hurts. Whole body is swollen, blood volume is reduced. I avoid it at all cost. The time they pester you is when you are doing the markings. Doctor please do a little of my thigh, little around my calf, can you do my arm pits are innocuous requests. I have fallen prey to them. I did mark those areas and patient later went on complaining that I did not do them as planned. I have a very clear record of the areas planned for suction and it saved my day.
- It is good practice to have someone stay the night with the patient, if she is going home. Once they leave your place, you have no control over their activity. It is not safe to self-drive the same evening and a driver or taxi is a good option.

PERSONAL EXAMPLE THREE

I was tricked once by a patient. He had a mega liposuction of 12 liters. He wanted to go home in the evening. He had done extremely well and he was not willing to stay at the clinic at all. He agreed to book a hotel 100 meters from the clinic. I had my driver leave him there. I took a full consent that he has been advised against leaving the clinic and is doing so against medical advice. This man went ahead, picked up his car and self-drove to Mumbai about 165 km away. Called me twice from toll booth to say he was doing fine. Updated me when he reached home. On follow-up, I scolded him, he said "you have done such good surgery that I did not feel a thing and decided to go home". I was happy that I had a valid consent before he left the clinic.

- Improper communication about the logistics of dressings, follow-up advice, compression garments, medication changes, dietary advice can create lot of unpleasantness. Advice should be clear, preferably written, cell numbers well-documented to keep track, SMS to alert them about changes delays in schedule can make it a more happy situation.
- Please remember that money is the cause generally of majority of litigation. When patients are discussing costs, the final draft should be your reference point. The patient should know clearly surgeons fees, hospitalization cost, anesthesia fees, costs of medication, dressing charges, visit charges, follow-up fees, etc.

One advantage of this split is that the patient understands how much goes to surgeon and how much to the hospital. The level of anger and dissatisfaction is linked to the amount of fees patient pays.

OTHER ASPECTS IN PATIENT CARE

- Pain management is crucial in liposuction. It is important to realize that liposuction surgery is significantly painful. The pain is present over a large surface area. The intensity of pain can be acute. Pain medication is must. We use Buprenorphine skin patch before starting surgery. The skin patch works on transcutaneous drug delivery. By the time patient comes out of anesthesia, the Buprenorphine starts to work and pain is well controlled. I also think the Norphine has a euphoric effect, which works very well for me. I have found that it reduces the need for oral medications, makes the stomach comfortable. Pain-free liposuction should be the goal.

We know that pain essentially is individual perception. I prepare the patients mind to expect some pain after surgery. Once they know that there is nothing wrong and pain is due to the liposuction and is to be expected, the perception changes. The agony becomes discomfort and discomfort becomes soreness! The patient must blame you for scaring her, A patient saying "Doctor it did not hurt me at all" is a well-counseled patient.

I warn them specifically that paresthesia may linger for several weeks. Shooting pains, insects crawling on the skin, and hyperesthesia are common after Vaser-assisted liposuction. This is due to the effect of ultrasound energy on fat in Schwann cell membrane.

- When discussing time for recovery, it is good to keep it as vague as possible. Several weeks are a very nice term. Months are difficult to digest but weeks are not so bad. Several weeks make it several months!! Never disown your patient. Take them through their recovery with firm reassurance, gentle persuasion, and with authority. I have found that explaining the healing response preoperative is very useful. The psych is primed for adverse events and their occurrence is accepted without getting angry. What must not be missed is that this process involves hours of talk time. It makes you a trustworthy doctor, who does not shy away from questions. A blunt "I do not know" makes you an honest, believable person.

CASE EXAMPLE 1: Case Law on falsely claiming Magical Remedy of Severe Obesity by Liposuction and Its Malpractice.

Case facts: Following an advertisement in newspaper, severely obese patient weighing 130 kg went for liposuction to surgeon. But instead, lipoplasty was done. The patient filed a complaint in police for medical negligence, and medicolegal report was made by the civil hospital doctor, which mentioned "the injury present on the both arms is grievous in nature as it may result in permanent loss of movement of both arms to some extent. It has caused disfiguration of the body. Liposuction should not invariably produce such scars".

Surgeon's advertisement as published, which is as under:

"Body Shaping by Liposuction (Go home the same day) Body contouring and treatment of:

Paunchy belly, bulging flanks, lower belly bulge, blouse bulge or chest rolls, upper thigh side bags, double chin, male breast, or gynecomastia. Any other fat spot to give smooth contour to body shape.

Ideal for: Hanging belly, fold after deliveries, remaining fatty bulges after losing weight."

Complainant: I expected 4-mm scar, instead had longitudinal scars on upper limbs. Informed consent was not documented well. Postoperative care was alleged to be low. Long cuts/scars on both of her arms. I immediately protested to the doctor that I had not only been cheated but also been injured grievously with deep cuts and scars and suffered severe mental agony as also disfiguring of her body.

I sought another surgeon's certificate of second opinion, which is as under "this is to certify that patient had liposuction of both arms on March 7th, 1997. By the end of April, she still had gaping wound 3 × 4 in size C induration and scarring of right arm and induration and scarring of left arm. She was referred to plastic surgeon. Who advised skin grafting of right arm or dressing of wound (approximate healing time 6–8 weeks). She could not perform active movements of right arm after 2 months, she still had discharge from the wound C and collection of fluid at multiple sites of scars and swelling. She was again referred to the plastic surgeon for needful. She also had disfigurement of both arms."

Defense: I am skilled person and expert in the line of treatment of liposuction and lipoplasty, and as surgeon in first meeting with patient itself, informed that she was suffering from Bat-Wings, which is a deformity of the upper arms. Patient was a lady who was very obese and who had huge deposits of fat all over her body. In such a condition of a patient, large volume of fat hangs down on the upper arm and is covered with thick and stretched skin. The complainant agreed for lipoplasty of arms, which is an additional procedure of liposuction and involves removal of stretched and hanging skin of arms as well. A consent was obtained from the complainant, whereby informing her that the procedure of lipoplasty/liposuction is not for weight reduction.

Court verdict: Surgeon held guilty for not explaining the process of lipoplasty properly and also its after effects and negligence in not taking proper postoperative care and causing mental agony and partial disfigurement due to which the complainant had to incur huge expenses. Surgeon was asked to pay compensation of ₹ 50,000 to patient.

Discussion: Information was inadequate regarding the procedure. The scars due to poor postoperative care caused severe distress to patient. This was due to false representation on the part of surgeon as the entire procedure, after effects and subsequent treatment for removal of scars or rectification of the disfigurement were not explained.

Source: Veena Sethi versus Dr JB Ratti, on November 4, 2008. Delhi State Consumer Disputes Redressal Commission. [Online] Available from: https://indiankanoon.org/doc/124768739/.

CASE EXAMPLE 2: Cardiac Arrest during Anesthesia for Liposuction.

Case: Alleged medical negligence causing death of patient in operation table during liposuction surgery. Patient had cardiac arrest due to anesthesia reaction and was shifted to ICU, diagnosed as "hypoxic brain damage" and subsequently resulted into vegetative state and his death after few days.

Misleading advertisement by hospital on pamphlet was given about detailed information of liposuction: "We trim your Fat, not your Wallet. Satisfaction Guaranteed, So Long as Your Goals are Realistic." Most people get attracted by such glorious advertisements and want to be good looking. Whether it is handsome or beautiful, people will do almost anything to enhance their looks. Some people choose painful and expensive routes. Many people suffer from unattractive fat build-up in certain areas of their bodies. Women tend to accumulate fat around the hips, thighs, abdomen, and buttocks. Men have problems with "love handles" and their abdomen. Few might have problems with their neck, chin, legs, arms, or breasts. Liposuction is a cosmetic surgery that contours and sculpts your body into a slimmer profile and removes unwanted excess fat."

Defense: Plastic surgeon was qualified and experienced in the practice of liposuction surgery. Anesthetist was a qualified anesthetist. The cardiac arrest is not a complication of liposuction procedure. The obesity itself is one of the causes of cardiovascular disease. The patient suffered cardiac arrest before starting the procedure of liposuction. Therefore, plastic surgeon is not responsible for the happenings thereon. The anesthesia was given as per standard protocol. There was no excess dose for anesthetic. Cardiac arrest was an unfortunate event, but it happened so without any negligence on the part of anesthetist. It was a case of contributory negligence from patient, it is apparent that there was a mistake on the part of patient as well as his wife, who did not disclose about thyroid status and the previous medical treatment to the surgeon. AIIMS medical board report cannot be relied upon, as no any doctor was a plastic surgeon with experience of doing liposuction, themselves.

Court decision: Surgeon and anesthetist held liable for negligence and deficiency in service, whereas, the hospital is vicariously liable. Accordingly, we direct them to pay the patient's wife a sum of ₹ 2,000,000/- toward loss of deceased's prospective income, plus ₹ 500,000/- toward mental agony from the date of pronouncement of this order. Further, they shall pay ₹ 50,000/- toward the litigation costs. The entire compensation should be paid by them in equal share, jointly and severally.

Discussion: Court has noted several lapses on the part of the surgeon who did not make proper selection of patient and the anesthetist failed to monitor the case, after induction of ketamine/anesthesia. Liposuction is a major surgical intervention and not the minor procedure (as mentioned in the records by the surgeon). The liposuction is not a short procedure instead it is a lengthy procedure. It required preoperative consultation and all the possible complications arising out of such procedure should have been explained to the patients and his attendants by the surgeon. There is no documented plan in the records as to how much fat was to be removed and from which sites. Anesthesia notes do not mention the details of vital signs such as pulse rate, blood pressure, respiratory rate, and oxysaturation. There is no tabular representation of pulse, blood pressure, electrocardiography (ECG) during the intraoperative period. There is no mention about change in respiration, i.e. any obstruction, shallow respiration, or respiratory arrest when patient developed bradycardia. Patient was given diazepam, ketamine, propofol infusion but no oxygen was administered until patient developed bradycardia. It is a standard of care to give oxygen to obese patient before start of procedure whenever any procedure is done under sedation, which was not done, was held as negligence. OT team also responsible for not prompt cardiopulmonary resuscitation (CPR). The anesthesia record contains no time sequence of the events occurring immediately after the cardiac arrest. AIIMS expert opinion clearly indicates that the massive brain damage sustained by the patient would not have occurred, if resuscitation had been as prompt and effective as the doctors indicated in their evidence. It was the mandatory duty to advise proper pre-esthetic investigations, including thyroid profile. Mere filling of pre-esthetic assessment form is not an excuse or exclusion for not doing essential laboratory investigations. Thus, it was a deficiency on the part of surgeon and anesthetist.

Source: National Consumer Disputes Redressal (OP/391/2001). Smt K Shyamala Murthy vs Dr Manoj Khanna and Others on February 9, 2016. https://indiankanoon.org/doc/150336851/.

CASE EXAMPLE 3: False Allegation of Medical Negligence during Laparoscopic Abdominal Liposuction.

Case: During liposuction, her sciatic nerves being sucked and damaged beyond repair resulting in paralysis as alleged by the complainant. The complainant alleged that she was paralyzed below the waist because of liposuction operation and had persistent paresthesia in both lower limbs.

Defense: Paresthesia is a common sequela of liposuction and normally recovers within 3–6 months. The complainant herself filed prescription of neurologist dated 2-1-2002 wherein the tests/magnetic resonance imaging (MRI) advised revealed that degenerative changes in the spinal cord were suspected. The complainant filed a chronological list of diagnosis, medication, and treatment, in which admittedly on 28-6-1993 findings revealed bilateral predominantly L5 preganglionic root lesion. This clearly shows that she was suffering from some disk problem, which is totally unrelated to the surgery in question. Patient was advised by doctors at AIIMS to get another postcontrast MRI scan for further evaluation on 8-10-2004 but on some personal grounds of health she refused to undergo the same. She could have easily got it done, if not that day, immediately thereafter. We find that she consciously has not got the tests done and this inaction does not reflect well on behalf to deny the opportunity given by AIIMS to prove her case. Complaint is that she was unable to move her lower limbs after operation until 24-6-1993, whereas the findings of the neurologist dated 26-6-1993 recorded that power in right lower limb is grade IV and left lower limb as grade IV + with no sensory deficit and all deep tender reflexes are normal. This finding clearly disproves the contention taken by the complainant.

Court decision: Judges were of considered opinion that the complainant did not justifiably prove her case of medical negligence on the part of plastic surgeon. Hence, the complaint is dismissed.

Discussion: In the present case, a Committee of experts constituted by AIIMS gave a clear opinion that the allegations of weakness in her limbs are not connected with the liposuction surgery done by plastic surgeon.

Q. Whether abdominal or trochanteric liposuction can cause any weakness or paralysis or loss of sensation in the lower limbs?
Ans. It is impossible and completely inconceivable that abdominal and/or trochanteric liposuction can cause any weakness or loss of sensation or paralysis of the lower limbs.

Q. Whether such a procedure can cause any injury to or disease of the spinal cord, or the nerve roots, specifically in the region of L-5?
Ans. It is impossible and completely inconceivable that abdominal and/or trochanteric liposuction can cause any injury to, or disease of the spinal cord or the nerve roots, specifically in the region of L-5.

Source: National Consumer Disputes Redressal. Mrs Noni Singh vs Dr PK Talwar on 16 December, 2009. [Online] Available from: https://indiankanoon.org/doc/107257296/.

LIPOSUCTION SAFETY

Who can do liposuction surgery, what is the training required?

We must remember that no surgery is minor, there are only minor surgeons! Every surgery needs to be taken seriously. Surgeon undertaking liposuction must not trivialize it as simple, harmless procedure. Liposuction is not hacking fat from the body. It is a proper surgical procedure with its risk and rewards. A plastic surgeon is most appropriately suited to perform liposuction, as we practice it today. Dermatology colleagues have contributed immensely to liposuction. Major liposuction involves general or regional anesthesia, fluid balance management, blood loss estimation, and replacement. A surgeon is trained to work with them. Understanding of anatomy and its variations, the fat distribution, and vital structures that are around the area calls for a trained surgeon. Plastic surgeons have a unique exposure in that they work on the entire body. From the scalp to the toes, the plastic surgeon is no stranger to any region. Liposuction is done almost all over the body and the anatomical comfort zone of the plastic surgeon is the widest of the medical specialties.

Currently plastic surgeons, dermatologists, dentists, ENT surgeons, aestheticians, general surgeons, and gynecologists perform liposuctions. Legally, the plastic surgeon is qualified and trained to perform liposuction. It must be understood that there are gray areas and work domains overlap significantly. It is up to the personal honesty and professional integrity of the surgeon before he decides to perform liposuction. Good training is absolute must.

Infrastructure and Equipment required for Safe Liposuction

Minimum Infrastructure Needed

The surgeon must choose an appropriate place to perform the surgery. High-volume liposuctions need to be performed in a major hospital setting. Small volumes can be done in smaller clinics or hospitals. Small clinic does not mean it is permitted to be poorly equipped.

An injection of local anesthesia can induce a vasovagal attack or an intense allergic response that can be fatal. In recent years, I have an arrangement with my anesthetist. I arrange cases so that he is almost always around when I do a case under local anesthesia. It is very calming to have a trained person to look after your patient. I invariably start an IV line, however, small the procedure may be. The operating room must be fully-equipped for any eventuality. This surgery is an elective procedure, aesthetic surgery and every effort is welcome to make it as safe as possible. Clean, air-conditioned atmosphere, proper surgical operation theater, adjustable operation table, good lights, good anesthesia workstation, pulse oximeters and blood pressure monitors and ECG display are mandatory. Sterilization has to be adequate and proper. Do not compromise on the quality of care by using poor-quality equipment. There should be a recovery room able to host the patient for his stay in the hospital and is tuned for lifesaving procedures.

The standard of care will vary from place-to-place, but there is no place for poorly equipped environment for liposuction surgery.

Supplies of Medicines

Sterile IV lines, angiocatheters, surgical adhesive tapes of all sizes, IV fluids such as saline, Ringer's lactate, dextrose, and plasma expanders for hypovolemia are must. Emergency medical crash cart is needed. Lifesaving medications such as adrenaline, atropine, dexamethasone, corticosteroids should be at hand. I keep at least 10 syringes of size 2, 5, 10 mL each next to the anesthesia trolley.

Infection Control

I advise all my patients to have a bath using povidone iodine surgical scrub for 3 days prior to surgery. In the OR, the patient is sprayed with betadine and lies on a sterile sheet on the table. Large areas of the body are exposed and draping is not easy. It is very useful measure. When we do a circumferential liposuction, the patient goes to the bathroom and the whole body is sprayed with betadine. We use a good garden spray for this purpose. Patient wraps herself with a sterile sheet and gets on the operation table. All patients have shampoo and are advised not to use hair oil.

Manpower Requirement

Human resource is the key to successful and trouble-free surgery. In an emergency situation, you need many people and trained staff can save many a lives: surgeon, anesthesiologist, female attendant, female nurse, and theater assistants form the team. When doing cases under local anesthesia on female patients, it is must to have one female attendant every single minute in the OR. Maximum privacy should be afforded to female patients to make them comfortable.

Common Causes of Liposuction Death and Complications

Liposuction is like any other surgery and there can be a fatality. In his years of working, this author has noticed a few predicaments that lead to complications. During the consultation, the patient is promised certain liters of lipoaspirate. The surgeon falls short of the target and is pushed into over-resection. Tumescence adds safety to the procedure on two counts. It reduces blood loss and it bloats the tissue. This adds invaluable centimeters to the safety margin. It prevents surface irregularity, keeps the cannula away from vascular structures.

I have observed that the volume of fat harvested and the IV infusion required to maintain homeostasis is difficult to decide. What comes out has to be replaced does not work. Patients can go into fatal fluid overload due to this strategy. It is also unclear the relationship between volume fluid used for tumescence and the volume of aspirate.

It is good practice to catheterize patients and monitor urine output to maintain fluid balance. Peripheral vasoconstriction after tumescence can lead to reduced urine output and the fact must be kept in mind. Blood pressure and urine output together should act as a guide for IV infusions.

The author makes a documented plan, and asks the patient very pointedly to describe the the areas which he wants to be treated and in order of priority. This priority order is noted down. Patient is told that the surgeon will try and follow the sequence, but for some reason if the surgeon needs to modify the plan, areas with low priority will not be treated.

Toxicity of lidocaine can cause cardiac arrest and is very difficult to revive. Dose of lidocaine should be well-titrated as per body weight and proposed dilution during tumescence. Tumescence can be done in stages and it is not necessary to inject all the fluids at one go. It helps to spread over the dose of lidocaine, reducing its peak concentration.

Patient with rectus divarication, hernia can sustain bowel injury leading to infection may be fatality. Good history and clinical examinations are must. The cannula is a strong hard tube and great caution needs to be exercised. The secret is "not to push the cannula" if you encounter resistance.

When using power-assisted devices, improper usage can cause severe damage to skin vascularity and skin loss.

CONCLUSION

Liposuction is a great advance in aesthetic plastic surgery. A thorough consultation that explains the risks and benefits of surgery, explains in simple terms the course of treatment, its ill effects, and complications is very useful. I suggest to avoid describing results in superlatives like fantastic, mind blowing, super, or excellent. A wrong message is conveyed. Keep the lines of communication open all times. Gently but honestly discuss complications at the earliest. Avoid rude shocks as patient may get disproportionately upset and angry. Promise less but deliver more and your patient will be happy.

SUGGESTED READING

1. American Society of Plastic Surgeons (2003). Practice Advisory on Liposuction: Executive Summary; Practice Advisory Approved by the ASPS Board of Directors, March 15, 2003. [online] Available from: www.plasticsurgery.org. [Accessed December, 2018]
2. College of Physicians and Surgeons of British Columbia (2017). Guidelines of Liposuction; Non-Hospital Medical and Surgical Facilities Accreditation Program College of Physicians and Surgeons of British Columbia approved on December 30, 2017. [online] Available from: https://www.cpsbc.ca/files/pdf/NHMSFAP-Liposuction.pdf. [Accessed December, 2018]
3. Mysore V. Tumescent liposuction: Standard guidelines of care. Ind J derm Ven Lepr. 2008; 74(7):54-60.
4. Svedman KJ, Coldiron B, Coleman WP 3rd, et al. ASDS guidelines of care for tumescent liposuction. Dermatol Surg. 2006;32(5):709-16.

CHAPTER 52

Tips and Pearls for Medicolegal Situations

Bhanuprakash

Story so far......
Medicine as a science is riddled with unpredictable outcome. Doctors operate where success cannot be guaranteed in every case and the final outcome depends upon factors beyond his control. On the one hand, *a relation based on trust and true professionalism exists between a doctor and patient.* The patient comes to the doctor innocently not knowing his illness, medical terms, concepts, need of treatment procedures, and fate. He expects the doctor to be ethical and honest,[1] it is no sin to say that he is looked upon as a demigod. On the other side, factors such as Insurance company's payments, a stressful urban life, changing lifestyles, information exposure in the internet regarding diseases, treatment and medicines, enhanced awareness among patients regarding incurable diseases, and investors investing with profitable motives in health industry are playing a major role in creating hurdles in this relation. This leads to patients getting dissatisfied with the outcomes, leading to mistrust and suspicion leading often to legal resort of seeking compensation (Box 1).

Prior to 80s, there were few cases filed against the doctors as the court fees was high and duration of cases going on in the courts was unpredictable. A major landmark was

BOX 1: Legal remedies available for the patient in questioning doctor's way of handling the patient.
- The Consumer Protection Act for deficiency in service.
- Civil Court for monetary compensation.
- The Law of Torts, Section 357 of Criminal Procedure Code, 1973, and also under section 1 (A) of the Fatal Accidents Act, 1855. If found guilty, the doctor may be sentenced to rigorous imprisonment.
- Sections 337 and 338 of Indian Penal Code, 1860 are also relevant as to Medical Negligence. Through the Indian Medical Council Act, 1956. The Medical Council of India (MCI) and the State Medical Councils regulate the medical profession by constituting the Code of Ethics and standards of Medical professional conduct and etiquette. *Medical practitioner violating these standards, amounts to misconduct and can be tried, but not legally.*

the passing of the Consumer Protection Act in 1986. The Supreme Court of India brought medical profession within the ambit of the Consumer protection Act, 1986.[2] Since then cases against doctors are on the increase helped by minimal court fees and early settlement of the case in the consumer courts.

Mahendra Kumar Bajpai has reported a 110% increase in the number of medicolegal cases in India every year. Till 1995, various judgments in different courts led to confusion as to whether medical services are covered under Consumer Protection Act or not. In 1996,[3] the apex Court clarified that medical services or medical profession fall under the coverage of Consumer Protection Act and patient can get relief against medical negligence of doctors, hospitals, etc. The Supreme Court decided that medical service would fall within the ambit of "service" as defined in Section 2(1)(o) of the Consumer Protection Act and patient can be considered as a consumer under the definition of "consumer" as defined in Section 2(1)(d) of the Act. The process of the medical negligence under the Consumer protection act is discussed elsewhere in detail.[4]

Since the beginning of the century, a huge rise in the number of cases filed as both civil and criminal cases may be noticed. The Court explained the distinction between simple negligence and gross negligence in Jacob Mathew case.[5] In Dr Suresh Gupta vs Government of NCT of Delhi and Anr (2004),[6] the apex court held that whenever a patient died due to medical negligence, the doctor was liable in civil law for paying the compensation and when the negligence was so gross and his act was so reckless as to endanger the life of the patient, criminal law for offence under Section 304A of Indian Penal Code (IPC), 1860 will apply. The Honorable Judges have clarified that for ordinary negligence, the doctors could not be held criminally liable. In Dr Suresh Gupta case and other cases,[7,8] the Supreme Court differentiated between degree of negligence and when cases can be tried under civil or criminal laws. It was only in gross negligence and recklessness, the doctors could be criminally held responsible.

Addressing the concerns of medical professionals In Martin D'Souza case,[9] the Supreme Court has directed that, "whenever a complaint received against a doctor or hospital by the consumer forum or by the Criminal Court then before issuing notice to the doctor or hospital against whom the complaint was made the consumer forum or Criminal Court should first refer the matter to a competent doctor or committee of doctors, specialized in the field relating to which the medical negligence is attributed and only after that doctor or committee reports that there is prima facie case of medical negligence should notice be then issued to the concerned doctor or hospital. This is necessary to avoid harassment to doctors who may not be ultimately found to be negligent".

In Poonam Verma vs Ashwin Patel case,[10] the Supreme Court distinguished between negligence, rashness, and recklessness. A negligent person is one who inadvertently commits an Act of omission and violates a positive duty. A person who is rash knows the consequences but foolishly thinks that they will not occur as a result of her or his Act. A reckless person knows the consequences but does not care whether or not they result from her or his Act. Any conduct falling short of recklessness and deliberate wrong-doing should not be the subject of criminal liability.

Thus a doctor cannot be held criminally responsible for a patient's death unless it is shown that she or he was negligent or incompetent, with such disregard for the life and safety of his patient that it amounted to a crime against the State.

The Court further warned the police officials not to arrest or harass doctors unless the facts clearly come within the parameters laid down in Jacob Mathew's case; otherwise the policemen will themselves have to face legal action.[11]

What is negligence?
According to Halsbury's Laws of England,[12] the definition of negligence is as under—
Negligence: Duties owed to patient. A person who holds himself out as ready to give medical (1) advice or treatment impliedly undertakes that he is possessed of skill and knowledge for the purpose. Such a person, whether he is a registered medical practitioner or not, who is consulted by a patient, owes him certain duties, namely, a duty of care in deciding whether to undertake the case—a duty of care in deciding what treatment to give; and a duty of care in his administration of that treatment (2) A breach of any of these duties will support an action for negligence by the patient (3).

How to establish the negligence of a doctor?
A doctor by agreeing to treat a patient implies that he is possessed of skill and knowledge and exercises a reasonable degree of care while treating the patient. This may vary according to the cadre (general practitioner, specialist, super specialist, etc.) or rank (resident, senior or junior consultant, etc.)

A professional can be considered to be negligent, when he fails to prove he has requisite skills and knowledge for treating or when he fails to exercise the same competency while treating the patient.

In spite of differing opinions, judgment in Bolam vs Friern[13] is considered as a standard in the definition of care and negligence. It is defined as follows—"The test is the standard of the ordinary skilled man exercising and professing to have that special skill. A man needs not possess the highest expert skill. It is well-established law that it is sufficient, if he exercises the ordinary skill of an ordinary competent man exercising that particular art".

A doctor can be implicated with two types of liabilities—(1) criminal and (2) civil.

1. **Criminal liabilities** arise when it is proved that a doctor has committed an Act, which is grossly negligent, and that Act has led to substantive damage or led to the patients' death. Then, under Section 304A of the IPC the doctor is punishable with imprisonment for a term which may extend up to 2 years or with a fine or both.

2. **Civil liabilities** arise under Section 73 and 74 of the Indian Contract Act. For liability to be established, the onus of the burden is on the patient to prove that. (1) There is a normal practice. (2) The defendant doctor has not adopted it. (3) The course adopted by the doctor is one which no professional man of ordinary skill would have taken, if he had been acting with ordinary care.

Damages are the monetary compensation awarded by law. This may be:

- **Pecuniary damages:** Amounts awarded for financial loss by the patient covering all medical expenses, nursing and recuperation cost, loss of earning capacity, etc.
- **Nonpecuniary damages:** Amounts awarded for indirect sufferings such as inability to participate in sports, drive vehicles, marital disharmony, mental agony, and other suffering.
  - **Vicarious liability:** Vicarious liability implies the master is answerable for the wrong doings of the staff engaged by him—provided that is done in

the course of the employment. The hospital that engages the doctors and supportive services housekeeping, nurses, technicians, pharmacist, physiotherapists, etc. have vicarious liability. Common examples of vicarious liability are a patient falling from a trolley while being carried by a ward boy, a patient falling on a slippery floor, etc.

- *Prerequisites for a doctor:*[14] The Supreme Court held that the duty of a doctor will include: (1) a duty of care in deciding whether to undertake a case and (2) a duty of care in deciding what treatment to give or a duty of care in administration of that treatment. Any breach of these duties gives a rise of action for negligent acts toward the patient. The Court also observed that the doctor has the discretion in choosing the treatment, which he proposes to give to the patient in one way or the other.

There are several clauses or sections of medical care in which the cases have been filed. Though these are beyond the scope of this article, effort is made here to bring the various clauses and classical case examples are listed for the readers to draw their conclusion. Readers should also be aware that the law and legal standards may not only vary from case-to-case, but also from jurisdiction-to-jurisdiction. It also must be brought to the notice of the readers that there are many contradictory judgments given on the same topic and is being listed. The authors themselves are not giving any opinion in this matter but to make the readers aware of the various judgments.

- *Ethics and doctors:* Generally, the courts have been very tough on doctors who have violated the basic ethos and ethics laid down by the Medical Council of India. Three important cases are listed here:
  1. Every doctor whether at a Government hospital or otherwise has the professional obligation to extend his services with due expertise for protecting life.[15]
  2. In the case of **Pravat Kumar Mukherjee vs Ruby General Hospital and Others (2005),**[16] an accident case came into the hospital. The hospital demanded an immediate payment of ₹ 15,000. Hospital discontinued treatment after 45 minutes. This leads to shifting of patient to other hospital from the current hospital. The patient died on the way. The National Commission allowed the complaint and the Opponent Ruby Hospital was directed to pay ₹ 1,000,000 to the complainant for mental pain agony. The commission observed that a human touch is necessary, that is their code of conduct, that is their duty, and that is what is required to be implemented. The court observed that in emergency or critical cases, a doctor must discharge their duty or social obligation of rendering service without waiting for fee or for consent.
  3. In **the case of Dr Laxman Balkrishna Joshi vs Dr Trimbak Bapu Godbole and Another,**[14] the duties, which a doctor owes to his patients came up for consideration and Supreme Court has passed guidelines on doctor's primary duty toward the patients and the society. The doctor does not have to adhere to the highest or sink to the lowest degree of care and competence in the light of the circumstance. A doctor, therefore, does not have to ensure that every patient who comes

to him is cured. He has to only ensure that he confers a reasonable degree of care and competence.
- **Burden of proof:** Generally, in cases of medical negligence, the patient must establish her or his claim against the doctor. In Kanhaiya Kumar Singh vs Park Medicare and Research Center,[17] it was held that negligence has to be established and cannot be presumed. In case of Calcutta Medical Research Institute vs Bimalesh Chatterjee,[18] it was held that the responsibility of proving negligence and the resultant deficiency in service were clearly on the complainant.
- However, in another judgment in Nizam's Institute of Medical Sciences vs Prasanth S Dhananka,[19] the Supreme Court held that "moreover, in a case involving medical negligence, once the initial burden has been discharged by the complainant by making out a case of negligence on the part of the hospital or doctor concerned, the onus then shifts on to the hospital or to the attending doctors and it is for the hospital through their records to show as to what care was given and satisfy the Court that there was no lack of care or diligence".
- Does giving free treatment provide immunity for a doctor from being filed claims against?
  - A totally free treatment in a place, which gives free treatment to everybody may not entitle the complainant to approach the Consumer Court. But he would still be entitled to approach the District Court by filing a suit for damages. In a case,[20] the Supreme Court observed that: (1) it was no defense that the treatment was gratuitous or free and (2) the State Government would be liable for negligence in such activities.
  - In a case related to All India Institute of Medical Sciences (AIIMS),[21] the hospital claimed that since the treatment was subsidized by the hospital, it would not be covered under the Act. The National Commission rejected this argument and held since the treatment was subsidized and not totally free; the hospital would be covered under the Consumer Protection Act.
  - In another case related to Employees' State Insurance (ESI) hospitals,[22] the complainant was ordered to be paid compensation. This case is significant because it lays down that the ESI hospitals, though Government run, are covered under the Consumer Protection Act.
- **Can the consumer court go into the propriety of the fees charged by a doctor or a hospital?** In[23] the complainant approached the Consumer Forum against exorbitant charges levied by the respondent cardiologist. *Though the Forum expressed its shock at the exorbitant charges leveled by the hospital, it held that it did not have the jurisdiction to go into the propriety of the fees charged by a doctor.*
- **Is a doctor responsible for the negligence of his nurse?**
  In[24] ***KG Krishnan vs Praveen Kumar (minor),*** the National Commission held that the nurse was the employee of the doctor and as such the doctor was vicariously liable for her negligence.
- **Is a hospital liable for the negligence of its doctors?**[25]
  Savita Garg vs The Director. The Supreme Court, in a landmark decision held the following—it was not necessary to join the treating doctors or nurses as parties as long as the hospital was made a party.

- Hospitals brazenly disown their liability, if something goes wrong in treatment of patients claiming assertively that they only provide the infrastructure like operation theatres and pathological and radiological support to doctors, who should be blamed for any mishap. This plea put forward by hospitals was set aside by the Supreme Court in the case.[26]
- **Whether hospitals' responsibility extends to a mishap, if any, involving attendants of the patient?**
  In the matter of,[27] the commission held that all clinics and hospitals will be held liable for any mishap not only to patients but also their attendants for any faulty services, whether medical or otherwise.
- **Does the failure to monitor dosage of drugs amount to negligence?[28]**
  In this case, the court has clearly said it is negligence on the doctor for not monitoring dosage of drugs while treating the patient. Proper monitoring of adverse effects also forms a role in the treatment by the doctor. This is especially true for dermatological medications. *Examples of when dermatologists have found themselves liable have involved drugs such as Accutane and oral and topical corticosteroids. In Cooper,[29] a dermatologist had prescribed dexamethasone in excessive dosages and duration for recurrent dyshidrotic eczema without appropriate monitoring. The patient eventually developed avascular necrosis that required hip replacement surgery. The dermatologist was held guilty of improper care. In Moyer,[30] a patient was prescribed retinoids by two consecutive physicians even when the baseline triglyceride and cholesterol levels were increased. The patient eventually developed cardiac disease requiring quadruple bypass surgery. The dermatologists were sued for malpractice and negligence. The case was ultimately dismissed based on statute of limitations issues, but not before a lengthy lawsuit.*
- **What happens when there is a difference of opinion amongst experts concerning the line of treatment to be adopted?[31]**
  The Supreme Court held that a difference of opinion amongst experts on procedure adopted by a doctor cannot be called negligence, if the procedure adopted is commonly in practice in an area.
- **Can a doctor charge for facilities he does not offer?[32]**
  In *RM Joshi vs Dr PB Tahilramani,* the State Commission ordered the recovery of bed charges when the patient was made to sleep on a table amounted to deficiency in service. In yet another case,[33] excessive charging—"deficiency in service", but not medical negligence. Hospitals and nursing homes must have proper protocols such as rechecking of bills, to avoid charging the patient erroneously. It is advisable that the printed bills have a specific clause stating that, "patients are advised to check the bill before paying".
- **Does the nonconduct of necessary preoperative tests amount to negligence?**
  In *SV Panchori vs Dr Kaushal Pandey,*[34] the commission held that omission to do a routine investigation constitutes deficiency in service. This was the issue before the National Commission in *Dr Kaligoundon vs N Thangamuthu.*[35] Similarly, relying on a 2-day-old investigation report of another laboratory and not repeating the same was held as negligence. It is, therefore, advisable that investigations are repeated and in case of reports from substandard laboratories reinvestigations become rather mandatory.[36]

- **Failure to identify a complication:** If a certain complication is a known risk, it should be on the consent form for the medical procedure. However, the consent form need not list every single complication that has ever occurred for that procedure. Often there are mistakes in communicating the complications. If, for example, the complication is known to occur 10% of the time during a given procedure but the consent form states that it occurs only 1% of the time, then the consent form was wrong.
- **Standard textbooks—the best weapon in a doctor's defense:** Authoritative medical texts are the best tools in a doctor's defense. Once the science of medicine endorses a particular Act of omission or commission by the doctor, courts usually accept the correctness of the Medical Act.[37]
- **Does the legally prescribed "accepted medical practice" include "prevailing practice"?**
  Prevailing practice contrary to principles of medical science constitutes negligence. Any Medical Act contrary to the science of medicine, even if it is commonly practiced by a Section of doctors or doctors from a specific area, cannot be a justification in a court of law.[38]
- **Law accepts that all doctors may not act similarly under similar circumstances.** Law accepts that different doctors will act differently in similar situations. Law takes into consideration the doctor's personal choice in choosing an alternative amongst the various that may exist.[39]
- **Medical practices followed in other countries—How much relevant in Indian courts?**
  A doctor is not negligent if he or she follows what is practiced by peers of his or her locality and specialty. Hence, there is no need to get unnecessarily conscious about what is followed at other places or by other doctors, though taking inspiration from others and making endeavors to improve. A doctor is not negligent if he or she follows what is practiced by peers of his or her locality and specialty.[40]
- **Can an MD medicine doctor practice as a cardiologist?[41]**
  Goyal Hospital and Research Center Pvt. Ltd., Jodhpur and Ors, vs Kishan Shukla (R.P. No. 4023/2011) As per Indian Medical Council (IMC) Regulations, 2002 Clause-B subclause 1.1.3, "no person other than a doctor having qualification recognized by Medical Council of India and registered with Medical Council of India or State Medical Council is allowed to practice Modern System of Medicine or Surgery. Even otherwise, undergoing several trainings and attending workshops in Cardiology did not confer qualification of cardiologist. Hence, it is not recognized by MCI or Rajasthan State Medical Council.
- **Doctor's right to take on-the-spot decisions—legally acceptable.** Doctors can take and must take on-the-spot decisions as and when the situation demands. But all such actions must be solely in the patient's interest, in accordance with the accepted medical practice and the reason(s) thereof must be duly recorded in the patient's records.[42]
- **Managing medical conditions with no standard protocol or guidelines:** Standard and acceptable guidelines or practices or protocols, if any, must be duly followed. In cases, where there is none for a medical condition, greater caution is required in deciding the course of treatment. Consult peers and refer to standard texts and commentaries.[43]

- ***Is proceeding on leave by doctor negligence?***
  A doctor going on leave in unexpected compelling situations is not negligence. However, in case where the absence is planned in advance, care must be taken in accepting or admitting patient who would require personal attention during the scheduled absence.[44]
- ***Patient's refusal for the best and opting for the next best option—precautions:*** In cases, where the patient refuses the first or best option and chooses another option, take detailed consent very specifically recording the first or best option suggested by the doctor, the fact that the same was refused by the patient and the patient's choice.[45]
- ***Seizure of medical records by police:*** Taking a photocopy advisable. Cases of police seizing medical records are frequently reported. Thanks to the long-drawn Indian criminal justice delivery system. Once the records are seized, it takes years to get them back. The concerned doctor or hospital faces problems on two fronts—in further. The concerned doctor/hospital faces problems on two fronts - in further management of the patient and in legal matters in the court.[46]
- ***Caution in assigning responsibilities to interns:*** Hospitals and nursing homes must be cautious in assigning duties to interns. Proper supervision by senior doctors is absolutely necessary. Interns must be properly informed about the scope of their duties and restrictions, if any. Strict instructions must be given regarding managing critical patients.[47]
- ***Failure or delay from the patient in performing investigations:*** In case a patient refuses or fails to perform the investigations advised, especially the ones that are mandatory, the said fact must be meticulously recorded in the medical records of the patient.[48]
- ***Inadequate follow-up: When there is a procedural lapse either on the part of the patient or from the doctor on follow-up from the patient, it can lead to problems. For example, not coming with advised investigations, not following post discharge care regarding food, medicines, cross-referrals, etc.*** Legal consequences of failure to mention review dates. Prescription notes, discharge card or summary must compulsorily mention the next date for review, if one is required. This protocol is all the more necessary in pregnant women and critical patients who require periodical review.[49]
- ***Checking the drugs purchased by patient—a prudent practice.*** It is advisable to direct the patient to show the medicines to the doctor after purchasing them from the medical store, especially in cases of sensitive drugs, critical drugs, look-alike drugs,[50] sound-alike drugs, wrong substitute dispensing. In India, it is an established fact that medical shops do not have a qualified pharmacist.[51]
- ***Document all hypersensitivities/allergies to medications in your practice.*** There are situations in which physicians were able to avoid liability for allergic reactions just because they had documented events correctly.[52,53]
- ***Is allergy testing before prescribing medication necessary?*** Courts have accepted the impracticality, economic unfeasibility to test all patients for possible drug reactions and have held it to be unnecessary.[54]
- ***Should a doctor disclose all the rarer side effects while prescribing medications?***

The much "rare" or "remote" side effects may not require to be disclosed by the physician. Several courts have opined that there was no requirement of warning about rare side effects.[55] In another case, when the patient was prescribed topical corticosteroid for psoriasis and patient developed cataracts. As there was no agreement regarding the length of use, potency of the molecule, and the development of cataract, the judgment tilted in favor of the physician.[56] Several other judgments have also supported the physicians in not disclosing the rarer and remote side effects of drugs prescribed.[57,58]

Which are the common and which are rarer side effects? There is no uniform guideline. This probably depends on the social class, educational status of patient, patient's disease, type of treatment planned (short-term or long-term therapy), and local legal issues. However, with the information explosion in internet, it is better to talk and record about more and significant side effects. The more information the physician gives the patient, the better for both the physician and the patient.

In emergency situations, some courts have held that found it justified for failing to warn the patient of the adverse effects. In Shinn[59] and Niblack[60] cases, **the court favored the physician citing the emergency condition of the patient and the likelihood of developing immediate complications, if not for the drug used. Care should be taken to warn of potential common and significant adverse effects. The severity of disease and necessity for treatment also have been a reason to excuse a duty to warn of an adverse effect. In Jackson,[61] the patient was prescribed isoniazid (INH) without being told of the risk of possible hepatitis. Though the patient later developed hepatitis and was put on trial, the court favored the physician and noted that a reasonable person in the patient's position would have consented to INH treatment even with the knowledge of the risk of hepatitis.**

- What precautions to be taken for off-label indications?

  Even if the drug is not approved by the US Food and Drug Administration (FDA), its recommendation if found in manufacturer's package insert or in People's Democratic Republic Physicians' Desk Reference (PDR) has been legally accepted by courts.[62] In some courts, an expert's testimony of its usage in the medical community is accepted. In other jurisdictions, this information is merely some evidence of a physician's standard of care, and in yet another, it has been determined to have no legal significance.[63] In many jurisdictions, however, it is likely that the expert's testimony will be what is relied on to determine the medical community's accepted application of the medication. Morlino,[64] In Hogle vs Hall,[65] however, it is essential to document the issues while prescribing and following guidelines as prescribed by the PDR.

- *Recognition of associated injuries is crucial in the patient management[66] Shridevi Hospital and Shridevi Diagnostic and Research Center, Tumkur vs P Subhash 2007 Med LR 314.*

  It was held by the court the medical man should be able to recognize the presence of complications or associated injuries like severe vascular insufficiency in limb injuries so that urgent steps can be taken to shift the patient and appropriate steps taken to save the patient from the sequelae.

PREVENTIVE STRATEGIES

Several of the suggestions are often common sense approaches to treating the patient, but unfortunately, are not always carried out. Dermatologists need to be familiar with common and potentially significant adverse effects of medications and should inform the patients while prescribing them. They should check out for the particulars such as allergies, pregnancy, and significant past medical history and document them. Documentation is very important to safeguard their interest.

It rests solely on the shoulders of the doctors themselves to prevent any legal issues arising in their professional work. It is better to always work with the idea that every patient is a potential litigant. Approach and communicate to the patient and attendants with care and concern, human approach, and absolute professionalism. Follow the principles of evidence-based medicine in making the diagnosis and follow standard treatment protocols or guidelines while instituting treatment. They can be used in medical negligence claims and in court.[67,68]

- **Documentation:** The entire sequence of events unfolding should be documented properly, sequentially, and accurately. Good documentation should help recall the events that happened months or years ago during the testimony in the Court later. Such a document always carries legal sanctity as it can be used in the Courts to prove doctors innocence and sincerity to the patient care. *Justification for every medical Act*—in medical records and medical science. Medical records and medical science must both justify a particular line of treatment or surgery or procedure. Case history, symptoms, investigations, diagnosis, and the like, must clearly justify each and every medical Act and must also be clearly and specifically recorded in the patient's medical.[69] The medical records must be factual and complete. Tampering of records should be avoided. If a patient refuses to accept the advice of his doctor, this fact should be recorded in writing. The contents, which should be recorded, are listed in the Box 2.
- **Consent:** Obtain informed consent of the patient after explaining the possible outcome of the treatment, side effects and anticipated risks, available alternatives, and the result to be anticipated, if nothing is done. The consent has to be "informed and legally valid". Denied consent should also be recorded. The consent should be obtained from the patient only, exceptions being mentally insane patient, children, etc. (Box 3).[70]

In another case,[71] the National Commission held that, where informed consent is taken on the printed form without any specific mention about the name of the surgery, or signatures are taken from patient or relative in mechanical fashion, much in advance of the date scheduled for surgery, such forms cannot be considered as informed consent.

BOX 2: Contents in medical records.

Identity of the patient: name, age or sex, address, occupation, etc. date of examination
- Chief complaints
- History of present illness
- Past history
- *Treatment history:*
  - Personal history including history of drug allergy if any
  - Other histories if significant
  - Examination findings include general physical and systemic examination.
- *Clinical diagnosis:*
  - Daily notes should include progress of the patient, response to treatment, recording of any untoward events, and plan in the coming days for investigations and treatment or procedures.
  - All notes should be recorded with date and time and signed with stamp.
  - While prescribing guidelines for rational prescription should be followed.

> **BOX 3:** Ideal consent.
> - Documented in a simple language, read and understood by the patient.
> - *Covers in detail:*
>   - Diagnosis made
>   - Available modes of treatment with pros and cones of each option
>   - *If surgical*: Procedure, anesthesia, risk, and probability of complications
>   - Effect on quality of life postsurgery
> - Form should be signed by the patient and two witness, specifying date and time after having given time to think and Act.
> - Ideal consent protocol need not be followed in emergencies
> - Oral consent suffices for procedures like administering injections, enemas, etc.

In M Chinnaiyan vs Sri Gokulam Hospital & Anr. (2007),[72] the complainant was advised to undergo hysterectomy for which the consent was obtained from the complainant. However, the complainant suffered from bleeding of uterus as a result two units of blood was transfused after the operation. The blood units were not tested for contamination. The patient suffered with Human immunodeficiency virus-acquired immunodeficiency syndrome (HIV-AIDS) after three and a half year of the transfusion and died. The hospital was held liable because complainant had given consent only for hysterectomy operation and not for transfusion of blood. In contrast to the above judgments, in Pravat Kumar Mukherjee vs Ruby General Hospital and Ors (2005),[16] the National Commission observed that since emergency treatment is required to be given to a patient who was brought in seriously injured condition there was no question of waiting for consent. In the authors view, it is better, in all such cases, to involve another senior colleague in making the decision and recording in detail the justification or circumstances under which the decision was taken.

Taking single composite consent on admission—illegal. A general consent obtained at the time of admitting a patient for undergoing treatment, investigations, and surgery cannot be a substitute for a specific consent required for a surgery or procedure. Even a separate consent for a specific procedure or surgery taken at the time of admission is a MLCD.[73]

In Dr PS Hardia vs Kedarnath Sethia 33 2004 3 CPJ 19. (NC). 220. 114,[74] the court held that simply taking signature on a form stating "to treat him at his own risk under expressive consent" did not absolve the doctor from taking a more detailed and direct consent especially when there was no emergency.[74]

When the doctors have failed to produce the consent form and they even failed to produce the detailed records of treatment in their Nursing Home despite the fact that the patient stayed in the Nursing Home on two different spells, adverse inference about medical negligence has to be drawn against the treating doctor and the Nursing Home.[75]

There are still many gray areas in the subject of consent as far as doctors are concerned. A review article covering the entire of subject is worth reading.[76]

- There are certain Sections under which a doctor can claim support and security for the professional work he has done when he has to defend himself in the court of law on charge of negligence (Box 4).
- *Contributory negligence*: When a patient by his/her own want of care, contributes to the damage caused in the process of treatment then they are said to be guilty

BOX 4: Sections beneficial to doctors while defending himself in court.

- *IPC Section 52*: (Good faith). The doctor has to prove that his Act was in the best interest of the patient.
- *IPC Section 80*: Accident in doing a lawful Act. An accident without any criminal intention in the doing of an Act with proper care and caution.
- *IPC Section 88*: Act not intended to cause death, done by consent in good faith for person's benefit. The section highlights the importance of acting on good faith and with informed consent of the patient.
- *IPC Section 89*: It is similar to IPC Section 88 with the point of view of consent in case of children below 12 years and persons with a mental disorder where a guardian is authorized to give consent.
- *IPC Section 92*: Act done in good faith for benefit of a person without consent.
- *IPC Section 93*: Communication made in good faith.

BOX 5: Preventive strategies while deciding to plan for procedures.

- Make a proper near total diagnosis.
- Plan the nature of treatment.
- Discuss the treatment planned, possible alternatives, and risks of the treatment, possible adverse effects and the costs involved.
- Put everything in writing or use educational leaflets or handouts, videos, etc. to convey these information. Get a signature from the patient and an attendant.
- Assess the patient expectations, and ensure the patient will not have unrealistic goals.
- Discuss and ensure that insurance companies footing the bills are sorted out before the procedure.

of contributory negligence. For example, if the patient refusing to carry out the remedial treatment recommended by the doctor or indulging in activities forbidden by the doctor further exacerbates the damage. When there is negligence of two or more persons toward the patient resulting in a particular damage, it is called composite negligence. They are jointly or severally held liable for the damages.[23]

- Before ***prescribing*** any medication, a physician should be aware of all medications the patient is taking, including over-the-counter drugs and alternative medicines. Physicians should reinforce the importance of taking the medications only as prescribed. Patients should be advised that if they feel any medication is not having its intended effect, they should immediately contact their physician. An important way to prevent inadvertent drug interactions is by working in concert with hospital pharmacists. Avoid handwriting prescriptions and utilize instead electronic medical recording with electronic prescribing.
- Update your knowledge by attending continuing medical education (CMEs) and keep an eye on medicolegal cases.
- It is important that the doctor understands that patients who come to him have certain rights and he has to ensure that these rights are well-met during the course of his treatment.

Preventive Strategies while Deciding to Plan for Procedures

Some of the important preventive strategies to be followed when planning for procedures is mentioned in Box 5.

CONCLUSION

Dermatologists must become with the various medicolegal issues arising not only in dermatology, but also in the field of medicine. This is because dermatologists: (1) deal with some of the most chronic conditions such as psoriasis, pemphigus, and vitiligo where many experimentations are done by the patients; (2) important drugs such as steroids, retinoids, methotrexate, biologics, etc. which potentially have life-threatening side effects; and (3) deal with cosmetology where the expectations of the patients will be unrealistically high. Law keeps changing constantly and therefore doctors should discuss with lawyers before taking any action.

REFERENCES

1. Divekar S. Doctor-patient relationship worsening in Indian Context. Int J App Res Studies. 2012;1(2):207.
2. Consumer protection Act, 1986 (2).
3. Indian Medical Service versus V.P. Shantha's case, AIR 1996 SC 550.
4. Rao SBJ. Medical negligence liability under the Consumer Protection Act: A review of judicial perspective. Indian J Urol. 2009;25(3):361-71.
5. Jacob Mathew vs State of Punjab, (2005) 6 SCC 1.
6. Suresh Gupta (Dr) vs Govt. of NCT of Delhi.
7. Malay Kumar Ganguly vs Dr Sukamar Mukherjee (2009).
8. V Kishan Rao vs Nikhil Super Specialty Hospital (2010).
9. Martin F D'Souza vs Mohd Ishfaq-AIR 2009 SC 2049.
10. Poonam Verma vs Ashwin Patel and Ors. (1996) 4 SCC 322.
11. Police in MLC.
12. Halsbury's Laws of England, 4th Edition (Vol. 26 and 30). Oxford: Butterworth; pp. 17-18.
13. In Bolam vs. Friern Hospital Management Committee (1957) 1 WLR 582.
14. Shelat. Dr Laxman Balkrishna Joshi vs Dr Trimbak Bapu Godbole & Another (1969) 1 SCR 206. [online] Available from: https://indiankanoon.org/doc/297399/ [Accessed 2018].
15. Rangnath M Pt. Parmanand Katara vs Union of India & Ors 1989 AIR 2039, 1989 SCR (3) 997. [online] Available from: https://indiankanoon.org/doc/498126/ [Accessed December, 2018].
16. National Consumer Disputes Redressal Commission. Pravat Kumar Mukherjee vs Ruby General Hospital and Ors, II (2005) CPJ35 (NC). [online] Available from: https://indiankanoon.org/doc/173553/ [Accessed December, 2018].
17. Kanhaiya Kumar Singh vs Park Medicare and Research Centre III (1999), CPJ 9 (NC).
18. Calcutta Medical Research Institute vs Bimalesh Chatterjee I (1999) CPJ 13 (NC).
19. Prasanath Dhanaka vs Nizam's Institute of Medical Sciences (NIMS), Hyderabad, I (1999) CPJ 43 (NC).
20. AS Mittal vs state of UP AIR 1989, SC 1570.
21. Sailesh Munja vs All India Institute of Medical Sciences (AIIMS)
22. Ranjit Kumar Das vs ESI Hospital
23. BS Hegde vs Dr Sudhanshu Bhattacharya,
24. Dr KG Krishnan vs Praveen Kumar (Minor) II (2003), CPJ 125 NC.
25. Savita Garg vs Director, National Heart Institute, (2004), 8 SCC 56.
26. Spring Meadows Hospital vs Harjot Ahluwalia 1998, CTJ 81 (SC) (CP).
27. Smt Nihal Devi vs Ravi Hospital, Delhi Gate, Agra.
28. Martin F D'Souza vs Mohd. Ishfaq, AIR 2009, SC 2049.
29. Cooper vs Bronx Cross County Medical Group, 259 AD 2d 410, 687 NYS2d 156 (1999).
30. Moyer vs Three Unnamed Physicians from Marion County and Delaware County, Indiana, 845 NE2d 252 (2006).
31. Vinitha Ashok vs. Lakshmi Hospital and Ors. (AIR 2001 SC 3914).
32. RM Joshi vs Dr PB Tahilramani 1993, 3 CPR 435.
33. MLCD. 2010;3(12):167-9.
34. SV Panchori vs Dr Kaushal Pandey, 1999, 1 CPJ 332.
35. Dr Kaligoundon vs N Thangamuthu.
36. MLCD. 2012;5(4):59-60.
37. MLCD. 2011;4(6):80
38. MLCD. 2011;4(7):95-6.
39. MLCD. 2011;4(2):21-2.
40. MLCD. 2011;4(5):65-6.
41. Goyal Hospital & Research Centre Pvt. Ltd., Jodhpur & Ors, vs Kishan Shukla (R.P. No. 4023/2011).
42. MLCD. 2011;4(6):81-2.
43. MLCD. 2011;4(8):109-10.
44. MLCD. 2010;3(9):119-20.
45. MLCD. 2010;3(11):150-1.
46. MLCD. 2012;5(6):84.
47. MLCD. 2011;4(12):176-7.
48. MLCD. 2012;5(1):13-4.

49. MLCD. 2010;3(10):137-9.
50. Look-alike drug.
51. MLCD. 2010;3(11):148-149.
52. Tangoro vs Matansky, 231 Cal App 2d (2nd Dist 1964).
53. Regan vs Gore, 670 So2d 268 (La App 3d Cir 1996).
54. Slack vs Fleet, 242 So2d 650 (La App 1970).
55. Watkins vs United States, 482 F Supp 1006 (MD Tenn 1980)
56. Akers vs Levitt, Ohio App LEXIS 300 (Ohio App. 1992).
57. Woods vs Pommerening, 44 Wash 2d 867, 271 P2d 705 (1954).
58. Bullock vs Sasso, Tex App LEXUS 602 (1998).
59. Shinn vs St. James Mercy Hospital, 675 F Supp 94 (WD NY 1987).
60. Niblack vs United States, 438 F Supp 383 (DC Colo 1977).
61. Jackson vs State, 428 So2d 1073 (La App 1983).
62. Mulder vs Parke Davis & Co., 181 NW2d 882 (Minn 1970).
63. Ramon vs Farr, 770 P2d 131 (Utah 1989); Grassis vs Retik, 521 NE2d 411(1988).
64. Morlino vs Medical Center of Ocean County, 12 NJ 563, 706 A2d 721 (1998).
65. Hogle vs Hall, 112 Nev 599, 916 P2d 814 (1996).
66. Shridevi Hospital and Shridevi Diagnostic & Research Centre, Tumkur vs. P. Subhash 2007 Med LR 314.
67. Hurwitz B. How does evidence based guidance influence determinations of medical negligence? BMJ. 2004;329:1024-8.
68. Davies J. Clinical guidelines as a tool for legal liability. An international perspective. Med Law. 2009;28:603-13.
69. MLCD. 2012;5(10):146-147.
70. Samira Kohli vs Dr. Prabha Manchanda and Ors 50I (2008), CPJ 56 (SC)
71. Dr Sathy M Pillai & Anr. vs S Sharma & Anr. (2007), CPJ 131 NC
72. M. Chinnaiyan vs Sri Gokulam Hospital & Anr. (2007), CPJ 228 NC
73. MLCD. 2012;5(2):17-19.
74. Dr PS Hardia vs Kedarnath Sethia 33 2004, 3 CPJ 19. (NC). 220. 114.
75. Dr Arul Rajvs. N Ramanathan and Others, 2007 Med LR 655.
76. Mathiharan K. Law on consent and confidentiality in India: A need for clarity. Natl Med J India. 2014;27:39-42.

Index

Page numbers followed by *b* refer to box, *f* refer to figure, and *t* refer to table.

A

Abdominoplasty 423, 427
Ablative radiofrequency equipment 140
Academic Investigator Initiated Research 189
Accident in doing lawful Act 234
Accreditation program 455*f*
Accurate documentation 404
Acid attack 441, 494
    burns 494
    child victim of 444
    compensation for 443
    incidences of 443
    law on 494
    victims of 442, 443
Acne scar
    consent form for 342
    revision 333
    surgeries 334
Acne surgery 246
Acquired immunodeficiency syndrome 114, 283, 553
    Act 101, 289
Acts of Self-Advertisement and Unethical Conduct 106
Adolescent's preoperative assessment 440
Adrenaline 540
Adult cardiac life support 523
Advanced life support 335
Advanced Robotic Hair Transplantation Center 121
Adverse drug reaction 277, 282, 286
    cutaneous 281*t*
    high-risk situations for 283*t*
    signs of serious 283*b*
Advertising in medical practice,
        ethical implications of 105
Aesthetic dermatology 307
Aesthetic medicine 247
Aesthetic plastic surgery 542
    revision surgery in 423
Aesthetic practice, understanding 384
Aesthetic procedures 89, 435
    classification of 385
    performance of 136

Aesthetic surgery 84, 410, 411*b*, 426, 435, 439, 509, 535
    latest legal role of 441
    part of 434
Aesthetic transformation, job of 425
Ails Medical Laws in India 165
Aldrete's scoring system, modified 521
All India Association of Chemists and Druggists 305
All India Institute of Medical Sciences 547
Allegations 68
Allergic reaction 323
Allergy 523, 550
Allopathic medicine 115, 117
Allopurinol 283
Ambu bag 523
American Academy of Dermatology code 25
American Consent Requirements 456
American Society for Aesthetic Plastic Surgery
        Members, survey of 311
American Society of Anesthesiologists 523
American Society of Plastic Surgeons 309
Analgesia 522
Anaphylactic syndrome 324
Anaplastic large cell lymphoma 437
Ancillary care 187
Androgenetic alopecia 320
Anesthesia 320, 324, 522, 538
    consent 528
    equipment for 519
    regional 466
    supply cart 519
Anesthetic gas scavenging system 520
Anesthetic technique 528
Angioedema 282
Angiotensin converting enzyme 282
Annual service visit 371
Antemortem burn 479, 499
Antibiotics 283
Antiepileptics 283
Antihypertensives 283
Antimalarial drugs 283
Antiretroviral drugs 283
Antitubercular drugs 283

Anxiety 151, 283
Appeals 65
Approvals and Ethics Committees 184
Arrhythmia 461
Arthralgia 283
Arthritis 283
    victim of 114
Artificial hair fiber 321, 330
    implantation 330
    rejection of 330
Association of Cutaneous Surgeons 34
Association of Dermatologists,
        Venereologists, and Leprologists 35
Association of Hair Restoration Surgeons 181, 320
Association of Medical Consultants 230
Association of Perioperative Registered Nurses 402
Association of Physicians 174
Atopic dermatitis 211
Atropine 540
Australian Medical Association 109
Autoclave 140
    equipment 140
    register 528
Autopsy in child victims 160
Ayurveda, practitioners of 116
AYUSH, authorities of 117
Azathioprine 268, 283, 354
    hematological toxicity of 283
    safely with 283

B

Bandaging, equipment for 523
Bariatric surgery for weight reduction 446
Baseline triglyceride 548
Basic dermatosurgery services 137
Basic life support 523
Beauty clinics 116
Becker's nevus 435, 438
Best interests test 436*b*
Biomedical waste
    disposal agency 141
    disposal system 141
    handling rules 526
    management 526
    segregation 146
Biopsy, specimen register for 528
Birth and death register 99
Bleeding 342
    diathesis 336
Blepharoplasty 420, 423, 427
Blood banking system, poor 82
Blood pressure 409, 539
    apparatus 140, 523

Body contouring 446
    procedures 402
Body cover 525
Body dysmorphic disorder 310, 311, 395, 405, 414,
        417, 419, 419*b*, 440
    diagnosis of 417, 418
Body temperature 409
Bolam test, position of 386
Bolam's test 20, 510
Bollywood influence 517
Botulinum toxin 357, 385, 439
    A injection, consent form for 361
    treatment 128
Bowel injury 541
Brachial plexus nerve repair 247
Brachioplasty 406
Brain surgery 55
Breast
    augmentation 247, 423, 427, 437, 440, 446
        revision in 433
    implant, reconstruction with 247
    reduction 427, 437, 440
        surgery 437
    surgery 403, 437
British Association of Aesthetic Plastic Surgeons 439
British Society for Allergy and
        Clinical Immunology guidelines 281
Broken hearts, trail of 112
Built-in social media services 194
Burn 486, 502
    accidental 479
    acute 479
    after roadside trauma 491
    blister 501, 505
    care, acute 247
    case victim 486
    homicidal 479
    infection 502
    injury 480
    misusing 500
    severity 491
        WHO assessment forms for 483*f*
    shock 502
    suicidal 479
    victims 492

C

Café-au-lait macules 438
Callings and employment rules 303
Canadian Association of Plastic Surgery 439
Cancer, victim of 114
Capsular contracture 434, 437
    treatment of 433

Index

Cardiac arrest 538
   urgent treatment of 335
Cardiac bypass surgery 446
Cardiac catastrophe 265
Cardiac disease requiring quadruple bypass
      surgery 548
Cardiopulmonary resuscitation 514, 539
Care and competence, reasonable degree of 547
Cataract, development of 551
Cautery burn during circumcision surgery 504
Central Clinical Establishment Act 165, 166
Central Consumer Protection Authority 50
Central Consumer Protection Council 50
Central Council for Indian Medicine Act 184
Central Drug Standard Control Organization 89
Central Ethics Committee on Human Research 184
Central Information Commission 94
Central Public Information Officer 94
Central Sterile Supply Department 527
Centralized accident and trauma services 159
Centrofacial erythema 283
Cephalosporins 264
Cerebral artery, middle 58
Cerebral palsy 442
Cerebrovascular accident 58
Charaka samhita 23
Cheatle forceps 140
Chemical 139
   antiseptics washing 520
   peel 140, 211, 246, 248, 440
Chest
   diseases 35
   wall burn 501
Chief Judicial Magistrate 47
Chief Justice of India 177
Chief Medical Officer 452
Child abuse 499
Child Abuse Prevention and Treatment Act 500
Cholesterol levels 548
Christian Marriage Act 294
Chronic suffering, prospect of 113
Civil and criminal offence 217
Civil court 17, 127
Civil law 509
Civil liability 545, 38
Civil negligence 38, 43, 236, 238
   case of 47
Civil surgeon 71
Claims, remainder of 401
Clinic staff, mandatory holidays for 145
Clinical dermatology 254, 270
Clinical Establishment Act 139, 140, 159
Clinical Trials Registry of India 185
Closed circuit television 304

Cocaine drops, sale of 112
Code of ethics 35, 108
   elaborately prohibits 107
Code of medical ethics, legal implications of 35
Codified Regulations and Conundrum 213
Collagen vascular diseases 283
Commission under Section 14 of Act 79
Communication 269, 350, 392
   appropriate forms of 109
   history of 193
   tips on 393
Compensation 65, 190
   concept of 78
Complaint 183
   made in State Medical Council 71
Complete blood count 266, 523
Compound annual growth rate 355
Comptroller and Auditor General report 241
Conception, products of 155
Concomitant drug intake 336
Conduct of Medical Council of India 298
Conduct Under Medical Council Rules and
      Regulations 452
Congenital defects 441, 441b
Congenital disorders 441
Consciousness 521
Consensus of American Academy of
      Cosmetic Surgery 309
Consent form 362
Consent, audiovisual recording of 186
Constitute negligence 511
Consultation, purpose of 138
Consumer complaint 50
Consumer Complaints Council 328
Consumer Court's Data 411
Consumer Disputes Redressal Agencies 38, 42
Consumer Disputes Redressal Forum 325
Consumer Forum 4, 236
Consumer Forum and Consumer Commissions 166
Consumer forum, expert opinion in 236
Consumer Protection Act 32, 42, 49, 60, 61, 63, 64,
      68, 74, 93, 94, 133, 135, 137, 318, 322, 517,
      543, 544, 547
Consumer Protection Law 50
Consumer Protection Regulations 229
Contamination, minimizing risk of 524
Control and supervision of experiments on animals,
      purpose of 189
Corneal eye shields for lasers 369
Corticosteroids 540
Cosmetic 122
   center 140
   clinic 119, 398
   dermatologist 34

esthetic surgery 421
gynecology 248
results 406
surgeon 34, 400
surgical procedures 246, 517
Cosmetic dermatology 247, 254, 355
treatments 248
Cosmetic surgery 35, 125, 410, 413, 414, 435, 446
affordable 412
elective nature of 400
focuses 416
number of 517
practice 401, 403
Cosmetologist 119
Cosmetology 247
Cosmetology Society of India 34
Council for Scientific and Industrial Research 190
Council on Ethical and Judicial Affairs 25
Court directs payment of compensation 132
Court of Chief Judicial Magistrate 47
Courts, hierarchy of 16
C-reactive protein 406
Cremation, case report of 501
Criminal Act 132
Criminal and professional liabilities 318
Criminal complaints 44
Criminal court 18, 127, 236
Criminal law Act 493, 495
Criminal law amendment Act 496
Criminal law amendment ordinance 158
Criminal liabilities 545
Criminal medical negligence and criminal liability 44
Criminal negligence 234, 236, 510
Criminal procedure, code of 18, 64, 117, 493, 497
Criminal prosecution 509
Crow's feet 356
Crucial medical decisions 82
Cryosurgery 246
Cryosurgical procedures 246
Cryotherapy 334
Custody, chain of 157
Cyclosporine 283
Cysts, removal of 333
Cytopenias 283
Cytotoxic drugs 281

D

Daily case register 142
Dapsone-induced liver failure 286
Death
after hair transplantation 324
cause of 488f
certificate 490

notification to police 490f
register 528
report 485f
Defamation 217, 218
Defendant's Act 510
Defensive medicine 81, 274, 278
Defibrillator machine 228
Deoxyribonucleic acid 150, 451, 486
Depressions 431
Dermabrasion 246, 440
Dermal fillers 248
Dermatologic care, delivery of 338
Dermatologic surgery 246, 338
Dermatologic surgical procedures 337
Dermatological surgeries 446
Dermatologist 119, 133, 138, 333, 540
engaging in social media 207
Dermatology 115, 253, 254, 257, 263
clinic 140
integral part of 88
practice
changing face of 253
of general 263
Dermatoscope 140
Dermatoscopy 268
Dermatosis papulosa nigra, removal of 310
Dermatosurgeon 34
Dermatosurgery 35, 88, 253
and aesthetic medicine, practice of 339
operation theater 337
Dermatosurgical interventions, use of 439
Dermatosurgical procedures 337, 339
advanced 334
Dermatotrichologist 248
Dermoscopy 206
Device quackery 113
Dexamethasone 540
Dextrose 540
Diabetes 336
Dietary supplements, category of 122
Direct health hazard 114
Director General of Health Services 102
Director General of Police 11
Disaster preparedness and management 527
Discharge after ambulatory surgery 522
Discharge cards 429
Discharge criteria 521
Discovery rule 74
Disinfection 524
Disposable device 525
Distress, emotional 401
District Consumer Disputes Redressal Forum 316
District forum 63, 64

Index

District magistrate 452
Doctor against Criminal Prosecution in
    Indian Penal Code, safeguards for 234
Doctor Protection Act 220
Documentation 315, 338, 397
Documents needed for clinic registration 141*b*
Domestic cruelty 496
Domestic violence 496, 497
    protection Act 496
Donor agency, multilateral 187
Donor dissection 320
Down's syndrome 441
Dowry death 496-498
Dowry prohibition Act 496
Dressing, equipment for 523
Drug
    administration, consent for 271
    and therapeutic agents 524
    contamination 241
    dispensing of 142
    high-risk 283*t*
    hypersensitivity syndrome 279
    induced toxic epidermal necrolysis,
        development of 78
    interactions relevant in dermatology 283*t*
    monitoring dosage of 548
    overdose 156*b*
    quality testing 241
    use of 136
Drug allergy
    history of 552
    management of 281
    relevant information regarding 336
Drug Controller and Licensing Authority 302
Drug prescription 227
    brand 227
    generic 227
Drugs and Cosmetics Act 6, 116, 141, 184, 190, 302
Drugs and Cosmetics Rules 141, 142, 306
Drugs and Magic Remedies Act 107, 215, 316
Drugs Controller General of India 184
Dry heat sterilization 525
Dying declaration format 492
Dystrophy, multiple 442

E

Ear
    lobe surgeries 335
    surgery 247
Economic hazards 115
Eczema
    palms 265
    soles 265

Edema 283
    bruising 535
Electric burn, amputation in 484
Electrical requirements 520
Electrocardiogram 506
Electrocardiography 523, 539
Electrocautery burn 504
    case report of 504
Electroconvulsive therapy 498
Electrohomeopathy 115, 116
Electromyography 504
Electronic health record 75
Electronic insurance 370
Electronic medical records 146
Embryo, study of 451
Emergency contact mechanisms, misuse of 312
Emergency drugs 140
Emergency equipment required 523
Emergency medical care 153, 154
Empathy 459
Employees' State Insurance 547
Employing precautions guarding
        against injury 510
Encephalopathy, hepatic 286
Endotracheal tube 486, 523
Energy based devices 365
Energy boosters 113
Enforcing consumer forum order 63
Entral line 486
Enzyme disorder 364
Enzyme-linked immunosorbent assay 291
Eosinophilia 283
Equipment delivery system cart 519
Equipment maintenance register 528
Erbium-doped yttrium aluminum garnet 433
Erythroderma 279
Essential dermatosurgical equipment 140
Essential Information about Protective Acts 220
Essential Services Maintenance Act 230
Essential Social Networks Worth Engaging 204
Establishing grievance cells 182
Ethical Advertising Board 110
Ethical misconduct, major 300
Ethics Committee 188, 235
Ethylene oxide 525
Even numbers Indian Penal Code 158*b*
Evidence-based medicine, principles of 552
Excess monetary cost 403
Expensive health care procedures 449
Explosion proof plugs, use of 520
Eye
    glasses, safety 369
    protection 525

F

Face lift 403, 427
    related risks 402
Facial edema 404
Facial injuries 57
Facial nerve injury 402
Facial plastic surgery
    major 441
    perceptions of 441
    procedures 420
Facial volumization 423
Facilitating medical tourism 445
Fake medical degrees, variety of 116
False allegation, case of 498
Fat grafting 248, 335
Federal Trade Commission 109
Federation of Indian Chambers of Commerce and Industry 306
Fever 283
Fibrous tissue, quantum of 432
Fight against quackery 118, 182
Financial consent 528
Fire and burglary insurance 370
Fire pipe 519
Fire safety guidelines 146
First information report 45, 72, 153, 501
Flap surgery 247
Foleys catheter 486
Follicular unit
    extraction, advent of 318
    transplantation 319, 320, 329
Folliculitis 323
Food and Drug Administration 119, 358, 385
Food and fluids, oral intake of 522
Foreign exchange transactions 451
Foreigner registration office 447
Fractional carbon dioxide 433
Fraternal ties 213
Fraudulent Criminal or Malicious Act 132
Fraudulent medical practices 112
Free medical treatment 443, 493
Frown lines 356
Full surgical scrub 520
Fumigation 524
    machine 524
    register 528
Fundamental rights 4
Fungal cultures 144
Future medical expenses 78

G

Gangrenous limb, amputation in 484
Garment advice 409

Gas sterilization 525
Gender affirmation surgery state 418
Gender modification surgery 446
General anesthesia 466, 532
General cosmetology 247
General Medical Council 439
Generic names of drugs, use of 27
Geriatrics 188
Gillies principle 430
Glassblower factory, working in 502
Glucometer 140
Glucose-6-phosphate dehydrogenase 266, 282
Good clinical practice
    guidelines for 186
    principles of 404
Goods and Service Tax 142, 145, 534
    registration certificate 303
Gossypiboma 402
    place of 402
Governmental healthcare spending 80
Gynecomastia 436

H

Habit forming drugs 306
Hair 88
    and Cosmetology Centers, unauthorized and unqualified 118
    care 247
    reduction 248
    removal laser treatment 313
    replacement therapy 440
Hair restoration 423, 427
    surgery 320
Hair transplant 247, 248
    consent 321
    illegal activities of 119
    surgeon 318, 331
    surgery, perform 326
Hair transplantation 89, 90, 121, 123, 300, 318, 333, 352, 403
    bad job of 325
    case of 128
    centers, multiple 120
    guidelines for 320
    multisession 328
    quackery in 120
Hammurabi, code of 23
Harmless procedure 540
Harrison Narcotics Act 112
Hazardous waste receptacle 519
Health
    hucksters 112
    literacy, role of 68

Index

related issues 115
services 119
status 529
Health Guidelines Revision Committee,
    members of 518
Health Insurance Portability and
    Accountability Act 209
Health Ministry Screening Committee 190
Health quackery 112
    hazards 114
Healthcare
    facilities, challenge for 218
    organizations 57
    services 225
    system 80
Heart 55
Hemangiomas 435
Hematological toxicity 283
Hematopoietic stem cell transplantation 321
Hepatic impairment 283
Hepatitis
    risk of 551
    virus 286
Hepatotoxicity 283
Herbal remedies 113
Hereditary genetic muscle disease, group of 442
Hernia 541
High Courts and Supreme Court of India 512
Hindu Marriage Act 292, 294
Hindu Succession Act 294
Histrionic personality disorder 310, 311
Hospital credibility, loss of 403
Hospital Protection Act 220
Hospitals and facilitating agencies 447
Human immunodeficiency virus 101, 121, 151, 289, 553
    infection 291
    patients, legal issues in 289
    status, disclosure of 290
    test 291
Human leukocyte antigen 283
Human organ transplant Act 239, 502*f*
Human resource 140
Human Rights Commission 127
Human waste, disposal of 521
Hyaluronic acid 364, 385
    filler treatment, consent form for 363
    injections of 363
Hydroxychloroquine 268
Hyperpigmentation 333
Hypersensitivities 550
Hypovolemia, plasma expanders for 540

I

Iatrogenic burns 501, 503, 505, 507
Iatrogenic organ injury 402
Ilizarov technique 413*b*
Import export code 370
Inadequate informed consent 402, 420
Income tax Act 145
India medicine Ayurveda, Yoga, practitioners of 122
Indian Association of Dermatologists,
    Venereologists and Leprologists 118, 133, 139, 174, 181, 255, 269, 319, 320, 335, 371
Indian Contract Act 545
Indian Council of Medical Research 184, 447
    guidelines of 32
Indian Evidence Act 491
Indian Medical Association 83, 118, 127, 174, 180, 215, 231, 248
Indian Medical Council 84, 142, 366
    Act 25, 53, 93, 116, 160
        relevant regulation of 99
    regulations 25, 316
Indian Medical Degrees Act 117
Indian medicine, practitioners of 115
Indian National Science Academy 189
Indian Nursing Council 139
    Act 139
Indian Orthopaedic Association 174
Indian Penal Code 19, 48, 58, 155, 217, 226, 234, 292, 323, 443, 477, 480, 502*f*, 544
    sections, clauses of 219*b*
Indian Plastic Surgeon Survey 463
Indian Railway Act 294
Indian Society of Anaesthesia Guidelines 523
Individually identifiable health information 449
Infant mortality rate 113
Infection 342
    control 541
        measures 524
    risks of postoperative 450
Infectious diseases 441
Information based Democratic Society 93
Information privacy laws regulate 93
Informed consent 315, 318, 333, 337, 395, 404, 421, 440, 471, 529
    components of 272*f*
    elements of 396
    for mole removal and biopsy 344
    process 421
    types of 271
Infrastructure 139, 518, 540
Injected fat, total loss of 431
Injury, emotional 421
Instant messenger consultations 208

Institute of Health and Management Studies 224
Institutional Ethics Committees 184
Instrument maintenance register 528
Insurance 61, 370
    policy 135
Insured's technical management 132
Integrated system of medicine, practitioners of 116
Intensive care unit 69, 286, 352, 406
Intentional burning 499
Internal carotid artery 58
International Code of Medical Ethics 23
International Conference on Harmonization 184
International Covenant on Civil and
    Political Rights 170
International Society of Aesthetic Plastic Surgery 309
International Society of Hair Restorations
    Surgeons 181
Internet and communication media 517
Intra-treatment negligence 421
Iontophoresis 433
Irritant contact dermatitis 247
Isoniazid 551
Itraconazole 283

J

Jacob mathew's case 545
Jaundice 283
Judgment
    claiming error of 74
    error of 74
Judgment of Indian Courts 120
Judicial system 80

K

Karnataka Private Medical Establishment Act 181
Karnataka Violence Act 8
Keloid 333
    treatment 246
Keloidal tendencies 336
Ketoconazole 283
Knee and hip replacement 446
Koh mount 144
Kushtha 294

L

Labiomental 406
Labor maintenance contract 370
Laboratory animals, use of 189
Language, use of 295
Laparoscopic abdominal liposuction 539
Laryngoscope 523

Laser 246, 248, 319, 365
    adaptation 522
    assisted hair-removal 506
    consent for 366
    pigment removal 246
    procedures 246
    scar revision 246
    skin treatments 440
    treatments, real sequel of 433
Laser burns 502, 505
    allegations of 506
Laser hair
    reduction 211, 246
    removal 435, 438, 438*f*, 440
        case of 128
        doctor for 183
Law enforcement 118
Law in negligence, process of 126
Law under Indian Constitution 292
Lawyers, costs of 132
Legal education and legal awareness 3
Legal guardians 440
Legal liabilities 84, 274
Legal principles 298
    in defense, use of 73
Legal restrictions, evasion of 27
Legal Services Act 295
Legal significance 551
Legislature judiciary 116
Leprologist 133
Leprosy 294, 441
    bill, persons affected by 295
    colonies 295
    legal aspects of 294
Leprosy Mission Trust India 295
Leukocyte count, differential 264
Levocetirizine 264
Liabilities, types of 545
Licenses 140
    to sell drugs 302
Licensing authority 187
Lichen planus 286, 354
Linen management 525
Linkedin 215
Lip surgery 247
Lipomas 334
Liposuction 89, 247, 333, 353, 423, 427, 440, 446, 531,
    534, 536, 538
    circumferential 541
    death, common causes of 541
    revision surgery in 431
    safety 540
    surgery 531, 536
    tumescent solution for 461

Index

Liquid waste 144
Litigation
    and payment of compensation, event of 132
    fear of 457
    prevention of 421
Liver 55
    function test 264
Loading autoclave 525
Local anesthesia 227, 466
    complication of 523
Local legal issues 551
Local municipal rules and regulations 140
Local sepsis 523
Long-Drawn Indian Criminal Justice
        Delivery System 550
Lovastatin 283
Lower motor neurone 429
Lung 55
Lupus erythematosus 268
Lymphadenopathy 283
Lymphatic drainage, manual 431

M

Madhya Pradesh Medical Council 215
Magical remedies 215
Magnifying lens 140
Maharashtra Medical Practitioners Act 323
Malaise 283
Malpractice Insurance Premium in Los Angeles 80
Malpractice lawsuit insight 438*b*
Manpower requirement 541
Manufacturer's instructions 141
Marriage prospects 411
Mastopexy 423
Materially misleading 61
Maturation, process of 432
Mayo stand 519
Mechanical ventilation duct delivers 519
Media trials and violence against doctors 218
Media, role of 254, 258
Medical accident 237, 241, 243
    corpus 240
    no negligence 238
    victim 82
Medical Act contrary 549
Medical advertising 212
Medical and Healthcare Services and Consumer
        Protection 49
Medical attendant visa 447
Medical Board opinion 407
Medical Code of Ethics 93
Medical Council 105, 107
    Acts 107

Medical Council of India 53, 107, 117, 144, 177, 213,
        227, 233, 246, 546, 235, 305, 319, 326, 366,
        475
    Act 174, 184
    Code of Ethics Regulations 299
    Ethics Code Regulation 7.20 120
    Permission of 120
    Regulations Guidelines 491
Medical data
    confidentiality of 318
    in diseases 93
Medical devices, studies with 189
Medical diagnostic laboratory 139
Medical education/training 225
Medical emergencies, life-threatening 335
Medical error 237
Medical Ethics 23
    Code of 3, 22, 26
    for dermatologists 25
Medical examination 151
Medical Health Authority 407
Medical Indemnity
    Insurance 140, 142
    Scheme 142
Medical Injury 237
    categories of 238
Medical institutions 225
Medical insurance penetration 80
Medical intervention 88
Medical laboratory technician 144
Medical law 223
Medical Literature and Case Laws 75
Medical malpractice 237
    insurance 339
    litigation, pathogenesis of 412, 412*b*
    occurring overseas 450
    system 82
Medical mishap 237
Medical negligence 126, 318, 502*f*
    concept of 4
    defenses in 67
    false allegation of 539
    in plastic surgery 512
    legal principles in 233
    process of 544
    tort of 57
Medical practice, legal regulations in 165
Medical Practitioner 511
    Act 119
    Professional Indemnity Insurance 70
    Registered 138
Medical profession 180
    professional conduct of 213
Medical quackery 113, 122

Medical records
   disclosure of 296
   in burn case 491
   maintenance of 26, 142
Medical Science Constitutes Negligence, Principles of 549
Medical technology 448
Medical Termination of Pregnancy 502*f*
   Act 156, 451, 499
Medical tourism
   dark side of 451
   ethical issues in advertising for 451
   legal issues in 445
   travelling long distances for 451
Medical tourist, mind of 445
Medical treatment occurs, result of 69
Medical visa 445, 446
   extension of 447
Medical waste disposal 143
Medical/clinical cosmetology 247
Medicare Service Personnel 9
Medication
   costs of 536
   error 279, 284
      components of 279
Medicine 528, 115
   evidence-based 384
   in India, systems of 116
   integrated system of 116
   original system of 116
   practice of 194
   recognized system of 138
   supplies of 540
   system of 117
Medicolegal aspects
   of hair practice 318
   of lasers 365
Medicolegal case 480
   discussion 413, 413*b*
   number of 544
   rising incidence of 254
Medicolegal cell 128, 182, 230
Medicolegal issues 301, 495
   in burns 479
   in cutaneous adverse drug reactions 277
   in dermatology, rising incidence of 258
   in liposuction 531
Medicolegal law 223
   knowledge of 225
Medicolegal problems, experience of 73
Medicolegal Report 94, 156, 158
   of Child Survivor of Sexual Violence 156
   Writing for Doctors 157
Medicolegal situation, warning signs of 125

Medicos legal action group 71, 230
Mental agony 168
   and physical pain, compensation for 78
Mental disorders, statistical manual of 311
Mental fitness of minors 441*b*
Mental Health Act 98
Mental retardation 162
Mentally ill burn victim, case law on 498
Mesotherapy 385
Messiah complex 432
Methotrexate 89, 283, 554
   with oral retinoids 283
   with sulfa drugs 283
Meticulous documentation 333
Microdermabrasion 248
Microsclerotherapy 440
Midlife crises 310
Minimal court fees 544
Minimal invasive treatments 88
Minipunch grafting 334
Ministry of Health and Family Welfare 89, 306, 323
Minocycline 264
Misusing law during false complaint 161
Modern medicine, drugs of 117
Modern minimally invasive surgical techniques 529
Moist heat sterilization 525
Mole 334
Monetary compensation, landmark case law for 494
Motor accidents claims 66
Motor Vehicle Act 66, 294
Mucosal exposure 527
Multiple sclerosis, victim of 114
Multisystem failure 324
Munchausen syndrome 499
Muscular dystrophy 442
Muslim Marriage Act 294

N

Nail 88
   biopsies 334
   procedures 335
   surgeries 246
Narcissistic perfectionists 311
Narcissistic personality disorder 310, 311
Narcotic drug abuse 306
Narcotic Drugs and Psychotropic Substances Act 306
Nasogastric tube 486
Nasopharyngeal airways 523
National Commission 63, 64, 135, 285
National Consumer Disputes Redressal Commission 59, 71, 101, 134, 284, 285, 512, 513
National Guidelines for Stem Cell Research 321
National Health Service 257

Index

National Law School 224
National Medical Commission Bill 93
Needlestick injuries 527
Negligence 545
    allegations of 38
    by doctors 242
    concept of 38, 233
    essentials of proof of 40
    ordinary 544
    per se 39
    proof of 39
    received by
        consumer forum, complaint of 236
        police, complaint of 235
Negligent Act 133
Neodymium-doped yttrium aluminum garnet 334
Neonatal intensive care unit 69
Nerve repair 247
Neurotoxins, injections of 248
Nevoid conditions, treatment of 438
Nevus of Ota 435, 438
Nipple sensation, possible loss of 437
No objection certificate 486
Nodulocystic acne 264
No-fault compensation 240
Nonallopathic doctors 120
Nonclinical cosmetology 247
Noncultured cellular grafting technique 439
Noncutaneous procedures 420
Nonexisting emergency response systems 82
Non-governmental organization 187, 230
Nonintact skin exposure 527
Non-Medical Council of India Recognized
        Institutions 120
Nonpecuniary damages 545
Non-resident Indian doctor 43
Nonsteroidal anti-inflammatory drugs 282, 283
Notifiable diseases 100
Nuremberg code 23
Nutrition 248
Nutritional quackery 113

O

Oath of Hippocrates 105
Obesity, childhood 437
Offence, cognizance of 10
Omalizumab 353
Online consultation 207, 216, 450
Online reputation management 207
Operating theaters, types of 519
Operation register 527
Operation theater 55, 517, 518, 526
    environment, quality control of 526
    in plastic surgery, set-up an 517

Operations, minor 138
Opioid register 528
Oral consent 272
Oral contraceptive pills 283
Ordinance 158
Organ transplants 446, 451
Otoplasty 435
Out of compassion 127
Out-of-court settlement 125-128, 130, 134
Overenthusiastic manner 130
Own medical records 449
Oxygen
    cylinders 523
    saturation 521

P

Paid news, case of 108
Pain 342
    management 536
    relief, morphine for 493
    severe 493
Painless surgery, simple 533
Panchanama 486
Panel of lawyers 182
Parameters laid down 545
Parliamentary Standing Committee 177
Patient confidentiality 213
Patient education and responsibility 240
Payment and insurance benefits 449
Pecuniary damages 545
Pecuniary jurisdiction 63
Pemphigus vulgaris, severe 266
Penal provisions of Pre-conception and Pre-natal
        Diagnostic Techniques Act 167
Periodic inspection, process of 522
Permanent injury 420, 421
Permanent restoration 321
Personal protective equipment, use of 525
Personal safety 44
Personality trait 312
Pharmaceutical company 187
    role of 254, 258
Pharmaceutical manufacturer, liability of 285
Pharmacist 546
    and chemist-based quackery 116
Pharmacy license 140, 141
Photographic documentation 300
Photography and law 298
Physical torture 502
Physical trauma to wrong surgery 50
Physician and non-physician operator
        qualification 366
Physician extenders 315, 338

Physicians Insurers Association of America 278
Physicians, duties of 27
Physiological dysfunction of vital organs 50
Pityriasis alba 266
Planned preventive maintenance and quality control 526
Plastic and cosmetic surgeons 54
Plastic and reconstructive surgeons 512
Plastic surgeons 247, 391, 392, 422, 432, 435
    instructions 402
    responsibility 412
Plastic surgery 247, 391, 397, 398, 401, 410, 411b, 413, 509, 531
    and cosmetic dermatology 49
    and day care surgery, set-up 517
    changing face of 391
    endoscopic 247
    multiple sittings of 443
Plastic surgical practice 399
Plastic syringes and excised body parts 144
Platelet rich plasma 248, 319
    for facelift 385
Poisoning 156b
Poland's syndrome 437
Police notification form at time of admission 484f
Pollution Control Board 137
Polyclinic 139
Polycystic ovarian disease 438
Polypharmacy 283
Portwine stain 439
Post-inflammatory pigmentation 333
Postmortem
    burns 479
    notification form 489f
    report 158
        copies of 94
        discrepancy in 489
Postprocedure care 315
Potential medicolegal case 125
Potential witnesses 96
Potentially significant adverse effects of medications 552
Power-assisted devices 541
Practicing surgeons 451
Practitioners of Indian medicine, nonentitlement of 116
Preanesthesia checkup 526
Pre-conception and pre-natal diagnostic technique 499, 502f
    Act 166, 167, 169, 451
Prevention of Begging Act 295
Prevention of Cruelty to Animals Act 189
Prevention of Legal Implications of Code of Medical Ethics 35

Prima facie evidence 511
Primarily prescription-based practice 137
Private healthcare system 225
Private Medical Practitioners Association, qualified 304
Procedural hand hygiene 520
Professional commitments, discharge of 131
Professional incapacity 237
Professional incompetence 237
Professional indemnity
    coverage 50
    insurance 130-132, 269, 397
    policy 135, 136
Professional life insurance 269
Professional misconduct 237
Professional need-based clients 310
Professional negligence 237
Professional services, payment of 27
Professional tax 303
    payment 145
Prohibition of discrimination 289
Prohibition of violence 10
Prohibitive costs of defense 127
Prophylaxis, post-exposure 292
Protection of Children from Sexual Offences 148, 151, 158
Protection of Children from Sexual Offences Act 148, 149, 153, 154, 156, 159-161, 163, 167, 292, 477
    in marital rape 161
    male victim in 164
    victim of rape under 161
Protection of Children from Sexual Offences
    amendment to 159
    case 164
Protection of Human Rights Act 170
Provisions Contained in Drugs Act 117
Provisions of Consumer Protection Act 314
Psoriasis 211, 266, 321, 352
Psychiatric history 312
Psychiatrist certificate 418, 419, 419b
Psychiatrist opinion 439
Psychological disorders 312
Psychological distress 401
Psychological evaluation 440
Psychological injury 421
Psychological recovery 521
Psychological support 434
Psychological trauma 438
Psychosocial analysis 405
Public Health Notification 99
Public information officers 94
Pulmonary embolism 451
Pulse oximeter 523
    with electrocardiography monitor. 228

Index

Pulse rate 409
Purchase contract 369
Purchase order 369

Q

Quack medicines 112
Quackery 111, 115
    gradual elimination of 113
    prevention of 118, 122
    survival of 113
Quacks
    training of 115
    types of 112
Quacksalver 112
Qualified auditor, advice of 146
Quasi-judicial authorities 130

R

Radiofrequency
    skin therapy 431
    treatments 431
Reaction, severe 523
Reconstructive surgery 509
Rectus divarication 541
Recurrent dyshidrotic eczema 548
Recurrent expenditure involved in running pharmacy 304
Referral system, proper 338
Regional and Religious Hindrances 91
Registration of clinical trial 185
Registration of Doctors 33
Registration under Respective Clinical Establishments Act 140, 141
Regular preplanned schedule 404
Regulatory bodies 174
    nonstatutory 174
    statutory 174
Regulatory clinical trials 184
Renal function 283
Renal impairment 283
Renal toxicity 283
Repeal and Amendment of Certain Laws 295
Replantation surgeries 247
Reproductive tourism 451
Research 75, 90
    institutions 188
Researchers 188
Respiration 521
Respiratory rate 409
Resuscitation 522
    kit 140
    medication 521

Retinoid 89, 281, 548, 554
Retributive justice 168
Retrograde cholangiopancreatography, endoscopic 68
Return of sensory 522
Revision rhinoplasty 432
Revision surgery 427, 434
    timing of 430
Revisional Jurisdiction 63
Rheumatoid arthritis 283
Rhinoplasty 89, 247, 403, 423, 427, 436, 440, 446
    of nagging celebrity. 425b
Rifampicin 283
Right of Mentally ill patients 98
Right to Confidentiality 93, 98
Right to Education 296
Right To Employment 295, 296
Right to Freedom of movement 295
Right to Health and treatment 296
Right to Information 93, 319
    Act 94, 184, 226
Right to Life and survival 152
Right to Movement 296
Right to Ownership of property 296
Right to Privacy 100, 153
Right to Protest 229
Right to Safety 153
Rights of Persons with Disabilities 295
    Act 441
Ringer's lactate 540
Road accidents, victims of 82
Road traffic accident 486

S

Safe liposuction 540
Safe surgery saves lives 337
Sanitary facility for staff 522
Sati (Prevention) Act 496
Scald burns 505
Scalp incisions 329
Scar 404
    and deformities, correction of 446
    examination 409
    hypertrophic 333
    management 248, 409
    presence of 437
    types of 404
Scar revision 90
    consent form for 346
    failure 429b
    surgery 247, 424, 432
Scientific misconduct 300
Sclerotherapy 334

Scrub suits and dresses 525
Sebaceous cysts 334
Second consultation 403
Seeking Compensation, Legal Resort of 543
Seeks cosmetic surgery 412
Seizure of medical records 550
Self-inflicted burn 501
    case report of 501
Self-inflicted Code of Conduct 105
Self-regulatory organization 174
Sensitive drugs, case of 550
Sensitive patient data 300
Septic shock 324
Service report and spares 370
Setting-up laser theater 366
Settlement of claims 133
Sex of examining health worker 151
Sexual assault
    survivors of 160
    victims of 443
Sexual behaviour, responsible 289
Sexual reassignment surgery 418
Sexual violence
    intoxication in survivors of 156b
    suspected poisoning with 157
Sexually transmitted
    disease 148
    infections 289
Shocking lack of qualified nurses 82
Short-term therapy 551
SIDDHA, practitioners of 116
Silicone sheets 405
Simvastatin 283
Single electrical source 520
Sjögren's syndrome 283
Skilled quackery 255
Skin and hair clinic 138
    minimum standards for 139
Skin biopsy 333
Skin clinics, smooth running of 137, 146
Skin diseases, quackery in treatment of 115
Skin grafting 247, 333
    procedures 246
Skin loss 541
Skin pigmentations 431
Skin punch grafting 246
Skin tenderness 283
Skin vascularity 541
Skin whitening injections 385
Slit skin smear 144
Small accumulation of tissue 363
Smile surgery for improving beauty 446
Snake oil 112
Social awareness 296

Social media 194, 194b, 197, 209, 211
    advertising on 108
    by doctors, utility of 198f
    chain reaction 207
    in clinical practice, role of 193
    in healthcare and medicolegal aspects,
        regulatory status of 212
    on healthcare 197f
    platforms 196f, 204f
    portals 210
    skill enhancement on 202f
    use in dermatology 208
Social network
    mediablogs, uses of 197
    penetration in India 196
    sites 197
Soiled linen container 519
Sonophoresis 433
Sound-alike drugs 550
Special interest group 371
Special leave petition 230
Special task force, creation of 118
Speech-language pathologists, survey of 457
Spill cleanup 524
Spine surgery 446
Standard assessment forms 246
Standard operating procedure 11, 464, 524
Standard preoperative guidelines 522
Starting surgery 537
State AIDS Control Society 102, 290
State Commission 63, 64, 135
    ordered 548
State Consumer Disputes Redressal
        Commission 506, 512
State Drugs Control Department 304
State Government Order 120
State Legislation 173
State Medical Acts 116
State Medical Council 26, 32, 144, 325, 475
State Medical Practitioner's Act 326
State Medical Register 33
State Policy, Directive Principles of 100
State Pollution Control Board 143
State's Nurses and Midwives Council 139
Statutory regulations 248
Stem cell 319
    therapy
        for hair regrowth 385
        for regeneration 446
Sterile forceps 140
Sterile gloves 140
Sterile scissors 140
Sterilization 524
Sterilizer 140

Index

Steroid 554
    abuse 255
Stethoscope 523
Steven-Johnson syndrome 80, 258, 280, 282
Still birth reports 487*f*
Storage cabinets for records 140
Straight jacket method 136
Student research 187
Suction apparatus 523
Suction equipment 523
Suicide tourism 451
Sulfa drugs, risk with 283
Sulfonamides 283
Summon of witness 157
Supporting documentation, submission of 449
Supportive services housekeeping 546
Surface irregularities 431
Surgeon liability 402
Surgeon signature 432
Surgery 88
    benefits of 542
    equipment for 519
    gravity of 535
    major 534
    multiple consultations for 417
    of international standards 445
    risks of 542
Surgical blade 525
Surgical Consumables Register 528
Surgical devices 241
Surgical field suction 519
Surgical instruments 522
Surgical intervention 88
Surgical mask 525
Surgical procedures 439, 446, 450
    multiple 417
    video consent in 88
Surgical techniques 247
Surrogacy 451
Sushruta Samhita 23, 294
Suturing, equipment for 523
Swelling 342
Systemic lupus erythematosus 283

T

Tamil Nadu Medical Council 121, 215
Tandoor murder case 489
Task force against quackery 255, 280
Taxable commercial enterprise 137
Taxpayer identification number 141
Technical Principles of Code of Medical Ethics 23
Technology in dermatology 255
    role of 254

Teledermatology 256
Telephonic consultation 450
Tenancy Act 295
Tendon transfer 247
Terbinafine 265
Termination from employment 290
Tertiary care medical intensive care unit 324
Theater complex 518, 522
Theater equipment 522
Therapeutic procedures 336
Thermometer 140, 523
Thiopurine methyltransferase 268
Third party administrator 394
Thoracoplasty, lateral 406
Tibb, practitioners of 116
Time-dictated surgery 536
Tissue
    behaviour, predictability of 427
    distortion 425
    start changing shape 430
Tongue depressor 140
Tonsillectomy 502
Topical steroids 433
Total leukocyte count 264
Tourist visa 445, 446
Toxic epidermal necrolysis 279, 282
    case of 125
    treatment of 264
Toxic shock syndrome, died of 324
Toxicity of lidocaine 541
Transcutaneous drug delivery 537
Transplantation of Human Organs Act 170
Transportation 370
Trauma 247, 441
Traveling across international borders, practice of 445
Trichiatrist 248
Trichologist 117, 248
Trichology 206, 248
Trichoscope 140
Tropical diabetic hand syndrome 503
Trouble-free surgery 541
Tuberculosis 35
Tumescent anesthesia 531
Tummy tucks 403, 446
Tumor 333
    cancer surgery for removal of 446
    necrosis factor 282

U

Ugliness, anatomy of 424
Unani, practitioners of 116

Unethical Acts 29
    advertising 29
    Code of Conduct for Doctors 30
    Human Rights 30
    Patent and Copyrights 29
    Rebates and Commission 29
Unethical Conduct, exposure of 27
Unfair trade practices 61
Unidirectional airflow system 519
Uninterrupted power supply 365, 368
United States Food and Drug Administration 320
Unnatural offences 292
Urticaria 282
    chronic 352

V

Vascular tumors 439
Vasculitis 284
Vein flow 486
Venereologists 133
Venous treatment 248
Verbal dying declaration 492
Vexatious complaints against doctors 59
Vicarious negligence 41
Victim 96
Video recording, procedure for 91
Violence 9
    against doctors 182, 254, 257
    against medical professionals and medical care establishments 12
Viral hepatitis 286
Visual diagnosis 207
Visual literacy 210
Vital reflexes, recovery of 521

Vital signs 529
Vitamin C 433
Vitiligo 266, 267, 321
    surgery 90, 206, 333, 335, 423, 435, 438
        consent form for 348

W

Weepy dressings 534
Weighing machine 140, 523
Welfare measures 296
West Bengal Clinical Establishment Act 165
West Bengal National University of Juridical Sciences 224
Western closet 522
Wetchler's and Kortilla's Guidelines 522
White blood cell 406
White patches 266
Wider social acceptance 412
Women's commission 127
Wonder drugs 266
Wood's lamp 140
World alliance for patient safety, program of 451
World Health Organization 23, 277, 291, 337, 451
Wound dressings 246
Wrongful surgical procedure 55

X

Xylocaine 461
    spray 523

Z

Zero-tolerance Policy 257